NEUROPSYCHOLOGY AND CARDIOVASCULAR DISEASE

NEUROPSYCHOLOGY AND CARDIOVASCULAR DISEASE

Edited by

Ronald A. Cohen
John Gunstad

OXFORD
UNIVERSITY PRESS
2010

OXFORD
UNIVERSITY PRESS

Oxford University Press, Inc., publishes works that further
Oxford University's objective of excellence
in research, scholarship, and education.

Oxford New York
Auckland Cape Town Dar es Salaam Hong Kong Karachi
Kuala Lumpur Madrid Melbourne Mexico City Nairobi
New Delhi Shanghai Taipei Toronto

With offices in
Argentina Austria Brazil Chile Czech Republic France Greece
Guatemala Hungary Italy Japan Poland Portugal Singapore
South Korea Switzerland Thailand Turkey Ukraine Vietnam

Published by Oxford University Press, Inc.
198 Madison Avenue, New York, New York 10016

www.oup.com

Library of Congress Cataloging-in-Publication Data

Neuropsychology and cardiovascular disease/ edited by Ronald A. Cohen and John Gunstad
p. ; cm.
Includes bibliographical references.
ISBN-13: 978-0-19-534118-8
ISBN-10: 0-19-534118-X 1. Cardiovascular system—Diseases—Complications.
2. Neurologic manifestations of general diseases. 3. Clinical neuropsychology.
I. Cohen, Ronald A., 1955– II. Gunstad, John, 1975–
[DNLM: 1. Cardiovascular Diseases—complications. 2. Aged. 3. Cardiovascular
Agents—adverse effects. 4. Cardiovascular Surgical Procedures—adverse effects.
5. Cognition Disorders—etiology. 6. Dementia, Vascular—physiopathology.
7. Neuropsychology—methods. WG 120 N493 2010]
RC669.N48 2010
616.8—dc22

2009046666

9 8 7 6 5 4 3 2 1

Printed in the United States of America
on acid-free paper

PREFACE

CARDIOVASCULAR DISEASE AND THE BRAIN: CONSIDERATIONS FOR THE DEVELOPMENT OF VASCULAR COGNITIVE IMPAIRMENT

Ronald A. Cohen

Heart disease remains the most significant health problem in this country and throughout the world. It has consistently led all other diseases with respect to mortality and morbidity rates among adults over the past century. A remarkable number of important advances have occurred in the medical sciences with the development of many new drugs and surgical interventions that are effective in treating coronary artery disease, myocardial infarctions, arrhythmias, and the various pathological processes associated with heart disease. People are now living longer than ever before as a result, though often with chronic cardiovascular disease. Despite a decline in mortality and morbidity associated with acute cardiac events, such as myocardial infarction, heart disease remains an insidious process that tends to eventually express itself as people reach advanced age. This is evident by the fact that the prevalence of heart failure continues to increase as the population ages, even though people are surviving longer following the diagnosis of coronary artery disease, even after myocardial infarction.

The evolution of cardiovascular disease in the context of modern medicine provides the backdrop and rationale for this book. As people are now living to more advanced age, they are subject to a gradual cardiovascular breakdown, but also changes in brain structure and function. Neuropsychological decline associated with advanced age is now well recognized. Historically, there has been a tendency for doctors to focus on specific systems of the body, such as the heart or brain, based on their medical specialty and according to the acute medical problem that was presenting itself. Yet, in recent years there has been increased emphasis on approaching physical health from a multisystem perspective, with recognition that problems occurring in one system are likely to influence other body systems as well. There is mounting evidence that age-associated systemic health problems, in particular vascular disease, contributes to the development of brain dysfunction and associated cognitive and behavioral problems in the elderly.

Not too many years ago, heart disease was thought to have only very limited effects on the brain. Contributing to this belief is the fact that the cerebrovascular system is able to maintain hemodynamic regulation in the face of transient reductions in cerebral blood flow. This is in fact true for most healthy young people. Yet, with advanced age, cerebral hemodynamic function begins to breakdown, potentially exacerbating other age-associated changes in brain function.

Accordingly, there has been a growing interest in the neuropsychology of cardiovascular disease, and the influence cardiac and systemic vascular disease on the development of cerebrovascular disease and brain dysfunction. Historically, neuropsychological analysis of cerebrovascular disease primarily focused on the effects of stroke caused by infarction of large cerebral vessels. Acute stroke typically produces specific cognitive syndromes (e.g., aphasia, apraxia, agnosia) depending on the vascular territory affected by infarction. In such cases, the cerebrovascular event is focal, involving a specific cerebral artery or arteriole. As will be reviewed later in the book, this type of acute focal cerebral infarction is often cardiogenic in origin and reasonably well understood at this point in time. Yet, many people with heart disease report changes in cognitive function even though they have not experienced a large vessel stroke. For these individuals, the cognitive problems that they report are often not abrupt in onset, but rather insidious with gradual worsening over time. Are these cognitive problems real or simply a byproduct of the emotional distress that often occurs as one tries to cope with worsening health? Alternatively, are cognitive changes actually occurring in certain elderly people coincident with their heart disease, but due to other neurodegenerative brain conditions, such as Alzheimer's disease? If so, to what extent does systemic vascular pathology contribute to this brain neurodegeneration?

Interest in the neuropsychology of cardiovascular disease has coincided with an increased focused on vascular dementia (VaD) and awareness in the fields of neurology and neuropsychology that not all patients who develop dementia have Alzheimer's disease. There is still not consensus on whether Alzheimer's disease is a single disorder, or a common pathological pathway that may occur as a result of a variety of different etiological influences. Given that cerebrovascular disease underlies the development of vascular dementia, and that heart disease and cerebrovascular disease are strongly linked, neuropsychological inquiry into the contribution of cardiovascular disease to brain dysfunction and ultimately dementia in the elderly seems essential at this point in history.

While VaD is a logical important endpoint when one considers the effects of vascular disease on the brain, by the time that patients are diagnosed with VaD, their brains are typically too severely damaged and cognitive function too impaired to offer great insight into how specific vascular factors affect the brain and cognition. Studying the more subtle brain disturbances and neurocognitive impairments associated with cardiovascular disease provides an important window into how systemic vascular disease affects the brain. Beyond the scientific value of neuropsychological study of cardiovascular disease, there are important clinical reasons for such inquiry. Many elderly people have mild cognitive impairments that were first observed following a cardiac events or cardiothoracic surgery. They are often eventually referred for clinical neuropsychological assessment to determine the nature and extent of these impairments, and whether they are associated with their vascular disease. Accordingly, neuropsychologists, neurologists, psychiatrists, and other medical professionals should be aware of the existing clinical and scientific literature regarding the effects of heart disease on brain function. These were among the considerations that motivated the writing of *Neuropsychology and Cardiovascular Disease*.

This book looks to provide an integrated review of what is known about how heart and systemic vascular disease affect the brain and to also provide clinicians with insights on how to approach the neuropsychological assessment and treatment of patients with cardiovascular disease. The broad objectives of the book include:

- Provide a primer and overview of cardiovascular disease for neuropsychologists, neuroscientists, and clinicians of psychology, psychiatry and neurology.
- Consider how cardiovascular disease fits into the broader continuum of vascular cognitive impairment (VCI).
- Review current clinical and research evidence regarding the neuropsychological manifestations of cardiovascular disease, through individual chapters focusing on specific issues, such as heart failure, cardiac surgery, and cardiogenic stroke.
- Present recent research regarding the influence of specific vascular risk and etiological factors on development of brain dysfunction.
- Provide insights for the clinical neuropsychological assessment and treatment of patients with heart disease.
- Review findings from the emerging fields of structural and functional brain neuroimaging regarding the brain abnormalities associated with cardiovascular disease and the influence of specific vascular factors on the development of neuropsychological dysfunction.

To accomplish these goals, the book is organized into three sections. Part I begins with an introduction to the neuropsychology of cardiovascular disease. We then discuss the levels of analysis from which one can approach the neuropsychological study of cardiovascular disease. The epidemiology of cardiovascular disease and associated brain dysfunction is reviewed. The next chapter reviews current thinking regarding vascular dementia and the continuum of vascular cognitive impairment. This is followed by a chapter reviewing basic concepts from the field of cardiology that are a prerequisite for neuropsychologists working with patients who have heart disease, including a review of vascular and cardiac physiology, pathology, and etiologies. This is followed by discussion of cardiac rehabilitation, including how neurocognitive function impacts on these efforts. The final chapter in this part reviews aspects of behavioral medicine in cardiovascular disease.

Part II includes a chapter on important clinical considerations in assessment of neuropsychological function and treatment of cardiovascular disease. The neuropsychological effects of specific forms of cardiovascular disease are then reviewed, including blood pressure, metabolic syndrome, cardiosurgical interventions, and heart failure.

Part III reviews the systemic and cerebrovascular mechanisms that contribute to vascular cognitive impairment . This part begins with a discussion of cardioembolic stroke and its cerebrovascular impact. It continues with a description of the impact of reduced systemic perfusion on neurocognitive outcome. The next three chapters highlight the importance of impaired vascular function to vascular cognitive impairment, including measures of endothelial function, vascular reactivity and cerebral hemodynamic autoregulation. This is followed by a discussion of the mechanisms by which neurological conditions may adversely impact cardiac function. Two chapters then present the recent advances in neuroimaging and their contribution to understanding the neurocognitive consequences of cardiovascular disease, including both structural and functioning imaging. Finally, the impact of white matter pathology on cognitive function is reviewed.

We believe that this book is unique in its approach to this topic. It is our hope that the integration provided in this book will enable readers to achieve greater understanding of how cardiovascular and systemic vascular factors affect the brain, stimulate neuropsychological researchers interested in studying vascular brain effects, and provide insights for clinicians working with heart disease patients, when there is concern about possible vascular cognitive impairment.

CONTENTS

CONTRIBUTORS

Louise Allan
Newcastle University

Andreana Benitez
Kent State University

Jeffrey Browndyke
Duke University Medical Center

Elizabeth C. Casey
Kent State University

Ronald A. Cohen
Brown Medical School

Istvan Csapo
Brigham and Women's Hospital

Jeffrey Dewey
Brigham and Women's Hospital

E. Jesus Duffis
University of Massachusetts Medical School

Marc Fisher
University of Massachusetts Medical School

Daniel E. Forman
Brigham and Women's Hospital and Veterans' Administration Medical Center

W. Kin Fung
Brown University School of Medicine

Tania Giovannetti
Temple University

John Gunstad
Kent State University and Summa Health System

Andreana P. Haley
University of Texas

William G. Haynes
University of Iowa

Karin F. Hoth
National Jewish Health and University of Colorado, Denver

Joel W. Hughes
Kent State University and Center for Cardiopulmonary Research, Summa Health System

Brian E. Hunt
Wheaton College

Farzin Irani
University of Pennsylvania

Lynn Kakos
Kent State University

Melissa Lamar
King's College London

Elizabeth M. Lane
University of Missouri–St. Louis

David J. Libon
Drexel University

Susan E. Maloney
University of Missouri–St.Louis

G. M. MacQueen
McMaster University and St. Joseph's Healthcare Hamilton

Daniel McCaffrey
Brigham and Women's Hospital

William P. Milberg
Harvard Medical School, Brigham and Women's Hospital

Ivy N. Miller
University of Iowa

David J. Moser
University of Iowa

Robert H. Paul
University of Missouri–St. Louis

Athena Poppas
Brown University School of Medicine

Cate C. Price
University of Florida

Jared Price
Brigham and Women's Hospital

Troy Russell
Brigham and Women's Hospital

Ekta Sem
Brigham and Women's Hospital

Jorge M. Serrador
Harvard Medical School, Beth Israel Deaconess Medical Center

Patrick Smith
Duke University Medical Center

Kelly Stanek
Kent State University

Jose A. Suaya
Brandeis University

Lawrence H. Sweet
Brown Medical School

Rod Swenson
University of North Dakota Medical School

Ashley Szabo
Kent State University

David F. Tate
Brigham and Women's Hospital

V. H. Taylor
McMaster University

Suhrida Yadavalli
Kent State University

Part I

OVERVIEW

THE NEUROPSYCHOLOGY OF CARDIOVASCULAR DISEASE

INTRODUCTION

Ronald A. Cohen

Cardiovascular disease (CVD) remains the leading cause of death in the United States, causing over 700,000 deaths per year. CVD prevalence increases dramatically with advanced age, such that significant CVD is present in over 70% of people aged 75 years or older, and is the leading cause of mortality and morbidity in Western society—84.7% of people who die of CVD are age 65 or older. With improved survival from acute cardiac events, older adults are often faced with the prospect of living with chronic heart problems, including severe CVD. Besides its obvious effects on physical well-being, CVD causes significant psychological, social, and economic hardship and contributes to depression and psychiatric problems.

CVD predisposes people to cerebrovascular disease, which eventually may lead to cognitive dysfunction. Many patients with CVD experience cognitive impairments, though these have historically received less attention than CVD-associated psychosocial problems. There is compelling evidence that cognitive functioning is an important determinant of health status, quality of life (QOL) and ultimately functional ability. These effects limit the ability of the elderly to age successfully. We have previously shown that even subtle cognitive problems among CVD patients affect their QOL, their ability to benefit from treatment (e.g., cardiac rehabilitation), and may also be harbingers of more serious problems. Resulting cerebrovascular disease may eventually lead to functional impairments and even vascular dementia (VaD). This scenario provides a compelling reason to study the biobehavioral mechanisms underlying the development of brain dysfunction and cognitive impairments secondary to CVD in the elderly.

The relationship between CVD and brain dysfunction is not yet fully understood. While CVD and cerebrovascular disease share common pathophysiology and comorbidity, the cause of CVD-associated cerebrovascular changes and brain dysfunction is often difficult to determine, except in cases where acute stroke has occurred. Yet, as we will review subsequently, there is considerable evidence that such changes can develop when there is chronic cerebral hypoperfusion and/or microvascular disease associated with CVD.

Cardiovascular disease and cerebral perfusion

The brain requires a constant supply of blood to sustain the neural functions that underlie cognitive functioning. Cerebral blood flow provides a continual source of glucose and oxygen and enables the elimination of heat and the brain's metabolic by-products. Cessation of cerebral blood flow produces a rapid change in cellular metabolism and physiological disruption as cerebral glucose metabolism declines within seconds of complete cessation of blood flow. Within one minute, glucose metabolism is less than 10% of its normal level. A cascade of biochemical events begins during this period and escalates in association with ischemia duration. This cascade involves the entry of extracellular water, calcium, and sodium into the neuron, and acidosis. Within seconds, these cellular responses lead to a loss of hemodynamic autoregulation, a breakdown of ionic channels across the neuronal membranes, and reduced electrophysiological response. The resting potential becomes isoelectric by 30 seconds following complete ischemia, and presynaptic vesicles are affected within a few minutes, resulting in abnormal transmitter release and further neural disruption. This cascade has a snowballing effect, resulting in tissue damage or necrosis the longer it continues.

We describe this pathological cascade associated with cerebral ischemia to highlight how critical sustained cerebral circulation is for sustaining brain function. The heart is essential to this process, as it pumps the blood that supplies the brain. Remarkably, the heart maintains adequate cerebral circulation in healthy people so that there are rarely complete cessations of blood for more than a few seconds for most of childhood and the adult years. While there are continual changes in cerebral blood flow over time in all people, the cerebrovascular system is usually able to adjust to these fluctuations and to main normal brain physiological function. Nonetheless, this reliable functioning occurs against of backdrop of a requirement that sustained cerebral blood flow continue with no major interruptions and with blood levels that remain within a circumscribed range.

Neuropsychological impairments evolve over time among people who have experienced a disruption of cerebral blood flow. The most obvious example of this occurs in response to acute stroke, following occlusion or hemorrhage of a cerebral artery. While impairments may be evident from the onset, they typically increase during the acute phase of the stroke and reach greatest severity when an infarction has formed and it, along with associated edema, has developed to its full volume. Although many of the effects of focal cerebral ischemia may be reversible within one hour after occlusion, as the ischemic period continues, brain tissue becomes infarcted and functional recovery becomes less likely. The first few hours following a stroke are most critical in the transition from ischemia to complete infarction, although histological changes may continue for days after the event. Given that cognitive dysfunction is a function of the duration of ischemia and the eventual size of the infarction, a distinction needs to be made between the acute and chronic manifestations of stroke. Issues related to cardiogenic stroke will be discussed in much greater detail elsewhere in this text. For now, this consideration of how large-vessel strokes evolve provides a useful window into the development of neurocognitive dysfunction associated with cerebral ischemia.

Cardiovascular Disease and Stroke

For many years, clinicians concerned with the neurological manifestations of heart disease primarily focused on stroke caused by cardioembolism. Strokes with embolic origins are very common and typically produce focal lesions, depending on the cerebral vessel that is occluded. The neuropsychological manifestations of embolic stroke are now well understood, and in fact constitute much of the clinical foundation upon which the field of neuropsychology was based in its early years. Strokes of this type often result in specific neurocognitive syndromes (e.g., aphasis, apraxia, agnosia), depending on the vascular territory that is infarcted.

Both embolic and thrombotic stroke, in which cerebral blood flow is compromised due to occlusion, remain important for understanding the neuropsychology of cardiovascular disease. Yet brain dysfunction can occur due to heart disease for a variety of other reasons. In particular, global cerebral ischemia secondary to cardiac arrest often causes severe brain dysfunction. The neurocognitive impairments associated with global ischemia differ dramatically from those observed following focal stroke. Even in the absence of acute global cerebral ischemia secondary to cardiac arrest, there is now strong reason to believe that brain dysfunction may occur as a result of chronic cerebrovascular disease, accounting for the development of neurocognitive impairment among patients with cardiovascular disease who have not experienced clinical stroke.

Continuum of Vascular Cognitive Impairment

Presumably, the development of cognitive impairments associated with cardiovascular disease is attributable to cerebrovascular abnormalities occurring among certain patients. Severe cerebrovascular disease may ultimately cause major brain changes and profound cognitive change, resulting in vascular dementia (VaD). Yet the transition from CVD to cerebrovascular brain dysfunction is often ambiguous and requires some consideration. See Fig. I-1 below.

VaD may result from the cumulative effect of multiple large cortical infarctions from sequential strokes, single strategic infarction, diffuse small-vessel disease, or global cerebral hypoperfusion. Impairment severity is generally a function of the amount of brain volume that is damaged. For example, the severity of VaD-associated impairments has been shown to directly relate to total volume of damaged brain tissue on positron emission tomography (PET). Lesion location is also critical, as damage to critical brain regions can have enormous consequences.

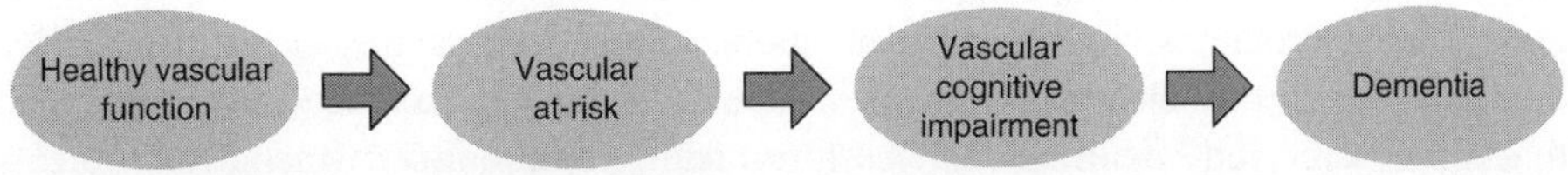

Figure I-1 Vascular cognitive impairment (VCI)

Functional disturbances that occur in response to occlusion or hemorrhage of a cerebral artery and the infarction of brain tissue that follows are the bread and butter of neurologists who specialize in stroke. When a large vascular territory and strategic brain areas are affected by a single stroke, severe cognitive dysfunction can occur, with some people exhibiting major changes in functional capacity (i.e., VaD). Alternatively, people who experience a series of large-vessel strokes over time may experience multi-infarct dementia, a common VaD subtype of vascular dementia. This is the most well recognized and understood form of VaD.

While large-vessel infarction is the most clear-cut basis for vascular dementia, clinicians have long recognized that brain disorders could also result from tissue damage associated with chronic cerebrovascular disease. This might involve either the aggregation of small areas of tissue damage due to ongoing microvascular infarctions, or chronic hypoperfusion. While these conditions are less well understood than large-vessel stroke, they attracted considerable research attention over the past two decades, in part because of the vulnerability of cerebral white matter and subcortical areas to this pathology. Furthermore, it is now generally accepted that the types of cerebrovascular disturbances that result in VaD are also capable of producing milder forms of cognitive impairments. Accordingly, the effects of cerebrovascular disease must be viewed on a continuum of vascular cognitive impairment (VCI) that ranges from subtle deficits associated with vascular risk factors and subclinical cerebrovascular disease, to VaD, which at its end stage can be very difficult to differentiate from Alzheimer's disease (AD) on the basis of cognitive presentation. The clinical and neuropsychological manifestations of VCI will be discussed in greater detail in subsequent chapters.

Efforts to better detect and treat "at-risk" patients led to the observation that mild cognitive impairments (MCI) usually precede the onset of dementia. About 10% to 15% of patients with MCI convert to dementia each year. While it was initially viewed as a precursor of AD, there is now considerable evidence that patients with VaD also exhibit MCI (VCI) prior to developing more severe dementia. Hachinski and his colleagues proposed that a continuum of cerebrovascular cognitive disorders exists, ranging from "at-risk" conditions to VaD. Within this VCI continuum are patients with significant cognitive and functional problems, whose impairments are subclinical and do not meet the criteria for dementia. Patients with circumscribed cognitive impairments, without global dysfunction, exemplify VCI. Patients who have cerebrovascular risk factors, without clinically identified cognitive symptoms, constituted the "at-risk" group at the mildest end of the severity continuum.

VCI is a logical starting point for our consideration of the neuropsychology of cardiovascular disease. Most people who develop cognitive problems in association with heart disease do not exhibit global dementia. Patients or their families are more likely to notice subtle problems with learning and memory retrieval, fatigue, effortful cognitive operations, and difficulty focusing and sustaining attention. They are often concerned that these perceived cognitive changes foreshadow more ominous memory problems and eventual dementia. For some of these patients, their concerns reflect anxiety and their sensitivity to the changes in their health status. However, patients with CVD who go on to experience cerebrovascular disturbances also develop VCI, which may affect their functional capacity and their quality of life. Furthermore, VCI represents the early stages of VaD for an unfortunate subset of individuals.

Heart Disease: A Window into VCI

Elderly people are vulnerable to cerebrovascular disease, as it is the third leading cause of death in this country. Acute stroke resulting in large-vessel infarction is now relatively well understood and will not be reviewed in detail. Less is known about the effects of small-vessel disease in the brain, though it is now widely recognized that a proportion of patients who develop VaD have large quantities of cerebral white matter infarctions rather than discrete cortical infarctions.

The effects of chronic cerebral hypoperfusion caused by reductions in overall blood supply to the brain are less well understood. Uninterrupted cerebral perfusion is essential for maintaining functional brain integrity. This depends on cardiac output and intact peripheral endothelial function, which is not the case for patients with severe CVD. Presumably, patients with severe CVD may experience chronic insufficiencies of cerebral perfusion, even if they have not had discrete stroke. The transition from chronic cerebral hypoperfusion to cerebral ischemia and eventual brain dysfunction is very complex when compared to infarction due to acute large-vessel stroke. Chronic hypoperfusion may cause subacute cerebrovascular abnormalities and contribute to microvascular disease and other brain abnormalities, even when there is not evidence of large-vessel infarction. Whereas large-vessel stroke typically evolves over a short time period, microvascular events and the effects of chronic cerebral hypoperfusion may occur without detection, making this an important area of clinical study.

From the perspective of the past line of research of our neuropsychological laboratory at Brown University, the reasons for focusing on the neuropsychological manifestations of cardiovascular disease were not entirely clinically based. They were also driven by our efforts to better understand the development of vascular dementia. For our research group, vascular dementia was the starting point. Our early work focused on differentiating vascular dementia from Alzheimer's disease. We observed subtle differences in neuropsychological test performance between Alzheimer's and vascular dementia patients in some of our studies. Yet, when we conducted well-controlled studies of vascular dementia that involved careful exclusion of patients with possible Alzheimer's or mixed dementia, it was extremely difficult to differentiate groups on the basis of their cognitive performance on standard neuropsychological tests.

The lesson seemed to be that by the time patients with VCI had worsened to the point of meeting criteria for vascular dementia, they were globally impaired, and their cognitive presentation was not particularly helpful in trying to sort out the development of their dementia. It was apparent that, to achieve a full understanding of how vascular dementia develops in patients who have not experienced large-vessel stroke, it would be necessary to begin studying people earlier in their vascular disease course, at a time when their brains were not severely damaged by the effects of a large volume of lesions.

Studying patients with heart disease who did not have clinical evidence of dementia or significant cognitive problems would enable an examination of how specific risk and vascular etiological factors contribute to structural and functional brain changes and the development of cognitive dysfunction. Furthermore, assessing heart disease patients over an extended period offered us the possibility of being able to determine the relative contribution of specific vascular factors to the development of VCI.

Cardiovascular Disease Affects Quality of Life

There is now a relatively large clinical literature, including studies by our group and others, providing compelling evidence that poor functional outcome among elderly CVD patients is partly attributable to cognitive problems. There are various ways by which cognitive impairments may affect QOL in CVD patients. In modern society, intact cognition is increasingly important for mastery of various instrumental activities of daily living. Cognitive ability also proves to be an important determinant of self-esteem related to mastery in one's environment, and ultimately one's emotional experience. Furthermore, cognitive impairment is directly associated with reduced health status, as the brain disturbances associated with cognitive impairment often reflect broader physical problems, and also because cognitive problems limit the ability of people to care for themselves.

Neurocognitive Effects of Cardiovascular Disease

Besides reducing QOL, psychosocial functioning, and self-care, neurocognitive impairments interfere with people's ability to learn and modify their behavior and lifestyle. Barclay and colleagues found that about 70% of patients in cardiac rehabilitation (CR) had significant cognitive impairments, and 35% were unable to manage their own medications. Our prior studies support this observation, as CR patients had significant learning, attention, and executive deficits that adversely impacted their functional outcome, even when they had no prior diagnosis of neurological brain disease. These impairments suggested cerebrovascular dysfunction secondary to CVD, and motivated us to conduct larger-scale longitudinal studies to examine the effects of heart disease on the brain and cognitive functioning in the elderly.

There is now a plethora of clinical evidence that many people with severe heart disease experience brain dysfunction and cognitive problems. This evidence will be reviewed in considerable detail later in the book. Various etiological factors associated with heart disease are now known to contribute to cardiovascular-associated brain dysfunction. For example, chronic hypertension has long been known to cause cerebrovascular disturbances. Cognitive dysfunction among patients with heart failure was also described many years ago and was generally attributed to the effects of reduced cerebral blood flow secondary to impaired cardiac output. Our first studies of neurocognitive dysfunction among patients in cardiac rehabilitation demonstrated that both chronic hypertension and impaired ventricular ejection fraction (EF) were factors associated with cognitive impairments, as well as reduced quality of life and health status.

Cardiac Output

Cerebral perfusion ultimately depends on the heart's pumping capacity. Left ventricular ejection fraction is the most widely used clinical measure of pumping efficiency, with EF < 40% being clinically significant. Cardiac output can also be measured and reflects the actual volume of blood expelled by the heart. The Framingham Study data show dramatic increases in heart failure in the elderly. Whereas only one to two new heart-failure cases per 1000 occur in adults under age 54, 13 to 14 cases per 100 occur among those 75 to 84 years of age, with a four- to sixfold increase in those over 85 years. This has enormous societal implications and is an important contributor to morbidity and mortality in the elderly. Exercise intolerance is compounded by the natural muscle atrophy (sarcopenia) and weakening with normal aging, resulting in a vicious cycle of infirmity exacerbating a cascade of deconditioning as measured by functional indices such as VO2 peak, six-minute walk distance, and eventual mortality. Reduced EF and cardiac output both impact cognitive impairment. Work from our laboratory points to the importance of reduced cardiac output in CVD-associated cognitive impairment, but additional research is needed to better understand this effect.

Systemic Vascular Contributions

The effects of heart failure (HF) on cerebrovascular and cognitive dysfunction in the elderly are not ubiquitous. Some HF patients continue to function well despite reduced cardiac function, while others have major cognitive problems. This seems to depend on whether cerebral hypoperfusion results from reduced cardiac output in a particular patient, which in turn depends on the ability of the cerebrovascular system to compensate for perfusion changes. Cardiac disease was once thought to have little bearing on brain function because of cerebral hemodynamic autoregulation and the efficiency of collateral circulation. This is largely true for young, relatively healthy adults, though with advanced age and the co-occurrence of systemic vascular disease, these autoregulatory processes break down, and the brain can not compensate for hypoperfusion.

Two factors appear to be particularly important in this regard: *(1)* endothelial function and *(2)* atherosclerotic burden. As endothelial function becomes impaired, cerebral vessels lose their ability to react to hemodynamic changes. The biochemical bases of these effects are quite complex and beyond the scope of the current discussion. However, the critical issue is that many of the factors that contribute to CVD and HF also contribute to systemic endothelial dysfunction. Atherosclerotic burden appears to be very important in this regard, both affecting characteristics of vascular smooth muscle and also contributing to reduced luminal diameter.

Vascular Burden

Atherosclerosis causes the narrowing of coronary, systemic, and cerebral blood vessels, including the cerebral arteries, leading to thrombosis and the occlusion of large vessels, and structural changes of penetrating arteries and arterioles that branch from these large vessels (arteriosclerosis). Atheromatous deposits in the subintima may affect the small vessels, with lipohyalinosis when both arterial and arteriolar processes occur in arteriosclerosis, with altered membrane permeability. A vicious cycle develops in the elderly, as hypertension caused in part by increased peripheral resistance causes damage to the arterial walls with an increase in quantities of collagen and a decrease in elastin, which in turn leads to vessel hypertrophy, with associated thickening and stiffening. Vascular stiffening contributes to altered baro-receptor response and impaired autoregulation in the elderly, making the cerebral vasculature less able to adapt to changes in blood pressure, blood flow, and oxygen supply. Subcortical structures, such as the basal ganglia and deep subcortical and periventricular white matter are very vulnerable to the effects of arteriosclerosis due to poor collateral blood supply, whereas the subcortical U fibers, the corpus callosum, and cortical structures are usually spared. Small-vessel narrowing can cause chronic hypoperfusion leading to demyelination, gliosis, and softening of the white matter. Advancing age, chronic hypertension, past cerebral ischemic events, and diabetes mellitus are major risk factors for these changes, which ultimately cause hypoperfusion and probably contribute to cognitive changes. Accordingly, we will continue to examine longitudinal changes in carotid intimal thickness and stiffness as a measure of cerebral vascular burden.

Endothelial Reactivity

Vascular endothelial function often becomes impaired with aging and CVD. The ability of the endothelium to react to hemodynamic changes and reduced cardiac output is essential to the maintenance of cerebral blood flow and brain functions. Such reactivity is dependent on the integrity of autoregulatory mechanisms. Hemodynamic dysregulation increases with age and with it the ability to compensate for perfusion variability. Cerebral vasoreactivity is difficult to directly measure in clinical situations, in large part because of anatomic (e.g., skull) and physiological constraints. Flow-mediated brachial artery response has been studied extensively as a measure of endothelial responsivity. It is robust and relatively easy to measure reliably. It will be used in this book as a proxy for cerebrovascular vessel reactivity and impairment of autoregulation. Impaired vascular reactivity has been related to cerebrovascular dysfunction.

Hypertension (HTN)

Hypertension prevalence increases among people over the age of 70, occurring in more than 85% of elderly CVD patients. Chronic HTN induces small-vessel stiffening due to progressive replacement of media by collagen (hyalinization) and altered permeability to circulating proteins and fibrinoid changes, which makes it an important systemic vascular factor. Spikes in systolic pressure and blood pressure variability can contribute to hypoperfusion, fluid exudation, and increased water content in subcortical regions, as seen as hyperintensities on T-2 weighted MRI. HTN causes cerebral microvascular damage and hypoperfusion, and reflects cerebrovascular dysregulation. As it is also among vascular factors associated with diminished neurocognitive performance in the elderly, HTN remains an important predictor of age-associated functional outcome in CVD.

Cerebral Blood Flow/Perfusion

Delineating the link between cardiac and systemic vascular function and the development of cerebrovascular-associated brain dysfunction requires direct examination of how systemic vascular function relates to cerebral hypoperfusion. Cerebral perfusion abnormalities are associated with stroke and frank cerebrovascular disease. Perfusion-weighted MRI (PWI) provides a means of measuring cerebral blood perfusion in specific regions of interest (ROI) using fast-gradient or spin-echo pulses to detect magnetic field inhomogeneities. Arterial spin labeling (ASL) is a noninvasive MRI method that involves manipulating proton spins in blood prior to its flow into a specific ROI. Perfusion indices are derived based on cerebral blood volume, flow, and transit time. Image contrast in ASL is obtained by magnetically labeling blood water spins flowing into the slice of interest. The flowing spins exchange with the tissue water in the slice, thereby altering the measured magnetization (signal to be measured). Two images are acquired; one with the flow labeling present and one with labeling absent. The labeled image is then subtracted from the non-labeled image, and the resulting image is converted to cerebral blood flow in units of (ml blood)/(ml tissue)/min from measured blood spin-lattice relaxation time and the relaxed magnetization of arterial blood are known.

Arterial Spin Labeling (ASL)

Arterial spin labeling has been applied to various neurological disorders, including stroke and AD, and also normal functioning, though cerebral ischemia has been the most frequently studied neuropathy using perfusion weighted imaging. These studies have shown that ASL is useful in the diagnosis of stroke, the identification of ischemic tissue, the prediction of infarct volume, and the evaluation of treatment outcome. Specifically, increased CBF, increased cerebral blood volume, and decreased mean transit time suggest acute ischemia, while CBF and cerebral blood volume have been shown to predict final infarct volume. In individual unilateral stroke patients, ASL values from the affected hemisphere are often compared to these measures from the unaffected hemisphere to identify and determine the volume of ischemic tissue. When the PWI-identified abnormal tissue volume exceeds the volume identified by DWI, the excess tissue has been shown to be in danger of permanent infarct. Thus ASL can be used in addition to DWI to identify ischemic tissue in danger of infarct, and when combined, both methods are more sensitive and specific than either alone. Perfusion weighted imaging using ASL has been shown to have unique value in identifying transient ischemic attacks and subarachnoid hemorrhage. Reduced subcortical perfusion has also been found in patients with small-vessel disease compared to healthy controls. In sum, there is now compelling reason to believe that ASL may be of value in measuring cerebral perfusion secondary to cardiovascular disease. This method, together with DTI and structural MRI, provides a means of identifying ischemic brain tissue as evidenced in its growing use in clinical settings. It may identify ischemic events not identified by DTI images and have special value when studying brain effects of cardiovascular disease.

Structural Brain Abnormalities in Cardiovascular Disease

In vivo MRI measurement is widely used to identify brain abnormalities. The most obvious MRI finding associated with CVD is large-vessel infarction, occurring following an acute cardiac event. The detection of discrete cortical infarctions with 24 hours of stroke onset is relatively straightforward, and requires little discussion. Efforts to characterize structural brain changes from chronic hypoperfusion and microvascular disease need to account for these larger infarctions. There is accumulating evidence that beyond acute cerebral infarction, structural brain changes occur in patients with CVD, related to different risk and etiological factors. Most notable is the occurrence of MRI hyperintensities involving the white matter.

White Matter Hyperintensities (WMH)

White matter hyperintensities are common among patients with cerebrovascular disease, with extensive volumes indicating subcortical and periventricular white matter disease. Detection of WMH is relatively easy, though determining its severity is more challenging, as small quantities of WMH are common among elderly people without known disease. Confluent areas of high WMH are associated with varying degrees of fiber loss, with large areas often reflecting WMD and microcystic infarcts.

Considerable research has focused on determining the significance of WMH in the elderly in a large number of prior studies. Studies by our group and others have evidence that WMH is associated with both cerebrovascular disease and CVD, with its severity strongly associated with cognitive function, particularly psychomotor and information-processing speed, attention, and executive control. A preponderance of vascular changes in frontal-subcortical white matter probably accounts for this deficit pattern. When specific subcortical nuclei (e.g., caudate and putamen of basal ganglia and thalamus) are affected, greater impact on higher cognitive functions occurs.

Regional Volume Loss

Interestingly, our studies have shown that WMH does not relate as strongly to other cognitive functions, such as language and memory, but that changes in whole brain and cortical volume also occur in patients with VaD and VCI that are associated with declines in these functions. Other investigators have also found evidence of reduced regional brain volumes in patients with CVD. Therefore, it seems very likely that, beyond the occurrence of infarctions, chronic cerebrovascular disease causes brain volume loss in particular regions that may be of functional importance. Large MRI morphometric databases have been developed by our group and others, enabling normative comparisons of MRI findings across the lifespan. Such normative MRI data are important, as they help provide a means of determining whether reductions in the volume of specific brain structures or other MRI findings are abnormal in patients with suspected brain disorders, including CVD.

Diffusion Imaging Approaches

One of the most significant methodological neuroimaging developments to affect the study and assessment of cerebrovascular disease, and consequently on the neuropsychology of cardiovascular disease, was the discovery that information about the diffusion of water across brain tissue could be derived using MRI techniques. Initially, diffusion-weighted imaging (DWI) methods were established that enabled the measurement of changes in the penumbra, the rim of mild to moderately ischemic brain tissues that surround the core infarction. As described in the chapter on cardioembolic stroke, DWI provides the ability to characterize the evolution of an infarction relative to the penumbra during stroke. DWI data are novel in that they characterize the physiological health of brain tissue for circumscribed brain regions of interest. Therefore, it is a hybrid technique that couples physiological and structural neuroanatomic information, which is extremely useful in the context of studying cerebral ischemic changes.

Diffusion imaging methods have been extended to enable measurement of diffusion across different spatial orientations (tensors) within the brain. The resulting method, diffusion tensor imaging (DTI), enables the identification of tissue that is organized in specific spatial orientations, which is particularly useful for assessing white-matter pathways in the brain and characterizing their structural integrity. DTI provides information that can be interpreted in parallel with WMH abnormalities on structural MRI. It has the potential for showing early microstructural changes occurring before the expression of larger and more permanent lesions. Based on this rationale, we have begun to use DTI methods to study white-matter changes among patients with chronic cardiovascular disease. This work will be described in greater detail in a later chapter.

Functional Brain Imaging in Cardiovascular Disease

Diffusion and perfusion MRI provide methods for assessing alterations in cerebral blood flow and subtle changes in the structural integrity of brain tissue in patients with cardiovascular disease. Functional brain imaging is a potentially important adjunct to these methods, providing physiological correlates of cognitive and behavioral processes.

Two methods have received greatest attention in recent years: functional magnetic resonance imaging (FMRI) and positron emission tomography. The relative merits of each of these methods have been well described in other texts and will only be briefly discussed here.

Given its strong temporal and spatial resolution, flexibility for use with various cognitive paradigms, and compatibility with other MR-based methods (e.g., DTI and ASL), our group has focused on the use of FMRI for the study of cardiovascular disease. This work is described in greater detail elsewhere in this text. These studies are summarized here to illustrate how FMRI could be used to link brain structure and function with measures of systemic vascular function in cardiovascular disease. In a series of studies published over the past three years, cardiovascular patients underwent FMRI while performing a working memory task (n-Back). The intensity and extent of brain activation during the working memory task was found to be significantly associated with the volume of cardiac output and also carotid IMT. These two measures reflect cardiac function and systemic vascular load, respectively. These results suggest that cardiovascular patients with greater cardiac and systemic vascular impairment also have greater abnormality of functional brain activation. In another study, Haley et al. found that, even among adults without cardiovascular disease or hypertension, those with a family history of hypertension differed in the FMRI response compared with patients without such a family history.

These results suggest that functional brain response differences among people may exist based on genetic differences, even in the absence of active vascular disease. This line of research is likely to prove very valuable in studying and eventually assessing the brain functioning of patients with cardiovascular disease.

CVD Causes CNS Inflammatory Responses

Inflammation is most likely a key element of CVD neuropathogenesis, occurring in response to cerebral ischemia. In the previous section, the cascade of cellular biochemical processes following ischemia was discussed. A critical aspect of this process is cytokine release, which both signals inflammatory processes occurring in response to ischemia and also has direct neurotoxic effects associated with the glutamate system. Many cytokines and inflammatory markers have been identified that may influence this process. Our data and the work of others led us to focus on five inflammatory markers: C-reactive protein (CRP), homocysteine, amyloid-β, tumor necrosis factor (TNF-α), and interleukin-6 (IL-6).

Homocysteine is a sulfur-containing amino acid derived from methionine and associated with increased risk for arteriosclerosis and stroke. It is known to promote endothelial dysfunction and alter blood coagulation systems. Homocysteine has more recently been associated with increased risk for Alzheimer's disease, vascular dementia, and poorer cognitive performance in non-demented samples.

C-reactive protein is an acute phase reactant that indicates low-grade inflammatory activity. CRP is known to predict CVD events. Its pro-inflammatory effects on the endothelium are known to result in altered nitrous oxide synthesis. Findings from our laboratory and others link CRP to cognitive dysfunction and dementia.

*TNF-*α is a pro-inflammatory cytokine that coordinates the synthesis and activity of other cytokines. *IL-6*, a pro- and anti-inflammatory cytokine, plays a key role in the immune response and hematopoiesis. Persons with dementia exhibit significant cytokine dysregulation, and higher cytokine levels are associated with cognitive dysfunction, especially in individuals with cardiovascular disease.

Amyloid beta (Aβ) protein peptide is deposited throughout the brain in response to ischemia and helps characterize Alzheimer's disease pathology. It is found in both healthy and demented older adults. Aβ deposits trigger an inflammatory response, resulting in neuronal dysfunction and neurodegeneration. Circulating levels of Aβ and its precursor (amyloid precursor protein) are associated with poor cognitive function and predict conversion to dementia.

Model of Heart Disease and the Brain

Our efforts to address these questions began with an initial study of patients enrolled in cardiac rehabilitation. We found that considerable variability existed among patients. While some were entirely normal with respect to cognitive function, others exhibited significant impairments, particularly in learning efficiency and certain aspects of executive functioning. We also observed that patients with the poorest cognitive status at baseline also showed poor functional outcome from the rehabilitation efforts and reported reduced quality of life and health status at completion of cardiac rehabilitation compared with patients with strong baseline cognitive functions. These findings, together with observations from our studies of vascular dementia, led to a National Institutes of Health-funded R01 study, "Heart Disease and Brain Dysfunction in Elderly," a project whose broad aim was to address these questions regarding the development of VCI in elderly people with heart disease.

As we planned how to best approach the question of how cardiovascular and systemic vascular disease leads to the development of VCI, it was necessary to first consider possible pathological mechanisms linking the heart and brain. It was readily apparent that there were many different ways of approaching heart disease, and that the level of analysis that we selected might greatly influence our findings. One could focus on specific cardiac events, such as myocardial infarction; or alternatively, cardiac procedures, such as coronary artery disease. Our overall hypothesis was that people who had the severest heart disease would be most vulnerable to the development of VCI. While this seemed intuitive, it was soon obvious that defining cardiovascular disease severity was not a simple matter, as there was not a single agreed-upon metric in cardiology for rating disease severity.

Given the fact that the heart is fundamentally a pump that is responsible for the perfusion of the blood throughout the body, and that chronic cerebral hypoperfusion was considered to be one etiological basis for the development of vascular dementia, it seemed reasonable to use some measure of the heart's ability to pump as a way of characterizing cardiac disease severity.

Summary and Integration

Mounting evidence indicates that CVD has adverse impact on the CNS with age. Elderly patients with severe chronic CVD, who have heart failure and endothelial dysfunction, often develop functional impairments. CVD-associated brain changes appear to increase over time. While there is compelling evidence that systemic vascular factors contribute to age- and CVD-associated brain metabolite abnormalities, further empirical work is much needed. See Fig. I-2 below.

In the following chapters, detailed information will be provided regarding the contribution of specific elements of the model described here. As one considers the neuropsychology of cardiovascular disease, it would be valuable to keep this model in mind, as it provides the conceptual basis for exploring heart disease from a neuropsychological perspective. For some readers, the neuropsychology of heart disease may seem far from the mainstream of traditional neuropsychology, which in the past typically focused on the effects of focal brain lesions on cognition or on neurodegenerative diseases such as Alzheimer's dementia. Why all the fuss about studying brain dysfunction associated with heart disease? In this regard, as the information in this book is considered, it would be useful to keep several key points in mind.

- Heart disease is the most common health problem among the elderly.
- Heart disease is strongly associated with the development of cerebrovascular disease.

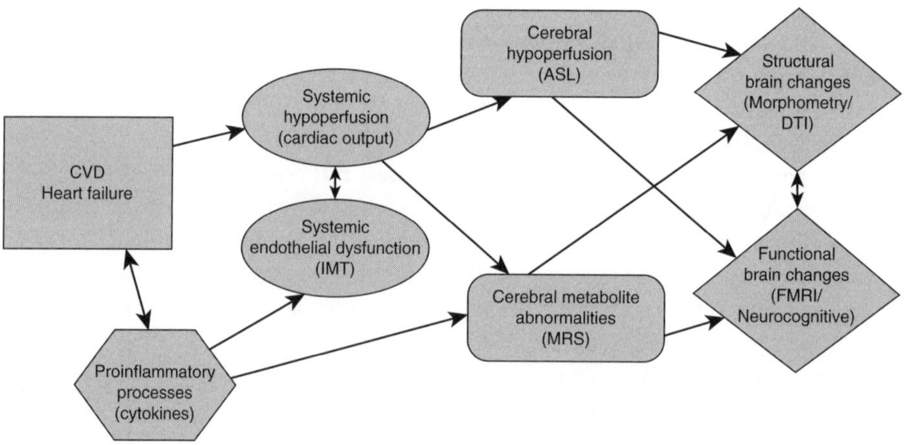

Figure I-2 Proposed model for the development of cognitive impairment in persons with CVD.

- Just as MCI is considered to be an antecedent of Alzheimer's and related dementias, there is now strong evidence that a continuum of vascular cognitive impairment exists, ranging from patients at risk to patients with severe vascular dementia. Heart disease should be considered in this context.
- Both heart and cerebrovascular disease share common risk factors, etiologies, and pathophysiology.
- Cerebrovascular disease is a risk factor for Alzheimer's disease.
- Systemic vascular dysfunction associated with chronic heart disease appears to be related to the development of cerebrovascular disease.
- Cognitive dysfunction occurs in many elderly patients with heart disease. In fact, in inpatient hospital settings, requests for neuropsychological consultations for mental status changes in patients with cardiovascular conditions are extremely common. Therefore it is important for clinicians to have an appreciation for the contribution of cardiovascular disease to neurocognitive outcome.
- Cognitive dysfunction among patients with heart disease hampers functional status, disease management, and cardiac rehabilitation.
- Heart disease patients who develop brain dysfunction are at increased risk for mortality and morbidity.
- The fields of behavioral and preventive medicine have traditionally focused on heart disease to a greater extent than on cerebrovascular disease. Yet much of what is known regarding heart disease has direct relevance to the clinical management of patients with cerebrovascular disease as well.
- While the conceptual basis for brain dysfunction secondary to heart disease may seem relatively straightforward, there is still much that is not known about how brain dysfunction develops over time in the context of chronic heart disease. Therefore, the neuropsychological study of heart disease has value from a neuroscientific perspective, beyond its clinical relevance.

In this regard, there are a number of open questions that we will discuss over the course of this book. While research is being conducted that is beginning to address some of these questions, we are still far from fully resolving important issues such as:

- How do CVD-associated cognitive problems progress to VCI (pre-dementia)?
- What CVD brain effects occur in the context of advanced age?
- How do systemic vascular factors relate to changes in cerebral perfusion and brain dysfunction?
- How do cardiac function and systemic hemodynamic function (endothelial function, atherosclerotic burden, etc.) interact to affect cerebral perfusion and brain dysfunction in CVD patients?
- To what extent do specific CVD risk and etiological factors influence these effects?

We hope that this book encourages further work into these and other key issues in the field. The growing proportion of older adults in many countries will undoubtedly increase the prevalence of multiple forms of CVD, ultimately increasing the prevalence of significant neurocognitive disorders. A clearer understanding of the mechanisms by which CVD adversely impacts the brain may identify effective prevention and treatment strategies to minimize both the financial and human costs of severe cognitive impairment.

1

NEUROPSYCHOLOGY OF HEART DISEASE

LEVELS OF ANALYSIS

Ronald A. Cohen

Neuropsychological inquiry into cardiovascular disease requires consideration of the various ways that heart disease can be characterized and the level of analysis that is chosen. Almost all adults have some familiarity with heart disease based on their knowledge of family members, friends, acquaintances, or their own personal experience. Early in life, this typically involves someone's being diagnosed with conditions that create cardiovascular risk, such as hypertension or hyperlipidemia. In midlife, many people know someone who has had a "heart attack" (i.e., myocardial infarction) who is undergoing a procedure to prevent this from reoccurring. In fact, there are many ways of classifying heart disease and also varieties of different pathological conditions that fall under the rubric of heart disease that differ in their significance to the development of brain dysfunction and our neuropsychological consideration.

The term *heart disease* is used to refer to pathological conditions that affect the heart's ability to pump blood to the rest of body. A healthy heart is capable of delivering sufficient quantities of blood on a consistent basis under normal physiological conditions. While the term "heart disease" is widely understood by both the lay public and medical community, heart disease is best thought of as an important component of cardiovascular disease—that is, pathology of the heart itself—as well as systemic and peripheral vascular functions that enable circulation of blood to all the body's organ systems. For reasons that will become clear throughout this book, neuropsychological consideration of the effects of heart disease is best framed in the broader context of cardiovascular disease. Heart disease tends not to occur in isolation, but rather is usually part of a larger disease process.

Cardiovascular Disease: A Precursor of Cerebrovascular Disturbance

Cardiovascular disease is typically distinguished from vascular disease affecting the brain's vasculature (i.e., cerebrovascular disease). To some extent this dissociation is arbitrary. Both cerebral and cardiovascular disease could be viewed as related pathologies involving vascular function. However, important differences do exist between cerebral perfusion and the circulation of blood throughout the rest of the body. The most obvious difference is the existence of the blood–brain barrier that limits access of external agents to the brain. There are also several important differences that distinguish vascular disease involving cerebral arterioles and capillaries from that involving the large cerebral vessels and arteries throughout the rest of the body. The distinction that is made between cerebrovascular and cardiovascular disease also recognizes the essential role that the brain plays in human functioning and the complexity of the brain as an organ system apart from others in the body.

This book focuses most of its attention on the effects of systemic and cardiovascular disease on the brain, and not the many types of primary cerebrovascular disease that can occur independently of cardiovascular disease. For example, certain people have cerebral arterial-venous malformations without any other appreciable history of vascular disease.[1] With this said, it is important to emphasize that cerebrovascular disturbances provide the interface between the heart and the brain. While problems with the cardiovascular function may cause other problems, such as renal or liver failure, that may affect the brain independently of cerebrovascular disease, this usually occurs primarily in the end stages of heart disease, or when there has been a cardiac crisis. More typically, the cardiovascular disease causes cerebrovascular abnormalities, which in turn result in neuronal and other cellular disturbances, and ultimately, brain dysfunction.

Furthermore, as we will discuss extensively throughout this book, cerebrovascular changes that occur in association with systemic and cardiovascular disease create conditions that make the brain more vulnerable to subsequent vascular events. With these considerations in mind, we will examine the various ways in which cardiovascular disease can be characterized, and the implications for different levels of analysis on neuropsychological inquiry. We will begin with a relatively global level of consideration.

Levels of Analysis

There are various ways that neuropsychologists could approach the study of the effects of cardiovascular disease on brain function. Levels of analysis can differ along many different dimensions, ranging from consideration based on the clinical setting or referral question, to specific cardiovascular conditions and risk factors, to the study of how particular vascular pathophysiological mechanisms affect the brain. Some of the important dimensions and levels of analysis that affect neuropsychological consideration of cardiovascular disease will be summarized in this chapter and then elaborated on throughout the rest of book. These dimensions include:

- Primary versus secondary effects of cardiovascular disease
- Acute versus chronic disease
- Cardiac versus cardiovascular and systemic vascular disease
- Risk factors
- Disorders

- Etiologies
- Procedures
- Clinical setting
- Clinical versus neuroscientific inquiry
- Neuropathophysiological level

Cardiovascular Effects on the Brain: An Overview

There are three primary routes by which cardiovascular disease can affect the brain, and at least three secondary or indirect routes (see Table 1-1). The two most acute and severe cerebrovascular disturbances that occur due to heart disease are: (1) cardioembolic stroke; and (2) global ischemia due to heart failure. These two routes are very different in their manifestations and brain effects. Whereas cardiogenic stroke is usually associated with an embolism that leaves the heart and travels to the brain, typically causing localized infarction with neurobehavioral syndromes and specific neurological signs and symptoms, cessation of heart function for even short periods of time affects the entire brain, though certain regions are more vulnerable to ischemic damage than others. We will discuss these routes in considerable detail in subsequent chapters.

The third primary route is more insidious and stems from the fact that cardiovascular and cerebrovascular disease share common risk factors and etiological underpinnings. For example, the atherosclerotic changes that affect the heart itself also tend to affect cerebral vessels.[2] Similarly, hypertension directly affects the heart and also contributes to related cerebrovascular problems, such as a breakdown in cerebral vascular membrane structure and function and the increased likelihood of microvascular events.[3]

There are several secondary routes to brain dysfunction. (1) Chronic cardiovascular disease leads to a breakdown of other organ systems of the body, such as the liver, pancreas, and kidneys, all of which play important roles in metabolic function.[4] (2) Patients are vulnerable to depression and other psychiatric problems, which are associated with neurophysiological brain disturbances in their own right and may

Table 1-1

Primary routes
Global cerebral ischemia
Cardiogenic stroke
Systemic vascular changes
Secondary routes
Metabolic changes from other organ disease
Psychiatric response to illness
Adverse treatment effects

contribute to longer-term brain dysfunction.[5] (3) Many of the drugs used to treat cardiovascular disease may affect the brain and cognition when used for long periods of time or at high doses.[6] (4) Surgical interventions are also known to have adverse neurobehavioral effects.[7] These secondary routes will be explored further in subsequent chapters.

Clinical Categories of Cardiovascular-associated Brain Dysfunction

Most patients exhibiting brain dysfunction secondary to cardiovascular disease fall into one of four major clinical categories that differ with respect to route of effects and neuropsychological presentation:

- Cardiovascular disease without cardiac arrest or cardioembolic stroke
- Cardiac arrest
- Co-morbid cardioembolic stroke
- Adverse post-surgical effects

The largest category of patients is those with cardiovascular disease but no prior history of stroke or cardiac arrest. This group is heterogeneous with respect to etiology and disease severity, ranging from individuals with coronary artery disease, but intact heart function, to those with severe chronic heart failure. Clinical considerations related to these four categories are discussed in greater detail elsewhere in this book.

Acute Versus Chronic Cardiovascular Conditions

Cardiovascular effects on the brain can be characterized in a number of other ways that help to elucidate important etiological issues. One of the most obvious but easily overlooked considerations is the distinction between acute cardiac events and chronic disease. We have already discussed this briefly with respect to the insidious effects of chronic vascular disease.

In general, acute cardiovascular effects on the brain are better understood and easier to diagnosis than chronic effects. Of course, acute events often occur in patients with chronic vascular disease, so this distinction has more to do with whether there is a discrete vascular event underlying the development of brain disturbance or not. It should also be noted that acute cardiovascular disturbance is also associated with the secondary effects of cardiothoracic surgical intervention[8].

The two primary routes discussed above constitute the basis for most acute cases of brain dysfunction in people with heart disease. Cardioembolic stroke is the basis for a significant percentage of stroke cases in this country each year.[9] People with heart disease are at risk for this type of stroke, particularly in the presence of certain types of cardiac arrhythmias[10]. While cardiogenic stroke is caused by cardiac events, it is an area of intense investigation by neurological researchers, and is usually considered from the perspective of the stroke field.

Acute global cerebral ischemia has historically received much less research inquiry. This is probably largely because cardiac arrest and the complete cessation of heart function for more than a very short period often results in either death or profound brain damage with victims lingering in vegetative states.[11] While historically this is certainly the case, there are many people who survive cardiac arrest and experience more subtle brain disturbances.[12] Also, neuropsychological consideration of acute global cerebral ischemia provides a window into the effects of chronic cerebral hypoperfusion, which as we will discuss subsequently is an increasingly important area of study.

The chronic effects of cardiovascular disease constitute most of the other bases for cerebrovascular-associated brain disturbance among people with heart disease. This includes the effects of chronic hypertension, atherosclerosis, reduced cardiac output, and a host of other conditions that can cause cumulative problems with brain function.

Cardiac Versus Systemic Vascular Bases of Brain Disturbance

An alternative level of consideration is whether impaired cardiac perfusion is central to the resulting brain disturbance or not. Of course the heart plays some role in all cerebrovascular functions, because of its central role in pumping blood. Yet an important distinction must be made between patients who are experiencing heart failure (i.e., failure to supply blood on a consistent basis throughout the body) versus people who have heart problems that are part of a broader matrix of vascular disturbance leading to cerebrovascular changes.

The important conceptual issue underlying this distinction is that heart failure constitutes only a subset of cases involving heart disease. For most people, their first encounter with heart disease is through symptoms of angina, which often reflect underlying coronary artery disease (CAD). In fact there is a tendency among some to use the terms *CAD* and *cardiovascular disease* interchangeably, though in reality they represent very different levels of specificity. CAD is an important component of cardiovascular disease. When untreated, CAD often leads to myocardial infarction and probably contributes to the slow development of heart failure among some people who have not experienced overt myocardial infarction.[13] Yet, from a neuropsychological perspective, CAD does not have the same significance as heart failure. Most patients with CAD who are treated effectively are unlikely to experience major neurocognitive disturbance from their heart disease, at least over the short term.[14] This fact probably accounts for the fact that, for many years, heart disease was not thought to be highly relevant to the brain, except in the context of stroke. The typical patient with CAD who is relatively healthy otherwise is able to sustain relatively intact cognitive functioning and normal activities of daily living as long as they have successfully adapted to the psychological and physical effects caused by their heart problems.

In contrast, brain function among people with chronic heart failure is at risk due to the effects of chronic cerebral hypoperfusion.[15] Heart failure by definition means that the heart is either not pumping a sufficient quantity blood regularly, or that its efficiency in doing so is reduced, so that the heart has to work much harder to sustain perfusion. In either case, the brain is susceptible to resultant drops in cerebral blood flow. Therefore, not all forms of heart disease are equivalent from a neuropsychological perspective. As we discuss in greater detail later in this book, heart failure should probably be considered the severest form of chronic heart disease.

For many years heart failure received relatively little attention by neuropsychologists. The fact that in the past most patients with heart failure did not survive very long probably was a major reason for this. However, as we will discuss in greater detail elsewhere, the brain's hemodynamic functions were once thought to be largely protected from changes in blood flow as a result of autoregulatory mechanisms. While this seems to be true for most healthy adults, there is increasing evidence that with advanced age and in the context of reduced overall vascular health, hemodynamic regulation breaks down.[16, 17] Therefore, understanding the link between cardiac and cerebral perfusion has become an important area of clinical neuroscience inquiry.

Risk Factors, Etiology, Disorders, and Procedures

Perhaps the most obvious way of classifying cardiovascular disease and its effects on the brain is to do so with respect to the presence of underlying vascular risk factors, etiologies, and specific disorders and procedures. In fact, most neuropsychologists interested in cardiovascular effects on the brain first approach the field by addressing one of these topics. The difficulty in this approach, however, is that risk factors, etiologies, and procedures are often overlapping. Since these bases for brain dysfunction among cardiovascular disease patients will be reviewed in subsequent chapters, we will now only briefly summarize what is meant by each of these terms.

Vascular Risk Factors

Neuropsychological researchers have long focused on the effects of certain vascular risk factors on brain structure and function. The most obvious example of this is hypertension, for which there is now a large neuropsychological literature. Increasingly, there has been interest in the contribution of other risk factors, such as dyslipidemia and impaired glucose metabolism.

Some caution needs to be exercised when considering vascular risk factors, as they may or may not be associated with actual cardiovascular disturbance at a given point in time. While some cardiologists and other clinicians consider people with certain risk factors to have cardiovascular disease, others are more inclined to view these factors as precursors of heart disease, but to keep risk factors quite separate from cardiac pathology. From a neuropsychological perspective, consideration of risk factors is important in its own right because they independently contribute to the development of cerebrovascular abnormalities and may be important in determining cognitive outcome among heart patients.[18]

Specific Disorders of the Heart

As discussed earlier, there are many disorders of the heart that influence the overall health of a particular patient, the risk of worsening cardiac function, and also the likelihood of developing cerebrovascular disease. Symptoms of angina and shortness of breath during exertion are among the most common symptoms to occur among patients with CAD whose arteries are becoming severely occluded.[19] While these symptoms are clinically significant, they are not particularly relevant to whether a patient is likely to have brain dysfunction secondary to their heart disease. Similarly, the presence of CAD is important because it points to the presence of significant atherosclerotic disease and increased risk for stroke, but in its own right it is not strongly predictive of brain dysfunction in most adults.

Even myocardial infarction (MI), the cardiac condition most commonly identified as an indicator of severe heart disease among lay people, is not strongly associated with cognitive dysfunction when considered relative to other cardiological factors.[20] In a recent analysis of the contribution of specific risk and etiological factors to neurocognitive impairment and MRI brain abnormalities among people with cardiovascular disease (Cohen, 2008), we found that myocardial infarction was not among the factors most significantly associated with abnormalities. This is not to say that brain dysfunction does not occur in some cases of MI. Yet, in the absence of cardiac arrest, MI tends not to be associated with major brain dysfunction relative to other risk and etiological factors.[20] If the heart is infarcted but continues to pump blood without major disruption, brain function typically is preserved in spite of damage to the heart.

In contrast, when there is cessation or major reduction in cardiac output, the likelihood of brain dysfunction increases. Most notably, heart failure is strongly associated with brain dysfunction for reasons summarized earlier. When the valves of the heart become diseased, there also tends to be an increased likelihood of cognitive problems, again because of problems with consistent cardiac output.

Cardiac arrhythmia is the other major condition that is strongly associated with brain dysfunction. The reason for this is that when heart rhythm breaks down, there is an increased risk of cardiogenic stroke.[10] This is particularly true for people with uncontrolled atrial fibrillation. Other than this increased cardiogenic stroke risk, the effects of chronic arrhythmia on brain function are much like the effects of CAD; the effects have more relevance to the health of the heart itself than to whether a patient is likely to have cognitive problems.

Cardiac Procedures

The effects of cardiac surgical procedures on brain function and cognition have received considerable attention over the past 25 years. With improvements in surgical technique, the prevalence of neurocognitive problems secondary to heart surgery has decreased, though certain patients continue to experience significant impairments, particularly after complicated coronary bypass surgery, transplantation, and certain types of valve surgery.[7] The current literature on these effects will be reviewed in greater detail in a later chapter.

Treatment Setting

From a clinical neuropsychological perspective, it is important to distinguish between heart disease patients seen in the hospital, in outpatient clinics, and in cardiac rehabilitation programs. For clinicians who have worked in hospital consultation-liaison services, this distinction may seem obvious. The mental status of hospitalized inpatients has to be viewed in the context of the acute medical factors that have led to their being hospitalized. Among the most common reasons for neuropsychological referral from hospital inpatient units is the assessment of patients with heart disease who have experienced alterations in their mental status. Frequently, the question is whether the particular patient is experiencing dementia or delirium. Analysis of mental status results from patients referred to the consultation-liaison service at our teaching hospital during a one-year period revealed a mean Mini Mental Status Examination (MMSE) = 18.5. While some of these patients were in fact demented, a significant proportion showed major improvements in function once they left the hospital and had time to recover.

In contrast with hospitalized cardiac patients, the cognitive presentation of people with heart disease who present in outpatient clinics typically does not differ greatly from that of the general population, except in cases of severe disease. Similarly, patients in cardiac rehabilitation (CR) programs are usually quite motivated and on average may not appear to have major cognitive problems. Yet, when the cognitive functions of the cardiac rehabilitation cohort are compared to healthy controls, evidence of mild impairments may be apparent.[21] Perhaps more important, nurses and other clinicians working with CR patients commonly note that certain patients seem to have significant cognitive problems that impede their ability to benefit from the intervention. This observation was supported by an early study by our group a number of years ago that looked at quality of life and health status as a function of cognitive status among patients in cardiac rehabilitation.[22]

Neuropathophysiological Perspective

An alternative way of characterizing heart disease patients for purposes of neuropsychological consideration is to place primary emphasis on cardiac and systemic vascular functional status, independent of the specific cardiovascular condition that a particular patient presents with. The rationale for this approach is that the fundamental consideration when considering whether or not cardiovascular disease is either actively or "at risk for" affecting brain function is the extent to which certain vascular functions are impaired. Among the cardiac and systemic functions that we have examined in our work are measures of cardiac function (ejection fraction and cardiac output), measures of atherosclerotic burden (e.g., carotid intima medial thickness), and blood pressure variability, as well as measures of endothelial function (e.g., brachial artery reactivity). Members of our research team have helped elucidate the contribution of some of these factors to the presence of cognitive dysfunction and MRI abnormalities among patients with heart disease. This work is laid out in greater detail in the chapters that follow.

Several considerations motivated our neuropsychological consideration of cardiovascular disease from this level of analysis. Perhaps most important is the fact that efforts to link cardiovascular disease with the development of brain dysfunction ultimately depend on demonstrating associations between specific vascular factors, such as cardiac output, and evidence of cerebrovascular disturbance as measured by brain imaging methods, such as perfusion and diffusion weighted–MRI and functional imaging (e.g., functional magnetic resonance imaging (FMRI) and positron emission tomography (PET)). By focusing on severity of cardiac output dysfunction as well as systemic vascular health, it is possible to examine factors that are most closely tied to cerebrovascular function.

Several other issues also provide support for this approach when conducting neuropsychological studies of cardiovascular disease. While it is possible to isolate populations of heart disease patients who have a single vascular risk or etiological problem, in the real world, patients with cardiovascular disease are a very diverse group. Many effects of factors such as hypertension that are known to have influence on cognitive status in large epidemiological studies tend to get washed out when considered in the context of the heterogeneous set of vascular problems that typically exists among patients with heart disease. While it makes sense to dichotomize patients with heart disease on certain dimensions, such as the presence or absence of heart failure, or whether they have undergone a particular procedure, such groupings make less sense when considering other cardiac conditions. Studying patients on the basis of the extent of disturbance in certain key dimensions of vascular function, such as cardiac output and endothelial health, links heart disease more closely to the mechanisms that are likely to contribute to cerebrovascular-associated brain abnormalities. This approach is reflected in the topics of many of the chapters that follow.

Summary

The levels of analysis that have been discussed may provide a useful means of organizing research efforts for neuropsychologists and other brain scientists interested in the study of vascular effects on the brain as well as in the approach taken by clinicians who are assessing or treating patients with heart disease who are suspected of having brain dysfunction. These levels of analysis are by no means exhaustive. There are probably other ways that cardiovascular disease can be conceptualized from a neuropsychological perspective. The important take-away message from this review is that the impact of heart disease on the brain is ultimately a function of the effect of the integrity of cardiac output over time and the ability of the brain to adjust to changes or disruptions in cerebral blood flow. Cardiovascular conditions that affect these two factors are likely to affect brain function, whereas conditions that affect the heart, but do not directly influence cerebral blood flow, may have relevance to the eventual development of cerebrovascular disease, but most likely are not directly responsible for major brain disturbance, except in cases of acute cardiovascular events, such as global cerebral ischemia due to heart failure, or stroke associated with cardiac conditions and procedures. On this note, we will move on to a consideration of the epidemiology of cardiovascular disease, cerebrovascular disturbance, and cognitive disturbance among patients with heart disease.

Notes

1. National Institute of Neurological Disorders and Stroke. Arteriovenous malformations and other vascular lesions of the central nervous system fact sheet. Available at: http://www.ninds.nih.gov/disorders/avms/detail_avms.htm. Accessed: August 9, 2008.
2. Diehm C, Kareem S, Lawall H. Epidemiology of peripheral arterial disease. *Vasa*. 2004; 33(4):183–9.
3. Pleşea I.E., Cameniţă A, Georgescu CC, et al. Study of cerebral vascular structures in hypertensive intracerebral haemorrhage. *Rom J Morphol Embryol*. 2005;46(3):249–56.
4. American Heart Association. Diabetes, kidney and cardiovascular disease. Available at: http://www.americanheart.org/presenter.jhtml?identifier=3044857. Accessed: August 9, 2008.
5. Thomas AJ, Gallagher P, Robinson LJ, et al. A comparison of neurocognitive impairment in younger and older adults with major depression. *Psychol Med*. 2008;30:1–9.
6. Huffman JC, Stern TA. Neuropsychiatric consequences of cardiovascular medications. *Dialogues Clin Neurosci*. 2007;9(1):29–45.
7. Reichenberg A, Dahlman KL, Mosovich S, Silverstein JH. Neuropsychiatric consequences of coronary artery bypass grafting and noncardiovascular surgery. *Dialogues Clin Neurosci*. 2007;9(1):85–91.
8. Selnes OA, McKhann GM, Borowicz LM Jr, Grega MA. Cognitive and neurobehavioral dysfunction after cardiac bypass procedures. *Neurol Clin*. 2006;24(1):133–45.
9. Ogata J, Yutani C, Otsubo R, et al. Heart and vessel pathology underlying brain infarction in 142 stroke patients. *Ann Neurol*. 2008;63(6):770–81.
10. Savelieva I, Camm J. Update on atrial fibrillation: Part I. *Clin Cardiol*. 2008;31(2):55–62.
11. Hoesch RE, Koenig MA, Geocadin RG. Coma after global ischemic brain injury: Pathophysiology and emerging therapies. *Crit Care Clin*. 2008;24(1):25–44, vii–viii.
12. Maryniak A, Bielawska A, Walczak F, et al. Long-term cognitive outcome in teenage survivors of arrhythmic cardiac arrest. *Resuscitation*. 2008;77(1):46–50.
13. National Heart, Lung and Blood Institute. What is heart failure? Available at: http://www.nhlbi.nih.gov/health/dci/Diseases/Hf/HF_WhatIs.html. Accessed: August 9, 2008.
14. Selnes OA, Grega MA, Borowicz LM Jr, Royall RM, McKhann GM, Baumgartner WA. Cognitive changes with coronary artery disease: A prospective study of coronary artery bypass graft patients and nonsurgical controls. *Ann Thorac Surg*. 2003;75(5):1377–84; discussion 1384–6.
15. Vogels RL, Oosterman JM, Laman DM, et al. Transcranial Doppler blood flow assessment in patients with mild heart failure: Correlates with neuroimaging and cognitive performance. *Congest Heart Fail*. 2008;14(2):61–5.
16. Carey BJ, Eames PJ, Blake MJ, Panerai RB, Potter JF. Dynamic cerebral autoregulation is unaffected by aging. *Stroke*. 2000;31(12):2895–900.

17. Zhang R, Witkowski S, Fu Q, Claassen JA, Levine BD. Cerebral hemodynamics after short- and long-term reduction in blood pressure in mild and moderate hypertension. *Hypertension.* 2007;49(5):1149–55.
18. Cherubini A, Lowenthal DT, Paran E, Mecocci P, Williams LS, Senin U. Hypertension and cognitive function in the elderly. *Am J Ther*. 2007;14(6):533–54.
19. Cleveland Clinic. Coronary artery disease—Symptoms. Available at: http://my.clevelandclinic.org/heart/disorders/cad/cadsymptoms.aspx. Accessed: August 9, 2008.
20. Silbert BS, Scott DA, Evered LA, Lewis MS, Maruff PT. Preexisting cognitive impairment in patients scheduled for elective coronary artery bypass graft surgery. *Anesth Analg*. 2007;104(5):1023–8.
21. Moser DJ, Cohen RA, Clark MM, et al. Neuropsychological functioning among cardiac rehabilitation patients. *J Cardiopulm Rehabil*. 1999;19(2):91–7.
22. Cohen RA, Moser DJ, Clark MM, et al. Neurocognitive functioning and improvement in quality of life following participation in cardiac rehabilitation. *Am J Cardiol*. 1999;83(9):1374–8.

2

EPIDEMIOLOGICAL FACTORS IN THE NEUROPSYCHOLOGY OF CARDIOVASCULAR DISEASE

John Gunstad, Andreana Benitez, Suhrida Yadavalli, and Ashley Szabo

The societal impact of cardiovascular disease (CVD) is difficult to overestimate. Roughly one in three American adults has some form of CVD. Age-related changes raise the prevalence rates to more than 80% of men and 90% of women over the age of 80.[1,2] CVD is the leading cause of death in the United States for both men and women, accounting for approximately 700,000 deaths annually.[3] Total costs of CVD (including health services and lost productivity) for 2008 are estimated at $448.5 billion,[1] and CVD is a leading contributor to poor quality of life and disability.[3]

As described throughout this book, multiple forms of CVD also adversely impact cognitive function. It is well established that persons with CVD are at elevated risk for Alzheimer's disease and vascular dementia.[4,5] Work from recent years demonstrates that CVD produces cognitive changes long prior to the development of these conditions. For example, it has been estimated that CVD adds approximately four years of "brain age," with deficits in attention, executive function, and psychomotor speed being among the most commonly reported.[6–8] Recent sociodemographic trends suggest the interplay between CVD and neurocognitive outcome may have even greater societal impact in coming years. Between 1970 and 2000, the life expectancy of the average American increased by six years—with four years of that increase attributable to reduced CVD mortality.[9] This extended lifespan increases the possible development of conditions like Alzheimer's disease.[10] Similarly, prevalence rates for CVD risk factors like obesity have also increased over time,[3] which may also further increase the eventual neurocognitive consequences of CVD.

The goal of the current chapter is to provide introductory information for several of the most common forms of CVD and neurocognitive disorders to facilitate reading of the subsequent chapters. To do so, basic epidemiological information and known interactions with other disorders are briefly presented, as well as important implications for further work.

Review of Epidemiological Terms and Methods

A thorough review of the terms and methods employed in epidemiological studies is well beyond the scope of this chapter. However, to facilitate the interpretation of work presented in this and other chapters, several key items are briefly discussed below.

An important series of epidemiological terms refers to the occurrence of disorders. "Incidence rates" can be defined as the number of new cases of a given disorder within a specified period, and this value is often adjusted for the size of the population being studied. "Prevalence rates" indicate the number of cases of a given disorder at a specified point in time. To use a hypothetical example, the total number of individuals who newly develop high blood pressure during a period would establish the incidence rate, whereas the total number of persons with high blood pressure (i.e., new onset and existing cases) would compose the prevalence rates. Closely related are studies that seek to determine the factors that make developing a given disorder more likely typically using measures of relative risk such as the Odds Ratio or Risk Ratio. Although computations and appropriate uses differ, both Odds Ratios (OR) and Risk Ratios (RR) estimate the likelihood of a given disorders in one group of persons relative to another in case-control studies, such that a value >1 indicates increased risk of having the disorder.

Although these values indicate how one disorder might be statistically related to another, determining causation often involves an understanding of the possible explanations for their co-occurrence in one individual—often termed *comorbidity*. Neal and Kendler (1995) provide an excellent review of the different models for comorbidity, several of which appear relevant to understanding the frequent co-occurrence of CVD and poor neurocognitive outcome, such as Alzheimer's disease (AD):[11]

- Simple chance, due in part to high base rates of these disorders
- One disorder causes the other (e.g., CVD causes Alzheimer's disease [AD] or Alzheimer's disease causes CVD)
- Reciprocal causation (e.g., both CVD and Alzheimer's disease cause each other)
- Both disorders are manifestations of a single disorder (e.g., both CVD and AD result from a higher-order process)

A final epidemiological consideration involves sampling issues that may distort the observed patterns of comorbidity. A common concern is found in the use of clinical samples to estimate comorbidity rates, as these samples often have a greater number of more severe symptoms. Similarly, "Berkson's bias" reminds us that persons with multiple disorders are more likely to be part of a clinical sample.

With these considerations in mind, basic epidemiological factors of many common forms of CVD and neurocognitive disorders, with particular emphasis on their comorbidities, is presented below.

Cardiovascular Disease

In its broadest definition, CVD refers to all conditions of the heart and vascular system. This definition encompasses conditions with a wide range of physiological mechanisms and hypothesized risk for adverse neurocognitive outcome. In this section, we will briefly introduce three common forms of CVD that are linked to cognitive dysfunction through empirical evidence and clinical experience; namely: (1) hypertension; (2) myocardial infarction; and (3) heart failure.

Hypertension

Hypertension is typically defined as having a systolic blood pressure of ≤140 mmHg, diastolic blood pressure ≤90 mmHg, or a prescription for antihypertensive medication.[1] It is one of the most common medical conditions, as nearly one-third of adult Americans meet these criteria—including more than 50% of people over 60 years of age.[12, 13]

Hypertension will likely become even more prevalent in coming years through multiple factors, including: (1) the rise in obesity rates; (2) the growing proportion of older adults in America; and (3) the 37% of Americans meeting criteria for prehypertension (systolic blood pressure 120–139 mmHg, diastolic 80–89 mmHg).[1, 14, 15]

As a result, medical conditions that are caused or exacerbated by hypertension may also become more prevalent, including end-stage renal disease, atrial fibrillation, and congestive heart failure.[16, 17] Such conditions contribute to the nearly $70 billion in estimated costs for hypertension in 2008 alone.[1]

The increased prevalence of hypertension may also result in greater numbers of persons with poor neurocognitive outcome. Hypertension is a known risk factor for stroke, vascular dementia, and Alzheimer's disease.[18, 19] It is associated with many adverse brain changes, including greater atrophy and the development of white matter disease.[20, 21] In terms of cognitive performance, hypertensive individuals exhibit cognitive deficits long prior to the onset of stroke or dementia, particularly on tests of attention, memory, and psychomotor speed.[7, 22–26] Interestingly, recent work suggests that blood pressure (BP) variability may be even more closely associated with structural brain changes and cognitive function than hypertension alone.[27, 28]

Myocardial Infarction

Myocardial infarction (MI) also referred to as acute myocardial infarction (AMI) or heart attack, results from an interruption of blood flow to the heart. It most often results from the occlusion of a coronary artery after the rupture of a vulnerable atherosclerotic plaque, which is an unstable collection of lipids and white blood cells in the wall of an artery. The resulting ischemia and oxygen shortage can cause infarction of the myocardium if it is left untreated for a sufficient period. The acute rupture of a plaque may also lead to an acute myocardial infarction.[1]

This year an estimated 770,000 Americans will have a new MI and another 430,000 will have a recurrent attack.[1] It is estimated that an additional 190,000 silent first heart attacks occur each year.[1] Men typically have their first heart attack at a younger age (65 years) than women (70 years).[1] Depending on gender and clinical outcome, people who survive the acute stage of a heart attack have a chance of further illness or death that is 1.5 to 15 times higher than that of the general population.[1] The risk of another heart attack, sudden death, angina pectoris, heart failure, and stroke is substantial for both men and women.[1] Not surprisingly, depression is common in patients recovering from a myocardial infarction and is an independent risk factor for early mortality.[29–32]

Cognitive impairment is common in patients with MI and is associated with poor outcome. Persons suffering an MI demonstrate greater white matter lesions and more frequent brain infarction on MRI.[33] MI patients are at an increased risk of dementia, as women with a history of a single MI are up to five times more likely to develop dementia.[33, 34] Given these findings, it is perhaps not surprising that MI is independently associated with cognitive impairment even without development of dementia or stroke.[35]

MI patients can exhibit deficits in nearly all cognitive domains, including global cognitive function, attention, processing speed, and memory.[36] Cognitive impairment is particularly prevalent in MI patients with comorbid depression.[37] This depression often has important functional implications for the lives of MI patients. Patients with depression following an acute MI are less likely to adhere to recommended behavior and lifestyle changes intended to reduce the risk of subsequent cardiac events.[38] This tendency may help explain why depression is associated with poor long-term prognosis in patients recovering from an MI.[38]

Many different physiological processes may link MI and cognitive impairment. Cardiac arrest can sometimes be triggered by an MI and can result in severe reduction in cerebral blood flow and thus significant ischemia.[39, 40] There is substantial evidence that cerebral blood flow may be disrupted in MI in the absence of cardiac arrest and may lead to cognitive deficits in this population.[41] Sudden elevation of blood pressure due to chronic hypertension is also associated with incidence of MI and cognitive deficits.[42, 43]

Heart Failure

Despite advances in treatment, the incidence of heart failure has remained stable or increased during the past two decades.[12] Approximately 1% to 2% of adults have HF, with the prevalence increasing to 6% to 10% of persons older than 65 years of age.[44–46, 54, 80, 85] HF is the single most costly cardiovascular disease in the United States, with estimated costs of nearly $30 billion for 2006 alone.[12, 47] Much of this cost is attributable to the high rates of disability in HF patients, as 22% of male and 46% of female heart attack victims will be disabled with HF within 6 years.[12, 47] HF patients are six to nine times more likely to suffer sudden cardiac death, and 20% will die within

12 months following discharge.[12] Given these findings, it is perhaps not surprising that HF is also associated with significant depression, anxiety, and poor quality of life.[48–50]

Cognitive impairment is common in patients with HF and associated with poor outcome. Though estimated prevalence rates typically range from 35% to 50%, cognitive dysfunction has been found in up to 80% of HF samples.[51, 52] Cognitive impairment is believed to exist in more than one million HF patients in the United States alone, with more than 50% of HF patients showing cognitive deficits severe enough to meet diagnostic criteria for dementia.[53, 54] Although cognitive deficits are most prevalent in older adults with HF, even young HF patients (average age = 41 years) exhibit significant impairment on testing.[55–57]

HF patients exhibit deficits in nearly all cognitive domains. Recent reviews demonstrate that impairments in attention, working memory, executive function, memory, and language abilities can be found on testing.[55, 56, 58–61] In turn, this cognitive impairment is associated with many adverse outcomes. In older adults with HF, cognitive impairment is associated with a five times greater risk of mortality and sixfold risk of reduced functional abilities.[62–64] These risks are often attributed to reduced ability to adhere to prescribed medical regimens and lifestyle changes prescribed by physicians.[65–67] For example, only 55% of HF patients can name their current medications, and just 36% can identify what time of day to take them.[65] In addition to these functional difficulties, the cognitive dysfunction of HF is also associated with reduced quality of life and impairment in social, work, and leisure activities.[51, 68]

The cognitive dysfunction found in HF patients is believed to result from multiple factors. Substantial evidence indicates that brain pathology and reduced cerebral blood flow are common in HF and probably contribute to reduced neuropsychological function.[69]

Conditions Frequently Comorbid to CVD

Recent years have seen considerable research devoted to the association between conditions frequently comorbid to CVD and poor cognitive outcome. Examination of the neurocognitive impact of disorders such as type 2 diabetes, obesity, and sleep apnea indicates persistent adverse impact. The growing prevalence of these conditions encourages continued work to identify the underlying neurological mechanisms for impairment and improved interventions for them. A brief introduction to these findings is presented below.

Type 2 Diabetes

Diabetes mellitus is a group of metabolic diseases characterized by high blood-sugar levels, which result from defects in insulin secretion, or action, or both. Elevated levels of blood glucose (i.e., hyperglycemia) lead to spillage of glucose into the urine. Normally, blood glucose levels are tightly controlled by insulin, a hormone produced by the pancreas. Insulin lowers the blood glucose level. When blood glucose elevates (for example, after eating food), insulin is released from the pancreas to normalize the glucose level. In patients with diabetes, the absence or insufficient production of insulin causes hyperglycemia. Diabetes is a chronic medical condition, meaning that although it can be controlled, it lasts a lifetime.[1] A fasting blood sugar level of 126 mg/dL or higher is consistent with either type 1 or type 2 diabetes when accompanied by classic signs and symptoms of diabetes—increased thirst or hunger, frequent urination, weight loss, or blurred vision.[9] There are two types of diabetes mellitus—type 1 and type 2. Type 1 diabetes is an autoimmune disease that results in the permanent destruction of insulin-producing beta cells of the pancreas. Type 2 diabetes (formerly called non-insulin-dependent diabetes mellitus or adult-onset diabetes) is a metabolic disorder that is primarily characterized by insulin resistance, relative insulin deficiency, and hyperglycemia.[70]

Diabetes mellitus affects an estimated 6% (one in 17 people) of the population of the United States, about half of whom are undiagnosed. Incidence is greater in females and rises with age. Type 2 diabetes accounts for 90% of cases.[71] 798,000 new cases of type 2 diabetes are diagnosed per year.[71] Of the 16 million Americans who have type 2 diabetes, only about 7.2 million have actually been diagnosed with it.[72] 11.8% of African American women over 20 and one in four African American women over the age of 55 have type 2.[71] Of Native Americans over 19, 12.2% have type 2; 50% of Pima Indians aged 30 to 64 and 25%% of Hispanic-American women are living with type 2.[71] There are 1.2 million Hispanic Americans of both sexes diagnosed with type 2 diabetes.[71]

Having type 2 diabetes increases one's risk for many serious complications, including cardiovascular disease, retinopathy, neuropathy, and nephropathy. Among patients with type 2 diabetes, depressive symptoms are associated with greater diabetes symptom reporting, poorer physical functioning, and less adherence to exercise regimens and diet.[73] Children who develop type 1 diabetes before they are five years old have been reported to have intellectual impairment,[74–76] and older persons with type 1 diabetes have also been found to have cognitive deficits.[77] Even short-term mild hypoglycemia can cause subtle abnormalities in cognitive function.[78] There is also evidence for an elevated risk of both vascular dementia and Alzheimer's disease in type 2 diabetes with strong interaction of other factors such as hypertension, dyslipidaemia, and apolipoprotein E phenotype.[79] Diabetes is associated with lower levels of cognitive function and greater cognitive decline among older women.[79, 80] Type 2 diabetes and longer duration of diabetes mellitus are similarly related to cognitive impairment and decline in men and women.[81] Type 2 diabetes is associated with diminished cognitive function in different cognitive domains[82] including memory and verbal fluency,[80] executive function,[83] working memory, attention, and processing speed.[84]

Neuropathological studies of neonates have shown that hypoglycemia can cause lesions similar to those caused by hypoxia,[85] and autopsies of adults have shown that nearly twice as many persons with diabetes mellitus have atherosclerosis as those who do not have this disorder.[86] Proliferative lesions of cerebral parenchymal vessels are 25 times more common in persons with diabetes.[87] These patients also have increased blood viscosity[88] and cerebral vessel reactivity.[89] It is well known that diabetes mellitus causes peripheral neuropathies and autonomic neuropathies.[90–93] Neuropsychological deficits have been found in patients with peripheral neuropathies.[94] Diabetes is also associated with disruption in blood-brain barrier function, which can cause neurological and cognitive dysfunction.[95]

Obesity

Nearly two-thirds of American adults are overweight or obese, an increase of 110% over the past two decades.[96–98] Approximately 31% of people between 20 and 74 years of age are obese (BMI $\geq$ 30), with 5% meeting criteria for extreme obesity (BMI $\geq$ 40).[97]

Obesity is a leading preventable cause of death, accounting for an estimated 400,000 deaths each year.[99] Some researchers predict obesity will cause the first decline in life expectancy in 100 years.[100, 101] This risk is largely attributable to the many health consequences of obesity, including cardiovascular disease, type 2 diabetes, sleep apnea, and cancer.[102, 103] For example, obese adults are five times likelier to have high blood pressure and 40 times likelier to have type 2 diabetes than their normal-weight peers.[14, 104–106] Given these associations, it is perhaps not surprising that an elevated body mass index (BMI) is also linked to greater risk of disability.[107, 108]

Though less frequently examined than other medical consequences, there is growing evidence that obesity is associated with poor neurocognitive outcome. Elevated BMI is associated with stroke, Alzheimer's disease, and other forms of dementia.[103, 109–111] Structural brain abnormalities in obese older adults have also been identified, including greater temporal atrophy and white matter disease.[112, 113]

A growing number of studies have directly examined the relationship between obesity and cognitive function. These studies show obesity is associated with poorer cognitive test performance.[114, 115] Obesity is inversely related to global intellectual abilities in children and adults.[116–118] Attention deficit hyperactivity disorder (ADHD) is found in 27% of persons presenting for obesity treatment, including 43% of those with a BMI $\geq$ 40.[119] Candidates for bariatric surgery show reduced executive function and psychomotor speed.[120] Obesity is independently related to reduced memory, executive function, and abstract reasoning.[22, 121, 122]

Sleep Apnea

Obstructive sleep apnea (OSA) is defined as a decrease or cessation of airflow at the nose and mouth during sleep, and is often concurrent with disruptive snoring, excess body weight, and excessive daytime sleepiness.[123] OSA is prevalent in 3% to 7% of the general population[124] and in as many as 42% of older adults, composing an estimated total of 15 million Americans.[125] Gone untreated, OSA costs tens of billions of dollars to the economy due to increased health-care utilization, reduced work performance, and a high rate of occupational and driving accidents.[2, 126–128] Individuals who delay treatment have significantly higher health-care expenses[129] and are at greater risk of developing vascular diseases.[130] At least 30% of patients with heart failure have OSA,[131, 132] while half of the individuals with OSA are likely to develop hypertension[133] or congestive heart failure,[134] and are three times more likely to experience a stroke.[135] Many pathophysiological mechanisms that underlie OSA, including heightened sympathetic activation, cardiovascular variability, and inflammation, purportedly account for the consequent development of cardiac disease and stroke.[123] Furthermore, studies that have shown associations between OSA and dementia that point towards a common diathetic allele, APOE4, which is also implicated as a marker for cerebrovascular disease.[136]

Due to the effects of sleep fragmentation and hypoxemia, patients with OSA exhibit impairments in many cognitive domains including attention and vigilance, executive functions, memory, psychomotor speed, and visuoconstruction.[137, 138] Neuroimaging studies of brain injuries in OSA revealed that changes in vascular structure and function,[123] white matter hyperintensities in the frontal lobes,[139] and hippocampal atrophy[140] promote these deficits. The prevailing treatment for OSA is continuous positive airway pressure (CPAP), a respiratory ventilation device that delivers a stream of compressed air to splint the airway, enabling unobstructed breathing. Studies point towards partial reversibility of cognitive dysfunction in OSA patients after CPAP use, though these findings await further validation.[140, 141]

Neurocognitive Disorders

Any discussion of the possible neurocognitive consequences of CVD is incomplete without brief mention of the epidemiology of common neurological and psychiatric conditions. Conditions like stroke, Alzheimer's disease, and depression are prevalent and have long been associated with CVD. Although the relatively high base rates of these conditions may contribute to the observed co-occurrence, there is growing evidence that CVD is an independent risk factor for their development.

Stroke

A "stroke" is the rapidly developing loss of brain functions due to a disturbance in the blood supply to the brain. Stroke can result from either ischemia (lack of blood supply) caused by thrombosis or embolism; or hemorrhage, typically described as an ischemic stroke or a hemorrhagic stroke.[1] In both cases, the affected brain regions are unable to function normally, producing dramatic neurological symptoms such as hemiplegia, hemiparesis, aphasia, and visual neglect.[1]

Approximately 780,000 people suffer a stroke each year.[1] Of this number, approximately 600,000 of these are first attacks, and 180,000 are recurrent stroke.[1] A number of demographic and medical factors moderate an individual's risk for stroke. The chance of having a stroke approximately doubles for each decade of life after age 55.[3] The female population not only carries a higher burden of stroke during their lifespan—women also account for most stroke deaths.[12] Men typically have a higher incidence of stroke than women up to the age of 75 years, when the incidence in women becomes higher.[12] New data, however, indicate that the incidence of stroke in women in the midlife years might be increasing—women aged 45 to 54 years are around twice as likely to have a stroke as men of the same age.[142] One potential explanation for this finding is that women in this age group are transitioning to menopause, a time when cardiovascular risk factors appear or existing risk factors worsen.[8] Interestingly, there is an interaction between gender and race, as the age-adjusted stroke incidence rates at ages 45 to 84 are 6.6 per 1000 population in black males, 3.6 in white males, 4.9 in black females, and 2.3 in white females.[1] Risk factors for stroke include advanced age, hypertension (high blood pressure), previous stroke or transient ischemic attack (TIA), diabetes, high cholesterol, and atrial fibrillation.[1] High blood pressure is the most important modifiable risk factor of stroke.[1] Other modifiable risk factors include smoking, which almost doubles a person's risk for ischemic stroke, independently of other risk factors and obesity.[143]

Stroke causes considerable physical and psychosocial impairments. Depression after stroke is common, with an estimated prevalence rate of 5% to 70%.[144–146] Although different opinions exist about the definition, diagnosis, and measurement of outcomes related to depression after stroke, there is little debate about their impact on stroke survivors and their families: namely, a longer hospital stay.[147] Depression after stroke has long been recognized as a common condition with many adverse consequences in the post-stroke period, but more recently it has also been identified as an independent stroke risk factor through increased autonomic arousal and neurotransmitter dysregulation.[148] Depression may increase stroke risk through heightened adrenergic activity[148, 149] or through neuroendocrine and immunological effects.[124, 150, 151] It has also been suggested that platelet activation may be a factor explaining the depression–stroke connection.[152, 153] It is also possible that depression operates indirectly by increasing the risk of other diseases that may in turn increase the risk of stroke.[154–156]

Cognitive impairment is common after stroke. Though the specific nature of cognitive impairment varies as a function of the location and size of the infarct, impairments are most commonly reported in attention, executive function, memory, language, and motor functions.[157–159] The pattern of deficits is further modified by a number of premorbid factors, including demographic characteristics, medical conditions, and prior brain pathology.[160] For example, white matter hyperintensities, generalized brain atrophy, and brain infarcts on MRI are associated with steeper decline in processing speed and executive function in stroke patients.[161] Recent work also demonstrates that persons receiving tissue plasminogen activator (t-Pa) within three hours of stroke onset show significant cognitive benefits,[162] further encouraging rapid intervention.

Dementia

Dementia is an increasingly common diagnosis in our aging population. Among individuals aged 71 and older in the United States, 13.9% of individuals have been estimated to have dementia.[163] An estimated 24.3 million individuals have dementia worldwide, with an additional 4.6 million new cases occurring every year.[164] The substantial decline in functional abilities results in staggering costs for care and treatment. Direct costs of dementia worldwide in 2003 were estimated to be between $129 to $159 billion U.S. dollars, with 92% of this expense spent in advanced countries.[165] Although institutionalization represents the largest proportion of expenses,[166] the behavioral and psychological symptoms that manifest throughout the disease course significantly contribute to caregiver burden and overall costs of care.[167] Furthermore, these costs will only continue to climb, as the prevalence of Alzheimer's disease is expected to quadruple by 2050.[168]

Alzheimer's disease and vascular dementia (VaD) have been identified as the most common subtypes of dementia, with an estimated 4.5 and 1 million individuals with these diagnoses in the United States, respectively.[169, 170] The diagnoses of AD and VaD are usually rendered using the criteria of the *Diagnostic and Statistical Manual of Mental Disorders*, (4th ed.) (DSM-IV),[171] the *National Institute of Neurological Disorders and Stroke—Alzheimer Disease and Related Disorders* (NINDS-ADRDA), and the NINDS *Association international pour la recherche et l'enseignement en neurosciences* (AIREN) criteria.[172, 173] The DSM-IV-TR criteria require the presence of severe memory loss and impairment in at least one other cognitive domain (as a result of cerebrovascular disease, for VaD) as well as evidence of interference in social function or activities of daily living. The NINDS-ADRDA and NINDS-AIREN clinical criteria do not require evidence of impaired social or occupational functioning but support a probabilistic diagnostic approach, where a definite diagnosis of AD or VaD is only rendered upon histopathological confirmation from biopsy or autopsy.

With regard to cognitive functioning, AD patients exhibit severe memory loss and rapid forgetting, as well as difficulties in language, executive functioning, semantic knowledge, and visuospatial abilities.[148] These cognitive deficits have been etiologically linked with the presence of amyloid plaques and neurofibrillary tangles, although this hypothesis has been challenged due to its lack of specificity.[174] In contrast, cognitive impairment associated with VaD is characterized by loss of executive function, psychomotor slowing, milder memory loss compared with AD, and a stepwise progression of deficits in the context of confirmed cerebrovascular lesions.[175]

Though both AD and VaD have been researched extensively, only recently has more attention been paid to the co-occurrence of these disorders, often termed *mixed dementia* (MD). While its actual prevalence remains unknown, it is estimated that MD occurs in 4.5% of the elderly population,[176] although this is likely to be an underestimate. Considering the methodological dissimilarities across epidemiological studies, the lack of established criteria for the identification of MD, and the variegated onset and progression of neurodegenerative and vascular pathology in individuals identified to have MD, the prevalence of MD may be as high as 20% to 40% among autopsy-confirmed dementia cases.[177] Although some studies have attempted to differentiate MD from AD and VaD, the results differ in the extent to which the cognitive profile observed in MD is more similar to AD,[178, 179] or VaD,[180] or is a unique, discrete entity.[181] However, a recent study by Zekry and colleagues suggests that identifying the location of the cerebrovascular infarcts may have a role in identifying the type and extent of the cognitive impairment.[182] Further research is needed to delineate the diagnostic criteria for MD to ascertain its true prevalence and disease course.

Depression

Depression afflicts people of all ages, genders, and nationalities, and is frequently comorbid with medical conditions. Worldwide estimates of the prevalence of depression vary greatly; in a recent survey by the World Health Organization, the presence of mood disorders ranged from 0.8% (Nigeria) to 9.6% (United States) among the populations sampled.[183] Epidemiological studies in the United States have indicated that as many as 4.9% of individuals meet criteria for major depression, with a lifetime prevalence estimate reaching 17.1%.[184] Depression is also associated with a high economic burden, costing as much as $83.1 billion to the US economy in 2000 due to medical costs and loss of workplace productivity.[185]

Depression and cardiovascular disease Among individuals with cardiovascular disease, unipolar depression is prevalent[186] and has been shown to predict disease progression,[187, 188] severity,[189] and mortality.[189, 190] Reviews have identified depression as a risk factor in the etiology of cardiovascular disease,[29, 190] prompting behavioral health specialists to promote and create standards for the assessment and treatment of depression in these patients.[191] Biological and psychosocial mechanisms that may account for this causal relationship have been proposed, including hypothalamic-pituitary-adrenocortical (HPA) axis and sympathoadrenal hyperactivity,[192] increases in serum cortisol,[193] chronic stress,[194] and lack of social support.[195]

Nonetheless, the unidirectional relationship between depression and cardiovascular disease remains tentative.[196] For instance, it is possible that cardiovascular disease may precipitate depressive syndromes due to restricted cerebral blood flow resulting from ischemic lesions in key areas of the brain, particularly in older adults.[197, 198] Alternatively, psychosocial (i.e., stress) and genetic (i.e., S and L alleles) etiologies common to both cardiovascular disease and depression have been hypothesized to potentially account for the high rate of comorbidity between these conditions,[196, 199] though these studies are preliminary and warrant further investigation. Examination of alternative mechanisms and causative relationships appears necessary, as extensive clinical trials have shown that treating patients for depression after myocardial infarction have only, at best, modestly minimized recurrence and mortality.[200, 201]

Depression and cognitive function Depression, specifically major depression, has been associated with cognitive difficulties across a variety of domains. Suppressed performance in attention, memory, language, and visuospatial functioning have been observed in depressed individuals compared to controls,[202–205] as well as notable impairments in executive functions.[205, 206] However, there is a lack of consensus regarding the extent to which these difficulties are accounted for by depression subtype (e.g., melancholic vs. non-melancholic, early- vs. late-onset), disease severity, or comorbid psychopathology.[202–204, 207–209]

Neuroanatomical correlates of depression are similarly diffuse, but studies largely identify the prefrontal cortex, the anterior cingulate, and the limbic system as activated in patients with unipolar depression and cognitive dysfunction.[210, 211] Further research associating these structures with the various features of depressive disorders, while taking into account comorbid medical and neurological pathologies, may better delineate cognitive correlates and improve the specificity of measures used to assess these domains.

Summary and Conclusions

CVD is prevalent and associated with cognitive dysfunction long prior to the development of Alzheimer's disease or vascular dementia. Medical conditions that are frequently comorbid to CVD (e.g., obesity, sleep apnea) adversely impact cognitive function and are likely to interact with CVD to have even greater neurological consequences. Continued work is needed to better understand complex heart–brain connections, as the growing proportion of older adults suggests such interactions will become more prevalent and have greater societal impact in coming years. For example, recent work demonstrates that people with Alzheimer's disease exhibit silent ischemia and arrythymias, even without a history of coronary artery disease.[212] Such findings suggest that heart–brain connections are more complicated than typically believed and require further investigation.

Notes

1. Heart Disease and Stroke Statistics—2008 Update. A report from the American Heart Association statistics committee and stroke statistics subcommittee (cited 2008 November 23); Available from: http://circ.ahajournals.org/cgi/reprint/CIRCULATIONAHA.107.187998.
2. Young T, et al. The occurrence of sleep-disordered breathing among middle-aged adults. *N Engl J Med.* 1993;328(17):1230–1235.
3. Heart disease facts and statistics. Centers for Disease Control and Prevention. (cited 2008 November 23); Available from: http://www.cdc.gov/heartdisease/statistics.htm#reports.
4. Duron E, Hanon O. Vascular risk factors, cognitive decline, and dementia. *Vasc Health Risk Manag*. 2008;4(2):363–381.
5. Newman AB, et al. Dementia and Alzheimer's disease incidence in relationship to cardiovascular disease in the Cardiovascular Health Study cohort. *J Am Geriatr Soc*. 2005;53(7):1101–1107.
6. Roman GC, et al. Vascular cognitive disorder: A new diagnostic category updating vascular cognitive impairment and vascular dementia. *J Neurol Sci*. 2004;226(1–2):81–7.
7. Waldstein SR, et al. Neuropsychological correlates of hypertension: Review and methodologic considerations. *Psychol Bull*, 1991;110(3):451–68.
8. Matthews KA, et al. Changes in cardiovascular risk factors during the perimenopause and postmenopause and carotid artery atherosclerosis in healthy women. *Stroke*. 2001;32(5):1104–1111.
9. Heart Disease Fact Sheet. National Institutes of Health (cited 2008 November 23); Available from: http://www.nih.gov/about/researchresultsforthepublic/heartdisease.pdf.
10. Fratiglioni L, et al. Prevalence of Alzheimer's disease and other dementias in an elderly urban population: Relationship with age, sex, and education. *Neurology*. 1991;41(12):1886–1892.

11. Neale MC, Kendler KS. Models of comorbidity for multifactorial disorders. *Am J Hum Genet*. 1995;57(4):935–953.
12. Thom T, et al. Heart disease and stroke statistics–2006 update: a report from the American Heart Association Statistics Committee and Stroke Statistics Subcommittee. *Circulation*. 2006;113(6):e85–151.
13. National Heart Lung and Blood Institute. Disease and Conditions Index (cited 2008 November 23); Available from: http://www.nhlbi.nih.gov/health/dci/Diseases/Hbp/HBP_All.html.
14. Harris MM, et al. Associations of fat distribution and obesity with hypertension in a bi-ethnic population: The ARIC study. Atherosclerosis Risk in Communities Study. *Obes Res*. 2000;8(7):516–524.
15. Merck Institute of Aging and Health: *The State of Aging and Health in America*.
16. Heist EK, Ruskin JN. Atrial fibrillation and congestive heart failure: Risk factors, mechanisms, and treatment. *Prog Cardiovasc Dis*. 2006;48(4):256–269.
17. Johnson DW, Usherwood T. Chronic kidney disease—management update. *Aust Fam Physician*. 2005;34(11):915–923.
18. Peila R, et al. Reducing the risk of dementia: Efficacy of long-term treatment of hypertension. *Stroke*. 2006;37(5):1165–1170.
19. Posner HB, et al. The relationship of hypertension in the elderly to AD, vascular dementia, and cognitive function. *Neurology*. 2002;58(8):1175–1181.
20. DeCarli C. Prevention of white-matter lesions through control of cerebrovascular risk factors. *Int Psychogeriatr*. 2003;15 Suppl 1:147–151.
21. Gianaros PJ, et al. Higher blood pressure predicts lower regional grey matter volume: Consequences on short-term information processing. *Neuroimage*. 2006;31(2):754–765.
22. Elias MF, et al. Lower cognitive function in the presence of obesity and hypertension: The Framingham heart study. *Int J Obes Relat Metab Disord*. 2003;27(2):260–268.
23. Harrington F, et al. Cognitive performance in hypertensive and normotensive older subjects. *Hypertension*. 2000;36(6):1079–1082.
24. Knopman D, et al. Cardiovascular risk factors and cognitive decline in middle-aged adults. *Neurology*. 2001;56(1):42–48.
25. Morris MC, et al. Association between blood pressure and cognitive function in a biracial community population of older persons. *Neuroepidemiology*. 2002;21(3):123–130.
26. Ostrosky-Solis F, Mendoza VU, Ardila A. Neuropsychological profile of patients with primary systemic hypertension. *Int J Neurosci*. 2001;110(3–4):159–172.
27. Gunstad J, et al. Blood pressure variability and white matter hyperintensities in older adults with cardiovascular disease. *Blood Press*. 2005;14(6):353–358.
28. Kanemaru K, Kanemaru A, Kuwajima I. Antihypertensive therapy in patients with stroke. *Nippon Rinsho*. 2001;59(5):945–948.
29. Frasure-Smith F. Lesperance, Reflections on depression as a cardiac risk factor. *Psychosom Med*. 2005;67 Suppl 1:S19–25.
30. Frasure-Smith N, Lesperance F, Talajic M. Depression following myocardial infarction. Impact on 6-month survival. *JAMA*. 1993;270(15):1819–1825.
31. Strik JJ, et al. One-year cumulative incidence of depression following myocardial infarction and impact on cardiac outcome. *J Psychosom Res*. 2004;56(1):59–66.
32. Romanelli J, et al. The significance of depression in older patients after myocardial infarction. *J Am Geriatr Soc*. 2002;50(5):817–822.
33. Ikram MA, et al. Unrecognized myocardial infarction in relation to risk of dementia and cerebral small vessel disease. *Stroke*. 2008;39(5):1421–1426.
34. Aronson MK, et al. Women, myocardial infarction, and dementia in the very old. *Neurology*. 1990;40(7):1102–1106.

35. Singh-Manoux A, Britton AR, Marmot M. Vascular disease and cognitive function: Evidence from the Whitehall II Study. *J Am Geriatr Soc*. 2003;51(10):1445–1450.
36. Vinkers DJ, et al. Generalized atherosclerosis, cognitive decline, and depressive symptoms in old age. *Neurology*. 2005;65(1):107–112.
37. Vinkers DJ, et al. Temporal relation between depression and cognitive impairment in old age: Prospective population-based study. *BMJ*. 2004;329(7471):881.
38. Ziegelstein RC, et al. Patients with depression are less likely to follow recommendations to reduce cardiac risk during recovery from a myocardial infarction. *Arch Intern Med*. 2000;160(12):1818–1823.
39. Eisenberg MS, Mengert, TJ. Cardiac resuscitation. *N Engl J Med*. 2001;344(17): 1304–1313.
40. Irwin RS, Rippe JM. *Irwin and Rippe's Intensive Care Medicine*, 6th ed., 2008 (p. 2336). Philadelphia: Lippincott Williams & Wilkins.
41. Dolan RJ, et al. Regional cerebral blood flow abnormalities in depressed patients with cognitive impairment. *J Neurol Neurosurg Psych*. 1992;55(9):768–773.
42. dos Santos MG, et al. Risk factors for the development of atherosclerosis in childhood and adolescence. *Arq Bras Cardiol*. 2008;90(4):276–283.
43. Laskarzewski P, et al. The relationship of parental history of myocardial infarction, hypertension, diabetes and stroke to coronary heart disease risk factors in their adult progeny. *Am J Epidemiol*. 1981;113(3):290–306.
44. Ho KK, et al. The epidemiology of heart failure: The Framingham study. *J Am Coll Cardiol*. 1993;22(4 Suppl A):6A–13A.
45. Massie BM, Shah NB. Evolving trends in the epidemiologic factors of heart failure: rationale for preventive strategies and comprehensive disease management. *Am Heart J*. 1997;133(6):703–712.
46. O'Connell JB, Bristow MR. Economic impact of heart failure in the United States: Time for a different approach. *J Heart Lung Transplant*. 1994;13(4):S107–112.
47. Lithell H, et al. The study on cognition and prognosis in the elderly (SCOPE): Principal results of a randomized double-blind intervention trial. *J Hypertens*. 2003;21(5): 875–886.
48. Moser DK, Doering LV, and Chung ML. Vulnerabilities of patients recovering from an exacerbation of chronic heart failure. *Am Heart J*. 2005;150(5):984.
49. Lesman-Leegte I, et al. Depressive symptoms are prominent among elderly hospitalised heart failure patients. *Eur J Heart Fail*. 2006;8(6):634–640.
50. Gott M, et al. Predictors of the quality of life of older people with heart failure recruited from primary care. *Age Ageing*. 2006;35(2):172–177.
51. Almeida OP and Tamai, S. Congestive heart failure and cognitive functioning amongst older adults. *Arq Neuropsiquiatr*. 2001;59(2-B):324–329.
52. Zuccala G, et al. Use of angiotensin-converting enzyme inhibitors and variations in cognitive performance among patients with heart failure. *Eur Heart J*. 2005;26(3):226–233.
53. Roman GC. Brain hypoperfusion: A critical factor in vascular dementia. *Neurol Res*. 2004;26(5):454–458.
54. Cacciatore F, et al. Congestive heart failure and cognitive impairment in an older population. Osservatorio Geriatrico Campano Study Group. *J Am Geriatr Soc*. 1998;46(11):1343–1348.
55. Gorkin L, et al. Assessment of quality of life as observed from the baseline data of the studies of left ventricular dysfunction (SOLVD) trial quality-of-life substudy. *Am J Cardiol*. 1993;71(12):1069–1073.
56. Schmidt R, et al. Brain magnetic resonance imaging and neuropsychological evaluation of patients with idiopathic dilated cardiomyopathy. *Stroke*. 1991;22(2):195–199.

57. Trojano L, et al. Cognitive impairment: A key feature of congestive heart failure in the elderly. *J Neurol*. 2003;250(12):1456–1463.
58. Almeida OP, Flicker L. The mind of a failing heart: A systematic review of the association between congestive heart failure and cognitive functioning. *Intern Med J*. 2001;31(5): 290–295.
59. Bennett SJ, Sauve MJ. Cognitive deficits in patients with heart failure: A review of the literature. *J Cardiovasc Nurs*. 2003;18(3):219–242.
60. Zuccala G, et al. Left ventricular dysfunction: A clue to cognitive impairment in older patients with heart failure. *J Neurol Neurosurg Psychiatry*. 1997;63(4):509–512.
61. Ware J, Sherbourne C. The MOS 36-item short-form health survey (SF–36) I. Conceptual framework and item selection. *Med Care*. 1992;*30*:473–483.
62. Barclay LL, et al. Unrecognized cognitive impairment in cardiac rehabilitation patients. *J Am Geriatr Soc*. 1988;36(1):22–28.
63. Konstam MA. Progress in heart failure management? Lessons from the real world. *Circulation*. 2000;102(10):1076–1078.
64. Zuccala G, et al. The effects of cognitive impairment on mortality among hospitalized patients with heart failure. *Am J Med*. 2003;115(2):97–103.
65. Cline CM, et al. Non-compliance and knowledge of prescribed medication in elderly patients with heart failure. *Eur J Heart Fail*. 1999;1(2):145–149.
66. Karlsson MR, et al. A nurse-based management program in heart failure patients affects females and persons with cognitive dysfunction most. *Patient Educ Couns*. 2005;58(2): 146–153.
67. Rogers AE, et al. Knowledge and communication difficulties for patients with chronic heart failure: Qualitative study. *BMJ*. 2000;321(7261):605–607.
68. Bennett SJ, Baker SL, Huster GA. Quality of life in women with heart failure. *Health Care Women Int*. 1998;19(3):217–229.
69. Bennett SJ, Sauve MJ, Shaw RM. A conceptual model of cognitive deficits in chronic heart failure. *J Nurs Scholarsh*. 2005;37(3):222–228.
70. Diabetes Information (cited 2008 December 2); Available from: http://www.diabetes.org/about-diabetes.jsp.
71. National Diabetes Statistics (cited 2008 December 2); Available from: http://www.diabetes.niddk.nih.gov/dm/pubs/statistics/#allages.
72. Frasure-Smith N, Lesperance F, Talajic M. Depression and 18-month prognosis after myocardial infarction. *Circulation*. 1995;91(4):999–1005.
73. Ciechanowski PS, et al. The relationship of depressive symptoms to symptom reporting, self-care and glucose control in diabetes. *Gen Hosp Psychiatry*. 2003;25(4):246–252.
74. Ack M, Miller I, Weil WB Jr. Intelligence of children with diabetes mellitus. *Pediatrics*. 1961;28:764–770.
75. Rovet JF, Ehrlich RM, and Hoppe M. Specific intellectual deficits in children with early onset diabetes mellitus. *Child Dev*. 1988;59(1):226–234.
76. Ryan C, Vega A, Drash A. Cognitive deficits in adolescents who developed diabetes early in life. *Pediatrics*. 1985;75(5):921–927.
77. Skenazy JA, Bigler ED. Neuropsychological findings in diabetes mellitus. *J Clin Psychol*. 1984;40(1):246–58.
78. Holmes CS, et al. Verbal fluency and naming performance in type I diabetes at different blood glucose concentrations. *Diabetes Care*. 1984;7(5):454–459.
79. Gregg EW, et al. Is diabetes associated with cognitive impairment and cognitive decline among older women? Study of Osteoporotic Fractures Research Group. *Arch Intern Med*. 2000;160(2):174–180.

80. Logroscino G, Kang JH, Grodstein F. Prospective study of type 2 diabetes and cognitive decline in women aged 70–81 years. *BMJ*. 2004;328(7439):548.
81. Okereke OI, et al. Type 2 diabetes mellitus and cognitive decline in two large cohorts of community-dwelling older adults. *J Am Geriatr Soc*. 2008;56(6):1028–1036.
82. van Harten B, et al. Cognitive impairment and MRI correlates in the elderly patients with type 2 diabetes mellitus. *Age Ageing*. 2007;36(2):164–170.
83. Stewart R, Liolitsa D. Type 2 diabetes mellitus, cognitive impairment and dementia. *Diabet Med*. 1999;16(2):93–112.
84. Sommerfield AJ, Deary IJ, Frier BM. Acute hyperglycemia alters mood state and impairs cognitive performance in people with type 2 diabetes. *Diabetes Care*. 2004;27(10):2335–2340.
85. Brierley J. Cerebral hypoxia. *Greenfield's Neuropathology third edition* (Corsellis, J & Blackwood, W., eds). 1976, London: Blackwood W.
86. Grunnet ML. Cerebrovascular disease: diabetes and cerebral atherosclerosis. *Neurology*. 1963;13:486–491.
87. Alex M, et al. An autopsy study of cerebrovascular accident in diabetes mellitus. Circulation. 1962;25:663–673.
88. Barnes AJ, et al. Is hyperviscosity a treatable component of diabetic microcirculatory disease? *Lancet*. 1977;2(8042):789–791.
89. Dandona P, et al. Cerebral blood flow in diabetes mellitus: Evidence of abnormal cerebrovascular reactivity. *BMJ*. 1978;2(6133):325–326.
90. Bergstrom B, et al. Autonomic neuropathy in type I diabetes: Influence of duration and other diabetic complications. *Acta Med Scand*. 1987;222(2):147–154.
91. Harati Y. Diabetic peripheral neuropathies. *Ann Intern Med*. 1987;107(4):546–559.
92. Reichel G. Autonomic symptoms in diabetic polyneuropathies. *Fortschr Neurol Psychiatr*. 1987;55(4):107–129.
93. Ziegler D, et al. Peripheral and autonomic nerve function in long-term insulin-dependent diabetes. *Diabetes Res*. 1987;4(1):9–14.
94. Lawson JS, et al. Neuropsychological function in diabetic patients with neuropathy. *Br J Psychiatry*. 1984;145:263–268.
95. Horani MH, Mooradian AD. Effect of diabetes on the blood brain barrier. *Curr Pharm Des*. 2003;9(10):833–840.
96. Flegal KM, et al. Overweight and obesity in the United States: Prevalence and trends, 1960–1994. *Int J Obes Relat Metab Disord*. 1998;22(1):39–47.
97. Flegal KM, et al. Prevalence and trends in obesity among U.S. adults, 1999–2000. *JAMA*. 2002;288(14):1723–1727.
98. Stein CJ, Colditz, GA. The epidemic of obesity. *J Clin Endocrinol Metab*. 2004;89(6): 2522–2525.
99. Mokdad AH, et al. Actual causes of death in the United States, 2000. *JAMA*. 2004; 291(10):1238–1245.
100. Flegal KM, et al. Excess deaths associated with underweight, overweight, and obesity. *JAMA*. 2005;293(15):1861–1867.
101. Olshansky SJ, et al. A potential decline in life expectancy in the United States in the 21st century. *N Engl J Med*. 2005;352(11):1138–1145.
102. Bray GA. Medical consequences of obesity. *J Clin Endocrinol Metab*. 2004;89(6): 2583–2589.
103. O'Brien PE, Dixon JB, Brown W. Obesity is a surgical disease: Overview of obesity and bariatric surgery. *ANZ J Surg*. 2004;74(4):200–204.
104. Chan JM, et al. Obesity, fat distribution, and weight gain as risk factors for clinical diabetes in men. *Diabetes Care*. 1994;17(9):961–969.

105. Colditz GA, et al. Weight gain as a risk factor for clinical diabetes mellitus in women. *Ann Intern Med.* 1995;122(7):481–486.
106. Rosenberg L, et al. Obesity and hypertension among college-educated black women in the United States. *J Hum Hypertens.* 1999;13(4):237–241.
107. Launer LJ, et al. Body mass index, weight change, and risk of mobility disability in middle-aged and older women. The epidemiologic follow-up study of NHANES I. *JAMA.* 1994;271(14):1093–1098.
108. Rissanen A, et al. Risk of disability and mortality due to overweight in a Finnish population. *BMJ.* 1990;301(6756):835–837.
109. Gustafson D, et al. An 18-year follow-up of overweight and risk of Alzheimer disease. *Arch Intern Med.* 2003;163(13):1524–1528.
110. Rosengren A, et al. Body mass index, other cardiovascular risk factors, and hospitalization for dementia. *Arch Intern Med.* 2005;165(3):321–326.
111. Whitmer RA, et al. Obesity in middle age and future risk of dementia: A 27-year longitudinal population based study. *BMJ.* 2005;330(7504):1360.
112. Gustafson D, et al. A 24-year follow-up of body mass index and cerebral atrophy. *Neurology.* 2004;63(10):1876–1881.
113. Gustafson DR, Steen B, Skoog, I. Body mass index and white matter lesions in elderly women. An 18-year longitudinal study. *Int Psychogeriatr.* 2004;16(3):327–336.
114. Jeong SK, et al. Interactive effect of obesity indexes on cognition. *Dement Geriatr Cogn Disord.* 2005;19(2–3):91–96.
115. Kilander L, et al. Cognitive function, vascular risk factors and education. A cross-sectional study based on a cohort of 70-year-old men. *J Intern Med.* 1997;242(4):313–321.
116. Halkjaer J, Holst C, Sorensen TI. Intelligence test score and educational level in relation to BMI changes and obesity. *Obes Res.* 2003;11(10):1238–1245.
117. Halkjaer J, Sorensen TI. Psychosocial and demographic determinants of regional differences in the prevalence of obesity. *J Biosoc Sci.* 2004;36(2):141–152.
118. Li X. A study of intelligence and personality in children with simple obesity. *Int J Obes Relat Metab Disord.* 1995;19(5):355–357.
119. Altfas JR. Prevalence of attention deficit/hyperactivity disorder among adults in obesity treatment. *BMC Psychiatry.* 2002;2:9.
120. Chelune GJ, Ortega D, Linton JC, Boustany MM. Personality and cognitive findings among patients electing gastroplasty for morbid obesity. *Int J Eat Disord.* 1986;5:701–712.
121. Gunstad J, et al. Obesity is associated with memory deficits in young and middle-aged adults. *Eat Weight Disord.* 2006;11(1):e15–19.
122. Gunstad J, et al. Elevated body mass index is associated with executive dysfunction in otherwise healthy adults. *Compr Psychiatry.* 2007;48(1):57–61.
123. Somers VK, et al. Sleep apnea and cardiovascular disease: An American Heart Association/American College of Cardiology Foundation scientific statement from the American Heart Association Council for High Blood Pressure Research Professional Education Committee, Council on Clinical Cardiology, Stroke Council, and Council On Cardiovascular Nursing. In collaboration with the National Heart, Lung, and Blood Institute National Center on Sleep Disorders Research (National Institutes of Health). *Circulation.* 2008;118(10):1080–1111.
124. Punjabi N. The epidemiology of adult obstructive sleep apnea. Proceedings of the American Thoracic Society. 2008(5):136–143.
125. Ancoli-Israel S, et al. Sleep-disordered breathing in community-dwelling elderly. *Sleep.* 1991;14(6):486–495.

126. AlGhanim N, et al. The economic impact of obstructive sleep apnea. *Lung*. 2008; 186(1):7–12.
127. Kapur V, et al. The medical cost of undiagnosed sleep apnea. *Sleep*. 1999;22(6):749–755.
128. Sassani A, et al. Reducing motor-vehicle collisions, costs, and fatalities by treating obstructive sleep apnea syndrome. *Sleep*. 2004;27(3):453–458.
129. Wittmann V, Rodenstein DO. Health care costs and the sleep apnea syndrome. *Sleep Med Rev*. 2004;8(4):269–279.
130. Pelletier-Fleury N, et al. Economic arguments for the immediate management of moderate-to-severe obstructive sleep apnoea syndrome. *Eur Respir J*. 2004;23(1):53–60.
131. MacDonald M, et al. The current prevalence of sleep disordered breathing in congestive heart failure patients treated with beta-blockers. *J Clin Sleep Med*. 2008;4(1):38–42.
132. Oldenburg O, et al. Sleep-disordered breathing in patients with symptomatic heart failure: A contemporary study of prevalence in and characteristics of 700 patients. *Eur J Heart Fail*. 2007;9(3):251–257.
133. Hla KM, et al. Sleep apnea and hypertension. A population-based study. *Ann Intern Med*. 1994;120(5):382–388.
134. Shahar E, et al. Sleep-disordered breathing and cardiovascular disease: Cross-sectional results of the Sleep Heart Health Study. *Am J Respir Crit Care Med*. 2001;163(1): 19–25.
135. Neau JP, et al. Habitual snoring as a risk factor for brain infarction. *Acta Neurol Scand*. 1995;92(1):63–68.
136. Bliwise DL. Sleep apnea, APOE4 and Alzheimer's disease, 20 years and counting? *J Psychosom Res*. 2002;53(1):539–546.
137. Aloia MS, et al. Neuropsychological sequelae of obstructive sleep apnea-hypopnea syndrome: A critical review. *J Int Neuropsychol Soc*. 2004;10(5):772–785.
138. Rourke SB, Grant AK, *The neuropsychological correlates of acute and chronic hypoxemia*, 2nd ed., p. 23. 1996. New York: Oxford University Press.
139. Zimmerman ME, Aloia., MS. A review of neuroimaging in obstructive sleep apnea. *J Clin Sleep Med*. 2006;2(4):461–471.
140. Gale SD, Hopkins RO. Effects of hypoxia on the brain: Neuroimaging and neuropsychological findings following carbon monoxide poisoning and obstructive sleep apnea. *J Int Neuropsychol Soc*. 2004;10(1):60–71.
141. Ferini-Strambi L, et al. Cognitive dysfunction in patients with obstructive sleep apnea (OSA): Partial reversibility after continuous positive airway pressure (CPAP). *Brain Res Bull*. 2003;61(1):87–92.
142. Towfighi A, et al. A midlife stroke surge among women in the United States. *Neurology*. 2007;69(20):1898–1904.
143. National Institute of Neurological Disorders and Stroke. (cited 2008 December 3); Available from: http://www.ninds.nih.gov/disorders/stroke/preventing_stroke.htm.
144. Astrom M, Adolfsson R, Asplund K. Major depression in stroke patients. A 3-year longitudinal study. *Stroke*. 1993;24(7):976–982.
145. Pohjasvaara T, et al. Frequency and clinical determinants of poststroke depression. *Stroke*. 1998;29(11):2311–2317.
146. Burvill PW, Johnson GA, Chakera TMH, Steward-Wynne E.G., Anderson CS, Jamrozik KD. The place and site of lesion in the aetiology of post-stroke depression. *Cerebrovascular Disease*. 1996;6:208–215.
147. Ebrahim S, Barer D, and Nouri F. Affective illness after stroke. *Br J Psychiatry*. 1987; 151:52–56.

148. Siever LJ, Davis, KL. Overview: Toward a dysregulation hypothesis of depression. *Am J Psychiatry*. 1985;142(9):1017–1031.
149. Ford DE, et al. Depression is a risk factor for coronary artery disease in men: The precursors study. *Arch Intern Med*. 1998;158(13):1422–1426.
150. Andreoli AV, et al. Depression and immunity: Age, severity, and clinical course. *Brain Behav Immun*. 1993;7(4):279–292.
151. Herbert TB, Cohen, S. Depression and immunity: A meta-analytic review. *Psychol Bull*. 1993;113(3):472–486.
152. Dwight MM, Stoudemire A. Effects of depressive disorders on coronary artery disease: A review. *Harv Rev Psychiatry*. 1997;5(3):115–122.
153. Musselman DL, Evans DL, Nemeroff CB. The relationship of depression to cardiovascular disease: Epidemiology, biology, and treatment. *Arch Gen Psychiatry*. 1998;55(7): 580–592.
154. Anda RF, et al. Depression and the dynamics of smoking. A national perspective. *JAMA*. 1990;264(12):1541–1545.
155. Camacho TC, et al. Physical activity and depression: Evidence from the Alameda County study. *Am J Epidemiol*. 1991;134(2):220–231.
156. Kaplan GA, et al. Psychosocial factors in the natural history of physical activity. *Am J Prev Med*. 1991;7(1):12–17.
157. Hochstenbach J, et al. Cognitive decline following stroke: A comprehensive study of cognitive decline following stroke. *J Clin Exp Neuropsychol*. 1998;20(4):503–517.
158. Pohjasvaara T, et al. Dementia three months after stroke. Baseline frequency and effect of different definitions of dementia in the Helsinki Stroke Aging Memory Study (SAM) cohort. *Stroke*. 1997;28(4):785–792.
159. Tatemichi TK, et al. Cognitive impairment after stroke: frequency, patterns, and relationship to functional abilities. *J Neurol Neurosurg Psychiatry*. 1994;57(2):202–207.
160. del Ser T, et al. Evolution of cognitive impairment after stroke and risk factors for delayed progression. *Stroke*. 2005;36(12):2670–2675.
161. Llewellyn DJ, et al. Framingham Stroke Risk Profile and poor cognitive function: A population-based study. *BMC Neurol*. 2008;*8*:12.
162. Kwiatkowski TG, et al. Effects of tissue plasminogen activator for acute ischemic stroke at one year. National Institute of Neurological Disorders and Stroke Recombinant Tissue Plasminogen Activator Stroke Study Group. *N Engl J Med*. 1999;340(23):1781–1787.
163. Plassman BL, et al. Prevalence of dementia in the United States: The aging, demographics, and memory study. *Neuroepidemiology*. 2007;29(1–2):125–132.
164. Ferri CP, et al. Global prevalence of dementia: A Delphi consensus study. *Lancet*. 2005; 366(9503):2112–2117.
165. Wimo A, Jonsson L, Winblad B. An estimate of the worldwide prevalence and direct costs of dementia in 2003. *Dement Geriatr Cogn Disord*. 2006;21(3):175–181.
166. Wimo A, Ljunggren G, and Winblad B. Costs of dementia and dementia care: A review. *Int J Geriatr Psychiatry*. 1997;12(8):841–856.
167. Herrmann N, et al. The contribution of neuropsychiatric symptoms to the cost of dementia care. *Int J Geriatr Psychiatry*. 2006;21(10):972–976.
168. Brookmeyer R JE, Ziegler-Graham K, Arrighi MH. Forecasting the global burden of Alzheimer's disease. *Alzheimer's and Dementia*. 2007:6.
169. Hebert LE, et al. Alzheimer disease in the U.S. population: Prevalence estimates using the 2000 census. *Arch Neurol*. 2003;60(8):1119–1122.
170. Roman GC, Vascular dementia may be the most common form of dementia in the elderly. *J Neurol Sci*. 2002;203–204:7–10.

171. *Diagnostic and Statistical Manual of Mental Disorders*, 4th ed. 2005. Washington DC: American Psychiatric Association.
172. McKhann G, et al. Clinical diagnosis of Alzheimer's disease: Report of the NINCDS-ADRDA Work Group under the auspices of Department of Health and Human Services Task Force on Alzheimer's Disease. *Neurology*. 1984;34(7):939–944.
173. Roman GC, et al. Vascular dementia: Diagnostic criteria for research studies. Report of the NINDS-AIREN International Workshop. *Neurology*. 1993;43(2):250–260.
174. Schneck MJ. Vascular dementia. *Top Stroke Rehabil*. 2008;15(1):22–26.
175. Castellani RJ, et al. Neuropathology of Alzheimer disease: Pathognomonic but not pathogenic. *Acta Neuropathol*. 2006;111(6):503–509.
176. Ritchie J, Nemeroff CB, *Stress, the hypothalamic-pituitary-adrenal axis, and depression. Stress, neuropeptides, and systemic disease*, ed. J. McCubbin J, Kaufmann PG, Nemeroff CB. 1991. San Diego: Academic Press. 181–197.
177. Zekry D, Hauw JJ, and Gold G. Mixed dementia: Epidemiology, diagnosis, and treatment. *J Am Geriatr Soc*. 2002;50(8):1431–1438.
178. Kurita A, et al. Relationship between cognitive status and behavioral symptoms in Alzheimer's disease and mixed dementia. *J Am Geriatr Soc*. 1993;41(7):732–736.
179. Schmidtke K, Hull M. Neuropsychological differentiation of small vessel disease, Alzheimer's disease and mixed dementia. *J Neurol Sci*. 2002;203–204:17–22.
180. Bowler JV, et al. Comparative evolution of Alzheimer disease, vascular dementia, and mixed dementia. *Arch Neurol*. 1997;54(6):697–703.
181. Rockwood K, et al. The diagnosis of "mixed" dementia in the Consortium for the Investigation of Vascular Impairment of Cognition (CIVIC). *Ann NY Acad Sci*. 2000;903: 522–528.
182. Zekry D, et al. The vascular lesions in vascular and mixed dementia: The weight of functional neuroanatomy. *Neurobiol Aging*. 2003;24(2):213–219.
183. Demyttenaere K, et al. Prevalence, severity, and unmet need for treatment of mental disorders in the World Health Organization World Mental Health Surveys. *JAMA*. 2004; 291(21):2581–2590.
184. Blazer DG, et al. The prevalence and distribution of major depression in a national community sample: The National Comorbidity survey. *Am J Psychiatry*. 1994;151(7):979–986.
185. Greenberg PE, et al. The economic burden of depression in the United States: How did it change between 1990 and 2000? *J Clin Psychiatry*. 2003;64(12):1465–1475.
186. Scott KM, et al. Depression-anxiety relationships with chronic physical conditions: Results from the World Mental Health Surveys. *J Affect Disord*. 2007;103(1–3):113–120.
187. Davis J, et al. Major depression associated with rates of cardiovascular disease state transitions. *Am J Manag Care*. 2008;14(3):125–128.
188. Goldston K, Baillie AJ. Depression and coronary heart disease: A review of the epidemiological evidence, explanatory mechanisms and management approaches. *Clin Psychol Rev*. 2008;28(2):288–306.
189. Rugulies R. Depression as a predictor for coronary heart disease. A review and meta-analysis. *Am J Prev Med*. 2002;23(1):51–61.
190. Wulsin LR. Singal BM. Do depressive symptoms increase the risk for the onset of coronary disease? A systematic quantitative review. *Psychosom Med*. 2003;65(2):201–210.
191. Davidson KW, et al. Assessment and treatment of depression in patients with cardiovascular disease: National Heart, Lung, and Blood Institute working group report. *Ann Behav Med*. 2006;32(2):121–126.

192. Rozanski A, Blumenthal JA, and Kaplan J. Impact of psychological factors on the pathogenesis of cardiovascular disease and implications for therapy. *Circulation.* 1999;99(16): 2192–2217.
193. Brown ES, Varghese FP, McEwen BS. Association of depression with medical illness: Does cortisol play a role? *Biol Psychiatry.* 2004;55(1):1–9.
194. Bunker SJ, et al. "Stress" and coronary heart disease: Psychosocial risk factors. *Med J Aust.* 2003;178(6):272–276.
195. Kuper H, Marmot M, and Hemingway H. Systematic review of prospective cohort studies of psychosocial factors in the etiology and prognosis of coronary heart disease. *Semin Vasc Med.* 2002;2(3):267–314.
196. Joynt KE, Whellan DJ, O'Connor CM. Depression and cardiovascular disease: Mechanisms of interaction. *Biol Psychiatry.* 2003;54(3):248–261.
197. Alexopoulos GS, et al. "Vascular depression" hypothesis. *Arch Gen Psychiatry.* 1997;54(10):915–922.
198. Doraiswamy PM, et al. Magnetic resonance assessment of cerebral perfusion in depressed cardiac patients: Preliminary findings. *Am J Psychiatry.* 1999;156(10):1641–1643.
199. Bondy B. Common genetic factors for depression and cardiovascular disease. *Dialogues Clin Neurosci.* 2007;9(1):19–28.
200. Berkman LF, et al. Effects of treating depression and low perceived social support on clinical events after myocardial infarction: The Enhancing Recovery in Coronary Heart Disease Patients (ENRICHD) randomized trial. *JAMA.* 2003;289(23):3106–3116.
201. Glassman AH, et al. Sertraline treatment of major depression in patients with acute MI or unstable angina. *JAMA.* 2002;288(6):701–709.
202. Burt DB, Zembar MJ, Niederehe G. Depression and memory impairment: A meta-analysis of the association, its pattern, and specificity. *Psychol Bull.* 1995;117(2):285–305.
203. Christensen H, et al. A quantitative review of cognitive deficits in depression and Alzheimer-type dementia. *J Int Neuropsychol Soc.* 1997;3(6):631–651.
204. Naismith SL, et al. Neuropsychological performance in patients with depression is associated with clinical, etiological and genetic risk factors. *J Clin Exp Neuropsychol.* 2003;25(6):866–877.
205. Veiel HO. A preliminary profile of neuropsychological deficits associated with major depression. *J Clin Exp Neuropsychol.* 1997;19(4):587–603.
206. Degl'Innocenti A, Agren H, Backman L. Executive deficits in major depression. *Acta Psychiatr Scand.* 1998;97(3):182–188.
207. Basso MR, Bornstein RA. Neuropsychological deficits in psychotic versus nonpsychotic unipolar depression. *Neuropsychology.* 1999;13(1):69–75.
208. Castaneda AE, et al. A review on cognitive impairments in depressive and anxiety disorders with a focus on young adults. *J Affect Disord.* 2008;106(1–2):1–27.
209. Smitherman TA, et al. The relation of depression and anxiety to measures of executive functioning in a mixed psychiatric sample. *Arch Clin Neuropsychol.* 2007;22(5):647–654.
210. Levin R, Heller W, Mohanty A, Herrington JD, Miller GA. Cognitive deficits in depression and functional specificity of regional brain activity. *Cognitive Therapy Research.* 2007;31:22.
211. Elliott R. The neuropsychological profile in unipolar depression. *Trends in Cognitive Sciences.* 1998:7.
212. Zulli R, et al. Increased prevalence of silent myocardial ischaemia and severe ventricular arrhythmias in untreated patients with Alzheimer's disease and mild cognitive impairment without overt coronary artery disease. *Clin Neurol Neurosurg.* 2008;110(8):791–796.

3

VASCULAR DEMENTIA

A CLINICAL CONUNDRUM

Elizabeth M. Lane, Susan E. Maloney, and Robert H. Paul

The impact of vascular disease remains an important area of clinical and research interest. Historically, severe cognitive impairment among older individuals was attributed to vascular disease in the brain. However, in the 1970s, interest became more focused on Alzheimer's disease (AD) as a primary etiology of significant age-related cognitive impairment. Interestingly, the attention of researchers has begun to shift once again towards a focus on vascular mechanisms associated with age-related cognitive impairment. Vascular dementia (VaD) is now believed to account for a significant percentage of dementia cases worldwide, and there is concern that vascular damage in the brain may serve as a catalyst for the development of other forms of degenerative brain disease. Our understanding of VaD continues to evolve, though the area of clinical and research focus remains complicated by an ever-changing nomenclature, uncertain neuropathological correlates, and questions regarding the clinical expression of the disease. This chapter will focus on these and other factors that are important considerations in the field of VaD. Specifically, the chapter will review challenges to the definition, diagnosis, neuropsychological expression, and imaging correlates associated with VaD. Additionally, new approaches to investigating the disease will be discussed. These sections cover the current state of knowledge in each area and provide recommendations for future areas of research.

Challenges in the Definition of Vascular Dementia

Dementia associated with vascular insult remains difficult to define objectively, despite data suggesting that VaD represents 8% to 15.8% of all dementias in Western societies.[1] Complicating the process of defining the condition is the fact that the nomenclature used to identify VaD has continuously changed since the 1950s. Originally branded *arteriosclerotic dementia*, it was later termed *multi-infarct dementia* and *post-stroke dementia*; and recently *vascular dementia* became the most widely recognized appellation.[1] Vascular cognitive impairment (VCI) is often used to describe cognitive decline resulting from vascular injury without a dementia diagnosis.[2] When this damage affects cognitive and behavioral systems, clinicians and researchers use terms like VCI, and when the clinical outcome of the damage reaches the criteria set forth for a dementia diagnosis, the term VaD is applied. Aside from nomenclature, the heterogeneity of the neuropathology that underlies VaD has complicated our understanding of the disease. Ultimately, cerebrovascular disease (CVD) represents the primary etiology of VaD and VCI. *Cerebrovascular disease* is a term that encompasses dysfunctions of the vascular system in the brain. This includes damage caused from hypertension or ischemic or hemorrhagic stroke. Primary risk factors for CVD include age, smoking, diabetes mellitus, cardiovascular disease, and obstructive sleep apnea, just to name a few. CVD is difficult to diagnose in its own right because some individuals suffering from CVD show no signs of damage, while others show only selective impairment depending on the site of damage, while still others may show more global dementia. It is important to understand that any vascular event in the brain falls under the rubric of CVD; therefore, VaD can be described as dementia secondary to CVD.[3]

Individuals may exhibit cognitive impairment due to a variety of CVD profiles, including large- and small-vessel disease and ischemic lesions that can be focal, multifocal, and/or diffuse.[1] The variety of anatomical locations of pathology that gives rise to the different clinical outcomes observed with VaD accounts for the heterogeneous nature of VaD. Large-vessel injury involves major arterial infarction, including the middle, anterior, or posterior cerebral arteries. One strategic focal infarct can result in sudden major neurological symptoms, such as aphasia, amnesia, visual agnosia, or neglect, typical of stroke patients.[3] Large-vessel infarction is most commonly the cause of the step-wise cognitive decline that sets some VaD patients apart from AD patients who exhibit slow and insidious cognitive decline.[4] Damage from large-vessel injury may involve a relatively clear temporal relationship between the infarction and clinical expression. However, it is critical to emphasize that this is not the most common form of CVD, and clinicians cannot reliably use a step-wise pattern as indicative of VaD vs. AD.

Strategic infarcts do not necessarily involve large vessels, and oftentimes occur in critical subcortical gray nuclei. Strategically located infarcts can occur in the small vessels of functionally important brain areas, such as the thalamus, hippocampus, basal forebrain, and angular gyrus, among others.[5] For example, when the basal forebrain areas are affected, the patient may experience cholinergic deficits because this area, home to much of the brain's cholinergic nuclei, is infused with arterioles that are susceptible to arterial hypertension.[3] Lesions here can also disrupt white matter connections with the cortex and amygdala.

As noted above, large-vessel infarction may present with a step-wise decline, and while this was originally believed to be the most common pattern of expression, current studies suggest that this is a less common subtype of VaD. Fisher et al.[6] found that only 34% of the patients with VaD displayed the typical step-wise deterioration, while 54% displayed an insidious onset with a progressive course of deterioration. Other studies have found similar patterns of expression, not just large-vessel pathology, suggesting that small-vessel disease exhibiting an insidious onset with a progressive course is the most common expression of VaD.[7, 8] Moreover, the most frequent course of cognitive decline in VaD is slow and insidious manner, due to progressive small-vessel damage.[3]

The most common areas of the brain affected are the white matter of the cerebral hemispheres and the subcortical nuclei, especially the striatum and the thalamus. Small-vessel disease, or multiple infarctions of the small vessels of the brain, can be expressed in the form of ischemic injury to white matter or cortical regions (less likely to involve the cortex), or lacunar infarction—damage to the deep tissue of the brain.[4] Multiple lacunar infarctions can cause a variety of cognitive deficits. Predominantly, a patient with this sort of damage may express apathy, and impaired executive and psychomotor function.[2] Lacunar infarction and ischemic damage to white matter that is extensive may cause cognitive impairment of sufficient severity to warrant a diagnosis of subcortical dementia. This type of damage interferes with the processing of information across frontal-subcortical circuits and results in difficulties with decision-making, processing speed, cognitive flexibility, abstraction, and learning efficiency.

VaD has been referred to as a subcortical dementia because the most common pathology occurs in the form of small-vessel disease, primarily in the white matter and subcortical areas, and because of the cognitive profile associated with this sort of damage. Many individuals, including healthy older adults, suffer silent lacunar infarcts that produce no initial cognitive or behavioral impairment. These asymptomatic insults have been associated with an increased risk for later development of cognitive impairment and dementia subsequent to a more clinically recognized cerebrovascular event, such as a stroke.[2] This finding is true for about 25% to 30% of individuals who suffer these events.[5]

Yet another form of VaD includes an inherited condition known as "cerebral autosomal dominant arteriopathy with subcortical infarcts and leukoencephalopathy" (CADASIL), which is a pure genetic form of VaD resulting from mutations in the NOTCH3 gene located on chromosome 19.[2] This disease manifests with the initiation of multiple small-vessel lacunar strokes when the patient is around 40 years of age. Unfortunately, clinicians and researchers have struggled to use this form of the disease as a template for the pathology or the cognitive and behavioral impairments of all forms of VaD because the vascular burden is so great in these individuals that it is difficult to determine precise relationships between the damage and the clinical outcomes.[3]

As can be determined from the complex picture of VaD described above, this form of dementia is very complicated to define and diagnose. Important pathological factors that play into determining a global definition of VaD include different aspects of damage such as the volume of brain destruction, and the location and number of lesions.[5] It is difficult to define a minimum of cerebral impact because of the polymorphic nature of the vascular pathology that produces VaD.[2] Location and size of lesions are probably the most important factors in determining a diagnostic scheme based on clinical expression; yet, unfortunately, such a scheme will be closely intertwined with and complicated by the factors of overall brain-volume destruction and the number of lesions in the broad spectrum of VaD.

Challenges with the Diagnosis of Vascular Dementia

At present there is no universally agreed-upon set of diagnostic criteria for VaD. Studies have shown that using different diagnostic criteria identifies inconsistent frequencies and clusters of VaD patients, and therefore the different sets of existing criteria are not interchangeable.[9, 10] Some require neuroimaging, while others do not; and some indicate VaD subtypes, while others do not. Currently, the most widely used diagnostic criteria are found in the Diagnostic and Statistical Manual, Fourth Edition (DSM-IV),[11] the Hachinski Ischemia Score (HIS),[12] the National Institute of Neurological Disorders and Stroke–Association Internationale pour la Recherche et l'Enseignement en Neurosciences (NINDS–AIREN),[13] the State of California Alzheimer's Disease Diagnostic and Treatment Centers criteria for ischemic VaD (ADDTC),[14] and the International Classification of Diseases, *10th Revision* (ICD-10).[15] These criteria were created by the observations of experts in the field of VaD, but were not based on studies completed among VaD patients.[16]

While most of the current criteria-sets require the presence of focal neurological symptoms and evidence of cerebral vascular disease, the majority do not require neuroimaging data to verify evidence of stroke. NINDS–AIREN and ADDTC criteria both require imaging data from either a CT or MRI scan for a diagnosis of VaD. In the case of a large cortical stroke or a strategically placed subcortical lesion, the imaging data must support a temporal relationship with the onset of dementia. In conjunction with imaging data, both sets of criteria provide different levels of certainty for the diagnosis being made: "possible," "probable," and "definite," with "definite" requiring autopsy evidence of VaD. However, not all strokes have an obvious temporal relationship. This is particularly the case for subcortical ischemic vascular disease, which may not present with an abrupt change in function. Imaging data are important in these situations to differentiate its presence from other diseases and to accurately diagnose the presence of VaD. Still, the decision of how much pathology on MRI is sufficient to render a diagnosis of dementia remains uncertain.

There is also no agreement between the diagnostic criteria on which cognitive domains must be involved to meet criteria for a diagnosis of VaD. Most (but not all) of the criteria require memory impairment to be present for a diagnosis of VaD, in addition to other domains. The requirement for memory impairment is a remnant of the VaD criteria's being derived from the criteria for AD, but it is not a universal feature of this form of dementia. The HIS is the least inclusive and does not give any description of the cognitive profile associated with the disease. The ADDTC is the most flexible, requiring any deficit in two or more cognitive domains. The other diagnostic criteria do not encompass the most common deficit associated with VaD—executive dysfunction—and because of this, many people may go undiagnosed until they reach a severe state of dementia.

Although several subtypes of VaD have been identified, many of the diagnostic criteria do not distinguish between the different types. The ICD-10 does provide several subtypes of VaD; however, it lacks operational criteria to make a differential diagnosis. Since strokes to different parts of the brain have different functional outcomes, future research should focus on creating different diagnostic criteria sets for each different subtype of VaD. Several different subtypes have been suggested over time based on lesion type, size, and location.[17–21] Without the use of subtypes, VaD appears to affect a heterogeneous population with a diverse expression and appearance. Additionally, thorough neuropsychological profiles need to be developed that define each of these subtypes.

The current criteria vary widely regarding their limits of sensitivity and specificity for diagnosis. In a review of the sensitivity and specificity of different diagnostic criteria for VaD conducted by Wiederkehr et al.,[22] the ADDTC criteria were the most sensitive criteria, and the NINDS–AIREN criteria were the most specific. The age of the patient affects the sensitivity and specificity rates of the different criteria, which show more sensitivity in older cohorts for the NINDS–AIREN and HIS, but lower specificity with the NINDS–AIREN, ADDTC, and HIS criteria.[23] Criteria that are both sensitive and specific need to be developed that are unaffected by age, education, and other important demographic factors.

The lack of agreement between diagnostic criteria emphasizes the necessity of further research in this area. Research studies are difficult to compare, because the criteria vary so widely. The clinical profile of subjects in one study diagnosed according to one set of criteria may be very different from that of subjects recruited using another diagnostic method. Additional factors that create problems in the VaD arena are the heterogeneous appearance of the disease, discrepancies between a smooth progression versus step-wise progression, the requirement of a memory deficit, and an absence of a gold standard for imaging correlates.

Patchy vs. Global Neuropsychological Impairment

VaD has been described as "patchy" in several publications,[24] though this view has recently been challenged. As was mentioned earlier, there are several different ways that VaD is expressed, depending on which area of the brain is affected. Strokes can happen anywhere in the brain, resulting in a diverse pattern of expression. A single strategic infarct in the cortex or in a vital region of the brain, such as the thalamus, can cause a striking loss in function—whereas a progression of small subcortical infarcts may not begin to affect the person until a functional threshold is reached, which differs from person to person.[25] This presents a problem when trying to establish a profile of the typical VaD patient. The diversity in expression has led many researchers to describe the neuropsychological profile of VaD as "patchy." However, different dementias express themselves differently in each individual and at each level of disease progression, not only in VaD.[4] For example, in the early stages of AD, many patients may exhibit episodic memory and language impairments, but have intact executive function and visuospatial skill (hence a "patchy" profile). Furthermore, work from our lab demonstrated that most patients with VaD exhibit global impairments, even in the more moderate stages of dementia. As dementia severity increased, the profile of impairment remained fairly global. As such, clinicians seeking islands of cognitive preservation to assist with a diagnosis of VaD would have little success relying on the neuropsychological profile alone.

Subcortical ischemic vascular disease (SIVD) has been shown to be the most common form of VaD. Many studies show impairments in executive functions and verbal fluency,[26] distinguishing this form of dementia from other forms of dementia, such as AD. Executive deficits are the hallmark of this form of SIVD. White matter lesions and lacunar infarcts cause a disruption of the frontal-subcortical circuits and are believed to be the culprits of the executive problems.[27] Sultzer et al.[28] found that subcortical lesions on PET scans cause lower metabolism in the frontal lobe in VaD patients that was directly related to the severity of the dementia. This grouping of VaD probably represents the best homogeneous subgroup of patients for pharmaceutical trials and related clinical interventions.[26]

Memory Deficit

As noted above, most diagnostic schemes for VaD require memory impairment as the core criterion. However, memory impairment is often not the central feature in cases of VaD, especially in the early stages when the disease may be controlled and further damage halted. The diagnostic criteria for VaD were created to distinguish it from AD,[29] still using memory impairment as the main criterion. However, problems with executive functions, psychomotor speed, and language fluency tend to be the central features associated with VaD.[4]

In the advanced stages of VaD, memory impairment is prevalent; however, the pattern of impairment may be very different from that of AD. Instead of having core impairments in encoding and consolidation as is the case with AD, the typical profile of a VaD patient is characterized by impaired working memory and learning efficiency, and more preserved recognition.[30] The ability to perform better on recognition tasks is likely to be due to the frontal lobe support provided by these tests.

While memory impairment is present in VaD, executive function impairment may be the most prominent feature of the disease. Most of the diagnostic criteria specify that memory plus other domains must be impaired for a diagnosis of VaD, but fail to specify a deficit in the area of executive functioning. Additionally, memory may not be significantly impaired until the later stages of the disease, while executive functions are affected at the initial onset of the disease.[31] Also, activities of daily living have been found to be most impaired due to deficits in executive function and may be impaired earlier than the onset of memory impairment; therefore, the patient's profile may not meet the criteria for dementia until late in the disease course when they are already severely disabled.[3] The exception to this is when there is a stroke in the hippocampus, effectively causing memory impairment that is similar to that seen in an AD patient.[32]

Absence of a Gold Standard with Imaging Correlates

Small subcortical infarcts and white matter lesions are common in the aged population and do not necessarily produce any sort of measurable deficits.[33] Currently, there are no set standards for the amount of damage that must be present from stroke for the diagnosis of VaD, and the diagnostic criteria do not provide a means to determine a diagnosis based on lesion type, size, or location. Our current understanding of VaD and the current radiological techniques are not sophisticated enough to specify a cutoff that defines a standard in the diagnosis of VaD. A lack of common language used to describe different types of lesions exacerbates the problem. Additionally, individual variations in education and life experience have been shown to affect each person's outcome affecting the development of CVD.

The variable anatomical pathology associated with VaD complicates the search for a "gold standard" of neuroimaging correlates. There is some general agreement that areas such as the thalamus, caudate, and putamen are critical centers for cognitive function, especially executive functions, since they are part of the frontal–striatal circuit.[26, 34] Additionally, varying degrees of white matter lesion and lacune damage have been found to cause dementia; however, there is no agreed-upon cutoff point that definitely warrants a diagnosis of dementia.

Individual differences in education level and life experience have also been shown to be a variant in determining the outcome of the affect of burden to the brain. Research has shown that there is lower cognitive performance and higher dementia rates among those with less education than in people who have a higher level of educational attainment.[35] People with more education have been found to be able to withstand a greater degree of white matter burden, while still maintaining a higher level of functioning.[36] The cognitive-reserve hypothesis states that activities that are geared toward "building" the brain, such as education, may be able to give an individual more synapses, the ability of a network in the brain to continue functioning after trauma, or the ability to recruit novel brain networks in response to pathology.[37] Thus, an older individual with lower cognitive reserves may exhibit cognitive (e.g., executive, learning efficiency) deficits at one stage of vascular burden, whereas another individual with higher cognitive reserves may exhibit no deficits in these areas when compared to age-matched controls. Many neuropsychological tests are not normed using education as a demographic correction, and even fewer tests are normed on clinical populations, and there is no reason to believe that cognitive reserve affects neuropsychological performance in clinical populations in the same manner or degree as it does in healthy populations.

New Approaches to Unraveling the Mystery

New Imaging Techniques

The most commonly used neuroimaging methods to identify VaD are computed tomography (CT) and MRI, but these methods are not remarkably sensitive to microvascular damage and metabolic disturbances. CT is the least sensitive method and is only capable of detecting areas of large infarction.[38] While MRI is superior to CT in its ability to detect infarcts, it may lack the necessary sensitivity to detect damage to the white matter pathways that make up most the brain, and it is unable to detect small areas of necrotizing tissue. More sensitive imaging methods are being developed to help us understand the impact of cardiovascular burden in the brain. These newer methods (reviewed below) are more sensitive to the white matter pathways and the effects of acute stroke. These new methods are important, because they may provide a more sensitive image that correlates better with functional outcome, providing insight into the area of VaD.

Diffusion weighted imaging (DWI) measures how water moves freely through the tissue of the brain in a particular region of interest. The movement of water in the brain is restricted by the physical characteristics of the brain tissue, such as cell membranes, size, shape, and the space between individual structures. The restriction of this movement, called *anisotropic motion*, is measured, providing information about the connectivity and integrity of the cells in the region of interest on an x, y, and z plane. This measurement is called the apparent diffusion coefficient (ADC). Studies using DWI have found damage in the white matter and gray matter that were undetectable by other imaging methods. Mayzel-Oreg and colleagues[39] found that high b-value q-space diffusion on DWI was more sensitive in detecting white and gray matter changes in VaD and was better at discriminating between tissue types than conventional MRI or diffusion tensor imaging (DTI). Additionally, DWI can be used to distinguish acute strokes that are asymptomatic, providing another path for investigating the mechanisms of disease progression in patients who are less severely affected.[40]

Diffusion tensor imaging is a perfusion method of imaging that examines tissue integrity, white matter connectivity, and directionality of connecting pathways. DTI is similar to DWI, but it allows at least six non-collinear directions to be examined at the same time, instead of just a single x, y, and z plane. This additional measurement allows for the direction and average magnitude of water diffusion to be determined. DTI measures the amount of the directional coherence, or fractional anisotropy (FA), in the white matter pathways. Since white matter pathways are highly organized and water moves faster parallel to the white matter tract than it does perpendicular, the integrity of these pathways can be measured. DTI can also measure the amount of anisotropy, or diffusion in a particular direction, giving a measurement of the structural integrity of the white matter fibers. Using DTI methods, a loss of neuronal integrity is associated with lower FA values and higher mean diffusivity.[41] Imaging correlates of executive function and VaD using MRI have shown only weak relationships at best, but DTI correlates show a strong relationship between the amount of damage and the executive function outcomes.[42] Additionally, DTI can detect subtle changes in normal-appearing white matter (NAWM) that are correlated with changes in cognition and may be able to differentiate between VaD and AD.[43] These findings are important, because many studies have shown no relationship, or a weak relationship at best, between vascular lesions on T2 weighted images on traditional MRI and cognitive status.[44]

Perfusion weighted imaging (PWI) echo pulse sequences observe the movement of a contrast agent called gadolinium diethylenetriaminepentaaceti acid through the vasculature of the brain. The contrast agent provides a magnetic field in the blood that can be visualized using MRI techniques, showing the volume of blood to tissue in the brain, or cerebral blood volume (CBV); the amount of blood that the brain tissue is receiving per minute, or cerebral blood flow (CBF); and the time it takes for the contrast to pass through the tissue, or mean transit time (MTT). These contrast agents have few side effects and are safer than other, more traditional methods that use radioactive contrast agents. One study using PWI in individuals with leukoaraiosis found reduced CBF in white matter, but no difference in gray matter areas of interest.[45]

Arterial spin labeling (ASL) involves methods similar to PWI's, except it uses electromagnetic manipulation of proton spin to give the arterial blood water a magnetic charge. The effects of perfusion are assessed using a comparison of the image with and without the arterial spin labeling. ASL is safer than the PWI method of imaging, since it is using an endogenous tracer instead of the exogenous tracer used with PWI, and this method may be repeated indefinitely without any risk to the patient. The same measures can be acquired using ASL that can be found using PWI. Studies using ASL have successfully visualized ischemic damage immediately after stroke and determined areas that are affected by reduced perfusion, by hyperperfusion, as well as areas of restored perfusion.[46]

Many studies have used a combination of these techniques to visualize the macrostructural and microstructural integrity of the brain with better results than using any one method independently.[39, 46–47] Relatedly, many of these techniques can be added to a traditional MRI sequence without adding significant amounts of time to the total imaging time. Further studies are needed to determine the significance of these imaging methods in relation to VaD, especially in the areas of PWI and ASL.

Consensus on a Standard Cognitive Battery to Examine VaD Expression

Efforts are now under way to develop a universal battery for the assessment of cognitive impairments associated with CVD. The development of a standard neuropsychological battery would provide a more sensitive measure to differentiate VaD from AD, give a deeper understanding of the changes that are happening pertaining to VaD, allow a comprehensive comparison of studies and in clinical comparison of patients, provide a standard template to compare individuals who are afflicted, and allow greater progress in multicenter studies. The Vascular Dementia Assessment Scale cognitive subscale[48] (VADAS–cog) was designed as revision to the Alzheimer's Disease Assessment scale[49] (ADAS–cog) to differentiate VaD from AD by adding several measures of executive functions to the original ADAS-cog. The largest move towards this end was a harmonization meeting of the National Institute of Neurological Disorders and Stroke (NINDS)–Canadian Stroke Network (CSN) Vascular Cognitive Impairment Harmonization Standards workshop in 2005.[50]

The VADAS–cog is a revised version of the ADAS–cog, used for assessing AD. The VADAS–cog was derived from the original ADAS–cog, with several measures of executive functions incorporated into the test battery to identify disruptions in frontal-subcortical circuitry. In a multinational, multicenter study done by Ylikoski et al.,[51] the VADAS–cog and the ADAS–cog were compared on subjects with leukoaraiosis. The study found that the VADAS–cog significantly differentiated between the different WMH groups, and the VADAS–cog may be a more sensitive measure for evaluating patients with vascular burden in the brain.

The harmonization workshop was attended by a large group of experts in the field of VaD who met to discuss the development of common standards associated with vascular cognitive impairment (VCI) and VaD. The goal of the workshop was to create a testing battery to attain a minimal data set that would accelerate progress and treatment, identify individuals at earlier stages of disease development, combine several researchers' understanding of the disease, and allow studies to be more comparable. Since risks for cardiovascular disease are reducible, this conglomerate effort is of special importance pertaining to VaD. The NINDS-CSN workshop made three suggestions for different neuropsychological testing batteries, each consisting of different time periods: 60 minutes, 30 minutes, and 5 minutes. These three different batteries would allow researchers and health practitioners to fit appropriate testing measures into any time period. Each battery was designed to include all cognitive domains, the 60-minute battery being the most comprehensive and dividing domains into separate tests; and the 5-minute battery being the fastest, with tests that overlap between domains, but still including all of them. All tests chosen were "conventional well-validated tasks" and were chosen on their ability to be time-efficient, while providing the best information about the domain or several domains at the same time.

Some multicenter studies have developed their own batteries to study the effects of VaD on cognition, with good results.[52] However, the development of a general battery that can be administered and compared across studies and patient populations would be of great importance to the field of VaD. Studies using the same battery would greatly increase the understanding and treatment of this disease, and the work from the harmonization meetings is an important step toward a unified approach.

Importance of Genetics to VaD

One rare form of VaD, CADASIL, has been successfully linked to the NOTCH3 gene located on chromosome 19.[53] Researchers have been able to develop mouse models of CADASIL that enable the study of the underlying pathology of this pure genetic form of VaD and initiate the genetic research into this disease.[54] This gene appears to be involved in cell development, more specifically the cell proliferation and differentiation, of vascular smooth muscle cells.[54] In the adult vascular system, expression of the NOTCH system is central in the events causing vascular damage, including apoptosis.[53]

It has been suggested that genes involved in AD may influence the tissue responses to CVD. This suggestion comes from the presence of vascular pathology in the brains of individuals with AD and the presence of plaques and tangles in individuals with VaD. Early onset forms of AD that have greater hereditary components also have mutations in the genes for the presenilin proteins.[54] These proteins are enzymes that are responsible for cutting amyloid precursor protein (APP) to create amyloid beta, which forms the amyloid plaques found in AD brains. Presenilins have been shown to interact with the NOTCH proteins, including NOTCH3,[55] suggesting an influence on vascular pathology. Mutation in the APP gene is directly responsible for hereditary cerebral hemorrhage with amyloidosis-Dutch type (HCHWA-D), a form of CVD. This mutation causes cerebral amyloid angiopathy, a build up of amyloid protein in the cerebral vascular system that causes hemorrhagic strokes and subsequent dementia.[54]

The ε4 allele of the apolipoprotein E (apoE) gene is a genetic biomarker for greater risk for AD. This allele also is associated with greater likelihood to develop atherosclerosis and coronary heart disease, conditions that can lead to cerebrovascular injury.[56] The presence of the ε4 allele has also been shown to be associated with reduced survival after intracerebral hemorrhage.[54] Davidson and colleagues[56] demonstrated that the apoE ε4 allele increases the risk of VaD. In another study, Baum and colleagues[57] found that this allele was associated with an increased risk of VaD when interacting with hypertension and diabetes. However, another study conducted by Orisitto and colleagues[58] found that the ε4 allele was present more often in individuals with AD than in those with VaD or no cognitive impairment, as was to be expected, but also that there was no difference found between individuals with VaD and individuals with no cognitive impairment.

Matrix metalloproteinases (MMPs) are involved in extracellular mechanisms such as receptor cleavage, apoptosis, and cell proliferation,[59] and an increased expression of these proteases due to genetic variation at the promoter regions of the responsible genes is associated with a number of different pathological conditions, including stroke and AD. A group of scientists in Italy investigated polymorphisms of the genes responsible for the expression of MMPs in individuals with VaD and AD, and normal controls.[59] The genotypes MMP-1 2G2G, MMP-1 1G2G, MMP-3 5A5A, and MMP-9 TT were found to be associated with VaD; however, independent of each other. This association was stronger in individuals who were carrying more than one version of the MMP gene. Polymorphisms of MMP genes were found to be associated with an increased risk of AD only in individuals with the ε4 allele of the apoE gene.

An increased genetic risk for VaD has been found specifically among females, and these genes are involved in cellular functions, just like the MMPs. Three of these genes include those for transforming growth factor-β1 (TGFB1), insulin-like growth factor-1 (IGF-1), and the LIGHT gene (homologous to *Lymphotoxins*, exhibits *Inducible* expression, and competes with herpes simplex virus *Glycoprotein* D for *Herpes* virus entry mediator, a receptor expressed by *T* lymphocytes). Transforming growth factor-β1 is an anti-inflammatory cytokine. This polypeptide is secreted to perform cellular functions such as cell growth, cell proliferation, cell differentiation, and apoptosis. Following ischemia, the expression of this protein is increased. Kim and Lee[60] found that the Pro10Leu polymorphism of the TGFB1 gene is associated with increased risk of VaD in females with small-vessel occlusion. Insulin-like growth factor-1 is a protein hormone that acts primarily as a potent stimulator of the AKT signaling pathway that inhibits apoptosis. This gene has been significantly associated with protecting neurons in brains with AD from oxidative stress.[61] The A allele of the IGF-1 receptor has been associated with VaD and suggested to be involved with the pathogenesis of this disease in females.[61] The T allele at the locus C-770T and the haplotype TTGA of the promoter region in the LIGHT gene may increase the susceptibility of females to VaD as well, by decreasing the overall expression of the LIGHT gene.[62] It has been suggested that this is only seen in females because these autosomal genes are linked to sex genes.

Researchers have just begun to scratch the surface of investigating genetic biomarkers of VaD. The heterogeneity of the pathology of this disease may make this search more difficult than that for other diseases. Ultimately newer, more sensitive neuromaging methods will be required to define the factors that determine the clinical expression of vascular-related brain dysfunction. Recent work with our collaborators incorporates genetic risks for both microvascular disease and central inflammation, along with indices of quantified diffusion tractography to determine the impact of vascular disease and its associated inflammation on white matter integrity in the brain. While the white matter is by no means the only brain region affected by microvascular disease, the white matter pathways are significantly involved, and the critical role these pathways play in the flow of information across brain systems highlights the importance of these brain regions. It is only through such interdisciplinary efforts that the questions about VaD will eventually lead to answers.

Summary

In the last 30 years there has a shift towards a renewed interest in vascular mechanisms of brain injury and the behavioral expression associated with these injuries. The field of CVD and VaD has been significantly advanced from both clinical and bench-science efforts to understand this condition, but much more work is required. Research focusing on defining homogenous subtypes of VaD, patterns of expression, clear neuroimaging signatures, and physiological correlates are needed to further our understanding and improve our effectiveness in diagnosing and treating VaD. As VaD may be the second most prevalent type of dementia in the United States, it is critical, with the aging population, that this disease be explored and understood.

Notes

1. Jellinger KA. Morphologic diagnosis of "vascular dementia"—A critical update. *J Neurol Sci.* 2008; doi:10.1016/j.jns.2008.03.006.
2. Knopman DS. Cerebrovascular disease and dementia. *Br J Radiol.* 2007;80:S121–S127.
3. Paul RH, Fortenbury S, Boyle P. Everyday functioning in vascular dementia. In Marcotte T and Grant I (Eds.), *Neuropsychology of activities of daily living*. In press.
4. Paul R, Garrett K, Cohen R. Vascular dementia: A diagnostic conundrum for the clinical neuropsychologist. *Appl Neuropsychol.* 2003;10(3):129–136.
5. Jellinger KA. Understanding the pathology of vascular cognitive impairment. *J Neurol Sci.* 2005;229–230:57–63.

6. Esiri MM, Wilcock GK, Morris JH. Neuropathological assessment of the lesions of significance in vascular dementia. *J Neurol Neurosurg Psychiatry*. 1997;63:749–753.
7. Jokinen H, Kalska H, Mantyla R, et al. Cognitive profile of subcortical ischaemic vascular disease. *J Neurol Neurosurg Psychiatry*. 2006;17:28–33.
8. Paul R, Moser D, Cohen R, Browndyke J, Zawacki T, Gordon N. Dementia severity and pattern of cognitive performance in vascular dementia. *Appl Neuropsychol*. 2001;8:211–217.
9. Pohjasvaara T, Mäntylä R, Ylikoski R, Kaste M, Erkinjuntti T. Comparison of different clinical criteria (DSM-III, ADDTC, ICD-10, NINDS-AIREN, DSM-IV) for the diagnosis of vascular dementia. *Stroke*. 2000;31:2952–2957.
10. Chui HC, Mack W, Jackson JE, et al. Clinical criteria for the diagnosis of vascular dementia. *Arch Neurol*. 2000;57:191–196.
11. American Psychiatric Association on Nomenclature and Statistics. *Diagnostic and Statistical Manual of Mental Disorders (DSM-IV), Fourth Edition*. Washington, D.C.: American Psychiatric Association; 1994.
12. Hachinski VC, Iliff LD, Zilhka E, et al. Criteria for the diagnosis of ischemic vascular dementia proposed by the state of California Alzheimer's disease diagnostic and treatment centers. *Neurology*. 1992;42:473–480.
13. Román GC, Tatemichi TK, Erkinjuntti T, et al. Vascular dementia: diagnostic criteria for research studies. *Neurology*. 1993;43:250–260.
14. Chui HC, Victoroff JI, Margolin D, Jagust W, Shankle R, Katzman R. Criteria for the diagnosis of ischemic vascular dementia proposed by the state of California Alzheimer's disease diagnostic and treatment centers. *Neurology*. 1992;42:473–480.
15. World Health Organization. *The ICD-10 Classification of Mental and Behavioral Disorders: Clinical Descriptions and Diagnostic Guidelines*. Geneva, Switzerland: World Health Organization; 1992:50–51.
16. Erkinjuntti T. Vascular dementia: Challenge of clinical diagnosis. *Int Psychogeriatr*. 1997; 9:51–58.
17. Brun A. Pathology and pathophysiology of cerebrovascular dementia: Pure subgroups of obstructive and hypoperfusive etiology. *Dementia*. 1994;5:145–147.
18. Verhey FR, Lodder J, Rozendaal N, et al. Comparisons of seven sets of criteria used for the diagnosis of vascular dementia. *Neuroepidemiology*. 1996;15:166–172.
19. Gold C, Glannakopoulos P, Montes-Piaxao JC, et al. Sensitivity and specificity of newly proposed clinical criteria for possible vascular dementia. *Neurology*. 1997;49:690–694.
20. Erkinjuntti T, Inzitari D, Pantoni L, et al. Limitations for the diagnosis of vascular dementia in clinical trials. Is a focus on subcortical vascular dementia a solution? *Ann N Y Acad Sci*. 2000;903:262–272.
21. Wallin A, Milos V, Sjögren M, Pantoni L, Erkinjuntti T. Classification and subtypes of vascular dementia. *Int Psychogeriatr*. 2003;15:25–37.
22. Wiederkehr S, Simard M, Fortin C, van Reekum R. Validity of the clinical diagnostic criteria for vascular dementia; A critical review. Part II. *J Neuropsychiatry Clin Neurosci*. 2008;20:162–177.
23. Baccetta J, Kövari E, Merlo M, et al. Validation of clinical criteria for possible vascular dementia in the oldest-old. *Neurobiol Aging*. 2007;28:579–585.
24. McPherson SE, Cummings JL. Neuropsychological aspects of vascular dementia. *Brain Cogn*. 1996;31:269–282.
25. Boone KB, Miller BL, Mehringer CM, Hill-Gutierrez E, Goldberg MA, Berman NG. Neuropsychological correlates of white-matter lesions in healthy elderly subject. A threshold effect. *Arch Neurol*. 1992;49:549–554.
26. Vataja R, Pohjasvaara T, Mäntyla R, et al. MRI correlates of executive dysfunction in patients with ischaemic stroke. *Eur J Neurol*. 2003;10:625–631.

27. Sultzer DL, Mahler ME, Cummings JL, Van Gorp WG, Hinkin CH, Brown C. Cortical abnormalities associated with subcortical lesions in vascular dementia. Clinical and positron emission tomographic findings. *Arch Neurol.* 1995;52:773–780.
28. Rockwood K, Wentzel C, Hachinski V, Hogan DB, MacKnight C, McDowell I. Prevalence and outcomes of vascular cognitive impairment: Vascular cognitive impairment investigators of the Canadian study of health and aging. *Neurology.* 2000;54:447–451.
29. Bowler JV, Hachinski V. Criteria for vascular dementia: Replacing dogma with data. *Arch Neurol.* 2000;57:170–171.
30. Libon DJ, Price CC, Garrett KD, Giovannetti T. From Binswanger's disease to leukoaraiosis: What we have learned about subcortical vascular dementia. *Clin Neuropsychol.* 2004;18: 83–100.
31. Bowler JV, Eliasziw M, Steenhuis R, et al. Comparative evolution of Alzheimer disease, vascular dementia, and mixed dementia. *Arch Neurol.* 1997;54:697–703.
32. Stark CEL, Squire LR. Hippocampal damage equally impairs memory for single items and memory for conjunctions. *Hippocampus.* 2003;13:281–292.
33. De Leeuw FE, de Groot JC, Achten E, et al. Prevalence of cerebral white matter lesions in elderly people: A population-based magnetic resonance imaging study. The Rotterdam Scan Study. *J Neurol Neurosurg Psychiatry.* 2001;70:9–14.
34. Pohjasvaara T, Mäntylä R, Salonen O, et al. How complex interactions of ischemic brain infarcts, white matter lesions, and atrophy relate to post-stroke dementia. *Arch Neurol.* 2000;57:1295–1300.
35. Doufouil C, Alperovitch A, Tzourio C. Influence of education on the relationship between white matter lesions and cognition. *Neurology.* 2003;60:831–836.
36. Deary IJ, Bastin ME, Pattie A, et al. White matter integrity and cognition in childhood and old age. *Neurology.* 2006;66:505–512.
37. Stern, Y. What is cognitive reserve? Theory and research application of the reserve concept. *J Int Neuropsychol Soc.* 2002;8:448–460.
38. Wahlund LO, Barkhof F, Fazekas F, et al. A new rating scale for age-related white matter changes applicable to MRI and CT. *Stroke.* 2001;32:1318–1322.
39. Mayzel-Oreg O, Assaf Y, Gigi A, et al. High b-value diffusion imaging of dementia: Application to vascular dementia and Alzheimer disease. *J Neurol Sci.* 2007;257:105–113.
40. O'Sullivan M, Rich PM, Barrick TR, Clark CA, Markus HS. Frequency of subclinical lacunar infarcts in ischemic leukoaraiosis and cerebral autosomal dominant arteriopathy with subcortical infarcts and leukoencephalopathy. *Am J Neuroradiol.* 2003; 24:1348–1354.
41. Moorhouse P, Rockwood K. Vascular cognitive impairment: Current concepts and clinical developments. *Lancet Neurol.* 2008;7:246–255.
42. Nitkunan A, Barrick TR, Charlton RA, Clark CA, Markus HS. Multimodal MRI in cerebral small vessel disease: Its relationship with cognition and sensitivity to change over time. *Stroke.* 2008;39:1999–2005.
43. Sugihara S, Kinoshita T, Matsusue E, Fuji S, Ogawa T. Usefulness of diffusion tensor imaging of white matter in Alzheimer disease and vascular dementia. *Acta Radiol.* 2004;45: 658–663.
44. O'Sullivan M, Morris RG, Huckstep B, Jones DK, Williams SCR, Markus HS. Diffusion tensor MRI correlates with executive dysfunction in patients with ischaemic leukoaraiosis. *J Neurol Neurosurg Psychiatry.* 2004;75:441–447.
45. Markus HS, Lythgoe DJ, Ostegaard L, O'Sullivan M, Whilliams SC. Reduced cerebral blood flow in white matter in ischaemic leukoaraiosis demonstrated using quantitative exogenous contrast-based perfusion MRI. *J Neurol Neurosurg Psychiatry.* 2000;69:48–53.

46. Chalela JA, Alsop DC, Gonzalez-Atavales JB, Maldjian JA, Kanser SE, Detre JA. Magnetic resonance imaging in acute ischemic stroke using continuous arterial spin labeling. *Stroke*. 2000;31:680–687.
47. Hendrikse J, van Osch MJP, Rutgers DR, et al. Internal carotid artery occlusion assessed at pulsed arterial spin-labeling perfusion MR imaging at multiple delay times. *Radiology*. 2004;233:899–904.
48. Ferris SH. General measures of cognition. *Int Psychogeriatr*. 2003;15:215–217.
49. Rosen WG, Mohs RC, Davis KL. A new rating scale for Alzheimer's disease. *Am J Psychiatry*. 1984;141:1356–1364.
50. Hachinksi V, Iadecola C, Peterson R, et al. National Institute of Neurological Disorders and Stroke–Canadian stroke network vascular cognitive impairment harmonization standards. *Stroke*. 2006;37:2220–2241.
51. Ylikoski R, Jokinen H, Anderson P, et al. Comparison of the Alzheimer's disease assessment scale cognitive subscale and the vascular dementia assessment scale in differentiating elderly individuals with different degrees of white matter changes. The Ladis Study. *Dement Geriatr Cogn Disord*. 2007;24:73–81.
52. Madureira S, Verdelho A, Ferro J, et al. Development of a neuropsychological battery for the leukoaraiosis and disability in the elderly study (LADIS): Experience and baseline data. *Neuroepidemiology*. 2006;27:101–116.
53. Bianchi S, Dotti MT, Federico A. Physiology and pathology of NOTCH signaling system. *J Cell Physiol*. 2006;207:300–308.
54. Leblanc GG, Meschia JF, Stuss DT, Hachinski V. Genetics of vascular cognitive impairment: The opportunity and the challenges. *Stroke*. 2006;37:248–255.
55. Sisodia SS, St. George-Hyslop PH. Gamma-secretase, NOTCH, amyloid beta and Alzheimer's disease: Where do the presenilins fit in? *Nat Rev Neurosci*. 2002;3:281–290.
56. Davidson Y, Gibbons L, Purandare N, et al. Apolipoprotein E ε4 allele frequency in vascular dementia. *Dement Geriatr Cogn Disord*. 2006;22:15–19.
57. Baum L, Lam LCW, Kwok T, et al. Apolipoprotein E ε4 allele is associated with vascular dementia. *Dement Geriatr Cogn Disord*. 2006;22:301–305.
58. Orsitto G, Seripa D, Panza F, et al. Apolipoprotein E genotypes in hospitalized elderly patients with vascular dementia. *Dement Geriatr Cogn Disord*. 2007;23:327–333.
59. Flex A, Gaetani E, Proia AS, et al. Analysis of functional polymorphirms of metalloproteinase genes in persons with vascular dementia and Alzheimer's disease. *J Gerontol*. 2006;61(10):1065–1169.
60. Kim Y, Lee C. The gene encoding transforming growth factor β1 confers risk of ischemic stroke and vascular dementia. *Stroke*. 2006;37:2843–2845.
61. Garcia J, Ahmed A, Wonnacott A, Sutcliffe W, Nägga K, Söderkvist P, Marcusson J. Association of insulin-like growth factor-1 receptor polymorphism in dementia. *Dement Geriatr Cogn Disord*. 2006;22:439–444.
62. Kong M, Kim Y, Lee C. Promotor sequence variants of LIGHT are associated with female vascular dementia. *J Biomed Sci*. 2008;15(4):545–552.

4

OVERVIEW OF CARDIOVASCULAR PHYSIOLOGY AND PATHOLOGY

W. Kin Fung and Athena Poppas

Cardiovascular disease represents a tremendous burden to society. The most recent statistics from 2004 through 2005 in the United States reveal that the prevalence of coronary artery disease was 7.3% (16 million people) and of heart failure was 2.5% (5.3 million). The mortality from all cardiovascular disease was 870,000 people, with over half of these deaths due to coronary artery disease and a third due to heart failure.

(1) In most developed countries, mortality rates for cardiovascular disease have fallen by 25%–50% over the past 30 years.

(2) This has been associated with reductions in both the incidence of disease due to aggressive risk-factor reduction, and in the case-fatality rate due to dramatically improved pharmacological and surgical treatments. Conversely, by 2020, cardiovascular disease will replace infectious disease as the world's number-one cause of death and disability, accounting for one in every three deaths worldwide.

(3) Most of this shift will relate to changes in developing economies as they transition to more urbanization through improved economic circumstances, radical changes in work-related activities, and lifestyle modifications—all of which may be detrimental to the population as a whole (e.g. smoking, unhealthy dietary regimens, decreased exercise, etc.). Cardiovascular disease is a chronic condition, which adversely affects the health of a significant proportion of our population, and this is expected to grow worldwide.

Cardiac Anatomy

The heart consists of four chambers and one-way valves that work in concert to pump blood through the pulmonary and peripheral circulation. The main "pumping" chambers are the right and left ventricles, which are filled by the right and left atria (see Fig. 4-1). The right heart chambers receive deoxygenated blood returning from the periphery and produce forward flow to the lungs for oxygenation. The left heart chambers receive this

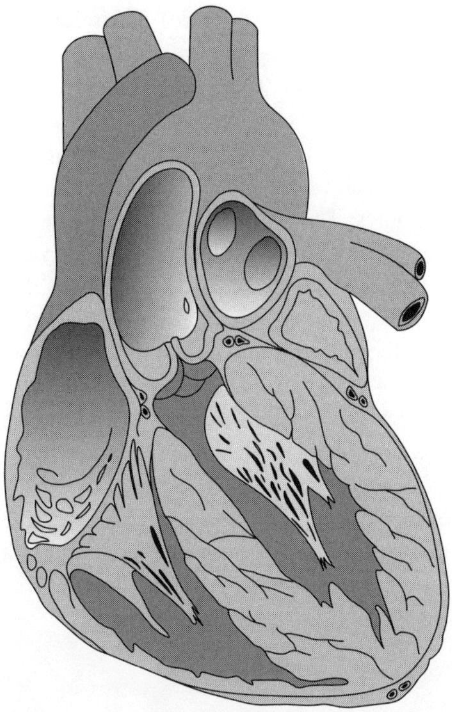

Figure 4-1 Diagram of heart and chambers.

newly oxygenated blood from the pulmonary vasculature and create forward flow to the body and all of its organs. Hence, the two sides of the heart work serially to create one circuit bridging both pulmonary and systemic circulations.

The cardiac cycle consist of a systole period of ventricular contraction and a diastolic period of ventricular relaxation. The cardiac cycle describes the rhythmic flow of blood through the heart. Deoxygenated blood returns from the head and upper extremities via the superior vena cava and from the lower extremities and abdominal organs via the inferior vena cava. Blood in these large-capacitance veins constantly flows under low pressure to the thin-walled right atrium. As the volume in the right atrium rises, the pressure rises causing the tricuspid valve to open, and blood is propelled forward into the right ventricle. During systole, the right ventricle contracts, closing the tricuspid valve and opening the pulmonary valve leading out to the pulmonary artery. The pulmonary vasculature branches out to the capillary level, and oxygen diffuses across the lung cells (alveoli) and is taken up by the red blood cells. Four pulmonary veins deliver the oxygenated blood to the left atrium. In response to rising left atrial volume and pressure, the mitral valve opens, and blood flows into the muscular left ventricle. During ventricular systole, the mitral valve closes and the aortic valve opens, propelling blood into the aorta and the systemic circulation.

Because the heart muscle contracts and relaxes, the pumping of blood is intermittent and rhythmic. In contrast to a tube with continuous flow, a cardiac pump requires valves that prevent reversal of flow during ventricular contraction (systole) and relaxation (diastole). The four cardiac valves separate the chambers and the great vessels, opening and closing to allow efficient forward output of blood. These valves are attached to a fibrous cardiac skeleton composed of dense connective tissue that serves as its supportive foundation. These are all one-way valves in non-diseased states and prevent the backflow of blood. During diastole, the mitral and tricuspid valves are open, and blood can flow freely from the atria to the ventricles. The aortic and pulmonary valves are closed so blood cannot leak back from the arteries to the ventricles while they are filling. Then, during ventricular systole, the mitral and tricuspid valves close so that blood cannot leak back from the ventricles to the atria, and the aortic and pulmonic valves open, allowing blood to be propelled into the systemic and pulmonic circulation, respectively.

Surrounding the heart is a protective structure, the pericardium. It consists of two layers: a strong, outer fibrous layer and an inner, serosal layer. The inner layer adheres to the epicardium of the heart and is termed the *visceral pericardium*. This visceral pericardium surrounds the heart and folds back onto itself, forming the second, outer layer, the *parietal pericardium*. Between the visceral and parietal pericardium is a small amount of pericardial fluid, which acts to reduce friction during every heartbeat.

Coronary Circulation

The heart pump is a muscle that needs energy to run. Oxygen and nutrients are delivered to the myocardium, and waste products are removed by the coronary circulation. There are three main coronary arteries, which arise from the aorta and are responsible for perfusing three distinct territories of the heart. The left main coronary artery divides into two of the three branches: the left anterior descending (LAD) artery and the left circumflex (LCx) artery. The LAD artery supplies oxygenated blood and nutrients to the anterior portion of the left ventricle and the septum that divides the two ventricles. The LCx artery delivers blood to the lateral wall of the left ventricle and infrequently (15%), the posterior-inferior regions of the heart as well. The right coronary artery (RCA) is the third main artery and perfuses the right-sided chambers of the heart and usually (85%), the inferior wall the left ventricle as well. There are respective cardiac veins that run along with the coronary arteries. Veins remove deoxygenated blood used by the cardiac myocytes and return it directly to the right side of the heart (right atrium) for oxygenation via the pulmonary circulation.

Conduction System of the Heart

The heart consists of specialized cells that have the ability to generate electrical (action) potentials and thus generate coordinated, cardiac muscle cell contraction. The main pacemaker of the heart is the sino-atrial (SA) node. It is located in the right atrium of the heart near the entrance of the superior vena cava and may be up to 3 cm in length. It is made up of modified cardiac myocytes, which cannot contract, but are able to spontaneously depolarize and initiate cardiac contraction. Normal depolarization rates range from 60 beats per minute (bpm) to 100 bpm, and this is termed *sinus rhythm.* Rates greater than 100 bpm or less than 60 bpm are termed *sinus tachycardia* and *sinus bradycardia,* respectively. Furthermore, although the SA node is the primary pacemaker of the heart, all cardiac myocytes can initiate depolarization and pace the heart. The rate of electrical depolarization depends on the location of the initial impulse generated. Sites higher up near the base of the heart are where the pacemaker rates are greatest, and this rate usually dictates the measured heart rate.

As the electrical impulse spreads from the SA node through both atria, it encounters the atrioventricular (AV) node, the electrical connection between the atrial and ventricular chambers. The AV node has a special property termed "decremental conduction," in which the more frequently the node is stimulated, the slower it conducts. This property is protective as it prevents extremely rapid atrial rhythms from conducting down to the ventricles, which would lead to underfilling of the ventricular chambers and systemic hypotension.

From the AV node, conduction spreads rapidly to the ventricles down to the Bundle of His in 0.03–0.04 seconds. The Bundle of His has the ability to become the backup pacemaker with an intrinsic rate of 40 to 60 beats per minute. The His bundles diverge into two bundle branches that continue distally within the interventricular septum; the right and left bundle. The left bundle is further divided into an anterior and posterior fascicle. The interventricular bundle branches give rise to thin filaments known as *Purkinje fibers*, which distribute the electrical impulse to the ventricular muscle. Together, the bundle branches and the Purkinje network make up the ventricular conduction system.

The heart and conduction system are under both sympathetic and parasympathetic control. Preganglionic sympathetic neurons from the upper thoracic spinal cord synapse in the cervical ganglia then travel to the heart via the recurrent cardiac nerve on the right and the ventrolateral cardiac nerve on the left. Preganglionic parasympathetic fibers from the dorsal motor nucleus of the medula travel to the heart via the vagus nerve. The vagus modulates cardiac sympathetic activity at the prejunctional and post-junctional sites by controlling norepinephrine release and inhibiting cyclic adenosine monophosphate (AMP) activity. There is a high density of vagal efferents to the SA and AV node, which modulate the initiation and rate of the electrical impulse generated as well as the speed of its conduction. There are vagal afferent fibers from the ventricular myocardium, which mediate cardiac reflexes.

Local and systemic catecholamines such as norepinephrine can directly stimulate cardiac myocytes. Sympathetic activation of β-one adrenergic receptors on the myocardial cell surface activates the G protein system, which increases production of cyclic AMP from Adenosine triphosphate (ATP). This augments cellular calcium influx, removal, and release to increase the force of contraction as well as enhance active relaxation. Parasympathetic vagal nerve inputs to the myocardial cells release acetylcholine, which inhibits the G protein system and counteracts the effects of sympathetic stimulation. In the myocardium, this cholenergic stimulation modestly reduces the force of atrial and ventricular contraction. In the conduction system, sympathetic stimulation increases the heart rate, and parasympathetic stimulation reduces the heart rate.

Cardiac Function

Histology

The chambers of the heart are made up of branching and anastamosing striated muscle cells: cardiac myocytes. The cardiac myocyte has five basic components: (1) cell membrane (sarcolemma) and T tubules, for electrical impulse conduction; (2) sarcoplasmic reticulum, a calcium reservoir necessary for electrical conduction and mechanical contraction; (3) myofibrils, the contractile elements; (4) mitochondria, high-energy phosphate stores; and (5) the nucleus. Cardiac muscle cells contain many more mitochondria than regular striated muscles do, this being consistent with their dependency on aerobic metabolism.

The myocardial cell is made up of parallel myofibrils, and within each myofibril are serial, connected sarcomeres. The sarcomere is the functional intracellular contractile unit of the cardiac myocyte. It consists of two overlapping contractile proteins—thick myosin filaments and thin actin filaments—and regulatory proteins, such as troponin and tropomyosin. The end of each sarcomere is demarcated by the Z-line, to which the thin filaments are anchored. Contraction occurs by the cumulative effect of sliding of the thin actin filaments between the thick myosin filaments toward the center of the sarcomere. The length of sarcomeres ranges from 1.6 to 2.2 micrometers. Shorter sarcomeres have considerable overlap between actin and myosin filaments with a consequent reduction in contractile force, while longer lengths increase the number of cross-bridges and thus contractility (see Fig. 4-2—Frank-Starling curve). Therefore, the force of contraction is dependent upon the initial length of the cardiac muscle fibers (isometric contraction). There is, however, an upper limit—with progressive lengthening, the sarcomere reaches a point where effective overlap is reduced, resulting in diminished contractile force. This may be seen in cases of dilated cardiomyopathy and heart failure.

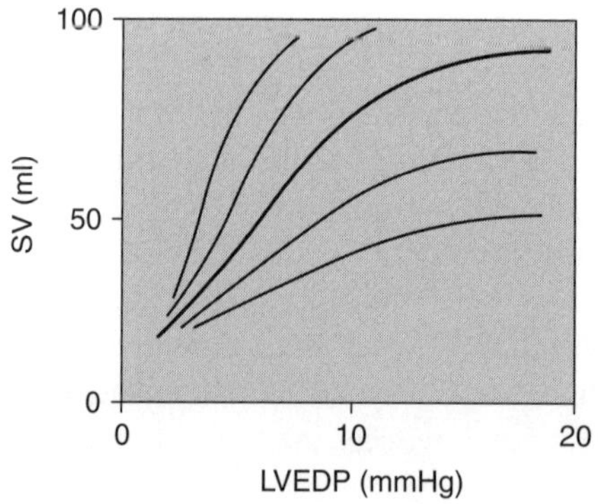

Figure 4-2 Frank-Starling curve.

Overall Cardiac performance

A measure of cardiac performance is "stroke volume," or the amount of blood ejected from the ventricle to the systemic circulation with each contraction. Cardiac output is a measure of total forward flow and is equal to the product of stroke volume and the heart rate.

In the intact heart, cardiac performance is therefore affected by three major factors: preload, afterload, and contractility. The increased venous return of blood to the ventricle is the preload, which affects passive myocardial fiber lengthening and isometric contraction; the greater the end-diastolic volumes, the greater will be the degree of stretching of the muscles before stimulation, and hence the greater will be the force of contraction. However, with further lengthening of the myocyte, it reaches a point at which positive inotropy is uncoupled, resulting in reduced contractile force (Fig. 4-3). Afterload (i.e., hypertension, aortic stenosis, etc.) and contractility also play a role in myocardial mechanical function. As can be seen from Fig. 4-2, with decreased afterload and/or increased contractility, the Frank-Starling curve shifts upward. The opposite occurs with increased afterload and/or decreased contractility. Thus, a change in venous return (preload) causes the ventricle to move along a single Frank-Starling curve that is defined by the existing conditions of afterload and inotropy.

Pathophysiology

Heart Failure Heart failure is a common cause of morbidity and mortality in the United States; there are over 5 million patients with heart failure and 550,000 new cases diagnosed each year.[1,4] It is a chronic disease seen more often in the elderly. Approximately 80% of all hospital admissions for heart failure occur in patients older than 65, and it is the most frequent discharge diagnosis in this population.[5] There are 56,000 deaths each year due to heart failure, resulting in a mortality rate of 20.2 per 100,000 persons.[6] With the aging population, economic impact of this condition is substantial and growing.

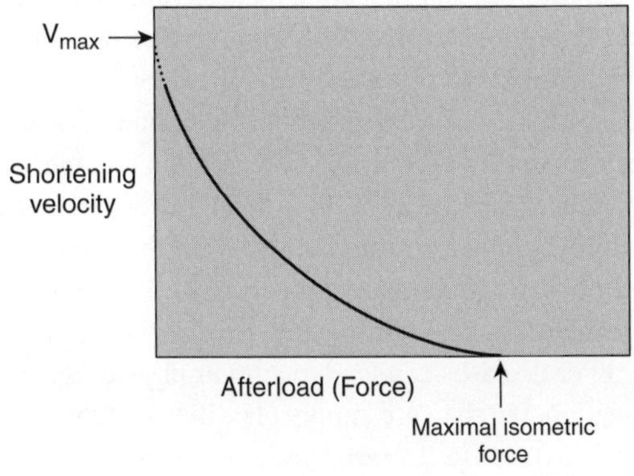

Figure 4-3 Length-tension curve.

In 2000, $3.5 billion was spent on Medicare beneficiaries for in-hospital management of heart failure, surpassing all other clinical conditions, including all cancers and heart attacks.[7, 8]

"Heart failure" is defined as the inability to produce an adequate forward flow at a pressure low enough to prevent pulmonary congestion. Heart failure is the final common disease complicating many, diverse cardiac pathologies, such as abnormalities of the heart muscle, cardiac valves, or epicardial coronary arteries. Systolic heart failure occurs when the left ventricular contractile function is reduced; diastolic heart failure occurs when the ventricle's ability to relax is abnormal and hence the chamber cannot fill adequately without elevation in pressures.[9]

The overall systolic function of the heart is governed by four primary factors: (1) the contractile state of the myocardium, (2) the preload of the ventricle (end-diastolic volume), (3) the afterload of the ventricle, and (4) the heart rate. Derangements in any one of these may lead to the clinical manifestations of heart failure. The most common cause of systolic dysfunction is depression of myocardial contractility due to prior myocardial infarction and loss of working tissue, toxins such as alcohol, or infectious processes such as the coxasackie virus. The ventricle can fail when subjected to acute or chronic volume overload, such as when one of the cardiac valves is diseased and leaking blood when it should be closed (see section below). The ventricle can fail when it is working against abnormally high afterload, such as a diseased and narrowed cardiac valve or elevated systemic blood pressure.

Diastolic heart failure results from abnormal and impaired filling of the ventricles. The systolic, contractile function is usually preserved.[10] Many epidemiological studies estimate that approximately 40% of congestive heart failure is due to diastolic dysfunction, and the prevalence is increased in older adults and women.[11] The impairment of ventricular filling may be related to slowed or incomplete relaxation and/or increase in stiffness of the chamber. This is seen in acute ischemia, restrictive cardiomyopathies secondary to infiltrative processes, and hypertrophied myocardium. The elevations in ventricular diastolic pressures will result in increases in atrial pressure and hence pulmonary venous pressure. The increase in pulmonary hemostatic pressures can drive fluid into the lung interstitium and alveoli. This pulmonary edema and congestion reduces oxygen exchange. In addition, not only can systolic and diastolic dysfunction manifest independently, but there are also clinical conditions where both systolic and diastolic dysfunction can be seen together, as in ischemic heart disease.

The taxonomy of the different diseases that cause heart failure is in flux. *Cardiomyopathy* is defined as a pathological process involving the myocardium, which is structurally and functionally abnormal, leading to heart failure. The European and American Cardiac Societies defines cardiomyopathy as primary diseases of the myocardium with particular morphological and physiological characteristics that are not due to systemic disorders of coronary artery disease, hypertension, valvular disease, or congenital heart disease. Importantly, these other diseases can lead to similar physiological derangements in systolic and diastolic function, but they are simply classified differently. Cardiomyopathies are classified into *dilated, hypertrophic, restrictive,* or *arrhythmogenic right ventricular dysplasia.*[12] The American Heart Association (AHA) definition is broader, adding abnormalities of the cardiac electrical system to their scheme.[13] Characteristics of *dilated* cardiomyopathy include dilation of cardiac chambers and diminished systolic function of the left ventricle or both ventricles. Measures of contractile function are reduced and may become progressively worse with time. In *hypertrophic* cardiomyopathy, ventricular size is normal but ventricular walls are markedly thickened, and individual myocytes are hypertrophied. Systolic function is normal, but end diastolic pressure is elevated because of reduced compliance. Similarly, in *restrictive* cardiomyopathy, cardiac chambers are normal in size or mildly dilated, and wall thickness is mildly increased. Systolic function is usually normal but diastolic pressure is elevated because of non-compliant walls due to fibrosis or infiltrative processes. Note that left ventricular diastolic pressure and therefore pulmonary capillary pressure are elevated in all three types of cardiomyopathies (albeit through different mechanisms), leading to pulmonary congestion.

The reduction in cardiac function and output triggers a series of compensatory mechanisms to maintain forward flow and adequate perfusion. The principal mechanisms include neurohormonal activation and ventricular hypertrophy and remodeling.[14] The lowered systemic perfusion is sensed in the periphery, and a neurohormonal response attempts to counteract the reduced flow. The activation of the renin-angiotensin-aldosterone system (RAAS) and the adrenergic system ensures adequate systemic perfusion by several mechanisms. The release of powerful vasoconstrictors increases arterial tone, which leads to increase in systemic pressure and improved perfusion to vital organs. There are also adrenergic receptors in the myocardium that increase the force of contraction (inotropy) and the heart rate (chronotropy). This sympathetic stimulation of myocardial cells leads to increased cardiac output and perfusion as well. The increased production of antidiuretic hormone leads to salt and water retention. This causes expansion of intravascular fluid volume, which serves to increase preload and hence, initially, improve cardiac performance. In time, these changes prove to be maladaptive and ultimately worsen cardiac performance and jeopardize the patient's survival.

The neurohormonal and mechanical adaptations are initially beneficial but over time are detrimental, leading to heart failure progression. By increasing peripheral resistance, the vasoconstriction response leads to increased afterload on the heart, and this may directly depress cardiac function as well as contribute to adverse ventricular remodeling: hypertrophy and dilation. Adrenergic stimulation leading to increased chronotropy and inotropy of the heart may result in ischemia and maladaptive remodeling. There is also down-regulation of the receptors, leading to reduced adrenergic sensitivity. Finally, there are data indicating that elevated neurohormones can directly cause or speed cell death (apoptosis).[15] The increase in circulating blood volume is not well tolerated by a dilated and stiff ventricle, leading to an increase in diastolic filling pressures, which is transmitted to the pulmonary vasculature. The increase in hydrostatic pressure causes transudation of fluid into the intercellular space, resulting in pulmonary congestion and shortness of breath, the pathonomonic signs and symptoms of heart failure. Current pharmacological treatment for heart failure is aimed at blocking the neurohormonal activation.

The clinical manifestations of heart failure reflect the pathophysiological effects on low forward blood flow and elevated filling pressures. The reduced perfusion of organs, reduced delivery of oxygen to tissues, and impaired removal of toxins results in kidney dysfunction and even failure. The skeletal muscles tire more easily, and even simple activities cause fatigue. The patient may have cool and cyanotic extremities due to maladaptive peripheral vasoconstriction. The metabolic demands of the organs cannot be met at increased workloads or ultimately even at rest. The elevated left ventricular and atrial filling pressures are reflected in the lungs, causing congestion and symptoms of shortness of breath. The elevated diastolic pressures on the right side cause congestion in the liver and lower-extremity edema. The abnormal myocardial cell function and scarring can lead to electrical short circuits and lethal rhythm disturbances such as ventricular tachycardia and fibrillation. Some 40% to 50% of heart failure mortality is due to arrhythmias and sudden cardiac death.[16]

There are two widely used classification schemes of disease severity. The New York Heart Association (NYHA) functional class (see Table 4-1—NYHA class) places patients in one of four categories, depending on their subjective symptoms in response to increasing levels of exertion. The NHYA class is the most established and has been shown to correlate with survival rates.[16] The 2001 classification scheme outlines the stages in the development of heart failure. It categorizes patients into those without overt symptoms, but who are at high risk (Stage A and B), and those with established symptoms of heart failure (Stage C and D; see Table 4-2). This second scheme was introduced to identify at-risk patients to initiate treatment aimed at the predisposing, established diseases such as hypertension or atherosclerosis before the appearance of overt structural heart disease, and thereby possibly prevent the onset of symptomatic heart failure. This ABCD staging system is useful to guide treatment algorithms depending on the severity and progression of disease.[16] The two classification schemes are complementary.

Table 4-1 NYHA functional classification

Class	
I	Patients with cardiac disease but without limitations of physical activity. Ordinary physical activity does not cause undue fatigue, palpitation, dyspnea, or anginal pain.
II	Patients with cardiac disease resulting in slight limitation of physical activity. They are comfortable at rest. Ordinary physical activity results in fatigue, palpitation, dyspnea, or anginal pain.
III	Patients with cardiac disease resulting in marked limitation of physical activity. They are comfortable at rest. Less than ordinary physical activity causes fatigue, palpitation, dyspnea, or anginal pain.
IV	Patient with cardiac disease resulting in inability to carry on any physical activity without discomfort. Symptoms may be present even at rest. If any physical activity is undertaken, discomfort is increased.

Table 4-2 Stages in the development of heart failure

Stage		Example—patients with:
A	At high risk for HF but without structural heart disease or symptoms of HF	Hypertension, atherosclerotic disease, diabetes, obesity
B	Structural heart disease but without signs or symptoms of HF	Previous MI, LV hypertrophy, low ejection fraction, asymptomatic valvular disease
C	Structural heart disease with prior or current symptoms of HF	Known structural heart disease *and* shortness of breath and fatigue, reduced exercise tolerance
D	Refractory HF requiring specialized interventions	Marked symptoms at rest despite maximal medical therapy. Recurrent hospitalizations or cannot be safely discharged without specialized interventions

Valvular Heart Disease

Aortic Stenosis Aortic stenosis is caused by degenerative changes affecting a trileaflet or congenitally bileaflet (bicuspid) aortic valve. The normally thin, pliable aortic leaflets become thickened, calcified, and stiff in response to various stimuli, resulting in reduced valve opening. The normal aortic valve area is 3–4 cm^2. In age-related or senile aortic stenosis, a normal trileaflet aortic valve develops changes that are similar to, and share common risk factors for, vascular atherosclerosis. There is endothelial damage resulting in inflammation, lipid accumulation, and active calcification, which progresses from the base of the leaflets to the tips.[17] A similar pathological process affects patients with congenitally abnormal valves, but due to the abnormal flow across these leaflets, the disease progresses more rapidly and presents clinically at younger ages. Rheumatic fever can cause aortic stenosis with leaflet thickening and commissural fusion early and calcification later. It is almost always associated with mitral valve involvement.

The pathophysiological consequences of aortic valve narrowing are felt by the preceding pumping chamber. The left ventricle must generate increased systolic pressure to drive the blood out across the narrowed aortic valve into the aorta and systemic circulation. The left ventricle myocardial wall will hypertrophy in response to the slowly progressing pressure overload. By LaPlace's relationship, where wall thickness is inversely proportional to wall stress, this compensatory response reduces wall stress and oxygen consumption, but at the expensive of increased ventricular stiffness. Therefore, patients with aortic stenosis will invariably have some degree of diastolic dysfunction. The natural history of aortic stenosis has a very prolonged latent period but with significant individual variability about hemodynamic disease progression. Once a valve develops severe obstruction, defined as aortic valve area less than 1.0 cm^2 or a mean transvalvular gradient of greater than 40 mm Hg, patients begin to develop sentinel symptoms that herald a precipitous decline in survival. The median survival after the onset of angina is five years; after exertional syncope it is three years, and after congestive heart failure it is two years.[18] These symptoms develop because the above compensatory response has been exhausted and/or become maladaptive. The treatment for severe, symptomatic aortic stenosis is surgical aortic valve replacement.

Aortic valve insufficiency Aortic valve insufficiency can be due to abnormalities of the valve leaflets or of the supporting structures: specifically, dilation of the aortic annulus and root. The most common valvular abnormalities are congenitally bicuspid valve, rheumatic heart disease, and infectious endocarditis. The most common causes of dilation of the aorta are congenital annulo-aortic ectasia, Marfan's syndrome, and degenerative aneurysm and dissection. The inability of the leaflets to close completely during diastole causes blood to leak from the aorta back into the left ventricle. Therefore, during each systolic contraction, the left ventricle must eject the regurgitant volume as well as the returning blood volume from the lungs via the left atrium. This places predominately a volume but also a pressure load on the ventricle. In chronic and progressive aortic valve insufficiency, such as congenital abnormalities and rheumatic disease, the ventricle compensates by chamber dilation. The ventricular dilation increases the compliance so that the increased volume can be accommodated at a lower ventricular filling pressure.

Mitral valve stenosis Mitral valve stenosis is a late sequelus of rheumatic fever. Recurrent inflammation as well as hemodynamic trauma to the deformed valve lead to leaflet thickening and calcification, fusion of the commissures between the two leaflets, and thickening and shortening of the submitral apparatus (chordae tendinea). The rigid and narrowed valve restricts diastolic filling of the left ventricle. A normal mitral valve area is 4–5 cm^2; when the valve area becomes less than 2 cm^2, left atrial pressure must be elevated for the same amount of blood to enter the left ventricle in the same time period. This elevation of left atrial pressures is transmitted into the pulmonary veins and capillaries and can lead to pulmonary edema and heart failure. The chronically elevated pressures cause changes in the pulmonary vascular bed leading to pulmonary artery hypertension. This elevation in load in turn can affect emptying of the right ventricle, leading to right ventricular hypertrophy and then pump failure. The limited filling of the left ventricle can lead to reduction in stroke volume and cardiac output when the filling time is decreased (increase in heart rate with exertion) or at rest when the valve narrowing is severe (MVA$<$1.0 cm^2 and mean gradient $>$10 mm Hg). The increased left atrial pressure in mitral stenosis leads to atrial enlargement. This in turn can produce atrial fibrillation (an abnormal heart rhythm) and thrombus formation. The thrombus can embolize and cause cerebral vascular occlusion (accidents or stroke). Most patients with symptomatic mitral stenosis can be treated with a percutaneous commissurotomy, in which a balloon is inflated across the narrowed valve, splitting the fused commissures. Other treatment options include surgical valve replacement.

Mitral valve regurgitation Mitral valve regurgitation, like aortic regurgitation, can be due to pathology of the valve leaflets or of the supporting structures, such as the papillary muscles and underlying ventricular myocardium. Common abnormalities that affect the closing function of the mitral valve leaflets include infection (endocarditis), myxomatous degeneration (prolapse), calcific degeneration, and rheumatic disease. Patients with dilated cardiomyopathy from any cause may develop mitral valve regurgitation due to displacement of the papillary muscles and resultant malcoaptation of the leaflets. Similarly, after a myocardial infarction, the scarred myocardium may affect papillary muscle function and hence leaflet closing force and/or position. With each ventricular contraction, a portion of the stroke volume is propelled backwards into the lower-pressure left atrium. This results in: (1) reduced forward or systemic cardiac output, (2) increased volume load on the ventricle as both the regurgitant volume and the normal pulmonary venous flow will be returned during diastolic filling, (3) increase in left atrial volume and pressure. Chronic changes in chamber size and myocardial function can maintain forward stroke volume, but in time, these adaptations are inadequate and heart failure occurs. Furthermore, increases in systemic vascular resistance (blood pressure) can cause increase in backward (regurgitant) volume and reduction in forward stroke volume. Also, with chronic volume loading, the left atrium adapts, becoming more compliant to accommodate the increase in volume without marked increase in pressure. Eventually, this compensatory change is inadequate, and pulmonary venous pressures rise, causing pulmonary edema (heart failure) and dyspnea. The treatment for chronic, severe mitral regurgitation is diuresis, and when symptomatic or the ventricular function deteriorates, surgical mitral valve repair or replacement.

Vascular Function

Normal Vasculature

The arterial wall is composed of three layers: the intima, the media, and the adventitia. The intima is composed of a thin layer of endothelial cells, which form an interactive barrier between the blood and the vessel. The media has varying proportions of elastic and contractile elements, depending on the type of vessel. The larger arteries have more prominent internal and external elastic laminae, which stretch and rebound with systole and diastole, respectively. The smaller arterioles have a more prominent smooth-muscle component, which constricts or relaxes in response to various stimuli to alter vascular tone (flow = pressure/resistance). The adventitia is the outer layer, which maintains external connections via blood vessels, lymphatics, and nerves.

Atherosclerosis

The most common arterial disease is atherosclerosis, in which a various stimuli produce an abnormal activity of cellular accumulation and changes within the intima and media. The predominant theory of atherogenesis supports inflammation as the primary initiating and perpetuating event.[19, 20] The atherosclerotic plaque begins with injury to the endothelium and lipid accumulation within the intima. Further oxidative stress releases cytokines, which recruit, bind, and further stimulate leukocytes and smooth muscle cells. Activated macrophages take up oxidized lipoproteins (LDL cholesterol), developing into foam cells, which, along with activated platelets and injured endothelial cells, release factors that further stimulate smooth muscle cells to migrate, proliferate, and produce extracellular matrix and connective tissue. All these components combine to form an atherosclerotic plaque in coronary, cerebral, and peripheral arteries.

Atherosclerotic plaques can slowly increase in size, causing lumenal narrowing and reduction in blood flow to the organ being supplied. A reduction in oxygen supply to and lactic acid removal from the brain, heart, kidneys, and legs produce the most common symptoms. Cardiac chest pain or angina results when an atherosclerotic plaque in one of the coronary arteries limits blood flow to the myocardium, producing myocardial ischemia. Normally, the coronary circulation can increase the delivery of oxygen and nutrients to meet an increase in metabolic needs, such as with exercise.

The balance between oxygen supply and demand can become deranged in patients with coronary artery disease. The supply is determined by the oxygen-carrying capacity of the blood and the rate of coronary flow. Oxygen-carrying capacity depends on the number of red blood cells and systemic oxygen acquired from the lungs. Unlike skeletal muscle, cardiac myocytes maximally extract oxygen at rest, and hence, any increase in demand requires an increase in blood flow. The rate of coronary flow is inversely related to the vascular resistance. The autoregulation of vascular resistance is mediated by three main factors: sympathetic neural control, local metabolites (i.e., adenosine), and the balance between endothelial factors that promote smooth muscle relaxation (i.e., nitric oxide) and vasoconstriction (i.e., endothelin-1). Atherosclerotic endothelium responds abnormally to the usual stressors such that inappropriate vasoconstriction may predominate.[21]

Atherosclerotic plaques can become unstable and rupture, leading to acute thrombosis with vessel occlusion.[19] The loss of blood flow to the organ quickly causes cell death in that vessel's territory. This is the etiology of a myocardial infarction (heart attack) or a cerebral infarction (stroke). When the fibrous plaque ruptures, it exposes the plaque's thrombogenic lipid core to the blood. Plaques with thinner caps are more likely to rupture and are termed "vulnerable plaques." Inside, they also have a higher concentration of inflammatory cells such as macrophages that contain powerful procoagulants.[20] Pharmacological treatment is aimed at stabilizing the plaques, reducing platelet aggregation, and dissolving clots. Acute percutaneous techniques can mechanically open the artery with balloons and stents.

There are six well-established risk factors for the development of atherosclerosis. The modifiable risk factors include hypertension, diabetes mellitus, cigarette smoking, and hyperlipidemia. The two major fixed-risk factors are advanced age and a family history of premature coronary artery disease (defined as disease in a first-degree male relative <55 years and female relative <65 years).[22] The levels of total cholesterol and low-density lipoprotein (LDL) have been shown to correlate with increased risk of atherosclerosis and ischemic heart disease. Decreasing these lipid levels by diet and medications has been shown to reduce the development of coronary artery disease. High-density lipoproteins (HDL) have the ability to remove intracellular lipids, reducing lipid accumulation in the vessel walls. They are therefore protective; blood levels of HDL have been shown to be inversely proportional to the incidence of atherosclerosis. There are a number of other putative risk factors that are under investigation, including markers of inflammation such as CRP.

Notes

1. American Heart Association: *Heart disease and stroke statistics—2004 update.* Dallas, TX: American Heart Association, 2003.
2. Cooper R, Cutler J, Desvigne-Nickens P, et al. Trends and disparities in coronary heart disease, stroke, and other cardiovascular diseases in the United States: Findings of the national conference on cardiovascular disease prevention. *Circulation* (online). 2000;102:3137.
3. Murray CJL, Lopez AD. *The global burden of disease.* Cambridge, MA: Harvard School of Public Health, 1996.
4. Massie BM, Shah, NB. Evolving trends in the epidemiologic factors of heart failure: Rationale for preventive strategies and comprehensive disease management: *Am Heart J.* 1997;133:703
5. Rich MW, Nease RF. Cost-effective analysis in clinical practice: The case of heart failure. *Arch Intern Med.* 1999; 159:1690.
6. Minino AM, Arias E., Kochanek KD, et al. Deaths: Final data from 2000. *National Vital Statistics Reports*, vol. 50, no. 15. Hyattsville, MD: National Center for Health Statistics, 2002.
7. Centers for Medicare and Medicaid Services. *2002 Data Compendium.* Baltimore, MD, 2002.
8. O'Connell JB, Bristow MR: Economic impact of heart failure in the United States: Time for a different approach. *J Heart Lung Transplant.* 13:S107, 1994.
9. Zile MR, Brutsaert DL. New concepts in diastolic dysfunction and diastolic heart failure: Part 1. *Circulation.* 2002;105:1387–1393.
10. Lester SJ, Tajik AJ, Nishimura RA, et al. Unlocking the mysteries of diastolic function: Deciphering the Rosetta stone 10 years later. *J Am Coll Cardiol.* 2008;51:679–689.
11. Owan TE, Hodge Do, Herges RM, et al. Trends in prevalence and outcome of heart failure with preserved ejection fraction. *N Engl J Med.* 2006;355:251–259.
12. Elliott P, Andersson B, Arbustini E, et al. Classification of the cardiomyopathies: A position statement from the European Society of Cardiology working group on myocardial and pericardial diseases. *Eur Heart J.* 2008;29:270–276.
13. Maron BJ, McKenna WJ, Danielson GK, et al. Contemporary definitions and classification of the cardiomyopathies. An American Heart Association scientific statement from the Council on Clinical Cardiology, heart failure and transplantation committee; Quality of care and outcomes research and functional genomics and translational biology interdisciplinary working groups and Council on Epidemiology and Prevention. *Circulation.* 2006;113:1807–1816.
14. Schrier RW, Abraham WT. Hormones and hemodynamics in heart failure. *N Engl J Med* 1999;341(8):577–585.

15. Communal C, Singh K, Pimentel DR, et al. Norepinephrine stimulates apoptosis in adult rat ventricular myocytes by activiation of the beta-adrenergic pathway. *Circulation.* 1998;98(13):1329–1334.
16. Hunt SA, Abraham WT, Chin MA, et al. ACC/AHA 2005 guideline update for the diagnosis and management of chronic heart failure in the adult. *J Am Coll Cardiol.* 2005;46: 1116–1143.
17. Bonow RO, Carbellow BA, Chatterjee K, et al. ACC/AHA 2006 practice guidelines for the management of patients with valvular heart disease: Executive summary. *J Am Coll Cardiol.* 2006;48:598–675.
18. Ross J Jr, Braunwald E. Aortic stenosis. *Circulation.* 1968;38(1 Suppl):61–67.
19. Fuster V, Moreno PR, Fayad ZA, et al. Atherothrombosis and high-risk plaque: Part I: Evolving concepts. *J Am Coll Cardiol.* 2005;46:937.
20. Libby P. Molecular basis of the acute coronary syndrome. *Circulation.* 1995;91:2844.
21. Davignon J, Ganz P. Role of endothelial dysfunction in atherosclerosis. *Circulation.* 2004;109(Suppl):III27032.
22. Lloyd-Jones DM, Leip EP, Larson MG et al. Prediction of lifetime risk for cardiovascular disease by risk factor burden at 50 years of age. *Circulation.* 2006;113:791.

5

CARDIAC REHABILITATION FOR ELDERLY CARDIAC PATIENTS

Daniel E. Forman and Jose A. Suaya

Prevalence of heart disease increases with age, but utilization of cardiac rehabilitation remains paradoxically low among older adults.[1–5] While cardiac rehabilitation offers many opportunities to moderate cardiac disease and age-related vulnerabilities among elderly, key obstacles limit its application. Ironically, there remains a paucity of data from randomized controlled trials to substantiate benefits of cardiac rehabilitation in relation to old age. Furthermore, cardiac rehabilitation entails a protracted commitment over many months, which for many older adults often amounts to daunting costs, logistics, and behavioral obstacles.

Nevertheless, the fact remains that senescence provokes a cascade of physiological changes that intrinsically predispose the elderly to cardiac disease.[6, 7] Moreover, prognoses for cardiac disease are worse in the elderly relative to young adults. Cardiac rehabilitation promotes healthful activity and life habits and provides opportunities to optimize medical management that can serve to moderate age-related physiological changes and cardiovascular vulnerabilities. Conceptual benefits include not only delayed mortality, but also reduced morbidity, increased function, and improved quality of life. Such benefits seem particularly compelling in the midst of demographic trends showing rapid growth of our elderly population. By 2004, an average 60-year-old was expected to live 22 more years, an average 70-year-old about 16 years, and an average 80-year-old about 9 years.[8] Cardiac rehabilitation provides an important opportunity to optimize health, vitality, and independence within this mushrooming population of susceptible elderly.

Prevalence of Coronary Heart Disease (CHD) and Major Clinical Implications

The U.S. Census Bureau estimates that there are 34.8 million Americans aged over 65 years (58.5% female) and 9.2 million aged over 80 years (65.7% female). By 2030, it is projected that there will be 70.3 million adults aged over 65 years, of whom more than 18% will be aged over 80.[9] The intrinsic age-related risk of cardiac disease is reflected in the fact that CHD prevalence is three times greater among adults aged 65 years and older than those aged 45 to 64 (22% vs. 7%).[10] Heart failure, arrhythmias, and hypertension similarly increase in association with typical aging.[6, 7]

Therefore, as the population of elderly people expands, implications of the fundamental age-related susceptibility to cardiovascular disease (CVD) are extensive. CVD-related mortality or non-fatal cardiac events (e.g., myocardial infarction, angina, congestive symptoms, and arrhythmias) and hospitalizations constitute a growing epidemic with staggering cost implications. Furthermore, diminished quality of life, functional capacity, and vascular-mediated neurocognitive capacity are also germane. CHD is an insidious disease of the vascular tree that leads to ubiquitous changes in organs and functions that depend on vascular perfusion. Diminished muscle perfusion can, for example, exacerbate physical weakening and functional decline.[11] Similarly, impeded cerebral perfusion is frequently manifested as vascular-mediated cognitive decrements.[12] Goals to moderate such widespread vascular-mediated vulnerabilities remain an important objective for which cardiac rehabilitation may be useful.

How Does Aging Affect Susceptibility to Cardiac Disease?

Normal senescence includes a constellation of cardiovascular changes that predispose old people to heart disease.[7] Senescent vessels stiffen as elastin fragments and calcium and collagen deposits increase,[6] increasing systolic blood pressure and cardiac workload.[13] Moreover, endothelial capacity to synthesize vital peptides for vascular homeostasis and vasomotor regulation declines with age,[14] leading to increased vulnerability to atheromatous lesions and plaque instability.[15] Coronary flow reserve (especially in the context of demand stressors) is also typically diminished, with even greater likelihood of cardiac ischemia.[7]

As the heart struggles to pump against stiffened vessels, there is a natural tendency for senescent myocytes to hypertrophy, a response that starts as a compensatory means to modify ventricular wall stresses, but that also predisposes them to individual myocyte degeneration in a process called *apoptosis*.[16, 17] Consequently, the senescent heart usually incurs mild hypertrophy along with progressive atrophy of individual cells, with associated fibrosis and stiffening of the myocardial walls. Consistently, hearts in older adults are relatively more vulnerable to diastolic filling impairment and impaired perfusion, i.e., in part due to ventricular stiffening and thickening, along with related susceptibility to subendocardial ischemia).[18]

Cerebral flow reserve is similarly constricted by intrinsic changes in the neurovasculature as well as by fluctuations in cardiac performance, especially in correlation to fluctuations in cardiac output that occur in context of age-related increases in systolic dysfunction, diastolic filling abnormalities, arrhythmias, and subendocardial ischemia.[19] Frontal lobe perfusion is particularly susceptible to changes in perfusion, and a growing body of literature highlights corresponding decrements in executive function.[12]

Such insights have led to a growing emphasis on therapies that enhance cardiac and vascular health, both as primary and as secondary disease-prevention priorities. Exercise training has been demonstrated to forestall and even reverse many aspects of cardiovascular aging and related propensity to disease.[20] Physical activity has been demonstrated to improve endothelial responses.[21, 22] Medication and lifestyle changes are synergistic, with trials showing that ACE inhibitors, statins, and vitamins can all bring about more healthful vascular endothelial responses.[23]

Cardiac Rehabilitation: The Original Program Design

The conceptual utility of cardiac rehabilitation in relation to age-related vulnerabilities represents a significant extrapolation from cardiac rehabilitation's original role in the medical armamentarium. Cardiac rehabilitation was formulated in the 1960s primarily as a means to initiate exercise among deconditioned and unstable patients after completed myocardial infarctions (MI). Until that time, therapeutic objectives for myocardial infarction mostly centered on prolonged bedrest and inactivity, as heart attacks were essentially observed by medical personnel as there were no therapies yet available to interrupt the progression of myocardial injury, myocyte cell death, and pro-arrhymogenic instability.[24, 25, 26] The discovery that early mobilization and exercise for MI survivors improved their prognoses startled the medical community, since these survivors were typically very infirm and unstable in terms of infarct expansion, arrhythmias, and further ischemia.

Herman Hellerstein pioneered the concept of cardiac rehabilitation (CR) when he proposed an organized intervention for the rehabilitation of patients recovering from a myocardial infarction.[27] The first phase (Phase I) occurs while the patient is hospitalized for a coronary event, and consists of early mobilization as soon as his clinical condition allows. The patient is then discharged with a set of instructions about type and intensity of activities to perform post-discharge. About one or two weeks thereafter, the second phase of CR (Phase II) is initiated and usually lasts for about six to eight weeks. Phase II emphasizes supervised exercise training. Finally, the third phase (Phase III), corresponds to unsupervised long-term exercise.[28]

Thereafter, cardiac rehabilitation was expanded into a comprehensive risk-reduction program. Blood pressure control, lipid reduction, smoking cessation, and healthy lifestyle behavior goals were integrated with exercise training as synergistic priorities.[29] Efficacy of cardiac rehabilitation as a comprehensive risk-reduction program was substantiated by two meta-analyses by O'Connor[30] and Oldridge[3] that demonstrated significant mortality benefits. These two meta-analyses served as the foundation for the clinical practice guideline for cardiac rehabilitation published by the Agency for Health Care Policy and Research (AHCPR) and the National Heart, Lung, and Blood Institute (NHLBI) in 1995.[31] Defined as comprehensive and customized to individual patients, CR services were described as a multifactorial set of interventions including exercise training, education, counseling, and behavioral interventions. This guideline became a milestone in the field of cardiac rehabilitation and was subsequently endorsed by the major cardiovascular professional associations.[32–35]

However, despite such formal changes, a great deal of programmatic heterogeneity has persisted. Many cardiac rehabilitation programs continue to emphasize primarily exercise training and receive referrals for adults who are predominantly deconditioned and frail. Other programs have morphed into risk-reduction programs and abandoned exercise training entirely, such that referral is more oriented to lipid lowering, weight loss, and medication compliance, with no exercise interventions. In the latter type of cardiac rehabilitation programs, many patients are referred primarily for education and behavioral reinforcement, and typical patients are relatively more robust and active at the onset.

Even more complicating, over the years since cardiac rehabilitation was established as a therapeutic tool for infirm myocardial infarction and cardiac surgery patients, therapy and techniques have markedly improved. Myocardial infarction patients are now routinely managed with emergent revascularization along with beta-blockers, aspirin, heparin, and other modalities that improve mortality and morbidity rates. Likewise, bypass surgery yields superior outcomes due to improved surgical techniques (e.g., smaller incisions, reduced blood loss, shorter hospitalizations, better adjunct therapy). In the context of these comprehensive improvements, it has become much more difficult to delineate morality benefits from cardiac rehabilitation thereafter.

Given all these dynamics, many third-party reimbursers have moved to eliminate or severely curtail disbursements for cardiac rehabilitation. Consistently, hospitals have moved to cut or shrink programs that are notoriously expensive (i.e., high overhead for exercise-training staff, medical supervision, equipment, and space). Today, one finds considerable regional heterogeneity and widespread uncertainty regarding the priority and application of cardiac rehabilitation.

Shifting Emphasis Within the World of Cardiac Rehabilitation

According to official guidelines, contemporary cardiac rehabilitation constitutes a comprehensive risk-reduction program. Blood pressure control, lipid reduction, smoking cessation, and healthy lifestyle behavior goals are coupled with exercise training goals as synergistic priorities.[35] Behavior modification goals are also prioritized as critical components to achieving long-term adherence to healthy life changes. In general, third-party payments for cardiac rehabilitation are restricted to secondary prevention for CHD or valvular heart disease; i.e., for those who have already endured a myocardial infarction, revascularization (percutaneous intervention or surgery), valve repair, or who have known CHD (based on a stress test). It remains particularly controversial that cardiac rehabilitation as primary prevention is not usually subsidized for those with multiple risk factors, including those with CHD equivalents (e.g., diabetes), but who have not been diagnosed with CHD. To the consternation of many, cardiac rehabilitation is also not subsidized for heart failure. Whereas older adults would clearly benefit from broadened eligibility for cardiac rehabilitation funding, specifically because age constitutes such a powerful promoter and predictor of CVD, in fact third-party disbursements are getting smaller, shorter, and often harder to attain.

In the midst of such financial tumult surrounding cardiac rehabilitation, the scientific/clinical rationale to promote cardiac rehabilitation as an ideal risk-factor-modification opportunity has been reinforced by evolving insights in the area of CV biology. Whereas clinicians were once riveted on a plumbing paradigm of cardiovascular management (revascularizing patients was the foremost endpoint for CHD), today there is more focus on overall vascular health. Diminished systemic inflammation, weight moderation, and sustained healthy life habits have all been demonstrated to achieve improved endothelial performance and healthful perfusion dynamics[36] to improve cardiovascular health as well as functional capacity, cognition, and a host of other advantages.

Cardiac rehabilitation provides a means to organize and guide risk-modification priorities. Moreover, such benefits not only apply to enfeebled myocardial infarction patients and bypass surgery patients, but also to a much broader population of CHD patients who may be more robust. Likewise, patients with peripheral arterial disease, heart failure, neurovascular events, and even patients with risk factors who have not yet had a specific cardiac event or formal diagnosis would also benefit, particularly because age adds to intrinsic vulnerability.

Such broad rationale for cardiac rehabilitation has contributed to a sense of financial tension and debate. Medicare and third-party payers have been reluctant to shoulder the costs for the broader base of patients who would be likely to benefit from cardiac rehabilitation. Hospitals have also been reluctant to allocate resources for expansive programming for all the patient candidates who would probably benefit from cardiac rehabilitation, especially given the uncertainties of third-party payers' reimbursements. Therefore, many regard cardiac rehabilitation as underemphasized for the expanding population of older adults, despite strong rationales for its application.

Amidst all these evolving insights, it seems quite remarkable that a 2005 American Heart Associaton (AHA) Scientific statement on cardiac rehabilitation emphasized only the exercise benefits of cardiac rehabilitation for elderly cardiac patients. "Elderly coronary patients have exercise trainability comparable to that of younger patients participating in similar exercise rehabilitation. ... Elderly patients of both genders should be strongly encouraged to participate in exercise-based cardiac rehabilitation," wrote its authors.[33] This important AHA positon paper on CR refers only to the merits of cardiac rehabilitation in terms of exercise training, but not as composite risk-modification. One might just as easily infer that a walking club, low-intensity aerobics, or other exercise-training programs could afford benefits as good as or better than cardiac rehabilitation, with perhaps even greater convenience and economy. Moreover, the inherent challenges of changing behavior, particularly among the elderly, is not emphasized, especially amidst the apprehensions created by exercise training in those of advanced age. Most important, comprehensive risk-reduction goals (lowering blood pressure, reducing cholesterol, and modifying lifestyle) in relation to advanced age are implicitly diminished in this CPC document.

Cardiac Rehabilitation and Survival

Many continue to assert that survival benefits are the most important endpoint in evaluating CR, and this result remains particularly hard to prove in reference to those who are elderly. To date, there have been five published meta-analyses of randomized control trials that focused on the survival benefits of CR. These have shown reductions in all-causes mortality ranging from 15% to 28%.[3, 30, 37–39] The first two meta-analyses, with 4347 and 4554 randomized patients, respectively, found a reduction in mortality rates of about 25% in a three-year follow-up after a myocardial infarction among middle-aged, low-risk men.[3, 30] The third meta-analysis, carried out by Jolliffe et al., included 7683 randomized patients (about 4000 additional patients from prior meta-analyses), and compared exercise-only CR programs with comprehensive, multi-factor programs. The analysis found reductions in all-causes mortality of 27% (OR 0.73, $p<0.05$) and 13% (OR 0.87, not significant), respectively. Both programs, however, showed reduction in cardiac-specific mortality rates of 31% (OR 0.69, $p<0.05$) in exercise-only programs, and 26% ($p<0.05$) in multi-factorial programs.[32, 38]

The two most recent meta-analyses, led by Taylor and Clark,[37, 39] included 8940 patients (from 48 trials) and 21,295 patients (from 63 trials), respectively, with a large share of randomized controlled trials (RCTs) performed since 1990. Taylor et al.'s analysis found reductions in all-causes mortality of 20% (OR 0.80, 95% CI: 0.68 to 0.93) and cardiac mortality of 26% (OR 0.74, 95% CI: 0.61 to 0.96).[39] Clark et al.'s analysis found that secondary prevention programs were associated with a reduction in all-causes mortality of 15% (RR 0.85, $p = 0.001$). Exercise-alone programs were associated with a reduction in all-causes mortality of 28% (RR 0.72, $p = 0.02$).[37]

Notably, the RCTs included in these meta-analyses had few or no women, racial/ethnic minorities, or individuals 65 years of age or older. Only two of 22 studies included in the two most cited meta-analyses on CR have included people over 65 years old, and no studies have been published on people over 70 years old.[3, 30] In addition, most studies excluded high-risk patients with severe congestive heart failure or cardiac arrhythmias. Therefore, extrapolations of CR benefits derived from RCTs to older populations or high-risk patients still need confirmation.

Specific Data on Cardiac Rehabilitation as a Composite Program in the Elderly

Most of the existing studies on cardiac rehabilitation are observational, primarily reporting that patients enrolled in secondary prevention programs derive significant improvements in exercise capacity.[40–42] In a 2001 review of 18 elderly-specific studies of CR consisting of 15 observational case series without control groups, two observational with control groups, and only one randomized controlled trial, Pasquali et al. identified the lack of robust data regarding cardiac rehabilitation in older adults and criticized the few elderly-specific trials for being predominantly observational (non-randomized) with only one including a non-exercise control group.[43] They asserted that the true benefits of cardiac rehabilitation cannot be determined without randomization, and that there is selection bias in studying only those referred to cardiac rehabilitation. Furthermore, while the studies ostensibly compared outcomes in young and old, the investigators did not account for baseline differences in clinical characteristics, diagnoses, or functional capacities, which may have further confounded the results. Nonetheless, they acknowledged that the studies showed consistent improvements in exercise capacity and quality of life, reduction in depression, universal safety, and modest improvements in lipids.[43]

Lavie et al. demonstrated improvements in exercise capacity, obesity indices, and lipids among older (age >65 years, mean 70) adults and indicated that the benefits are similar to those achieved in a younger cohort.[44] In a similar study, Lavie demonstrated improved HDL cholesterol, LDL/HDL ratio, body mass index, percent of fat, and exercise tolerance among older (age >65 years) cardiac rehabilitation participants.[41] In the second study, questionnaires were also used to show improvements in anxiety, depression, mental health, energy, general health, pain, function, well-being, and quality of life among the cardiac rehabilitation enrollees.

More recently, Lavie completed another study showing modest improvements in lipids, with marked improvements in exercise capacity, behavioral parameters, and quality of life among even older adults (age >75 years) who completed cardiac rehabilitation.[42] Balady et al. also showed improved exercise tolerance among patients enrolled in cardiac rehabilitation, including those aged over 75 years, and particularly among those with an initial peak metabolic equivalent (MET) level of less than five,[45] corresponding to severely reduced exercise capacity at the onset of the program.

In one of the only randomized controlled trials, Stahle et al.[46] analyzed adults aged over 65 years. Exercise tolerance, quality of life, physical activity, and fitness improved among those enrolled in cardiac rehabilitation compared with a control population.

Physiological Rationale for Cardiac Rehabilitation in the Elderly

A key appeal of cardiac rehabilitation for older adults is the fact it affords an individualized and comprehensive approach for vulnerable patients. This corresponds to the medical complexities inherent in age, the behavioral challenges in instilling new life patterns, and the potential for careful coordination with the primary care physicians. Issues of exercise training can be addressed with the almost inevitable likelihood that patients are dealing with hypertension, cholesterol, smoking, and diabetes as well as rhythm disorders, heart failure, and non-cardiac comorbidities (COPD, arthritis, incontinence). Likewise, complex factors like weight loss, compliance, safety, sleep, nutrition, and adherence can all be addressed in a comprehensive strategy.

Unfortunately, the valuation of such a program is not necessarily measured optimally by mortality endpoints, and it has also been relatively impossible to perform a randomized controlled trial to assess mortality in relation to old age. However, there have still been series of trials showing benefits of the components within a comprehensive cardiac rehabilitation in relation to older adults.

Exercise

Multiple training studies demonstrate the utility of aerobic and strength training to modify patterns of age-related decline with increased aerobic capacity and associated functional gains.[47–49] Physiological benefits include improved central cardiovascular performance (including improved diastolic filling and afterload reduction), improved peripheral vasomotor responsiveness (and perfusion), and improved metabolism, including improved glucose metabolism and other physiological benefits.[45, 50]

Exercise training among elderly cardiac patients is especially valuable in facilitating improved functional indices, with several studies highlighting increases in anaerobic thresholds and exercise tolerance.[51–53] Such benefits are particularly germane for a population that is notoriously prone to sedentary behaviors and deconditioning. Older adults are also particularly susceptible to heart failure (HF), a disease that is particularly likely to erode functional capacity due to its effects on the heart as well as peripheral muscle and vascular perfusion. While exercise training was once viewed as inadvisable among adults with impaired systolic function, a multitude of trials now indicate that low-intensity exercise training is well tolerated among HF patients and is associated with important functional gains,[54–57] despite relatively fixed cardiac output.

Recent investigations also emphasize the benefits of strength training in adults of all ages, including elders aged through their 90s.[58] In fact, strength training may exceptionally benefit older adults since it more directly helps allay customary age-related patterns of muscle wasting (sarcopenia)[59] and associated susceptibility to weakening and frailty. Multiple studies demonstrate the safety of strength training among cardiac patients and its value to stimulating muscle mass, endurance, and strength. In fact, cardiac rehabilitation guidelines[35] now recommend strength training as an elemental component in a combined aerobic–strength training regimen.

Hypertension

Systolic hypertension is common among elders, in large part due to the natural stiffening of vessels. Several large studies, including the Systolic Hypertension in the Elderly Program (SHEP),[60] the Systolic Hypertension in Europe Study (Syst-Eur),[61] and most recently, Hypertension in the Very Elderly (HYVET)[62] have consistently demonstrated that antihypertensive pharmacological therapy for older hypertensive patients reduces the risk of stroke, coronary heart disease events, and cardiovascular causes of deaths.[63] SHEP demonstrated that a diuretic regimen among patients aged over 60 years reduced stroke by 36%, and there was an overall 32% reduction of cardiovascular events.[60] Syst-Eur demonstrated that a calcium channel-blocker regimen reduced stroke by 42% and reduced all cardiovascular events by 31%.[61] Using primarily a diuretic, HYVET achieved a 30% reduction in fatal or nonfatal stroke, 39% reduction in deaths from stroke, 21% reduction in deaths from any cause, and 23% reduction in deaths from cardiovascular causes in a population aged 84+3 yrs. Antihypertensive therapy also exhibits a strong benefit in preventing incidental heart failure[64] as well as dementia.[65]

Among its many attributes, cardiac rehabilitation affords a unique opportunity to monitor blood pressure at rest and with exertion, and to titrate vital antihypertensive therapy. It also facilitates close hemodynamic and electrolyte monitoring, of key value since elderly hypertensives are also prone to orthostatic hypotension and electrolyte imbalances.[66] Cardiac rehabilitation also provides an opportunity to assess and modify lifestyle contributors to hypertension. Salt sensitivity increases in stiff senescent vasculature, and for most elders this becomes a liability when they are enticed by restaurants and processed foods that are overloaded with salt. Recently, the Trial of Nonpharmacological Interventions in the Elderly (TONE) Study[67] showed that rigorous sodium restriction (i.e., limiting sodium intake to 80 mEq/day, or 1.8 g of sodium/day) and weight reduction (by about 3.5–4.5 kg over 9 months) eliminated both recurrent hypertension and medication use in 44% of obese elderly patients, compared with 16% of the control population at 30 months. Cardiac rehabilitation provides a structure for education and reinforcement as lifestyle changes are nurtured.

Cardiac rehabilitation also provides opportunities to discover and begin to modify other lifestyle factors that often exacerbate hypertension among older adults. Alcohol use also can worsen hypertension, with alcoholism being a common geriatric problem. Likewise, nonsteroidal anti-inflammatory drug (NSAID) renal effects increase the propensity to hypertension,[68, 69] a problem for the many elders who rely on these medications for chronic pain relief. Finally, excess weight and inactivity are other well-known contributors to hypertension. All can be addressed and modified in a cardiac rehabilitation program.

Hypercholesterolemia

The National Cholesterol Education Program Adult Treatment Panel (NCEP ATP) III guidelines consider that, on the basis of age alone, older people should not be denied the benefits of cholesterol-lowering therapy that are offered to other age groups.[70] However, in a retrospective cohort study of 396,077 patients aged ≥66 years with a history of CVD or diabetes, Ko et al. reported that only 19.1% had been prescribed statins.[71] In patients aged 66 to 74 years with low, intermediate, and high baseline risk, the adjusted probabilities of statins' being prescribed were 37.7%, 26.7%, and 23.4%, respectively. Furthermore, for each year of age increase and each 1% increase in the predicted three-year mortality risk, the likelihood of statin prescription decreased by 6.4%.

The benefits of lipid-lowering statin therapy in reducing major coronary events have been demonstrated in a range of pivotal clinical trials in both primary and secondary prevention settings, and in high-risk patients. One pivotal trial, the PROspective Study of Pravastatin in the Elderly at Risk (PROSPER) specifically studied older adults (ages 70 to 82 years).[72] A total of 5804 individuals (mean age 75 years) with a history of, or risk factors for, vascular disease were randomized to receive pravastatin 40 mg/day or placebo. The mean follow-up for individuals who did not die or withdraw consent was 3.2 years. Compared with placebo, pravastatin reduced risk of coronary death, nonfatal MI, and/or stroke by 15% (P = 0.014), the risk of CHD death by 24% (P = 0.043), and the risk of coronary events by 19% (P = 0.006).

Subgroup analyses of clinical trials that have recruited subjects from broader age ranges have also demonstrated that statin therapy produces benefits for older adults. The Heart Protection Study (HPS) enrolled 20,536 subjects aged 40 to 80 years, of whom 5806 were ≥70 years old.[73] Trial participants had coronary disease, occlusive disease of non-coronary arteries, diabetes, or (if they were male and aged ≤65 years) treated hypertension—factors considered to constitute a substantial risk of death from CHD within five years. Subjects were randomized to receive simvastatin 40 mg/day or placebo. The mean duration of follow-up was five years, and the statin treatment produced a 24% reduction in the rates of nonfatal MI or coronary death, nonfatal or fatal stroke, and coronary or non-coronary revascularization, compared with placebo (P<0.0001). The authors reported that, allowing for non-adherence, use of this statin regimen for five years in the types of high-risk individuals studied should prevent between 70 and 100 people per 1000 from experiencing at least one of these major vascular events. The reduction in the event rate arising from statin treatment was similar and significant in various subcategories of participants, including those with baseline LDL-C <3.0 mmol/L (116 mg/dL), men, women, patients aged <70 years, and patients aged ≥70 years.

Similar benefits are consistently demonstrated in other major statin trials. The Scandinavian Simvastatin Survival Study (4S) enrolled 4444 patients with CHD, including 1021 patients aged ≥65 years.[74] A post-hoc analysis showed that, in this subgroup of older patients, simvastatin treatment conferred a 34% reduction in the risk of death (P = 0.009), compared with placebo, which was attributable to a 43% reduction in the risk of CHD mortality (P = 0.003) and a 34% risk reduction in major coronary events (P <0.001).

In the Treating to New Targets (TNT) trial, 10,001 patients who had clinically evident CHD and LDL-C <3.4 mmol/L (130 mg/dL) were randomized to receive atorvastatin 10 or 80 mg/day.[75, 76] A post-hoc analysis of patients aged ≥65 years (n = 3809) indicated that the intensive lipid-lowering regimen produced significant reductions in the relative risk for major cardiovascular events compared with the alternative, less intensive treatment (decrease of 19%; P = 0.03).[75, 76]

These clinical data are concordant with biological insights that have shifted from viewing cholesterol as a material that primarily clogs vessels, to a vascular constituent that affects endothelial function.[77] Low-density lipoproteins, especially when oxidized, promote endothelial dysfunction, in part due to the reduced availability of nitric oxide. Vasoconstriction, monocyte and platelet adhesion, thrombogenesis, and cytokine and growth factor stimulation are all effects of hypercholesterolemia, even amidst non-obstructive lesions.

In context of these insights, cardiac rehabilitation provides an excellent opportunity to emphasize and refine cholesterol reduction and to reinforce compliance with vital pharmacological adjuncts. Benefits for the elderly are not only likely to include reduced myocardial infarctions, heart failure, angina, strokes, and claudication, but may even include improved cognition and functional capacity. Given the notorious difficulty in achieving statin compliance even among younger adults, cardiac rehabilitation is particularly valuable for elderly candidates, especially since dietary modification is usually inherently complex. Low-cholesterol goals often must be coupled to low-salt and low-sugar diets. Moreover, a propensity to depression (especially after a cardiac event or surgery) often leads many clinicians to deemphasize dietary restrictions. Cardiac rehabilitation provides a better context to address these issues comprehensively and best clarify and reinforce eating and other lifestyle goals.

Smoking

While the prevalence of smoking declines with age, in part due to smoking cessation and in part due to earlier mortality among the smoking population, risks associated with smoking persist. In the Established Populations for Epidemiologic Studies of the Elderly (EPESE), 7178 persons 65 years of age or older were studied.[78] Current smoking was associated with a relative risk for cardiovascular death of 2.0 in men and 1.6 in women, independent of other risk factors. Adverse effect of smoking on mortality was greatest in men and women aged 65 to 74 years, but smoking was still associated with a survival disadvantage in seniors over 75 years. Similarly, a study of 316,099 men screened in the Multiple Risk Factor Intervention Trial (MRFIT) Research Group lead to the conclusion that the number of cigarettes per day is a significant predictor of CHD death in all age groups.[79] Therefore, smoking cessation is highly beneficial, even among adults aged ≥70 years.

Diabetes Mellitus

Prevalence of diabetes increases with age, approaching 20% in persons over 65 years of age, and relatively more common among men, and in African-Americans and Hispanics.[80] Sedentary lifestyles and increased body fat are both common with aging, and add to the predisposition of the elderly to diabetes. Diabetes is particularly worrisome in that the risks for and from resultant cardiovascular events are especially high in elderly. Framingham's data showed that the relative risk for coronary heart disease in diabetics over age 65 was 1.4 in men and 2.1 in women.[81] Furthermore, CHD risk increases with the duration of diabetes; i.e., generating increasing risk over time among the elderly.

The American Diabetes Association's clinical practice recommendations do not distinguish between younger and older patients.[82] Current recommendations stress the importance of diet (i.e., effective glucose control), exercise, and aggressive control of other cardiovascular risk factors, including hypercaloric intake in those who are overweight. Cardiac rehabilitation is well suited to all these objectives.

ACE inhibitors among diabetics are also strongly advised. HOPE (Heart Outcomes Prevention Evaluation) was a prospective study of 3577 diabetics over age 55 with vascular disease or at least one other cardiovascular risk factor who were randomized to ramipril 10 mg/day or placebo and followed for an average of 4.5 years.[83] Ramipril therapy was associated with a 26% reduction in a composite endpoint of cardiovascular death, nonfatal MI, or nonfatal stroke ($p = .0004$). Total mortality was reduced by 25%.

Cognition

Exercise in healthy older adults has been long been recognized to provide neurocognitive benefits, including improvements in both neuropsychological tests and key brain MRI indices.[84, 85] A study by Gunstad et al. demonstrated that exercise improves cognitive function in a heterogenous group of older cardiac patients, including improvements in psychomotor speed.[86] The potential of cardiac rehabilitation to induce cognitive improvements through exercise as well as enhanced medication supervision and lifestyle enhancements (e.g., diet, social interaction) constitutes a major potential benefit.

Projects are now under way to clarify specific mechanism(s) for these cognitive changes. In part, exercise-related enhancements of cardiac and vascular performance help improve neurocognitive capacity.[87] Exercise-related enhancement of autonomic nervous system (ANS) function also is important.[88]

Implications of neurocognitive decline are substantial. Older HF patients with cognitive impairment suffer a five-fold greater risk of mortality and a sixfold risk of functional impairment on the basis of cognition.[89–91] These risks have been attributed to reduced medication compliance as well as to intrinsic constitutional declines associated with cognitive impairments.[92]

Ironically, many cardiac rehabilitation programs regard dementia as a criterion for which referrals are declined, although many neurocognitively challenged patients may benefit from their participation. Furthermore, cardiac rehabilitation provides the opportunity to refine educational and behavior-modifying strategies to a format and style that respond to the needs of a population that is likely to be suffering with vascular and cardiac-mediated cognitive deficits.

Predictors of Cardiac Rehabilitation Participation

A review of the most important factors predicting participation in CR programs includes: age (less frequent referral of relatively older adults), gender (less frequent referral of females), race/ethnicity (less frequent referral of minorities), social deprivation (less frequent referral of those in lower socioeconomic strata), distance from the program (the longer the distance, the less likely a referral), and recommendation or referral from physicians.[93] Furthermore, even among those who begin a program, attrition is high. Carlson demonstrates high withdrawal[94] with attrition correlating to duration of participation (the longer participants were enrolled, the more likely they were to miss sessions or drop out.)[95] Depression also correlates to higher attrition from cardiac rehabilitation programs.[96] Paradoxically, increased coronary risk factors have also been correlated to higher cardiac rehabilitation attrition,[95] and higher risk in general among those with issues for which cardiac rehabilitation provides disproportionate benefit.[97]

Elderly patients are less often referred to, or participate in, CR programs than younger coronary patients.[32] However, the Behavioral Risk Factor Surveillance System Survey (BRFSS) in 2001 suggests that participation rates have modestly improved among the elderly since 1990. Twenty-nine percent of the people aged 65 to 79 and 22% of those aged 80 and older reported participation in CR after a myocardial infarction.[98] In 2005, based on a similar survey, about 37% of patients aged 65 and above participated in CR following a myocardial infarction.

A recent study analyzed CR use rates and predictors of use in a cohort of over 265,000 elderly Medicare beneficiaries after a hospitalization for a major coronary event. Only one in seven patients (13.9%) discharged from an acute myocardial infarction, and one in three patients (31%) who underwent coronary artery bypass graft surgery, received Phase II CR in 1997.[4] Whites, males, and younger patients were more likely both to receive CR and to have more CR sessions than non-whites, females, and older patients. Distance was also an important predictor of CR use—patients who lived closer to a CR facility were more likely to participate in CR than those living further away. Higher socioeconomic zip codes were also independent predictors of CR use. The number and type of comorbid conditions were additional predictors of participation in CR. For example, CR users had, on average, fewer comorbidities than non-users (2.1 versus 2.7), and patients with congestive heart failure, previous stroke history, diabetes mellitus, or chronic pulmonary disease were less likely to receive CR than coronary patients without these comorbid conditions.[4]

Future of Cardiac Rehabilitation in the Elderly

Given the escalating growth of the elderly population, and given the broadening understanding of how physiological changes of age exacerbate risks of cardiovascular disease, functional decline, and even cognition, incentives to enroll in cardiac rehabilitation are likely to rise. Cooper et al.[99] demonstrated the impact of patients' perceptions on their willingness to enroll in cardiac rehabilitation. As adults become more aware of the benefits of this preventive therapeutic program, they will probably be inclined to demand it. Similarly, while many now decry under-referral of women to cardiac rehabilitation,[100, 101] this will probably change as expectations among female patients evolve.

Summary

While cardiac rehabilitation originated primarily as a mechanism to mobilize patients after a myocardial infarction, it then evolved into a multifaceted risk-reduction program targeting predominantly middle-aged male cardiac patients. While some important research demonstrates that cardiac rehabilitation programs benefit the elderly, there is still no mandate to refer patients systematically for comprehensive exercise training and risk reduction. In contrast, today's growing insights into the mechanisms of disease and aging suggest that cardiac rehabilitation may be particularly germane to older men and women with specific biological and clinical implications. Critical research is needed to delineate the physiological effects and related clinical efficacy of a multifaceted risk-reduction program among older adults. Such inquiry will not only provide a stronger rationale for both patients and their doctors to consider this therapy, but will also facilitate refinements to best achieve the full potential of cardiac rehabilitation training, lifestyle, and pharmacological synergy.

It seems likely that cardiac rehabilitation constitutes a key opportunity to achieve cost-effective health care and a high quality of life for our elderly patients. Therefore, it is imperative that we explore strategies to increase the elderly patients' participation in CR. Examples of such strategies include: implementing performance measures based on referral to and delivery of CR;[102, 103] extending the use of pay-for-performance[104] or value-based purchasing incentives to CR referral or delivery; and assessing the resource costs and reimbursement rates associated with the delivery of CR to facilitate discussions about incentives for their use.[105]

Notes

1. Ades PA, Waldmann ML, Gillespie C. A controlled trial of exercise training in older coronary patients. *J Gerontol A Biol Sci Med Sci.* 1995;50A:M7–11.
2. Franklin BA, Hall L, Timmis GC. Contemporary cardiac rehabilitation services [editorial]. *Am J Cardiol.* 1997;79:1075–1077.
3. Oldridge NB, Guyatt GH, Fischer ME, Rimm AA. Cardiac rehabilitation after myocardial infarction. Combined experience of randomized clinical trials. *JAMA.* 1988;260:945–950.
4. Suaya JA, Shepard DS, Normand ST, Ades PA, Prottas J, Stason WB. Use of cardiac rehabilitation by Medicare beneficiaries after myocardial infarction or coronary bypass surgery. *Circulation.* 2007;116(15):1653–1662.
5. Centers for Disease Control and Prevention. Receipt of outpatient cardiac rehabilitation among heart attack survivors—United States, 2005. *MMWR.* 2008;57(04):89–84.
6. Lakatta EG, Levy D. Arterial and cardiac aging: Major shareholders in cardiovascular disease enterprises. Part II: The aging heart in health: Links to heart disease. *Circulation.* 2003;107(2):346–354.
7. Wei JY. Age and the cardiovascular system [*see comments*]. *N Engl J Med.* 1992;327: 1735–1739.
8. Arias E. United States life tables, 2004. *National vital statistics reports.* 2007;56(9):8–9.
9. Population Division, Population Projections Branch, U.S. Census Bureau. National Population Projections. Link: http://www.census.gov/population/www/projections/summarytables.html. Accessed on October 13, 2008.
10. Pleis JR, Lethbridge-Cejku M. Summary health statistics for U.S. adults: National Health Interview Survey, 2006. *Vital Health Stat.* 2007;10(235):1–153.
11. Duscha BD, Schulze P, Robbins JL, Forman DE. Implications of chronic heart failure on peripheral vascular and skeletal muscle before and after exercise training. *Heart Fail Rev.* 2008;13:21–37.
12. Hoth KF, Tate DF, Poppas A, et al. Endothelial function and white matter hyperintensities in older adults with cardiovascular disease. *Stroke.* 2007;38:308–312.
13. Chantler PD, Lakatta E.G., Najjar SS. Arterial-ventricular coupling: Mechanistic insights into cardiovascular performance at rest and during exercise. *J Appl Physiol.* 2008;105(4): 1342–1351.
14. Gerhard M, Roddy MA, Creager SJ, Creager MA. Aging progressively impairs endothelium-dependent vasodilation in forearm resistance vessels of humans. *Hypertension.* 1996;27: 849–853.
15. Versari D, Daghini E, Virdis A, Ghiadoni L, Taddei S. The aging endothelium, cardiovascular risk and disease. *Exp Physiol.* Sept. 19, 2008.
16. Edo MD, Andrés V. Aging, telomeres, and atherosclerosis. *Cardiovasc Res.* 2005;66(2): 213–221.
17. Libby P. Atherosclerosis: Disease biology affecting the coronary vasculature. *Am J Cardiol.* 2006;98(12A):3Q-9Q.
18. Kitzman DW, Daniel KR. Diastolic heart failure in the elderly. *Clin Geriatr Med.* 2007;(1): 83–106.

19. Jefferson AL, Poppas A, Paul RH, Cohen RA. Systemic hypoperfusion is associated with executive dysfunction in geriatric cardiac patients. *Neurobiol Aging.* 2007;28(3):477–483.
20. Arbab-Zadeh A, Dijk E, Prasad A, et al. Effect of aging and physical activity on left ventricular compliance. *Circulation.* 2004;110(13):1799–1805.
21. DeSouza CA, Shapiro LF, Clevenger CM, et al. Regular aerobic exercise prevents and restores age-related declines in endothelium-dependent vasodilation in healthy men. *Circulation.* 2000;102(12):1351–1357.
22. Franzoni F, Ghiadoni L, Galetta F, et al. Physical activity, plasma antioxidant capacity, and endothelium-dependent vasodilation in young and older men. *Am J Hypertens.* 2005;4(1): 510–516.
23. Tousoulis D, Antoniades C, Koumallos N, et al. Novel therapies targeting vascular endothelium *Endothelium.* 2006;13(6):411–421.
24. Brummer P, Linko E, Kasanen A. Myocardial infarction treated by early ambulation. *Am Heart J.* 1956;52:269–272.
25. Newman L, Andrews M, Koblish M. Physical medicine and rehabilitation in acute myocardial infarction. *Arch Intern Med.* 1952;89:552–561.
26. Pashkow FJ. Issues in contemporary cardiac rehabilitation: A historical perspective. *J Am Coll Cardiol.* 1993;21:822–834.
27. Bethell H. Cardiac rehabilitation: From Hellerstein to the millennium. *Int J Clin Pract.* 2000;54(2):92–97.
28. American Association of Cardiovascular and Pulmonary Rehabilitation. *Guidelines for cardiac rehabilitation and secondary prevention programs. Rehabilitation.* Champaign, IL: Human Kinetics, 2004.
29. Ades PA, Balady GJ, Berra K. Transforming exercise-based cardiac rehabilitation programs into secondary prevention centers: A national imperative. *J Cardiopulm Rehabil Prev.* 2001;21(5):263–272.
30. O'Connor GT, Buring JE, Yusuf S, et al. An overview of randomized trials of rehabilitation with exercise after myocardial infarction. *Circulation.* 1989;80:234–244.
31. Wenger N, Froelicher E, Smith L, et al. *Cardiac rehabilitation as secondary prevention. Clinical practice guideline, No. 17.* Rockville, MD: U.S. Department of Health and Human Services, Public Health Service, Agency for Health Care Policy and Research and National Heart, Lung, and Blood Institute, October 1995. AHCPR Pub. No. 96–0673.
32. Thompson P, Buchner D, Pina I, et al. Exercise and physical activity in the prevention and treatment of atherosclerotic cardiovascular disease: A statement from the Council on Clinical Cardiology (Subcommittee on Exercise, Rehabilitation, and Prevention) and the Council on Nutrition, Physical Activity, and Metabolism (Subcommittee on Physical Activity). American Heart Association. *Circulation.* 2003;107(24):3109–3116.
33. Leon A, Franklin B, Costa F, et al. Cardiac rehabilitation and secondary prevention of coronary heart disease: An American Heart Association scientific statement from the Council on Clinical Cardiology (Subcommittee on Exercise, Cardiac Rehabilitation, and Prevention) and the Council on Nutrition, Physical Activity, and Metabolism (Subcommittee on Physical Activity), in collaboration with the American Association of Cardiovascular and Pulmonary Rehabilitation. *Circulation.* 2005;111(3):369–376.
34. Smith S, Jr., Allen J, Blair S, et al. AHA/ACC guidelines for secondary prevention for patients with coronary and other atherosclerotic vascular disease: 2006 update: endorsed by the National Heart, Lung, and Blood Institute. *Circulation.* 2006;113(19):2363–2372.
35. Balady GJ, Williams MA, Ades PA, et al. Core components of cardiac rehabilitation/secondary prevention programs: 2007 update: a scientific statement from the American Heart Association Exercise, Cardiac Rehabilitation, and Prevention Committee, the Council on

Clinical Cardiology; the Councils on Cardiovascular Nursing, Epidemiology and Prevention, and Nutrition, Physical Activity, and Metabolism; and the American Association of Cardiovascular and Pulmonary Rehabilitation. *[Journal Article. Practice Guideline] J Cardiopulm Rehabil Prev.* 2007;27(3):121–129.

36. Tousoulis D, Antoniades C, Koumallos N, et al. Novel therapies targeting vascular endothelium. *Endothelium.* 2006;13(6):411–421.
37. Clark A, Hartling L, Vandermeer B, McAlister F. Meta-analysis: Secondary prevention programs for patients with coronary artery disease. *AnnIntern Med.* 2005;143:659–672.
38. Jolliffe J, Rees K, Taylor R, Thompson D, Oldridge N, Ebrahim S. Exercise-based rehabilitation for coronary heart disease (Cochrane Review). *Cochrane Database Syst Rev.* 2001;1(CD001800).
39. Taylor R, Brown A, Ebrahim S, et al. Exercise-based rehabilitation for patients with coronary heart disease: Systematic review and meta-analysis of randomized controlled trials. *Am J Med.* 2004;116(10):682–692.
40. Ades PA, Waldmann ML, Meyer WL, et al. Skeletal muscle and cardiovascular adaptations to exercise conditioning in older coronary patients. *Circulation.* 1996;94:323–330.
41. Lavie CJ, Milani RV. Effects of cardiac rehabilitation programs on exercise capacity, coronary risk factors, behavioral characteristics, and quality of life in a large elderly cohort. *Am J Cardiol.* 1995;76:177–179.
42. Lavie CJ, Milani RV. Effects of cardiac rehabilitation and exercise training programs in patients > or = 75 years of age. *Am J Cardiol.* 1996;78:675–677.
43. Pasquali SK, Alexander KP, Petersen ED. Cardiac rehabilitation in the elderly. *Am Heart J.* 2001;142:748–755.
44. Lavie CJ, Milani RV, Littman AB. Benefits of cardiac rehabilitation and exercise training in secondary coronary prevention in the elderly. *J Am Coll Cardiol.* 1993;22:678–683.
45. Balady GJ, Jette D, Scheer J, Downing J. Changes in exercise capacity following cardiac rehabilitation in patients stratified according to age and gender. Results of the Massachusetts Association of Cardiovascular and Pulmonary Rehabilitation Multicenter Database. *J Cardiopulm Rehabil Prev.* 1996;16:38–46.
46. Stahle A, Mattsson E, Ryden L, Unden A, Nordlander R. Improved physical fitness and quality of life following training of elderly patients after acute coronary events. A 1-year follow-up randomized controlled study. *Eur Heart J.* 1999;20:1475–1484.
47. Brechue WF, Pollock ML. Exercise training for coronary artery disease in the elderly. *Clin Geriatr Med.* 1996;12:207–229.
48. Fleg JL. Exercise therapy for elderly heart failure patients. *Heart Fail Clin.* 2007;3(4): 529–537.
49. Capodaglio P, Capodaglio E, Facioli M, Saibene F. Long-term strength training for community-dwelling people over 75: Impact on muscle function, functional ability and life style. *Eur J Appl Physiol.* 2007;100(5):535–542.
50. Schulman SP, Fleg JL, Goldberg AP, et al. Continuum of cardiovascular performance across a broad range of fitness levels in healthy older men. *Circulation.* 1996;94(3):359–367.
51. Coyle EF, Martin WH, Ehsani AA, et al. Blood lactate threshold in some well-trained ischemic heart disease patients. *J Appl Physiol.* 1983;54:18–23.
52. Lavie CJ, Milani RV. Effects of cardiac rehabilitation and exercise training on peak aerobic capacity and work efficiency in obese patients with coronary artery disease. *Am J Cardiol.* 1999;83(A7):1477–1480.
53. Yerg JE, Seals DR, Hagberg JM, Holloszy JO. Effect of endurance exercise training on ventilatory function in older individuals. *J Appl Physiol.* 1985;58:791–794.

54. Coats AJ. Exercise training for heart failure: Coming of age [editorial]. *Circulation.* 1999; 99:1138–1140.
55. Balady GJ. Exercise training in the treatment of heart failure: What is achieved and how? *Ann Med.* 1998;30(Suppl 1):61–65.
56. Clark AL, Poole-Wilson PA, Coats AJ. Exercise limitation in chronic heart failure: Central role of the periphery. *J Am Coll Cardiol.* 1996;28:1092–1102.
57. Belardinelli R, Georgiou D, Cianci G, Purcaro A. Randomized, controlled trial of long-term moderate exercise training in chronic heart failure: Effects on functional capacity, quality of life, and clinical outcome [see comments]. *Circulation.* 1999;99:1173–1182.
58. Brochu M, Savage P, Lee M, et al. Effects of resistance training on physical function in older disabled women with coronary heart disease. *J Appl Physiol.* 2002;92(2):672–678.
59. Evans WJ. Reversing sarcopenia: How weight training can build strength and vitality. *Geriatrics.* 1996(51):46–47, 51–43.
60. SHEP: Prevention of stroke by antihypertensive drug treatment in older persons with isolated systolic hypertension. Final results of the Systolic Hypertension in the Elderly Program (SHEP) [see comments]. *JAMA.* 1991; 265:3255–3264.
61. Fagard RH, Staessen JA. Treatment of isolated systolic hypertension in the elderly: The Syst-Eur trial. Systolic Hypertension in Europe (Syst-Eur) trial investigators. *Clin Exp Hypertens.* 1999;21:491–497.
62. Beckett NS, Peters R, Fletcher AE, et al. Treatment of hypertension in patients 80 years of age or older. *N Engl J Med.* 2008;358(18):1887–1898.
63. Ades PA. Cardiac rehabilitation in older coronary patients. *J Am Geriatr Soc.* 1999;47: 98–105.
64. Kostis JB, Davis BR, Cutler J, et al. Prevention of heart failure by antihypertensive drug treatment in older persons with isolated systolic hypertension. SHEP Cooperative Research Group. *JAMA.* 1997;278:212–216.
65. Forette F, Seux ML, Staessen JA, et al. Prevention of dementia in randomised double-blind placebo-controlled Systolic Hypertension in Europe (Syst-Eur) trial [see comments]. *Lancet.* 1998;352:1347–1351.
66. Lipsitz LA. Orthostatic hypotension in the elderly. *N Engl J Med* 1989;321:952–957.
67. Whelton PK, Appel LJ, Espeland MA, et al. Sodium reduction and weight loss in the treatment of hypertension in older persons: A randomized controlled trial of nonpharmacologic interventions in the elderly (TONE). TONE Collaborative Research Group. *JAMA.* 1998;279(11):839–846.
68. Field TS, Gurwitz JH, Glynn RJ, et al. The renal effects of nonsteroidal anti-inflammatory drugs in older people: Findings from the established populations for epidemiological studies of the elderly [see comments]. *J Am Geriatr Soc.* 1999;47:507–511.
69. White WB. Cardiovascular risk, hypertension, and NSAIDs. *Curr Rheumatol Rep.* 2007;9(1):36–43.
70. National Cholesterol Education Program (NCEP) Expert Panel. Third report on detection, evaluation, and treatment of high blood cholesterol in adults (Adult Treatment Panel III). *Circulation.* 2002;106(25):3143–3421.
71. Ko DT, Mamdani M, Alter DA. Lipid-lowering therapy with statins in high-risk elderly patients: The treatment–risk paradox. *JAMA.* 2004;291(15):1864–1870.
72. Shepherd J, Blauw GJ, Murphy MB, et al. Pravastatin in elderly individuals at risk of vascular disease (PROSPER): A randomised controlled trial. *Lancet.* 2002;360(9346):1623–1630.
73. Heart Protection Study Collaborative Group. MRC/BHF Heart Protection Study of cholesterol lowering with simvastatin in 20,536 high-risk individuals: A randomised placebo-controlled trial. *Lancet.* 2002;360(9326):7–22.

74. Miettinen TA, Pyorala K, Olsson AG, et al. Cholesterol-lowering therapy in women and elderly patients with myocardial infarction or angina pectoris: findings from the Scandinavian Simvastatin Survival Study (4S). *Circulation.* 1997;96(12):4211–4218.
75. LaRosa JC, Grundy SM, Waters DD, et al. Intensive lipid lowering with atorvastatin in patients with stable coronary disease. *N Engl J Med.* 2005;352(14):1425–1435.
76. Wenger NK, Lewis SJ, Herrington DM, Bittner V, Welty FK. Treating to New Targets Study Steering Committee and Investigators. Outcomes of using high- or low-dose atorvastatin in patients 65 years of age or older with stable coronary heart disease. *Ann Intern Med.* 2007;147(1):1–9.
77. Ray KK, Cannon CP, Cairns R, et al. PROVE IT-TIMI 22 Investigators: Relationship between uncontrolled risk factors and C-reactive protein levels in patients receiving standard or intensive statin therapy for acute coronary syndromes in the PROVE IT-TIMI 22 trial. *J Am Coll Cardiol.* 2005;46(8):1417–1424.
78. LaCroix AZ, Lang J, Scherr P et al. Smoking and mortality among older men and women in 3 communities. *N Engl J Med.* 1991;(324):1619–1625.
79. Neaton JD, Wentworth D. Serum cholesterol, blood pressure, cigarette smoking, and death from coronary heart disease. Overall findings and differences by age for 316,099 white men. Multiple Risk Factor Intervention Trial Research Group. *Arch Intern Med.* 1992;152(1):56–64.
80. Morley JE. Diabetes and aging: Epidemiologic overview. *Clin Geriatr Med.* 2008;24(3): 395–405.
81. Fox CS, Sulliven L, D'Agostino RB, Wilson PW. The significant effect of diabetes duration on CHD mortality: The Framingham Heart Study. *Diabetes Care.* 2004;27:704–708.
82. American Diabetes Association. 2007 clinical practice recommendations. *Diabetes Care.* 2007;30:S4–S41.
83. Investigators HOPES. Effects of ramipril on cardiovascular and microvascular outcomes in people with diabetes mellitus: Results of the HOPE study and MICRO_HOPE substudy. *Lancet.* 2000;355:253–259.
84. Erickson KI, Kramer AF. Exercise effects on cognitive and neural plasticity in older adults. *Br J Sports Med.* 2008;[Oct. 16, Epub, ahead of print].
85. Colcombe SJ, Erickson KI, Scalf PE, et al. Aerobic exercise training increases brain volume in aging humans. *J Gerontol A Biol Sci Med Sci.* 2006;61(11):1166–1170.
86. Gunstad J, Macgregor KL, Paul RH, et al. Cardiac rehabilitation improves cognitive performance in older adults with cardiovascular disease. *J Cardiopulm Rehabil Prev.* 2005;25(3):173–176.
87. Alagiakrishnan K, McCracken P, Feldman H. Treating vascular risk factors and maintaining vascular health: Is this the way towards successful cognitive aging and preventing cognitive decline? *Postgrad Med J.* 2006;82(964):101–105.
88. Kim DH, Lipsitz LA, Ferrucci L, et al. Association between reduced heart rate variability and cognitive impairment in older disabled women in the community: Women's Health and Aging Study I. *J Am Geriatr Soc.* 2006;54(11):1751–1757.
89. Barclay LL, Weiss EM, Mattis S, Bond O, Blass JP. Unrecognized cognitive impairment in cardiac rehabilitation patients. *J Am Geriatr Soc.* 1988;36(1):22–28.
90. Konstam MA. Progress in heart failure management? Lessons from the real world. *Circulation.* 2000;102(10):1076–1078.
91. Zuccalà G, Pedone C, Cesari M, et al. The effects of cognitive impairment on mortality among hospitalized patients with heart failure. *Am J Med.* 2003;115(2):97–103.
92. Cline CM, Björck-Linné AK, Israelsson BY, Willenheimer RB, Erhardt LR. Noncompliance and knowledge of prescribed medication in elderly patients with heart failure. *Eur J Heart Fail.* 1999;1(2):145–149.

93. Wyer S, Joseph S, Earll L. Predicting attendance at cardiac rehabilitation: A review and recommendations. *Coronary Health Care.* 2001;5(4):171–177.
94. Carlson J, Johnson J, Franklin B, VanderLaan R. Program participation, exercise adherence, cardiovascular outcomes, and program cost of traditional versus modified cardiac rehabilitation. *Am J Cardiol.* 2000;86(1):17–23.
95. Gutin B, Prince L, Stein R. Survey of cardiac rehabilitation centers in New York City. *J Community Health.* Aug 1990;15(4):227–238.
96. Casey E, Hughes JW, Waechter D, Josephson R, Rosneck J. Depression predicts failure to complete Phase-II cardiac rehabilitation. *J Behav Med.* 2008;31(5):421–431.
97. Dorn J, Naughton J, Imamura D, Trevisan M. Correlates of compliance in a randomized exercise trial in myocardial infarction patients. *Med Sci Sports Exerc.* 2001;33(7):1081–1089.
98. Centers for Disease Control and Prevention. Receipt of cardiac rehabilitation services among heart attack survivors—19 states and the District of Columbia, 2001. *MMWR.* 2003;52(44):1072–1075.
99. Cooper A, Lloyd G, Weinman J, Jackson G. Why patients do not attend cardiac rehabilitation: Role of intentions and illness beliefs. *Heart.* 1999;82:234–236.
100. Bonzheim KA, Franklin BA, Carpenter TA, Gordon SE. Cardiac rehabilitation participation: Motivators and barriers unique to women (abstract). *Med Sci Sports Exerc.* 1999;31:S339.
101. Mosca L, Grundy SM, Judelson D, et al. Guide to preventive cardiology for women. AHA/ACC Scientific Statement Consensus panel statement. *Circulation.* 1999;99:2480–2484.
102. Thomas R, Witt B, Lopez-Jimenez F, King M, Squires R. Quality indicators in cardiovascular care: The case for cardiac rehabilitation. *J Cardiopulm Rehabil Prev.* 2005;25(5):249–256.
103. Thomas RJ, King M, Lui K, Oldridge N, Piña IL, Spertus J. AACVPR/ACC/AHA 2007 performance measures on cardiac rehabilitation for referral to and delivery of cardiac rehabilitation/secondary prevention services. *Circulation.* 2007;116(14):1611–1642.
104. Remus D, Fraser I. Guidance for using the AHRQ quality indicators for hospital-level public reporting or payment. Rockville, MD: Department of Health and Human Services, Agency for Healthcare Research and Quality; 2004. AHRQ Pub. No. 04–0086-EF.
105. Office of the Inspector General. Review of Medicare outpatient cardiac rehabilitation provided by hospitals: Department of Health and Human Services. August 2005. A-05–03–00102.

6

DEPRESSION AND HEART DISEASE

CURRENT TREATMENT RECOMMENDATIONS AND FUTURE DIRECTIONS IN MECHANISM RESEARCH

Joel W. Hughes and Elizabeth C. Casey

One of the most prominent topics in behavioral medicine is the relationship between depression and cardiovascular disease.[1–4] Cardiovascular diseases are the leading causes of death in every industrialized nation, and depression is the leading cause of disability in the modern world. Cardiovascular disease and depression co-occur at rates far above chance and appear to be causally related. Depression has become an emerging risk factor for cardiovascular disease, and cardiovascular disease may likewise contribute to the development of depression.[5–8] Depression has been associated with an approximately 65% increase in risk of developing cardiovascular disease among persons initially free from heart disease, as well as a two- to fivefold increased risk of mortality in cardiac patients.[9] Therefore, depression is an important consideration in the clinical management of patients with cardiovascular disease, and care providers should be familiar with assessment and treatment recommendations. Furthermore, the nature of the association between depression and heart disease continues to receive scrutiny, as initial efforts to address this important public health problem have not been particularly successful.

Prevalence and Assessment of Depression in Heart Disease

Cardiac patients have a higher rate of depression than that observed in the general population.[10] For example, 15% to 20% of patients experiencing an acute myocardial infarction will qualify for a diagnosis of major depressive disorder after their heart attacks. In addition, the rate of minor depression, or clinically significant depression symptoms that do not meet the full criteria for major depressive disorder, is also about 15% to 20% among hospitalized cardiac patients. In total, about 30% of cardiac patients exhibit clinically significant depressive symptoms. Although it may seem counterintuitive, depression following an acute cardiac event is not merely attributable to the stress of experiencing a major medical event and its aftermath. For example, about 50% of the individuals enrolled in the Sertraline and Depression Heart Attack Randomized Trial (SADHART) were already depressed prior to their acute cardiac event[11] and a substantial proportion of patients continue to experience depression after they have been treated for and recovered from an acute event.

A recent science advisory from the American Heart Association (and endorsed by the American Psychiatric Association) recommended routine screening of cardiac patients for depression.[12] For screening in primary care and other settings, the Patient Health Questionnaire[13, 14] was recommended. An earlier National Heart, Lung and Blood Institute working group report made a number of recommendations regarding the assessment of depression in research settings.[15] For example, the Beck Depression Inventory[16] was recommended for epidemiological studies, and the Patient Health Questionnaire[14] was recommended to screen for eligibility for clinical trials. Of course, brief self-report measures often result in false positives, and possible cases identified using screening instruments should be verified with additional measures. In the context of a neuropsychological consult, a more comprehensive assessment would certainly be warranted, including a clinical interview yielding a diagnosis. Obviously, the possible effects of depression on neuropsychological test performance must be accounted for, and a thorough assessment should also include consideration of co-morbid problems such as anxiety and social support that may further complicate clinical management of the patient. Patients found to have significant depression should be referred for appropriate treatment, but here the evidential basis becomes more complicated.

Treatment of Depression in Heart Disease

In the 1990s, the evidence and reasoning appeared sound that depression should be treated to reduce cardiovascular risk, and the first step was treating depression in cardiac patients. However, psychotherapy and psychopharmacological treatments have not been shown to reduce mortality or recurrent cardiac events. For example, in the Enhancing Recovery in Coronary Heart Disease (ENRICHD) trial, psychological treatment did not reduce mortality rates[17] Although the Sertraline and Depression Heart Attack Randomized Trial was not designed with adequate statistical power to detect a reduction in mortality[11] sertraline was determined to be safe. The mortality results of the Canadian Cardiac Randomized Evaluation of Antidepressant and Psychotherapy Efficacy (CREATE) trial have not been reported at the time of this writing, but interpersonal psychotherapy for depression was not more effective than clinical management in the treatment of depression among patients with coronary artery disease.[18] Findings like these are disconcerting to behavioral medicine researchers and have been widely discussed. Future efforts to influence cardiovascular risk by treating depression will benefit from these landmark studies, and improved treatment strategies may yet ameliorate depression, improve quality of life, and reduce morbidity and mortality. Current treatment recommendations are also based on findings from these clinical trials, although some treatments that appear promising have not been fully evaluated in randomized studies.

Prominent Clinical Trials

The first large, randomized clinical trial designed to determine whether treating depression would reduce mortality following myocardial infarction (MI) was the ENRICHD trial.[19] The trial enrolled 2481 post-MI patients who were depressed or who reported a low level of perceived social support. Patients were randomized to usual care or individually administered cognitive behavioral therapy that was supplemented by group therapy and pharmacotherapy for patients who failed to adequately respond or who were severely depressed. Although therapy improved depression symptoms, the effect size was not much larger than that observed for the usual care control condition. Psychotherapy did not reduce patients' risk of mortality, although subgroup analyses revealed that Caucasian men may have benefited, and women may have had poorer outcomes in the psychotherapy arm of the trial.[20] On the basis of this trial, researchers concluded that cognitive behavioral therapy is effective for depression and improves quality of life[21] but that these effects are modest, and some cases of depression following MI appear to spontaneously remit (at least partially). A number of other notable findings have been reported from the ENRICHD trial, such as the fact that patients who failed to improve were at higher risk of eventual mortality.[22] Furthermore, self-reported exercise was associated with reduced risk of mortality[23] and the use of SSRI antidepressants was associated with reduced mortality[24] although these findings were not from randomized studies and must be considered suggestive until verified. In a sub-study of ENRICHD with a nondepressed control group, reduced heart rate variability partly explained the relationship between depression and mortality[25] which is strong evidence for involvement of the autonomic nervous system in the relationship between depression and cardiac mortality.

Occurring contemporaneously with the ENRICHD trial was another large multi-site clinical trial of treating depression in patients who had experienced an MI. The SADHART trial enrolled 369 post-MI patients with depression at a number of American and international sites to evaluate the use of sertraline in this population.[11] The SADHART trial was not powered to detect mortality effects, but was rather designed to test the safety and efficacy of sertraline. In the Cardiac Arrhythmia Suppression Trial (CAST)[26] tricyclic antidepressants had been found to be contraindicated for use in heart patients, so safety of antidepressants in patients with heart disease was important to establish. Patients were identified after an MI or hospitalization for unstable angina, and after a roughly two-week single-blind placebo washout, they were randomized to 24 weeks of sertraline or placebo during the double-blind treatment phase. Sertraline was found to be safe for cardiac patients, but it did not reduce depression symptoms in the full sample. Rather, sertraline was associated with a drop in depression scores only among patients with recurrent depression. Responder rates exceeded 50% for both sertraline and placebo; again supporting the hypothesis that many patients experience a partial remission in depression symptoms identified at the time of hospitalization for an acute coronary event. About half of the patients were depressed prior to hospitalization, so elevated depression in-hospital cannot be solely attributed to the psychosocial stress of a coronary event. Furthermore, responder rates were substantially better among patients with recurrent depression, suggesting that sertraline may be most effective when used with heart patients who have a prior history of depression.

The recent Canadian Cardiac Randomized Evaluation of Antidepressant and Psychotherapy Efficacy trial evaluated both citalopram and interpersonal psychotherapy for depression in 284 outpatients with established coronary artery disease and depression (Lesperance et al., 2007). Patients were randomized to a 2-by-2 factorial design that consisted of 12 weeks of either interpersonal psychotherapy or usual care, as well as 12 weeks of treatment with citalopram or placebo. Whereas citalopram was an effective treatment for depression, interpersonal psychotherapy for depression was not more effective than clinical management for depression among patients with coronary artery disease. The investigators concluded that sertraline or citalopram plus clinical management would be an appropriate treatment approach for patients with heart disease and depression. Although mortality results have not been reported at the time of this writing, it seems unlikely that interpersonal therapy for depression could affect prognoses given that it did not modify the putative risk factor.

Ongoing Clinical Trials

Additional randomized clinical trials evaluating treatment of depression among patients with heart disease are under way at the time of this writing. The Safety and Efficacy of Sertraline for Depression in Patients with CHF (SADHART-CHF) study will extend the basic rationale of the SADHART study to patients with heart failure and major depressive disorder. A total of 500 patients are expected to be enrolled and randomized to 12 weeks of sertraline or placebo, and a variety of endpoints such as depression, quality of life, and mortality will be assessed. The findings from the SADHART-CHF study may be available during 2009 and are particularly needed, given a recent report that sertraline was associated with increased risk of mortality or hospitalization among heart failure patients who were not selected on the basis of depression levels (i.e., antidepressant use may have been a marker for higher risk).[27]

We believe that the Understanding Prognostic Benefits of Exercise and Antidepressant Therapy for Persons with Depression and Heart Disease (UPBEAT) study[28] is particularly promising because it was designed to evaluate the effect of treatment on the mechanisms hypothesized to be responsible for the relationship between depression and outcomes in cardiovascular disease. James Blumenthal and his colleagues have been pioneers in advocating the use of exercise as a treatment for depression,[23, 29–31] and they reported that self-reported regular exercise was associated with a 50% reduction in mortality in the ENRICHD trial[23] Although the exercise analyses from ENRICHD were not from randomized groups, the findings prompted the UPBEAT study, which may yet lead to a large-scale, multi-site, randomized clinical trial of exercise for depression in heart patients. The UPBEAT study will enroll 200 outpatients with heart disease and depression, randomly assigning them to 16 weeks of sertraline or placebo, combined with exercise intervention. Although the trial is not powered for mortality effects, a number of intermediate endpoints will be assessed, including heart rate variability, baroreceptor functioning, endothelial function, platelet activation, and the inflammatory marker high-sensitivity C-reactive protein. These measures were chosen because they are associated with both depression and heart disease outcomes and are favorably modified by exercise.

In our view, the UPBEAT study represents a prescient departure from the strategy employed in other trials, in which it had been reasoned that targeting the risk factor (i.e., depression) would improve prognosis. For a number of reasons, convincing evidence that treating depression improves outcomes in patients with heart disease has not been forthcoming. Specifically, improvements in the risk factor have been modest or absent, thus decreasing the power to detect reductions in mortality. Furthermore, the mechanisms responsible for the relationship between depression and cardiac outcomes have not been fully elucidated, although much progress has been made in the literature since ENRICHD was initially conceived. Therefore, a more promising approach, which appears to be advocated by the UPBEAT study, would be to target directly the mechanisms responsible in order to improve outcomes.

Consider the historical example of the Type A behavior pattern, whose characteristics were thought to increase risk of cardiovascular disease during the 1960s and 1970s. However, the findings were not replicated in later research. One possible explanation, offered by Alexander Glassman, is that changes in the practice of cardiology (e.g., widespread use of beta-blockers) eliminated the association of Type A behavior and cardiovascular disease.[32] This reasoning could be applied to another example; namely, that anxiety and anger were not related to mortality among post-MI patients treated according to contemporary standards, even though epidemiological evidence suggests that anxiety and anger increase risk of cardiovascular disease.[33] Thus, the use of beta-blockers, anti-platelets, and other modern treatments may reduce the risk associated with anger and anxiety, even though anger and anxiety are not the focus of treatment. Following the same logic, it should be possible to attenuate or eliminate the risk associated with depression even if depression is not the sole focus of treatment. This approach is different from the traditional risk-factor-reduction approach, but it may be particularly useful for depression because depression is associated with a number of physiological mechanisms that are in turn predictive of cardiac morbidity and mortality.

Treatment Recommendations

Returning to the question of treatment recommendations for patients with heart disease and depression, the AHA/APA science advisory recommended SSRIs, cognitive behavioral therapy, and exercise (e.g., cardiac rehabilitation).[12] The advisory commends SSRI treatment on the basis of safety, relatively low cost, and possible effectiveness, although by now it should be clear that SSRIs are most likely to reduce depression symptoms among patients with a history of depression. Cognitive behavioral therapy has modest benefits for both reducing depression symptoms and improving perceived social support, but interpersonal therapy for the treatment of depression in patients with heart disease cannot be recommended at this time. Finally, exercise is a promising treatment for depression for a number of reasons, including its effectiveness in reducing depression symptoms in noncardiac samples[29, 30] evidence of improvement in cardiac outcomes from observational studies[23] and the fact that exercise directly targets modifiable mechanisms believed to account for the relationship between depression and cardiac disease.

There are also practical considerations that recommend exercise treatments for depression in patients with cardiac disease. Some patients perceive mental health treatments to carry a stigma, whereas exercise treatments are well accepted by patients. Mental health infrastructure is often inadequate at all but the best hospitals and academic medical centers, whereas cardiac rehabilitation is typically available (and underused). Depression can be a barrier to enrollment in and completion of cardiac rehabilitation programs[34–41] but this is not surprising, because depression appears to reduce adherence to a variety of recommendations and treatments.[42, 43, 48–50] Careful case management by a mental health provider may mitigate these concerns.

Future Directions

There may be future large-scale clinical trials of psychological and pharmacological interventions for depression in patients with heart disease. However, in our view, this approach to solving the public health problem of depression and heart disease has not been effective. Rather, we feel that the results of these clinical trials and subsequent ongoing studies underscore the importance of understanding mechanisms linking depression and cardiovascular disease. A number of mechanisms have been proposed[51–58] such as adherence to medical treatments; the association of depression with other established risk factors (e.g., smoking, hypertension, diabetes); and physiological mechanisms such as exaggerated platelet reactivity[54] increased inflammatory processes[55] and dysregulation of the autonomic nervous system (ANS).[56] It is likely that multiple and interrelated mechanisms are involved in the excess cardiovascular risk conferred by depression, as no single mechanism will fully explain the relationship between depression and cardiovascular disease. Research investigating these mechanisms continues and should lead to improved treatments, as well as a more complete understanding of the nature of the relationship between depression and heart disease.

The Cholinergic Anti-inflammatory Pathway

We believe that a relatively recently described physiological mechanism holds particular promise for helping to explain the relationship between depression and heart disease. The *cholinergic anti-inflammatory pathway* described by Kevin Tracey and his colleagues[59] is a physiological system by which the nervous system interacts with the immune system to inhibit potentially damaging inflammation.[60] The cholinergic anti-inflammatory pathway has implications for a number of diseases and conditions that involve chronic inflammation. With respect to the relationship between cardiovascular disease and depression, a broad array of evidence is collectively suggestive of its involvement. However, much of the evidence is circumstantial, and direct demonstrations are lacking.

Perhaps the potential importance of the cholinergic anti-inflammatory pathway is best appreciated by comprehending several major changes in our understanding of disease processes and of cardiovascular disease in particular. That is, the *cytokine theory of disease* has gained prominence in the last 20 years, and cardiovascular disease is now widely recognized to involve inflammatory processes.[61] Although atherosclerosis was formerly known only as a disease of lipid accumulation, it is now also considered to involve low-grade vascular inflammation.[62] Inflammatory markers, such as CRP, TNF, and IL-6, are independent predictors of the risk of cardiovascular events in healthy individuals.[63–68] Inflammatory markers also predict risk of a recurrent cardiovascular events and mortality in men and women who previously experienced a cardiac event.[69, 70]

The cytokine theory of disease focuses attention squarely on inflammatory processes in the initiation, progression, and endpoints of disease, which is a revolutionary departure from earlier pathogen theories of disease. Inflammation is of course a normal immune system response to injury or infection with the goal of destroying both the cause (e.g., microbes, toxins) and the consequences (e.g., necrotic cells and tissues) of injury.[71, 72] However, without proper regulation, inflammatory processes can potentially injure or kill the body's own tissues.[73] Cytokines, which are proteins produced by a variety of cell types such as lymphocytes and macrophages, mediate the process of inflammation by orchestrating the promotion and inhibition of inflammation.[71, 74] Thus, the cytokine theory of disease posits that high levels of pro-inflammatory cytokines, such as tumor necrosis factor-α (TNF-α), interleukin-1 (IL-1), and interleukin-6 (IL-6), can cause tissue damage and disease syndromes.[68, 75, 76]

A large body of evidence now supports the cytokine theory of disease. An effective inflammatory response requires a balance of pro- and anti-inflammatory cytokines. Inadequate levels of pro-inflammatory cytokines lead to immunodeficiency that limits the body's ability to fight infection, whereas high levels can result in chronic or systemic inflammation.[60, 73, 77] Chronic inflammation contributes to the initiation and progression of a number of disabling diseases such as rheumatoid arthritis, arthrosclerosis, tuberculosis, chronic lung disease, Crohn's disease, diabetes, Alzheimer's disease, multiple sclerosis, and cerebral and myocardial ischemia.[60, 71, 77] Research showing that drugs that inhibit inflammation can be used to treat inflammatory conditions, such as anti-TNF and IL-1 antagonist, also provides support for the theory.[60, 73, 77]

The Role of the Vagus Nerve

Tracey and his colleagues discovered that the central nervous system uses neural input to control cytokine overproduction, much like it coordinates other physiological functions such as heart rate, blood pressure, digestion, body temperature, organ perfusion, and blood glucose levels.[60] This was surprising because it had been previously believed that the immune system was regulated predominantly through circulating hormonal mechanisms. However, the vagus nerve turned out to be a key link between the brain and peripheral cytokine-mediated inflammatory responses. For example, vagus nerve stimulation inhibits production of TNF in the liver of rats injected with cytokine-producing lipopolysaccharide.[78] Furthermore, acetylcholine inhibited the production of pro-inflammatory markers, including TNF, IL-1, IL-6, and IL-8, but not the anti-inflammatory cytokine IL-10, in lipopolysaccharide-stimulated human macrophage cultures.[78] These and other experimental studies with animals provide strong empirical support for the role of the vagus nerve in inflammation regulation.

Depression and Inflammation

Depression is associated with elevated levels of inflammatory markers in cardiac and non-cardiac samples.[79–82] Depressive symptoms are associated with elevated levels of CRP in patients recovering from coronary heart disease[83] as well as elevated levels of TNF-α and IL-6 in patients with congestive heart failure.[84] The results of cross-sectional studies suggest that a relationship exists between depression and inflammatory markers, but this relationship may be attenuated when other variables, such as body mass index, age, smoking status, medications, or gender, are taken into account.[85–91] Additionally, the association between depression and inflammation often exists only among a subset of patients with high pro-inflammatory cytokine levels.[90, 92] This may be because the vagus nerve halts *overproduction* of inflammatory cytokines, as intact vagal function keeps inflammation to within about 30% of normal values, but does not depress inflammatory responses to lower than normal values. These are important caveats, and the need for additional research in cardiac patients is apparent.

Animal experiments show that injections of pro-inflammatory cytokine, such as IL-1β or TNF-α, induce depression-like behaviors.[93, 94] Pro-inflammatory cytokines have been found to induce alterations in brain function analogous to those in depressed patients, including cognitive impairment, increased activity of the hypothalamus-pituitary-adrenal axis, and altered neurotransmission.[95] Increasing inflammation (through methods such as injection of a mild, non-sickness-inducing vaccine, administration of recombinant human tumor necrosis factor [rH-TNF], or administration of lipopolysaccharide) also induces depressive symptoms in humans.[96–98] Furthermore, cancer patients tend to develop depressive symptoms after being exposed to high doses of inflammatory cytokines as part of their medical treatment, such as radiation or cytokine therapies.[99, 100] Thus, inflammation can cause depression in animals and humans. However, this direction of causality is reversed from how depression is typically understood in heart disease. That is, depression is considered to contribute to heart disease and poorer outcomes in patients with heart disease. Researchers do not generally believe that depression in heart disease is merely an epiphenomenon of underlying inflammation, although the evidence reviewed here suggests that individuals with a compromised ability to regulate inflammation may be more susceptible to depression or may recover less quickly or completely from depression.

With respect to the hypothesis that depression impairs inflammation regulation by altering vagal function, there is some evidence from animal and human studies that depression can induce inflammation. When exposed to anhedonia-inducing chronic mild stress, rats developed increased plasma levels of IL-1β and TNF-α.[101] In a human sample, an infectious challenge was used to assess the association of depression and inflammatory cytokine production in 41 patients with congestive heart failure.[102] Although depressive symptoms were not associated with inflammatory cytokine production, depression was associated with enhanced sensitivity to the anti-inflammatory properties of glucocorticoids, which led to increases in inflammatory cytokines, such as IL-6 and TNF-α. These results imply that the introduction or presence of depression could potentially hinder an individual's ability to properly regulate inflammation.

In summary, previous research provides support for a bidirectional relationship between inflammation and depression. Induction of depressed mood can lead to increases in inflammatory markers, and inducing inflammation in animals and humans who do not have heart disease tends to lead to development of depressed mood, or possibly an amplification of preexisting depressive states.[103] Of course it is also possible that a mutually shared third variable (such as genetic polymorphisms) contributes to both inflammation and depression.[103]

Depression, Vagal Function, and Inflammation

Depression is associated with several measures of autonomic (including vagal) function. These measures, such as reduced heart rate variability (HRV)[9, 104–108] resting heart rate, heart rate recovery, and baroreflex sensitivity, are predictors of cardiovascular mortality.[109–112] Indices of vagal function are also related to several established cardiovascular risk factors.[112] Finally, HRV was shown to partly mediate the relationship between depression and increased risk of mortality in cardiac patients.[113] Therefore, there is evidence supporting the assertion that depression alters autonomic function (including vagal activity), and that this helps explain the relationship between depression and prognosis in cardiovascular disease.

Reduced levels of HRV indices tend to be associated with elevated levels of inflammatory markers in non-cardiac samples.[114–117] But contrary to expectations, no or weak associations between HRV indices and inflammatory markers were present in studies of cardiac patients.[118–122] These conflicting results may be due to statin use's reducing inflammatory marker levels in cardiac patients[120] nonlinear relationships between HRV and blood levels of inflammatory markers[123] or other methodological concerns. Furthermore, although there is strong empirical support for the association between the vagus nerve and inflammation, the relationship between vagal control of the heart (as measured by HRV) and inflammatory markers is less clear. One crucial piece of missing information in this literature is the extent of the relationship between the vagal control of the cholinergic anti-inflammatory pathway and vagal control of the heart. That is, it is not now known how well vagus nerve activity in the heart, as reflected in some components of HRV, correlates with the activation of the cholinergic anti-inflammatory pathway in humans.[124] However, patients with diseases characterized by elevated levels of pro-inflammatory cytokines, such as severe sepsis, rheumatoid arthritis, lupus, and inflammatory bowel disease, do have reduced levels of various HRV indices.[124]

Inflammation, Depression, and Cardiovascular Disease

Prospective studies consistently report that depression and inflammation predict cardiac events.[125–131] But contrary to expectations, accounting for inflammation does not appear to attenuate the relationship between depression and cardiovascular disease, and inflammation does not have any additive effects in predicting cardiac events when combined with depression, although there were some conflicting results in studies that reported an interaction of depression and inflammation. For example, Frasure-Smith et al.[127] found that high CRP levels predicted cardiac events only in non-depressed patients, whereas Ladwig et al.[129] found that high CRP levels were predictive of cardiac events only in depressed patients.

Unfortunately, cross sectional studies do not allow inferences regarding whether inflammation accounts for the relationship between depression and cardiovascular disease, due to the lack of temporal precedence in these research designs. Although we believe that depression alters vagal function, which then impairs regulation of inflammation, alternative explanations remain. For example, inflammation could contribute to both depression and cardiovascular disease, or alternately cardiovascular disease could increase both depression symptoms and inflammation.[103] Studies assessing inflammation and depression at multiple time points may help clarify their roles in predicting cardiovascular disease and the direction of the effects.

Furthermore, inflammation and vagal control have not been examined extensively in cardiac populations.[132] Vagal control, inflammation, and depression have been examined together in only a few studies involving patients with cardiac disease. For example, the association between markers of inflammation and markers of reduced vagal functioning was recently assessed in a sample of 44 depressed patients with coronary heart disease. Higher levels of fibrinogen (a marker of inflammation and coagulation) were moderately correlated to lower HRV levels[121] IL-6 was also moderately negatively related to TP, VLF, and LF. Neither CRP nor TNF-α were related to HRV, which could be explained by lack of statistical power due to the small sample size. This is the only known study assessing inflammation and vagal functioning in a depressed cardiac sample, and conclusions could not be drawn regarding the role of depression due to the lack of a nondepressed control group.

Conclusion

We have argued in the second half of this chapter that the cholinergic anti-inflammatory pathway described by Tracey and colleagues may help explain the relationship between depression and cardiovascular disease. Specifically, vagal control of inflammatory processes may partly mediate a bidirectional relationship between depression and heart disease. The vagus nerve clearly plays a role in regulating inflammation, but support from studies in humans is limited. Inflammation can induce depression, and depression can promote inflammation. Inflammation predicts cardiovascular disease, but there is not yet any clear evidence that inflammation mediates the relationship between depression and cardiovascular disease. Reduced vagal control of the heart is related to depression and cardiovascular disease and probably helps account for the relationship between depression and cardiovascular mortality. There is also some evidence that reduced vagal control of the heart is related to increased inflammation and that the two may combine to better predict cardiovascular disease. However, in cardiac samples, HRV has not been related to inflammatory markers. Although reduced HRV and increased inflammation are associated in depressed patients, few studies have simultaneously assessed depression, HRV, and inflammation in patients with cardiovascular disease.

Nevertheless, we believe that the cholinergic anti-inflammatory pathway will prove central to understanding how depression contributes to risk of cardiovascular morbidity and mortality. First, research is necessary to clarify several issues. The functioning of the cholinergic anti-inflammatory pathway must be better understood, especially in humans. Investigating the immune system is notoriously complex, and there are likely to be methodological challenges rooted in the basic biology of inflammatory cytokines. For example, measuring plasma levels of inflammatory cytokines is not as informative as whole blood stimulation assays measuring immune responses to lipopolysaccharide.[133] That is, relationships between circulating levels of inflammatory cytokines and depression or vagal activity may be obscured unless the ability of the immune system to respond to a challenge is directly assessed.

Furthermore, research must address how other factors related to depression and cardiovascular disease, such as aging, gender, physical activity, and diet, impact the proposed role of the vagus nerve in the relationship between depression and cardiac disease. For example, a major implication of our model is that treatments targeting the vagus nerve may help reduce the risk of mortality associated with depression in patients with heart disease. That is, physical activity, aerobic exercise, and physical fitness are known to affect vagal function[134–139] and reduce inflammation in non-cardiac[140–142] and cardiac samples.[143, 144] The impact of pharmacological treatments on multiple risk factors of cardiovascular disease should also be assessed. For example, statin use, originally used to reduce low-density lipoprotein cholesterol levels, is related to improved HRV in rabbits with chronic heart failure[145] and reductions in inflammatory markers[91, 146] prevention of vascular events[147] and reduced risk of developing depression in humans.[148]

Finally, more studies comparing depressed and nondepressed individuals with heart disease in measurements of both HRV indices and inflammatory markers are warranted. In particular, prospective studies with repeated measurements of HRV and inflammation predicting cardiovascular outcomes for depressed and nondepressed individuals would possibly help clarify the complex relationships among vagal control, inflammation, depression, and cardiovascular disease.

Notes

1. Barth J, Schumacher M, Herrmann-Lingen C. Depression as a risk factor for mortality in patients with coronary heart disease: a meta-analysis. *Psychosom Med.* 2004;66: 802–813.

2. van Melle JP, De Jonge P, Spijkerman TA et al. Prognostic association of depression following myocardial infarction with mortality and cardiovascular events: a meta-analysis. *Psychosom Med.* 2004;66:814–822.
3. Carney RM, Freedland KE. Depression, mortality, and medical morbidity in patients with coronary heart disease. *Biological psychiatry.* 2003;54:241–247.
4. Rozanski A, Blumenthal JA, Davidson KW, Saab PG, Kubzansky L. The epidemiology, pathophysiology, and management of psychosocial risk factors in cardiac practice: the emerging field of behavioral cardiology. *Journal of the American College of Cardiology.* 2005;45:637–651.
5. Frasure-Smith N, Lesperance F. Recent evidence linking coronary heart disease and depression. *Canadian journal of psychiatry Revue canadienne de psychiatrie.* 2006;51:730–737.
6. Freedland KE, Carney RM, Lustman PJ, Rich MW, Jaffe AS. Major depression in coronary artery disease patients with vs. without a prior history of depression. *Psychosom Med.* 1992;54:416-421.
7. Glassman A, O'Connor C, Califf R et al. Sertraline treatment of major depression in patients with acute MI or unstable angina. *JAMA: the Journal of the American Medical Association.* 2002;288:701–709.
8. Frasure-Smith N, Lesperance F. Reflections on depression as a cardiac risk factor. *Psychosom Med.* 2005;67 Suppl 1:S19-S25.
9. Carney RM, Rich MW, teVelde A, Saini J, Clark K, Freedland KE. The relationship between heart rate, heart rate variability and depression in patients with coronary artery disease. *J Psychosom Res.* 1988;32:159–164.
10. Egede LE. Major depression in individuals with chronic medical disorders: prevalence, correlates and association with health resource utilization, lost productivity and functional disability. *General Hospital Psychiatry.* 2007;29:409–416.
11. Glassman AH, O'Connor CM, Califf RM et al. Sertraline treatment of major depression in patients with acute MI or unstable angina. *JAMA: the Journal of the American Medical Association.* 2002;288:701–709.
12. Lichtman JH, Bigger JT, Jr., Blumenthal JA et al. Depression and coronary heart disease: recommendations for screening, referral, and treatment: a science advisory from the American Heart Association Prevention Committee of the Council on Cardiovascular Nursing, Council on Clinical Cardiology, Council on Epidemiology and Prevention, and Interdisciplinary Council on Quality of Care and Outcomes Research: endorsed by the American Psychiatric Association. *Circulation.* 2008;118:1768–1775.
13. Kroenke K, Spitzer RL, Williams JB. The Patient Health Questionnaire-2: validity of a two-item depression screener. *Med Care.* 2003;41:1284–1292.
14. Kroenke K, Spitzer RL, Williams JB. The PHQ-9: validity of a brief depression severity measure. *Journal Of General Internal Medicine: Official Journal Of The Society For Research And Education In Primary Care Internal Medicine.* 2001;16:606–613.
15. Davidson KW, Kupfer DJ, Bigger JT et al. Assessment and treatment of depression in patients with cardiovascular disease: National Heart, Lung, and Blood Institute working group report. *Annals of behavioral medicine: a publication of the Society of Behavioral Medicine.* 2006;32:121–126.
16. Beck AT, Ward CH, Mendelson M, Mock J, Erbaugh J. An inventory for measuring depression. *Arch Gen Psychiatry.* 1961;4:561–571.
17. Berkman LF, Blumenthal J, Burg M et al. Effects of treating depression and low perceived social support on clinical events after myocardial infarction: the Enhancing Recovery in Coronary Heart Disease Patients (ENRICHD) Randomized Trial. *JAMA: the Journal of the American Medical Association.* 2003;289:3106–3116.

18. Lesperance F, Frasure-Smith N, Koszycki D et al. Effects of citalopram and interpersonal psychotherapy on depression in patients with coronary artery disease: the Canadian Cardiac Randomized Evaluation of Antidepressant and Psychotherapy Efficacy (CREATE) trial. *JAMA: the Journal of the American Medical Association*. 2007;297:367–379.
19. Berkman LF, Blumenthal J, Burg M et al. Effects of treating depression and low perceived social support on clinical events after myocardial infarction: the Enhancing Recovery in Coronary Heart Disease Patients (ENRICHD) Randomized Trial. *JAMA: The Journal of the American Medical Association*. 2003;289:3106–3116.
20. Schneiderman N, Saab PG, Catellier DJ et al. Psychosocial treatment within sex by ethnicity subgroups in the Enhancing Recovery in Coronary Heart Disease clinical trial. *Psychosom Med*. 2004;66:475–483.
21. Mendes de Leon CF, Czajkowski SM, Freedland KE et al. The effect of a psychosocial intervention and quality of life after acute myocardial infarction: the Enhancing Recovery in Coronary Heart Disease (ENRICHD) clinical trial. *J Cardiopulm Rehabil*. 2006;26:9.
22. Carney RM, Blumenthal JA, Freedland KE et al. Depression and late mortality after myocardial infarction in the Enhancing Recovery in Coronary Heart Disease (ENRICHD) study. *Psychosom Med*. 2004;66:466–474.
23. Blumenthal JA, Babyak MA, Carney RM et al. Exercise, depression, and mortality after myocardial infarction in the ENRICHD trial. *Med Sci Sports Exerc*. 2004;36:746–755.
24. Taylor CB, Youngblood ME, Catellier D et al. Effects of antidepressant medication on morbidity and mortality in depressed patients after myocardial infarction. *Arch Gen Psychiatry*. 2005;62:792–798.
25. Carney RM, Blumenthal JA, Freedland KE et al. Low heart rate variability and the effect of depression on post-myocardial infarction mortality. *Arch Intern Med*. 2005;165:1486–1491.
26. Preliminary report: effect of encainide and flecainide on mortality in a randomized trial of arrhythmia suppression after myocardial infarction. The Cardiac Arrhythmia Suppression Trial (CAST) Investigators. *N Engl J Med*. 1989;321:406–412.
27. Sherwood A, Blumenthal JA, Trivedi R et al. Relationship of depression to death or hospitalization in patients with heart failure. *Arch Intern Med*. 2007;167:367–373.
28. Blumenthal JA, Sherwood A, Rogers SD et al. Understanding prognostic benefits of exercise and antidepressant therapy for persons with depression and heart disease: the UPBEAT study—rationale, design, and methodological issues. *Clinical Trials (London, England)*. 2007;4:548–559.
29. Barbour KA, Blumenthal JA. Exercise training and depression in older adults. *Neurobiology of aging*. 2005;26 Suppl 1:119–123.
30. Blumenthal JA, Babyak MA, Doraiswamy PM et al. Exercise and pharmacotherapy in the treatment of major depressive disorder. *Psychosom Med*. 2007;69:587–596.
31. Brosse AL, Sheets ES, Lett HS, Blumenthal JA. Exercise and the treatment of clinical depression in adults: recent findings and future directions. 2002;32:741–760.
32. Glassman AH, Sheps D, Pepine CJ, O'Connor C. Cardiovascular Disease & Depression. *American College of Cardiology Webcast*. 2004.
33. Frasure-Smith N, Lesperance F. Depression and other psychological risks following myocardial infarction. *Arch Gen Psychiatry*. 2003;60:627–636.
34. Casey E, Hughes JW, Waechter D, Rosneck J, Josephson R. Depression Predicts Failure to Complete Phase-II Cardiac Rehabilitation. *Journal of Behavioral Medicinecase*. In press.
35. Hughes J., Bartley A. Casey E. Luyster F. Rosneck J. Waechter D. Josephson R. Depression Symptoms are not a Major Impediment to Enrollmentin Phase-II Cardiac Rehabilitation. Journal of CardiopulmonaryRehabilitation. 26, 255. 2006. Ref Type: Abstract

36. Blumenthal JA, Williams RS, Wallace AG, Williams RBJ, Needles TL. Physiological and psychological variables predict compliance to prescribed exercise therapy in patients recovering from myocardial infarction. *Psychosom Med.* 1982;44:519–527.
37. Glazer KM, Emery CF, Frid DJ, Banyasz RE. Psychological predictors of adherence and outcomes among patients in cardiac rehabilitation. *J Cardiopulm Rehabil.* 2002;22:40–46.
38. Lane D, Carroll D, Ring C, Beevers DG, Lip GY. Predictors of attendance at cardiac rehabilitation after myocardial infarction. *J Psychosom Res.* 2001;51:497–501.
39. Sanderson BK, Bittner V. Women in cardiac rehabilitation: outcomes and identifying risk for dropout. *Am Heart J.* 2005;150:1052–1058.
40. Turner SC, Bethell HJN, Evans JA, Goddard JR, Mullee MA. Patient characteristics and outcomes of cardiac rehabilitation. *J Cardiopulm Rehabil.* 2002;22:253–260.
41. Caulin-Glaser T, Maciejewski PK, Snow R, Lalonde M, Mazure C. Depressive symptoms and sex affect completion rates and clinical outcomes in cardiac rehabilitation. *Preventive cardiology.* 2007;10:15–21.
42. Glassman AH, Helzer JE, Covey LS et al. Smoking, smoking cessation, and major depression. *JAMA: the Journal of the American Medical Association.* 1990;264:1546–1549.
43. Carney RM, Freedland KE, Eisen SA, Rich MW, Jaffe AS. Major depression and medication adherence in elderly patients with coronary artery disease. *Health psychology: official journal of the Division of Health Psychology, American Psychological Association.* 1995;14:88–90.
44. Wang P, Bohn R, Knight E, Glynn R, Mogun H, Avorn J. Noncompliance with antihypertensive medications: the impact of depressive symptoms and psychosocial factors. *Journal of general internal medicine: official journal of the Society for Research and Education in Primary Care Internal Medicine.* 2002;17:504–511.
45. Gehi A, Haas D, Pipkin S, Whooley MA. Depression and medication adherence in outpatients with coronary heart disease: findings from the Heart and Soul Study. *Arch Intern Med.* 2005;165:2508–2513.
46. Bane C, Hughes CM, McElnay JC. The impact of depressive symptoms and psychosocial factors on medication adherence in cardiovascular disease. *Patient education and counseling.* 2006;60:187–193.
47. Morgan A, Masoudi F, Havranek E et al. Difficulty taking medications, depression, and health status in heart failure patients. *J Card Fail.* 2006;12:54–60.
48. Rieckmann N, Gerin W, Kronish IM et al. Course of depressive symptoms and medication adherence after acute coronary syndromes: an electronic medication monitoring study. *Journal of the American College of Cardiology.* 2006;48:2218–2222.
49. Ziegelstein RC, Fauerbach JA, Stevens SS, Romanelli J, Richter DP, Bush DE. Patients with depression are less likely to follow recommendations to reduce cardiac risk during recovery from a myocardial infarction. *Arch Intern Med.* 2000;160:1818–1823.
50. Romanelli J, Fauerbach JA, Bush DE, Ziegelstein RC. The significance of depression in older patients after myocardial infarction. *J Am Geriatr Soc.* 2002;50:817–822.
51. Carney RM, Freedland KE, Veith RC. Depression, the Autonomic Nervous System, and Coronary Heart Disease. *Psychosom Med.* 2005;67:S29–S33.
52. Carney RM, Freedland KE, Miller GE, Jaffe AS. Depression as a risk factor for cardiac mortality and morbidity: A review of potential mechanisms. *J Psychosom Res.* 2002;53: 897–902.
53. Gillespie CF, Nemeroff CB. Hypercortisolemia and Depression. *Psychosom Med.* 2005; 67:S26–S28.
54. Bruce EC, Musselman D. Depression, Alterations in Platelet Function, and Ischemic Heart Disease. *Psychosom Med.* 2005;67:S34–S36.

55. Kop WJ, Gottdiener JS. The Role of Immune System Parameters in the Relationship Between Depression and Coronary Artery Disease. *Psychosom Med.* 2005;67:S37–S41.
56. Freedland KE, Carney RM, Skala JA. Depression and Smoking in Coronary Heart Disease. *Psychosom Med.* 2005;67:S42–S46.
57. Rozanski A, Kubzansky LD. Psychologic Functioning and Physical Health: A Paradigm of Flexibility. *Psychosom Med.* 2005;67:S47–S53.
58. Thayer JF, Lane RD. The role of vagal function in the risk for cardiovascular disease and mortality. *Biological Psychology.* 2007;74:224–242.
59. Tracey KJ. Physiology and immunology of the cholinergic antiinflammatory pathway. *The Journal of clinical investigation.* 2007;117:289–296.
60. Tracey KJ. The inflammatory reflex. *Nature.* 2002;420:853–859.
61. Ross R. Atherosclerosis—an inflammatory disease. *N Engl J Med.* 1999;340:115–126.
62. Libby P, Ridker PM, Maseri A. Inflammation and atherosclerosis. *Circulation.* 2002;105: 1135–1143.
63. Ridker PM, Hennekens CH, Buring JE, Rifai N. C-reactive protein and other markers of inflammation in the prediction of cardiovascular disease in women. *N Engl J Med.* 2000;342: 836–843.
64. Ridker PM, Rifai N, Stampfer MJ, Hennekens CH. Plasma concentration of interleukin-6 and the risk of future myocardial infarction among apparently healthy men. *Circulation.* 2000;101:1767–1772.
65. Ridker PM. Clinical application of C-reactive protein for cardiovascular disease detection and prevention. *Circulation.* 2003;107:363–369.
66. Pradhan AD, Manson JE, Rossouw JE et al. Inflammatory biomarkers, hormone replacement therapy, and incident coronary heart disease: prospective analysis from the Women's Health Initiative observational study. *JAMA: the Journal of the American Medical Association.* 2002;288:980–987.
67. Cesari M, Penninx BWJH, Newman AB et al. Inflammatory markers and cardiovascular disease (The Health, Aging and Body Composition [Health ABC] Study). *The American Journal of Cardiology.* 2003;92:522–528.
68. Pearson TA, Mensah GA, Alexander RW et al. Markers of inflammation and cardiovascular disease: application to clinical and public health practice: A statement for healthcare professionals from the Centers for Disease Control and Prevention and the American Heart Association. *Circulation.* 2003;107:499–511.
69. Ridker PM, Rifai N, Pfeffer M, Sacks F, Lepage S, Braunwald E. Elevation of tumor necrosis factor-alpha and increased risk of recurrent coronary events after myocardial infarction. *Circulation.* 2000;101:2149–2153.
70. Volpato S, Guralnik JM, Ferrucci L et al. Cardiovascular disease, interleukin-6, and risk of mortality in older women: the women's health and aging study. *Circulation.* 2001;103:947–953.
71. Cotran RS, Kumar V, Collins T. Acute and chronic inflammation. *Robbins Pathologic Basis of Disease.* 6th ed. Philadelphia: W.B. Saunders Company; 1999:50–88.
72. Rankin JA. Biological mediators of acute inflammation. *AACN clinical issues.* 2004;15:3–17.
73. Tracey KJ. Physiology and immunology of the cholinergic antiinflammatory pathway. *The Journal of clinical investigation.* 2007;117:289–296.
74. Opal SM, DePalo VA. Anti-inflammatory cytokines. *Chest.* 2000;117:1162–1172.
75. Clark IA, Virelizier J, Carswel EA, Wood PR. Possible importance of macrophage-derived mediators in acute malaria. *Infection and Immunity.* 1981;32:1058–1066.
76. Fruchart, J.C. Atherosclerosis: an inflammatory disease? International Task Force for Prevention of Coronary Heart Disease: Task Force Symposium. 2-23-2003. Ref Type: Conference Proceeding

77. Tracey KJ. *Fatal sequence: The killer within.* New York: Dana Press; 2006.
78. Borovikova LV, Ivanova S, Zhang M et al. Vagus nerve stimulation attenuates the systemic inflammatory response to endotoxin. *Nature.* 2000;405:458–462.
79. Maes M, Meltzer HY, Bosmans E, Bergmans R. Increased plasma concentrations of interleukin-6, soluble interleukin-6, soluble interleukin-2, soluble interleukin-2 and transferrin receptor in major depression. *Journal of Affective Disorders.* 1995;34:301–309.
80. Suarez EC, Krishnan RR, Lewis JG. The relation of severity of depressive symptoms to monocyte-associated proinflammatory cytokines and chemokines in apparently healthy men. *Psychosom Med.* 2003;65:362–368.
81. Suarez EC, Lewis JG, Krishnan RR, Young KH. Enhanced expression of cytokines and chemokines by blood monocytes to in vitro lipopolysaccharide stimulation are associated with hostility and severity of depressive symptoms in healthy women. *Psychoneuroendocrinology.* 2004;29:1119–1128.
82. Panagiotakos DB, Pitsavos C, Chrysohoou C et al. Inflammation, coagulation, and depressive symptomatology in cardiovascular disease-free people; the ATTICA study. *European Heart Journal.* 2004;25:492–499.
83. Miller GE, Freedland KE, Duntley SP, Carney RM. Relation of depressive symptoms to C-reactive protein and pathogen burden (cytomegalovirus, herpes simplex virus, Epstein-Barr virus) in patients with earlier acute coronary sydromes. *American Journal of Cardiology.* 2005;95:317–321.
84. Parissis JT, Adamopoulos S, Rigas A et al. Comparison of circulating proinflammatory cytokines and soluble apoptosis mediators in patients with chronic heart failure with versus without symptoms of depression. *The American Journal of Cardiology.* 2004;94: 1326–1328.
85. Tiemeier H, Hofman A, van Tuijl HR, Kiliaan AJ, Meijer J, Breteler MMB. Inflammatory proteins and depression in the elderly. *Epidemiology (Cambridge, Mass).* 2003;14:103–107.
86. Kop WJ, Gottdiener JS, Tangen CM et al. Inflammation and coagulation factors in persons > 65 years of age with symptoms of depression but without evidence of myocardial ischemia. *The American Journal of Cardiology.* 2002;89:419–424.
87. Miller GE, Stetler CA, Carney RM, Freedland KE, Banks WA. Clinical depression and inflammatory risk markers for coronary heart disease. *The American Journal of Cardiology.* 2002;90:1279–1283.
88. Steptoe A, Kunz-Ebrecht SR, Owen N. Lack of association between depressive symptoms and markers of immune and vascular inflammation in middle-aged men and women. *Psychological Medicine.* 2003;33:667–674.
89. Whooley MA, Caska CM, Hendrickson BE, Rourke MA, Ho J, Ali S. Depression and inflammation in patients with coronary heart disease: findings from the Heart and Soul Study. *Biological Psychiatry.* 2007;62:314–320.
90. Glassman AH, Miller GE. Where there is depression, there is inflammation.. sometimes! *Biological Psychiatry.* 2007;62:280–281.
91. Lesperance F, Frasure-Smith N, Theroux P, Irwin M. The association between major depression and levels of soluble intercellular adhesion molecule 1, interleukin-6, and C-reactive protein in patients with recent acute coronary syndromes. *The American Journal of Psychiatry.* 2004;161:271–277.
92. Raison CL, Capuron L, Miller AH. Cytokines sing the blues: inflammation and the pathogenesis of depression. *Trends in Immunology.* 2006;27:24–31.
93. Anisman H, Merali Z, Poulter MO, Hayley S. Cytokines as a precipitant of depressive illness: animal and human studies. *Current Pharmaceutical Design.* 2005;11:963–972.

94. Dantzer R. Cytokine-induced sickness behavior: mechanisms and implications. *Annals of the New York Academy of Sciences*. 2001;933:222–234.
95. Capuron L, Dantzer R. Cytokines and depression: The need for a new paradigm. *Brain, behavior, and immunity*. 2003;17:119–124.
96. Wright CE, Strike PC, Brydon L, Steptoe A. Acute inflammation and negative mood: mediation by cytokine activation. *Brain, Behavior, and Immunity*. 2005;19:345–350.
97. Spriggs DR, Sherman ML, Michie H et al. Recombinant human tumor necrosis factor administered as a 24-hour intravenous infusion. A phase I and pharmacologic study. *Journal of the National Cancer Institute*. 1988;80:1039–1044.
98. Yirmiya R, Pollak Y, Morag M et al. Illness, cytokines, and depression. *Annals of the New York Academy of Sciences*. 2000;917:478–487.
99. Capuron L, Ravaud A, Dantzer R. Early depressive symptoms in cancer patients receiving interleukin 2 and/or interferon alfa-2b therapy. *Journal of Clinical Oncology*. 2000;18: 2143–2151.
100. Musselman DL, Lawson DH, Gumnick JF et al. Paroxetine for the prevention of depression induced by high-dose interferon alfa. *N Engl J Med*. 2001;344:961–966.
101. Grippo AJ, Francis J, Beltz TG, Felder RB, Johnson AK. Neuroendocrine and cytokine profile of chronic mild stress-induced anhedonia. *Physiology & behavior*. 2005;84:697–706.
102. Miller GE, Freedland KE, Carney RM. Depressive symptoms and the regulation of proinflammatory cytokine expression in patients with coronary heart disease. *J Psychosom Res*. 2005;59:231–236.
103. Shimbo D, Chaplin W, Crossman D, Haas D, Davidson KW. Role of depression and inflammation in incident coronary heart disease events. *The American Journal of Cardiology*. 2005;96:1016–1021.
104. Carney RM, Saunders RD, Freedland KE, Stein P, Rich MW, Jaffe AS. Association of depression with reduced heart rate variability in coronary artery disease. *Am J Cardiol*. 1995;76:562–564.
105. Carney RM, Blumenthal JA, Stein PK et al. Depression, heart rate variability, and acute myocardial infarction. *Circulation*. 2001;104:2024–2028.
106. Hughes JW, Stoney CM. Depressed mood is related to high-frequency heart rate variability during stressors. *Psychosom Med*. 2000;62:796–803.
107. Hughes J, Casey E, Luyster F et al. Depression symptoms predict heart rate recovery after treadmill stress testing. *Am Heart J*. 2006;151:1122–1126.
108. Stein PK, Carney RM, Freedland KE et al. Severe depression is associated with markedly reduced heart rate variability in patients with stable coronary heart disease. *J Psychosom Res*. 2000;48:493–500.
109. Bigger JT, Fleiss JL, Steinman RC, Rolnitzky LM, Kleiger RE, Rottman JN. Frequency domain measures of heart period variability and mortality after myocardial infarction. *Circulation*. 1992;85:164–171.
110. Klieger RE, Miller JP, Bigger JT, Moss AJ, The Multicenter Post-infarction Research Group. Decreased heart rate variability and its association with increased mortality after acute myocardial infarction. *The American Journal of Cardiology*. 1987;59:256–262.
111. La Rovere MT, Bigger JTJ, Marcus FI, Mortara A, Schwartz PJ. Baroreflex sensitivity and heart-rate variability in prediction of total cardiac mortality after myocardial infarction. ATRAMI (Autonomic Tone and Reflexes After Myocardial Infarction) Investigators. *Lancet*. 1998;351:478–484.
112. Thayer JF, Lane RD. The role of vagal function in the risk for cardiovascular disease and mortality. *Biological Psychology*. 2007;74:224–242.

113. Carney RM, Blumenthal JA, Freedland KE et al. Low heart rate variability and the effect of depression on post-myocardial infarction mortality. *Arch Intern Med.* 2005;165: 1486–1491.
114. Sajadieh A, Nielsen OW, Rasmussen V, Hein HO, Abedini S, Hansen JF. Increased heart rate and reduced heart-rate variability are associated with subclinical inflammation in middle-aged and elderly subjects with no apparent heart disease. *European heart journal.* 2004;25:363–370.
115. Sloan RP, McCreath H, Tracey KJ, Sidney S, Liu K, Seeman T. RR interval variability is inversely related to inflammatory markers: The CARDIA study. *Molecular Medicine.* 2007;13:178–184.
116. Sajadieh A, Nielsen OW, Rasmussen V, Hein HO, Hansen JF. C-reactive protein, heart rate variability and prognosis in community subjects with no apparent heart disease. *Journal of Internal Medicine.* 2006;260:377–387.
117. Dawood T, Lambert EA, Barton DA et al. Specific serotonin reuptake inhibition in major depressive disorder adversely affects novel markers of cardiac risk. *Hypertension research: official journal of the Japanese Society of Hypertension.* 2007;30:285–293.
118. Hamaad A, Sosin M, Blann AD, Patel J, Lip GYH, MacFadyen RJ. Markers of inflammation in acute coronary syndromes: association with increased heart rate and reductions in heart rate variability. *Clinical Cardiology.* 2005;28:570–576.
119. Janszky I, Ericson M, Lekander M et al. Inflammatory markers and heart rate variability in women with coronary heart disease. *Journal of Internal Medicine.* 2004;256:421–428.
120. Yue W, Schneider A, Ruckerl R et al. Relationship between electrocardiographic and biochemical variables in coronary artery disease. *International Journal of Cardiology.* 2007;119:185–191.
121. Carney RM, Freedland KE, Stein PK et al. Heart rate variability and markers of inflammation and coagulation in depressed patients with coronary heart disease. *J Psychosom Res.* 2007;62:463–467.
122. Lanza GA, Sgueglia GA, Cianflone D et al. Relation of heart rate variability to serum levels of C-reactive protein in patients with unstable angina pectoris. *The American Journal of Cardiology.* 2006;97:1702–1706.
123. Lanza GA, Sgueglia GA, Cianflone D et al. Relation of heart rate variability to serum levels of C-reactive protein in patients with unstable angina pectoris. *American Journal of Cardiology.* 2006;97:1702–1706.
124. Tracey KJ. Fat meets the cholinergic antiinflammatory pathway. *The Journal of experimental medicine.* 2005;202:1017–1021.
125. Arbelaez JJ, Ariyo AA, Crum RM, Fried LP, Ford DE. Depressive symptoms, inflammation, and ischemic stroke in older adults: A prospective analysis in the Cardiovascular Health Study. *Journal of the American Geriatrics Society.* 2007;55:1825–1830.
126. Empana JP, Sykes DH, Luc G et al. Contributions of depressive mood and circulating inflammatory markers to coronary heart disease in healthy European men: the Prospective Epidemiological Study of Myocardial Infarction (PRIME). *Circulation.* 2005;111: 2299–2305.
127. Frasure-Smith N, Lesperance F, Irwin MR, Sauve C, Lesperance J, Theroux P. Depression, C-reactive protein and two-year major adverse cardiac events in men after acute coronary syndromes. *Biological Psychiatry.* 2007;62:302–308.
128. Janszky I, Ahlbom A, Hallqvist J, Ahnve S. Hospitalization for depression is associated with an increased risk for myocardial infarction not explained by lifestyle, lipids, coagulation, and inflammation: the SHEEP Study. *Biological Psychiatry.* 2007;62:25–32.

129. Ladwig KH, Marten-Mittag B, Lowel H, Doring A, Koenig W. C-reactive protein, depressed mood, and the prediction of coronary heart disease in initially healthy men: results from the MONICA-KORA Augsburg Cohort Study 1984-1998. *European Heart Journal*. 2005; 26:2537–2542.
130. Redwine LS, Mills PJ, Hong S et al. Cardiac-related hospitalization and/or death associated with immune dysregulation and symptoms of depression in heart failure patients. *Psychosom Med*. 2007;69:23–29.
131. Vaccarino V, Johnson BD, Sheps DS et al. Depression, inflammation, and incident cardiovascular disease in women with suspected coronary ischemia. *Journal of the American College of Cardiology*. 2007;50:2044–2055.
132. Dickens C, McGowan L, Clark-Carter D, Creed F. Depression in rheumatoid arthritis: A systematic review of the literature with meta-analysis. *Psychosom Med*. 2002;64:52–60.
133. Marsland AL, Sathanoori R, Muldoon MF, Manuck SB. Stimulated production of interleukin-8 covaries with psychosocial risk factors for inflammatory disease among middle-aged community volunteers. *Brain, Behavior, and Immunity*. 2007;21:218–228.
134. Rosenwinkel ET, Bloomfield DM, Arwady MA, Goldsmith RL. Exercise and autonomic function in health and cardiovascular disease. *Cardiology Clinics*. 2001;19:369–387.
135. Carter JB, Banister EW, Blaber AP. Effect of endurance exercise on autonomic control of heart rate. *Sports medicine (Auckland, NZ)*. 2003;33:33–46.
136. Blumenthal JA, Sherwood A, Babyak MA et al. Effects of exercise and stress management training on markers of cardiovascular risk in patients with ischemic heart disease: a randomized controlled trial. *JAMA: the Journal of the American Medical Association*. 2005;293:1626–1634.
137. Stein PK, Ehsani AA, Domitrovich PP, Kleiger RE, Rottman JN. Effect of exercise training on heart rate variability in healthy older adults. *American Heart Journal*. 1999;138: 567–576.
138. Pichot V, Roche F, Denis C et al. Interval training in elderly men increases both heart rate variability and baroreflex activity. *Clinical autonomic research: official journal of the Clinical Autonomic Research Society*. 2005;15:107–115.
139. De Meersman RE, Stein PK. Vagal modulation and aging. *Biological Psychology*. 2007; 74:165–173.
140. McFarlin BK, Flynn MG, Campbell WW et al. Physical activity status, but not age, influences inflammatory biomarkers and toll-like receptor 4. *The Journals of Gerontology Series A, Biological Sciences and Medical Sciences*. 2006;61:388–393.
141. Stewart LK, Flynn MG, Campbell WW et al. The influence of exercise training on inflammatory cytokines and C-reactive protein. *Medicine and Science in Sports & Exercise*. 2007;39:1714–1719.
142. King DE, Carek P, Mainous AGI, Pearson WS. Inflammatory markers and exercise: differences related to exercise type. *Medicine and Science in Sports & Exercise*. 2003;35: 575–581.
143. Adamopoulos S, Parissis J, Kroupis C et al. Physical training reduces peripheral markers of inflammation in patients with chronic heart failure. *European heart journal*. 2001;22: 791–797.
144. Conraads VM, Beckers P, Bosmans J et al. Combined endurance/resistance training reduces plasma TNF-alpha receptor levels in patients with chronic heart failure and coronary artery disease. *European Heart Journal*. 2002;23:1854–1860.
145. Pliquett RU, Cornish KG, Zucker IH. Statin therapy restores sympathovagal balance in experimental heart failure. *Journal of Applied Physiology*. 2003;95:700–704.

146. Ridker PM, Rifai N, Clearfield DO et al. Measurement of C-reactive protein for the targeting of statin therapy in the primary prevention of acute coronary events. *N Engl J Med.* 2001;366:1959–1965.
147. Ridker PM, Danielson E, Fonseca FA et al. Rosuvastatin to prevent vascular events in men and women with elevated C-reactive protein. *N Engl J Med.* 2008;359:2195–2207.
148. Young-Xu Y, Chan KA, Liao JK, Ravid S, Blatt CM. Long-term statin use and psychological well-being. *Journal of the American College of Cardiology.* 2004;42:690–696.

Part II

NEUROPSYCHOLOGICAL EFFECTS OF CVD

7

CLINICAL CONSIDERATIONS IN THE NEUROPSYCHOLOGICAL ASSESSMENT OF PATIENTS WITH CARDIOVASCULAR DISEASE

Ronald A. Cohen, John Gunstad, and Andreana Benitez

The field of clinical neuropsychology has traditionally focused on the assessment of patients with neurological brain disorders. Historically, study was directed at the effects of focal brain lesions, typically resulting from cerebral infarction, penetrating wounds, or surgical interventions. Subsequently, there was also emphasis placed on the evaluation of brain disorders in which there was not a strongly localized presentation, such as progressive neurodegenerative diseases like Alzheimer's disease (AD), and closed head injury. These types of neurological brain disorders continue to be a central focus in the field, though increasingly there has been interest in the effects of diseases that affect the body beyond the central nervous system (CNS) and ultimately brain function. Neuropsychological consideration of cardiovascular disease is an example of this evolution.

As discussed earlier in the book, interest in the neuropsychological assessment of people with cardiovascular disease is a logical outgrowth of the clinical significance of cerebrovascular disease, and in particular, acute stroke. Given that cardiovascular and cerebrovascular disease share common risk and etiological factors and often co-occur; a natural pathophysiological relationship exists between them. From a clinical perspective, patients who have experienced an acute stroke often have a history of heart disease, and in many cases had subclinical cerebrovascular disease prior to experiencing an acute clinical stroke. The high prevalence of "silent stroke" in the elderly reflects this fact.[1]

For clinical neuropsychologists working in outpatient settings, it is common for elderly patients to be referred who do not have identified neurological disease or evidence of the global functional deterioration indicative of Alzheimer's disease or other related dementias. The term *mild cognitive impairment* (MCI) was coined by researchers in the AD field to characterize these individuals based on the observation that a proportion of people with such impairments convert to more global dementia in the years that follow baseline assessment. Yet, not all patients identified with MCI go on to develop AD, nor is the presentation of a primary amnestic syndrome evident in many elderly people who experience subtle cognitive problems. Given the incidence of cardiovascular disease in the general population, many people coming to neuropsychology clinics for evaluation have a medical history that is significant for cardiovascular disease, and an even greater proportion have risk factors for developing vascular disease. Accordingly, clinicians conducting outpatient assessments are likely to be confronted with the question of whether a particular patient's heart disease is a contributing factor affecting their cognitive presentation.

Neuropsychologists and other clinicians working in inpatient hospital settings are even more likely to be confronted with questions regarding the reasons for cognitive changes among patients admitted for cardiovascular conditions. The scope of these referrals ranges from elderly patients who have chronic heart disease who appear confused and disoriented during their hospitalization, to cases of acute mental status change following cardiac procedures. In many of these cases, there is no known history of neurological disease. Furthermore, the family may report that the patient seemed to be functioning "normally" prior to the hospitalization.

Another compelling factor motivating neuropsychological inquiry into the effects of cardiovascular disease stems from the fact that there is increasing evidence that brain function is strongly influenced by general health. As the field of medicine became increasingly specialized in the middle of the twentieth century, there was a tendency to focus on specific body systems to the exclusion of others. Cardiologists were focused on the heart, neurologists on the nervous system, and psychiatrists on the "mind." There is now much greater awareness that the systems of the body are highly integrated, and their health is dependent on the integrity of other organ systems. This shift in *zeitgeist* has made it more difficult to consider the brain in isolation. Understanding the development of neurodegenerative conditions may ultimately require factoring in the effects of pathology, such as vascular disease, that extend well beyond the boundaries of the brain. If a clinician hopes to fully characterize functional decline occurring over time, it is essential that changes in overall physical health be considered, and in this regard the cardiovascular system is a dominant factor.

These issues provide the backdrop for clinical consideration of the neuropsychology of cardiovascular disease. This chapter departs from most of the others in this book in that it primarily aims to outline factors that should be considered by clinicians working with cardiovascular disease who are attempting to sort out these effects. We offer recommendations for how to approach the assessment, clinical management, and psychological treatment of these individuals from the perspective of our clinical experience.

Neuropsychological Presentation

Given these objectives, an obvious starting point is to consider the neuropsychological presentations associated with cardiovascular disease. Several essential points should be made from the onset. Because of its systemic nature, patients with cardiovascular disease are very heterogeneous in both their presentation and clinical history. Furthermore, since cardiovascular disease really consists of a spectrum of different conditions affecting the heart and systemic vascular function, it is impossible to define a single neuropsychological profile common to all patients. To make neuropsychological consideration more manageable, it will be useful to distinguish between four broad categories of clinical presentation that account for the vast majority of cases: (1) heart disease with no prior evidence of stroke or cardiac arrest; (2) heart disease with stroke; (3) cardiac arrest with severe heart failure; and (4) cardiovascular disease with adverse postsurgical outcomes. While some of these categories have similar clinical neuropsychological manifestations, overall they are sufficiently different to warrant separate consideration.

Cardiovascular Disease Without Stroke or Cardiac Arrest

Patients falling into this category constitute the majority of cases likely to be seen by most neuropsychologists in outpatient settings, except for practices in which there are many referrals of stroke patients. This group also represents the purest group from the standpoint of examining the effects of chronic cardiovascular disease on brain function. Patients in this category have not experienced the effects of complete cessation of heart function, or the focal effects of clinically evident prior stroke. Therefore, any changes in brain function presumably relate to effects of the vascular dysfunction associated with heart disease or its underlying risk factors and pathology.

Among this group, significant cognitive dysfunction is not a given. In fact, brain disturbances would not be expected among most people with very mild cardiovascular disease who do not have a history of heart failure. The occurrence of brain abnormalities in such cases could reflect the presence of comorbid cerebrovascular disease, which has not resulted in a stroke that is clinically evident, but which is still having some effect on cerebral perfusion. Alternatively, clinicians should consider other factors not associated with vascular disease as a basis for observed cognitive problems.

As the severity and chronicity of vascular disease increases, particularly in the context of advanced age, there is an increased likelihood that cardiovascular factors may be contributing to observed neurocognitive impairments. In such cases, while heterogeneity of presentation exists, the neurocognitive profile will tend to mirror that observed in patients with vascular cognitive impairment (VCI) who have subcortical white matter disturbances. Table 7-1 summarizes the cognitive domains most likely to be affected, versus those least likely to be affected.

Table 7-1 Cognitive functions likely and unlikely to be affected among elderly patients with chronic moderate to severe cardiovascular disease, but no history of large vessel stroke, neurodegenerative disease, cardiac arrest, or major complications of cardiothoracic surgery. The functions likely to be affected are listed in order of their prevalence

Typically affected	Not usually affected
Information processing speed	Language
Psychomotor speed	Visual perception
Focused and sustained attention	Visual spatial functions
Executive functions	Reasoning and judgment
Learning efficiency	Global cognitive/intellectual level
Memory retrieval	

One of the most robust findings from our previous research on cardiovascular disease effects is the presence of diminished speed of psychomotor and information processing.[2] Slowing is likely to be observed on tests of fine motor speed and dexterity, such as the Grooved Pegboard. Furthermore, there is likely to be slowing on other timed tests of executive and attentional functioning, such as Trail Making, Digit Symbol Coding, or the Stroop test. We have found that processing speed on measures of sustained attention, such as the adaptive rate continuous performance test (ARCPT) is particularly sensitive to the extent of impairment as assessed by measures such as cardiac output, ejection fraction, blood pressure variability, and thickening and stiffening of blood vessels (e.g., Intima media thickness and brachial artery response).[2] These findings are discussed elsewhere in the book. Measures of simple and complex reaction time on tests such as the California Computerized Assessment Package CALCAP[3] may also be affected.

The domains of higher-order executive functions, including generative ability on tasks such as the controlled oral word-association test, and also learning and memory retrieval efficiency, are the next most vulnerable to impairment in patients with chronic cardiovascular disease. However, it is not entirely clear that impairments in these domains can be completely disassociated from deficits caused by the effects of slowed processing. Often when speed is factored in, the degree of observed impairment decreases. Deficits in the domain of executive function associated with VCI are discussed in much greater detail by Dr. Libon and colleagues (Chapter 20).

Visual motor deficits may also be observed in this population, though primary impairments of visual perception, spatial processing, and higher-order visual integration are uncommon. Again, processing speed and difficulty with organizational efficiency in the face of effortful demands and fatigue often seem to play a role when deficits are observed on tasks, such as copying a complex figure. Primary language disturbances should generally not be expected with this category of cardiovascular disease. Accordingly, the presence of aphasia, severe anomia, or other language syndromes of this type should alert the clinician to the likelihood of other problems beyond the cumulative effects of cardiovascular disease. Similarly, comprehension, reasoning, and "intellectual" functions tend to be preserved, except to the extent that patients may show subtle problems with abstraction or other types of problem solving that require considerable attentional effort and executive capacity.

From the standpoint of subjective symptoms, among the most significant complaints by many patients with chronic cardiovascular disease are fatigue and the feeling that they must make a greater effort to accomplish not only physical tasks, but also cognitive tasks. Problems with sustained attention and persistence of responding tend to go hand-in-hand with these complaints among some patients, though there is not always a strong correspondence between these subjective complaints and their objective performance. We will discuss the issue of subjective complaints to a greater extent later in this chapter.

Cardiovascular Disease with Evidence of Prior or Secondary Stroke

As discussed throughout this book, cardiovascular disease and stroke share a high rate of comorbidity. Among patients with a prior history of cerebral infarction or evidence of a recent cardioembolic stroke, the size and strategic location of the infarction, as well as their clinical and functional history prior to the current assessment should take precedence. If there is evidence of a significant language disturbance and evidence of an old left-hemisphere infarction, the working hypothesis should be that this infarction is making a significant contribution to the observed impairments. Clinicians should follow the general rules of syndrome analysis that have been established in the field of neuropsychology, which are well described in a number of classic texts.[4, 5] Furthermore, for patients exhibiting either severe focal symptoms, or evidence of aphasia, apraxia, agnosia, amnesia, or other well-defined brain syndromes, should almost always undergo brain neuroimaging to determine whether a cerebral infarction or some other focal brain disturbance exists. More extensive neurodiagnostic workup is usually indicated. Readers are encouraged to review Chapter 12 for a discussion of key issues related to the neurology of cardioembolic stroke.

Cardiac Arrest

Given that the brain requires a constant supply of blood to sustain neuronal function, cessation of blood flow to the brain for even a few seconds has significant physiological consequences. Complete cessation of cerebral blood flow for longer periods of time is often catastrophic, eventually resulting in severe global brain dysfunction and death. The severity of impairment that is observed is a function of the duration of global ischemia.

Cardiac arrest is usually fatal. Only between 2% and 8% of people admitted to hospitals following cardiac arrest survive. While a larger percentage (8%–22%) can be resuscitated at the time of hospital admission, more than half of these patients die during their hospitalization. The primary determining factor governing survival is whether a rhythm can be documented early. Cardiopulmonary resuscitation (CPR), along with defibrillation, intubation, and drug administration aimed at stimulating the heart are the standard treatments, though outcome is usually poor unless the factors driving the arrest have been identified and treated as well. Some causes of cardiac arrest have better outcomes associated with them than others, though prognosis for most etiologies is poor. Cardiac arrest caused by hypothermia has one of the best rates of survival, in large part because decreasing the body temperature slows metabolic activity. Among the most common reasons for cardiac arrest are: (1) myocardial infarction involving thrombosis of the coronary arteries, (2) pulmonary embolism, (3) hypovemia in which there is severe blood and fluid loss, often due to bleeding caused by severe trauma, and (4) cardiothoracic trauma in which severe damage to the heart occurs. Arrest due to myocardial infarction now has improved survival rates if anti-thrombolitic agents, can be administered soon enough, whereas the outcome following trauma, severe blood loss, and pulmonary embolism is much poorer.

Other common causes include: (1) alterations in plasma pH balance (acidosis) due to drug, alcohol, or solvent ingestion; (2) anoxia due to obstructed air flow, poisoning, or respiratory failure; (3) severe electrolyte imbalances; (4) severe hypoglycemia or hyperglycemia; (5) buildup of blood or fluids in the pericardium causing an inability of the heart to beat (cardiac tamponade); (6) tension pneumothorax caused by excessive air in the pleural cavity causing kinking of the vena cava and disruption of blood return to the heart; and (7) overdose of barbituates, opiates, or other drugs that depress the CNS. Prognosis varies across these etiologies, though in all cases, rapid intervention with correction of the underlying cause of the cardiac arrest is a key to survival.

While death is very common following cardiac arrest, a small percentage of patients survive. Among these individuals, severe and global brain dysfunction is common. There are numerous well-known cases in the news during the past several years of patients who survived cardiac arrest, but with severe coma or in vegetative states. Examination of the cortex through neuroimaging often reveals severe cortical atrophy and other major structural brain abnormalities. In these unfortunate cases, the person may be functionally decorticate and profoundly demented.

Cognitive Impairments

Other people who survive cardiac arrest due to rapid intervention fare better. Yet clinicians should approach these cases with the expectation that significant cognitive dysfunction is likely to exist. Because of the vulnerability of the hippocampus and proximal limbic/paralimbic structures to anoxic injury, amnestic disorder is often present. Because the actual rate of tissue damage may vary from patient to patient, along with the temporal dynamics of the event and underlying etiology, heterogeneity in cognitive presentation exists. However, global cognitive dysfunction is a likely outcome among many patients who survive. Accordingly, neuropsychological assessment should be directed at initially assessing for dementia, followed by a comprehensive evaluation of all cognitive domains if the patient is not globally demented.

It is worth noting that the term *cardiac arrest* is often misunderstood by the general public. Many patients report that they have experienced cardiac arrest, even though there is no indication of such an event in their medical history. This happens for several reasons. Many people equate myocardial infarction (i.e., heart attack) with cardiac arrest, and confuse the terms. Others are told that they have congestive heart failure, which usually causes reduced cardiac output, but does not imply complete cardiac arrest, unless the patient is in the end stage of their disease. In yet another subgroup of patients, their heart was stopped momentarily during a cardiac procedure, often intentionally as cross-clamping of vessels was being done. This becomes a notable life event in the memory of patients when told of this by their doctors or family. Finally, many patients with myocardial infarction experience marked arrhythmia along with a severe disruption of cardiac function, though without a complete loss of heart rhythm. While cardiac arrest has not occurred in these cases, alterations in consciousness may have occurred, and the patient's interpretation may be that they "died" or had a near-death experience.

Adverse Postsurgical Outcome

The fact that some patients who undergo cardiothoracic surgery such as coronary bypass graphing and valve replacement experience poor functional outcome is indisputable.

There is an extensive clinical research literature going back over forty years, describing the incidence of stroke and secondary brain disturbances following coronary artery bypass grafting (CABG) and other types of open-heart surgery.[6, 7] Yet considerable controversy has occurred in recent years regarding how common such adverse effects are in this day and age, given the remarkable advances that have occurred in surgical methods. This general topic is the focus of Chapter 10, and will not be reviewed in detail now. However, several conclusions can me made that may affect clinical decision-making.

An important point that should be made is that while functional outcomes associated with cardiothoracic surgery have improved dramatically, some patients do experience poor cognitive outcomes. Accordingly, it is necessary to consider each patient's case without applying general rules regarding whether or not impairments have occurred post-surgery. The assessment conducted for patients undergoing cardiothoracic surgery should largely follow the logic and decision rules governing comprehensive neuropsychological evaluation of other types of cardiovascular patients. However, it is strongly advised that a preoperative assessment be conducted to provide a baseline for comparison.

The most difficult challenge facing most clinicians assessing patients postsurgically is that they often do not have such baseline data to use as a reference to characterize change. Unfortunately, obtaining presurgical neuropsychological testing on patients is often difficult. In certain medical centers in which the cardiologists are particularly tuned into and interested in these types of effects, such testing may be routinely ordered. However, even in these settings, not all surgeons want to have their patients tested before surgery. Historically, there was even some resistance to routinely getting this type of information, based on the reasoning that saving the patient's life was the essential issue. Information that might suggest that a particular patient might be at risk for a poor outcome based on pre-morbid status would only confound decision-making on the medical issues in the case. Fortunately, in recent years there has been greater attention given to neurological status in the context of cardiothoracic surgery, though this still varies across centers. When the opportunity exists, neuropsychologists working with these patients should try to foster a relationship with the surgeons to promote presurgical assessment on patients whenever possible.

A somewhat related, though separate, issue stems from the fact that even though there may be a plan in place to obtain presurgical baseline testing, often events happen very quickly in specific cases, so that the evaluation cannot be initiated prior to the surgery. Even when there is some time available, the patient may be undergoing a large number of other procedures that interfere with the ability to do an extensive evaluation. Also, many patients are anxious and focusing on the upcoming surgery and would rather not be assessed for cognitive function, unless it is really mandated by their primary doctors. Sometimes the nursing staff may be reluctant to call for this assessment, given their sensitivity to the patient's anxiety and medical status prior to the surgery. Also, some patients are too sick to fully engage in the assessment. In light of these issues, it is recommended that efforts be made to obtain presurgical testing, with the understanding that it may not always be possible, and that in some cases premorbid functioning will have to be estimated from demographic, psychosocial, and normative data.

Given these constraints, a premium often needs to be placed on brevity, particularly with respect to the presurgical assessment. Furthermore, because a follow-up assessment is often desired a few months after surgery, it is best to use tests that can be repeated without sacrificing validity. The inclusion of an instrument that can provide a brief, comprehensive and repeatable assessment (e.g., Repeatable Battery for the Assessment of Neuropsychological Status: RBANS[8]) can serve this purpose and can be supplemented by other measures aimed to provide more thorough assessment of learning and memory, attention-executive functions, and measures sensitive to processing speed impairments.

For clinicians working on inpatient consultation-liaison services, it is common to be referred patients who are experiencing prolonged delirium following surgery. While there may be a tendency by some clinicians to dismiss doing neuropsychological assessment during the early postsurgical period, information from this type of assessment is often valuable so that recovery over the following weeks can be better quantified. Often patients undergo brief mental status assessment at this point in the recovery process, which is more qualitatively based, making it difficult to judge what the nadir of the patient's mental status postsurgically. There is some evidence that severity and duration of postsurgical delirium is predictive of subsequent outcome.[9]

Age and Pre-Morbid Cognitive Status

As is the case with neurological and other medical conditions, the likelihood and extent of brain disturbances that occur secondary to cardiovascular disease is a function of age. The elderly tend to experience greater cardiovascular-associated brain dysfunction than younger adults. Middle-aged people with coronary artery disease, but adequate cardiac output and only mild-to-moderate systemic vascular dysfunction are likely to have little cardiovascular cognitive impairment in the absence of prior stroke or adverse surgical outcome. As people reach more advanced age (>70 years), the possibility that cardiovascular disease is contributing to some cognitive deficits increases, though this is likely to be most evident with respect to psychomotor and information-processing speed, learning efficiency, and attention-executive functioning. Accordingly, most young patients coming for outpatient neuropsychological evaluation would be unlikely to have significant cognitive impairments that can be clinically distinguished from other potential comorbid factors if they have only moderate risk factors and coronary artery disease.

Even among elderly patients, it is unlikely that cardiovascular disease alone would account for global dementia, unless there is evidence of comorbid stroke, cardiac arrest, or a poor outcome from cardiac surgery. The exception to this occurs in the context of heart failure, as chronic problems with cardiac output tend to affect cerebral perfusion, particularly among elderly patients with impaired systemic hemodynamic function, who may have reduced cerebral hemodynamic autoregulatory capacity. While the exact relationship between duration of illness and age has not been fully determined in controlled studies, clinicians should begin to give increased weight to the potential contribution of cardiovascular disease when they are evaluating elderly patients with a long-standing history of vascular disease and impaired heart function.

The same general rule exists for patients in the other three categories discussed earlier, though their impairments are influenced to a greater extent by the nature of the circumstances surrounding a particular case. For example, cardiac arrest is likely to cause significant brain dysfunction due to cessation of cerebral blood flow, irrespective of age. Similarly, cerebral infarction during cardiac surgery or as a comorbid condition tends to produce a pattern of cognitive dysfunction consistent with the vascular territory affected. In such cases, age is likely to influence the patient's recovery of function following the event (i.e., serving as one of several contributors to cognitive and neuronal reserves).

Neuropsychological Assessment

As discussed above, the assessment approach taken with a patient depends on a number of factors, such as the clinical setting and category of cardiovascular disturbance that is being evaluated. The breadth and depth of the test battery may vary accordingly. Perhaps the most important consideration is that tests be included that are sensitive to psychomotor and information-processing speed, with some weighting of the battery towards tests of attention and executive function. Impaired learning efficiency rather than primary memory disturbance is likely, so tests that have sufficient encoding and retrieval demands are best.

Otherwise, it is important to have enough breadth in the test battery to provide information about functioning across all cognitive domains. The extent to which tests of language, visual, and intellectual function are emphasized depends on whether the patient is presenting with some evidence of stroke or major cardiac event. Assuming these criteria are met, there are several possible test batteries that could be employed. The most important issue is how hypothesis-testing and decision-making is done based on the findings that are obtained.

The specific test battery that we have used in our prior research and clinical work is shown in Table 7-2. Most of the tests included in this battery are widely used neuropsychological measures for which there are extensive normative data and strong reliability and validity in the field. For comprehensive outpatient assessment, we typically administer the Dementia Rating Scale[10, 11] to obtain a measure of the degree of global impairment and screen for dementia. Rather than administer the entire Weschler Adult Intelligence Scale-IV (WAIS-IV), we typically use the Wechsler Abbreviated Scales of Intelligence (WASI), with the inclusion of all four subtests (Vocabulary, Similarities, Block Design, and Matrix Reasoning).[12] In addition, the Digit Span and Symbol Coding subtests of the WAIS-IV are included to provide greater coverage of attention span and processing speed and efficiency.[13] Memory assessment includes the California Verbal Learning Test (CVLT-II)[14] and Brief Visual Memory Test Revised (BVMT-R)[15] to cover both verbal and nonverbal learning. In elderly patients (>75 years), we typically substitute the Hopkins Verbal Learning Test (HVLT)[16] for the CVLT-II. Language assessment is limited to the Boston Naming Test[17] and fluency measures, including the Controlled Oral Word Association Test (COWAT).[18, 19] To provide an adequate sampling of motor performance over time, the Grooved Pegboard Test is included.[20] We have also included the CALCAP to provide measures of simple and complex reaction time.[3]

Table 7-2 Recommended measures for neuropsychological assessment in persons with cardiovascular disease

Domain	Measures
Global Cognitive Function	Dementia Rating Scale-2 Wechsler Abbreviated Scale of Intelligence Repeatable Battery for the Assessment of Neuropsychological Status
Attention/Executive Functioning	Digit Span Digit Symbol Coding Letter Number Sequencing California Computerized Assessment Package Reaction Time Trail Making Test A and B Stroop Color Word Test Wisconsin Card Sort Test Adaptive Rate Continuous Performance Test
Memory	California Verbal Learning Test-II Brief Visual Memory Test-Revised Hopkins Verbal Learning Test Logical Memory I and II
Language	Boston Naming Test Controlled Oral Word Association Test Animal Naming
Visuospatial	Complex Figure Test Hooper Visual Organization Test
Motor	Grooved Pegboard
Depression	Beck Depression Inventory-2 Geriatric Depression Scale
Health-Related Quality of Life	Medical Outcomes Study 36-Item Short Form Health Survey (SF-36)
Fatigue and Apathy	Frontal Systems Behavioral Scale Neuropsychiatric Inventory Apathy Evaluation Scale Fatigue Severity Scale

The domains of attention and executive function are heavily weighted with Trail Making,[21] the Stroop test,[22, 23] COWAT,[18, 19] Wisconsin Card Sort Test (WCST),[24, 25] and Tower of Hanoi.[26] As discussed earlier, the Adaptive Rate Continuous Performance Test (ARCPT)[27] has been highly sensitive to various vascular functions in our past studies of cardiovascular disease. While other versions of the CPT can be used as well, it is important that they contain adequate measures of processing speed and performance inconsistency, beyond the standard signal-detection measures.

It is important that the battery be planned with respect to the need for repeated assessment. In standard outpatient cases, the battery described above is probably adequate if repeat assessment is planned for over 12 months post-baseline. However, when conducting evaluations in the context of cardiac surgery or when shorter-term follow-up is required, some of the lengthy sections of the comprehensive battery may be eliminated in favor of a briefer repeatable test battery. We have used the Repeatable Battery for the Assessment of Neuropsychological Status (RBANS[8]) in such cases as it provides some coverage of neuropsychological domains. The tests of attention and executive function described above are included along with the RBANS. If major impairments of specific cognitive domains are found at baseline, more extensive testing is conducted to fully assess that domain.

Delirium Assessment

For clinicians working in an inpatient hospital setting, patients with delirium represent one of the more common and challenging types of referral. Frequently, the question that is raised as part of the referral is whether the patient is experiencing delirium (i.e., a transient severe change in mental status and cognitive function) versus dementia, or some other more permanent brain disorder. The assessment of delirium has been well described in a number of other texts, and will not be reviewed in detail here. However, there are several key points worth mentioning.

1. Delirium should be suspected for patients exhibiting significant alterations in level of consciousness with lethargy or stupor.
2. This alteration is typically transient and fluctuating, which if evident should increase the weighting given to the possibility of delirium.
3. The presence of disorientation, agitation, aggressiveness, or psychosis in a patient with no prior psychiatric history following a procedure or cardiac event should also raise the specter of delirium.
4. When delirium is suspected, close monitoring of the patient's mental status should occur to document the temporal variation in their symptoms.
5. Since medication side effects are a common reason for delirium, particularly in the elderly, a review of possible pharmacological bases for these changes should be conducted, with the patient reassessed as drugs are withdrawn or doses changed. Similarly, metabolic functions should be monitored closely to determine whether a metabolic encephalopathy is responsible for the delirium.

Psychological Manifestations of Cardiovascular Disease

Beyond the potential effects on brain function, cardiovascular disease has significant psychological, social, and economic consequences. These effects are strongly associated with changes in perceived health status and lead to reductions in quality of life (QOL) among significant percentage of patients. These changes can occur regardless of the severity of the disease. For example, a middle-aged person who is functioning adequately in their occupation and family life will often find the discovery that they have significant heart disease to be extremely traumatic. It raises issues of mortality and the possibility of changes in the quality of life going forward.

In Table 7-2, a number of inventories are included for the assessment of the psychological, social, and functional manifestations of cardiovascular disease. We have found that perceived health status and QOL are influenced by both cognitive and emotional status. While cognitive function proved to be the strongest indicator of functional outcome in our study of patients enrolled in cardiac rehabilitation, depression was the second most important factor.[28]

Affective Disorder

Patients who are experiencing significant depression in association with the cardiovascular conditions may experience problems with psychomotor and cognitive slowing, reduced attention, and poor effort secondary to their affective disorder.[29] Accordingly, an assessment of depressive symptoms is imperative for all patients. If significant depressive symptoms are present, then conclusions regarding subtle cognitive findings primarily related to effort and psychomotor slowing should be withheld until there has been treatment of the symptoms and reduction in depression severity. There are many depression assessment measures that can be used for this purpose. The Beck Depression Inventory-II and Geriatric Depression Scale are most widely used.[30, 31, 32]

While depression is a significant concern among patients with chronic cardiovascular disease, it is not a ubiquitous finding. In our cardiovascular disease research cohorts, only about 15% of patients had elevated scores suggestive of moderate depression. It should be emphasized that, in these studies, patients with a history of chronic, intractable affective disorder were excluded, which may contribute in part to the low prevalence, though those cases have typically undergone psychiatric intervention apart from their cardiovascular disease experience.

Health Status and Quality of Life

While major depression is not present in most patients with heart disease, emotional distress is quite common, along with perceived changes in changes in both physical and psychological health status. This often involves changes in social or occupational roles as a result of their illness. To assess these changes, the SF-36 is a useful instrument for monitoring both overall perceived health status and underlying factors contributing to health status and QOL.[33] There are also many specific QOL inventories that are useful in this regard, and these should be included in a comprehensive assessment.

Fatigue and Apathy

Neuropsychiatric symptoms are also important to assess. In particular, apathy and fatigue are quite common. There are several possible reasons for these symptoms. Obviously, the contribution of comorbid major depression should be given strong weighting when present. In many cases, though, there may be no mood disturbance or severe psychological distress. Instead, patients may exhibit apathy, fatigue, psychomotor slowing, and other "vegetative" symptoms. Late-life presentation of such symptoms among people with no prior history of affective disorder (i.e., "late life depression") has been associated with vascular cognitive impairment and frontal-subcortical dysfunction secondary to white matter disturbance tied to microvascular disease. Accordingly, if a patient shows these symptoms without the other mood disturbances of major depression, the possibility that these symptoms relate to the cardiovascular-associated brain dysfunction should be given stronger consideration.

It is important in such cases to correlate these symptoms with neurocognitive findings from tests of attention, executive functioning, and processing speed, and also evidence of possible microvascular disease as evidenced by white matter hyperintensities on brain MRI. An alternative that should also be considered among patients who primarily report fatigue and problems with effort is that they are experiencing these symptoms because of the severity of their heart disease (i.e., reduced cardiac output and deconditioning). Therefore, clinicians should determine whether the patient's fatigue relates to systemic physical status and generalized weakness, as opposed to having brain origins. To assess apathy and related behavioral disturbances, the Frontal Systems Behavioral Scale (FRSBE[34]) is included in our battery. The Neuropsychiatric Inventory[35] may also be useful in this regard. There are also several good measures of apathy and fatigue that may be clinically useful, including the Apathy Evaluation Scale[36] and the Fatigue Severity Scale.[37]

Psychological Experience of Cardiovascular Disease

Apart from specific symptoms, such as depression, apathy, and fatigue, patients who are diagnosed with cardiovascular disease tend to experience some degree of anxiety and uncertainty about their future. Feelings of loss of control are very common, and their manifestation depends on factors such as internal or external locus of control and individual coping strategies.

There are often several issues that the individual may try to work through, such as finding an attribution for their disease. A grief process may also occur, which sometimes involves anger, despair, and eventual acceptance. These psychological adaptations to chronic illness have been well described in the field of health psychology and will not be reviewed in detail now. Our general approach to assessing for these factors is to use the clinical interview as a vehicle for exploring the individual patient's feelings and thoughts about their illness.

Self-Perceived Cognitive Impairment

One of the intriguing findings from our previous studies of cardiovascular disease is the relationship between self-perceived cognitive difficulties and objective findings of impairment based on neurocognitive assessment. While some patients are very sensitive and accurate with respect to their cognitive difficulties, this is not generally the rule. Gunstad et al. found that patients who reported the most cognitive impairment during baseline assessment tended to have greater emotional distress and poorer perceived qualify of life.[38] In contrast, patients with severe cognitive impairment often lack insight into their problems.[39] This tendency is well recognized in the neuropsychological literature.

Interestingly, our recent findings suggest that patients' self-report of cognitive symptoms at baseline actually corresponds more strongly to decline in functioning over time than to baseline performance. This suggests that, besides reflecting emotional distress, many patients may be picking up on very subtle deficits that are not clinically significant at baseline, but are vulnerable to change. Accordingly, the relationship between self-report and objective findings requires additional study.

From a clinical perspective, cognitive complaints should not be dismissed as only an indicator of emotional distress. They should be taken seriously, with efforts to relate the subjective and objective findings. If there is a large discrepancy, then the possibility of psychological factors' contributing to the patient's self perceptions should be factored in, though with an openness to the possibility that they may be tuning into subtle, early problems. Furthermore, the presence of heightened concern about cognitive decline should be viewed as an important piece of clinical information that often should lead the clinician to consider referral for psychotherapy to address the functional effects of the patient's illness on their life.

Clinical Neuropsychological Decision-Making for Cardiovascular Disease

Summary of Important Clinical Considerations

1. *Why is the patient being referred to you?* This is an essential question to be considered prior to conducting any neuropsychological assessment. It is important to know whether the patient has requested the evaluation because of their own concern; whether family or clinicians are concerned about their mental status changes (even though the patient is not) or whether the referral is coming as part of a standard protocol. Patients who are self-referred because of concerns about cognitive changes associated with their heart disease often have a much greater level of awareness than those who have impairments, but lack such awareness. For self-referred patients, the issues discussed in the previous section should be considered. For patients being referred because of family or physician concern, it is essential to determine what aspects of the person's functioning have been particularly troubling and whether there have been changes in functional capacity in everyday living. Please see Fig. 7-1.
2. *What is the clinical context?* Neuropsychological assessments conducted in inpatient hospital settings usually differ substantially from those conducted in outpatient clinics. Requests for assessment in inpatient settings are usually made because there is concern that a patient's hospital course is not proceeding as expected, and the clinicians involved with the case are seeking help with planning subsequent care. Often there is an underlying question about whether a particular patient needs to go to a rehabilitation hospital prior to returning home.

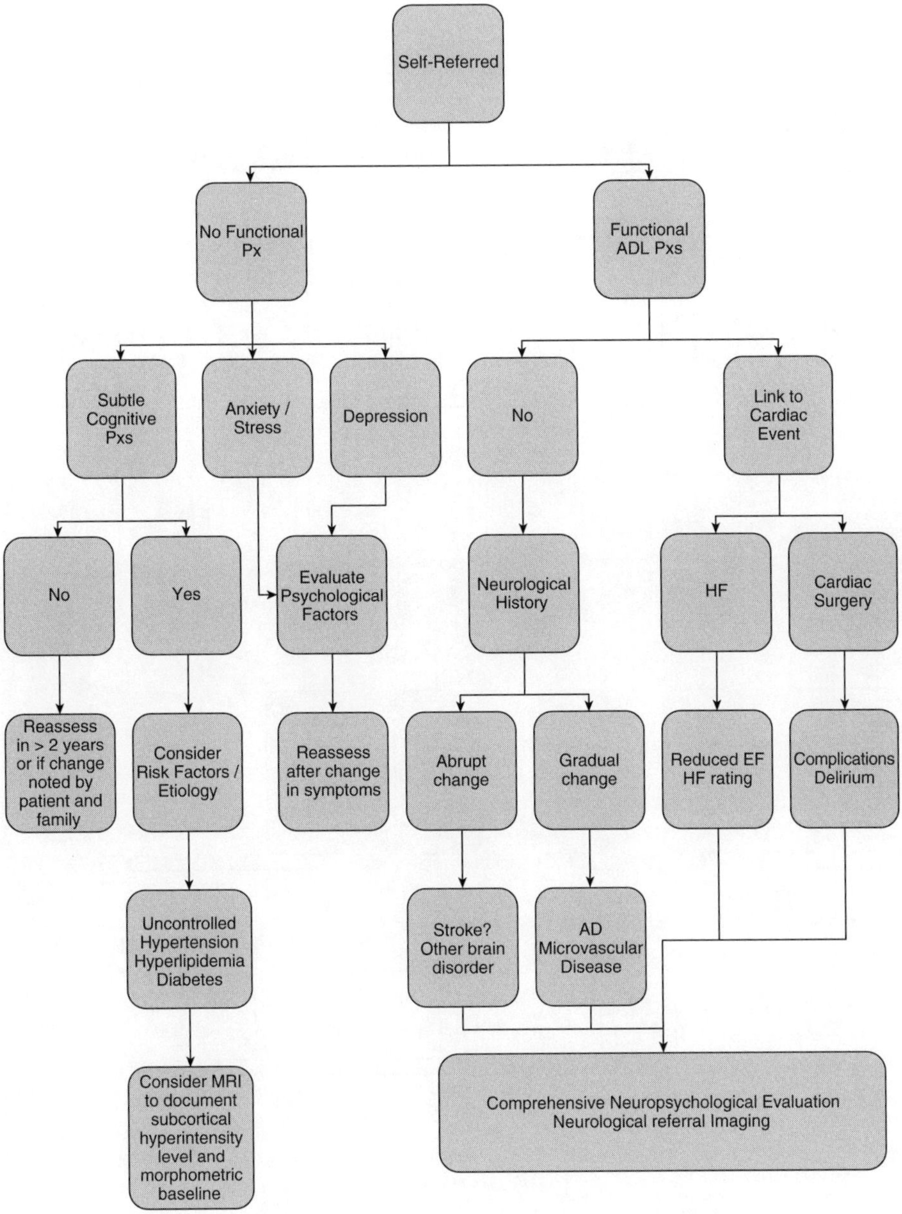

Figure 7-1 Decision tree for self-referred outpatients with CVD.

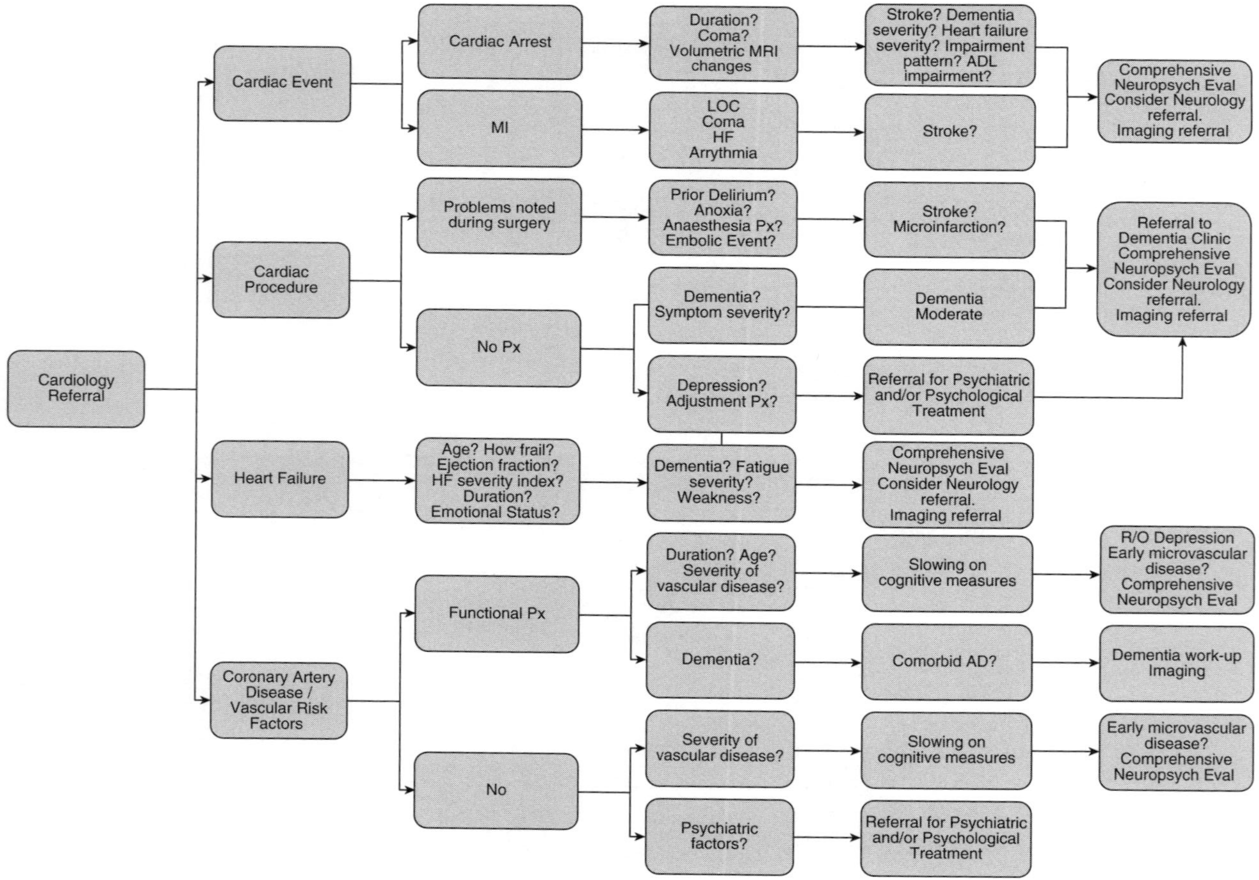

Figure 7-2 Decision tree for outpatients with CVD referred by a cardiologist.

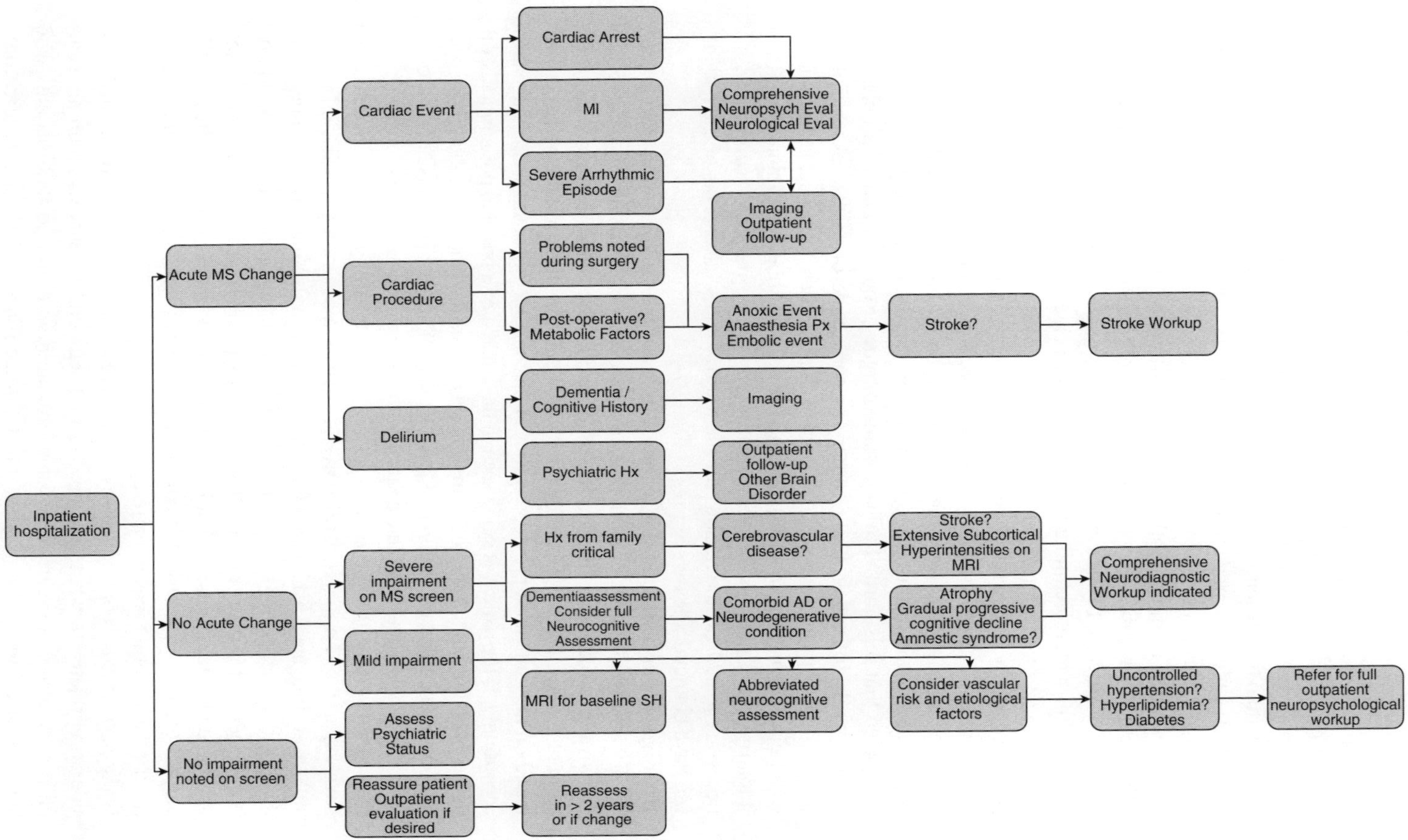

Figure 7-3 Decision tree for inpatients with CVD.

In other cases, the question relates to distinguishing between dementia and delirium in a patient who is confused during the hospitalization. Behavioral or emotional changes that make the patient difficult to manage often drive the referral more than the presence of subtle cognitive changes, even though such changes may exist. Unless the mental status change is very dramatic, there is a tendency to not focus on this issue, given the other medical concerns that may exist. Requests for assessment of more subtle cognitive dysfunction in the hospital setting usually occur when either the patient or their family has observed some change that has raised concern. In such cases, a brief screening evaluation may be initiated in the hospital with a recommendation that more extensive assessment be done on an outpatient basis after the elapse of some recovery time so that the results will more accurately reflect the patient's typical cognitive status post-illness.

In contrast, cardiovascular patients who are referred for outpatient assessment typically are experiencing some problems in daily functioning or their cognitive experience that is disturbing to them or their family. Often the patient has been counseled that it is normal to have some fatigue or other cognitive problems for a short while following major surgery or some type of cardiac event, but that they should improve over time. Concern builds when the patient continues to experience cognitive problems. Beyond the need to obtain an evaluation of these impairments, it may not be clear what is driving the referral. Accordingly, it is necessary to address the reasons for the referral and what aspects of the patient's life have changed. Please see Figs. 7-2 and 7-3.

3. *What type of cardiovascular condition exists; what level of analysis is appropriate?* As discussed in Chapter 1, an important consideration for the neuropsychology of cardiovascular disease is the level of analysis that one employs when considering particular cases. It is recommended that clinicians consider formulating hypotheses based on the guidelines provided earlier in this chapter and categorizing the patient accordingly. If the patient is being seen in the context of a pre- and postsurgical evaluation, then this should trigger a different set of questions than if a patient is presenting post-myocardial infarction and has a history of stroke. The consideration of the level of analysis should influence many of the other issues discussed subsequently.
4. *Has there been a specific cardiac event?* Distinguishing between patients that have experienced a major cardiac event, such as a severe myocardial infarction, and those that have a history of chronic, low-grade symptoms is important, as those with episodes of reduced cardiac output are at higher risk for neurocognitive impairment. However, caution also needs to be applied in this regard. Events that have affected the heart, but have not impaired cardiac function (i.e., cardiac output) are less likely to have contributed to cognitive problems than if cardiac function and output was impaired.
5. *Is the patient experiencing heart failure?* This is a more narrowly defined consideration related to what was previously discussed. Patients with chronic heart failure are at much greater risk for neurocognitive problems than patients who have coronary artery disease, but intact cardiac function. The effects of chronic

heart failure on cognitive function appear to be particularly strong among elderly people who are frail. In fact, this should be considered an important risk factor for worsening cognitive function.

It is noteworthy that no single measure of cardiac disease severity exists that is universally accepted; nor is there even agreement among all cardiologists over what disease severity means in this regard, or on the basis for defining severity. This issue relates directly back to the different levels of analysis that are possible when considering cardiovascular disease. However, certain rating scales have been developed to provide indices of the extent of heart failure (e.g., New York Heart Association Classification; Minnesota Heart Failure Scale). Such ratings provide a reasonable way of determining severity, at least as related to heart failure and its functional impact.

6. *How chronic and severe are underlying risk factors?* While in their own right risk factors are not sufficient basis for assuming cardiovascular-associated brain dysfunction, there is now considerable evidence that patients with long-standing uncontrolled blood pressure and hyperlipidemia are at much greater risk for developing cerebrovascular problems than patients with controlled risk factors, apart from their cardiac function. The reasons for this, which are discussed in detail in other sections of the book, generally relate to the fact that vascular risk factors contribute to the development of atherosclerosis, endothelial dysfunction, and a general breakdown in cerebral hemodynamic function. Vessels thicken and become stiff and inelastic, unable to respond to changes in perfusion. When considering patients presenting with significant white matter abnormality on MRI, but no other specific neuroimaging findings, consideration should be given to the possibility that microvascular changes are occurring, and vascular risk factors are contributory. However, it then becomes important to monitor changes in vascular function, risk factors, and cognitive function over time to see if MRI changes correspond to worsening of vascular function and cognitive status.
7. *Is there a history of chronic uncontrolled diabetes?* This should be considered a red flag to clinicians. Diabetes increases the risk of cerebrovascular disturbance and specifically, microvascular disease. Diabetes frequency emerges as one of the strongest predictors of poor cognitive outcome among patients with cardiovascular disease.
8. *Does the patient report past cardiac arrest? Do records substantiate this?* Definitive evidence that cardiac arrest has occurred should be weighted strongly and is likely to influence the interpretation of neuropsychological findings from the assessment. For example, if a patient exhibits dementia and evidence of brain atrophy, along with a history of cardiac arrest, conclusions regarding the possibility of Alzheimer's disease should be made with greater caution. The possibility that the patient has experienced a vascular dementia secondary to global cerebral hypoperfusion must be given strong consideration.
9. *Is the patient experiencing atrial fibrillation? What type of arrhythmia exists?* While the presence of cardiac arrhythmia is not in is own right an indicator or direct cause of cognitive problems, certain arrhythmias are associated with

increased stroke risk. Therefore, among patients with chronic problems with heart rhythm, the possibility of prior embolic stroke should be considered. Prospectively, these patients should be monitored for this possibility as well and strongly encouraged to seek treatment to control the arrhythmia.

10. *Are the reported cognitive problems occurring postsurgically?* In such cases it is very important to obtain as much information as possible regarding any adverse events that occurred during the surgery, and whether major postoperative mental status changes were observed. In the absence of early problems, it is unlikely that patients will exhibit major problems when they are well into their recovery. However, there is one important caveat. This conclusion depends on whether the patient, their family, or the medical staff was inclined to be concerned about mild to moderate cognitive difficulties early on. In some cases, these problems may have been dismissed as "within normal limits," and only became burdensome when the patient returned to their home or occupational setting.
11. *What type of procedure was conducted?* Historically, the greatest risk for cognitive sequelae occurred with valve replacement surgery, followed by CABG. However, statistics regarding these risks are continually changing as new methods are developed. Therefore, it is important for clinicians working with these patients to stay abreast of new developments in the field of cardiothoracic surgery and their impact on stroke risk and neurological outcome. In contrast to open-heart surgical procedures, angioplasty and procedures associated with angioplasty are safer from a neurocognitive perspective, though there remains some risk that emboli could be released into the bloodstream by the catheter dislodging plaque or fat.
12. *Are findings obtained during the acute illness phase subject to transient effects?* If so, neurocognitive assessments conducted during this period need to be framed with respect to the underlying question to be addressed and the goals of the assessment. In cases involving assessment post-CABG or valve replacement, cognitive difficulties are relatively common in the days following surgery, so monitoring should be done in the days and weeks that follow, with a more comprehensive reassessment after three months, or when the patient has returned home and is concerned about continuing problems.
13. *Longitudinal assessment should be considered routinely.* For cases involving cardiovascular disease without stroke, cardiac arrest, or postsurgical sequelae, this assessment should probably be done 12 to 24 months after the initial workup, or sooner if perceived changes in functioning are observed. If a patient exhibits relatively intact cognitive function on baseline assessment, is young, and has coronary artery disease, with relatively mild, well-controlled risk factors and no evidence of heart failure, then they probably can forgo reassessment, with such evaluation conducted primarily if there is any indication of a functional change.

Unresolved Clinical Issues

In this final section, we will review several unresolved questions related to the neuropsychological assessment of cardiovascular disease patients. Some of these questions may surface in the inquiries or concerns of patients or their families when feedback is given regarding the assessment results. Others are of greater relevance for neuropsychologists or other clinicians when conceptualizing findings from cases.

1. *What is the temporal course of brain effects among patients with severe chronic cardiovascular disease?* While there is now compelling evidence of an association between cardiovascular disease and neurocognitive function, how these effects on brain function evolve and progress among patients with chronic severe cardiovascular disease is not yet known. Some studies of post-CABG cognitive outcome suggest that over a three-year period patients who have undergone surgery do not worsen appreciably relative to controls.[40] However, patients undergoing CABG in these studies typically do not have chronic heart failure and are not necessarily the patients most susceptible to decline. Long-term prospective studies of neurocognitive function among patients with severe cardiovascular disease have not been conducted yet to address this question.
2. *Are patients with severe and chronic cardiovascular disease likely to develop vascular dementia due to chronic hypoperfusion?* This was a primary question that motivated our research to date. Most of the evidence that we have collected on patients over the short term (i.e., less than 48 months of follow-up) suggests that the systemic vascular factors associated with heart disease correspond to problems with attention and executive functioning, particularly speed of processing. Whether these problems eventually evolve into a more global dementia in these patients is not clear.
3. *Do the white matter abnormalities observed on MRI among patients with cerebral microvascular disease eventually lead to cortical changes, such as atrophy?* This question relates to the previous one, and needs to be resolved to achieve greater understanding about the effects of chronic cardiovascular disease on the brain. While the extent of white matter hyperintensities on MRI relates strongly to the severity of attention, executive, and processing-speed deficits observed on neuropsychological assessments, it is not clear how this pathology results in more global dementia if the disease progresses. In our past studies of VaD, white matter abnormalities did relate to impairments in these same cognitive domains, whereas the severity of dementia was associated with overall cortical volume. Given that chronic cerebral hypoperfusion is considered to be one basis for vascular dementia, more information is needed to determine whether these effects occur first with respect to cerebral white matter, with cortical changes resulting from diaschesis, or some other process.
4. *Does chronic cardiovascular disease contribute to the development of, or exacerbate the progression of Alzheimer's disease or other neurodegenerative disorders?* Cerebrovascular disease typically emerges as a risk factor for the development

of Alzheimer's-type dementia. Yet the extent to which vascular pathophysiology actually contributes to the underlying neuropathology and progression of the neuronal disturbance underlying AD remains an open question, and one for which there are strong viewpoints on both sides of the argument. It is possible that cerebrovascular disturbances associated with heart disease exacerbate the cognitive disturbances associated with AD by reducing cognitive and brain reserves without directly affecting the underlying neurodegenerative condition. This remains an important area for further investigation. At this point, clinicians should probably counsel patients that a direct link between cardiovascular disease and AD has not been established, but that vascular and other risk factors that affect the brain beyond AD are likely to have adverse consequences.

5. *To what extent can these vascular brain effects be prevented or slowed through programs of exercise and reconditioning, diet, or increasing cardiac output and cerebral perfusion through other forms of treatment?* This is obviously an important question for patients and their families and one that often emerges when the results of the assessment are discussed. Intuitively, it seems that there should be benefit from this approaches, though the verdict is still out and clinical trials treating cognitive function as the outcome are necessary.

In sum, there are many unresolved questions regarding the extent to which the brain changes associated with cardiovascular disease are a direct result of reduced blood flow to the brain versus the combined effect of hypoperfusion and other pathological processes that are co-occurring. The extent to which improving cardiovascular health improves neurocognitive and functional outcome requires additional study. Cardiovascular disease patients and their families should be encouraged to do whatever is possible to sustain optimal heart function, with potential benefits for the brain connected to the broader importance of such intervention for overall health and quality of life.

Notes

1. Vermeer SE, Koudstaal PJ, Oudkerk M, Hofman A, Breteler MM. Prevalence and risk factors of silent brain infarcts in the population-based Rotterdam Scan Study. *Stroke*. 2002;33:21–25.
2. Cohen RA, Poppas A, Forman DE, et al. Vascular and cognitive functions associated with cardiovascular disease in the elderly. *J Clin Exp Neuropsychol*. 2008;16:1–15.
3. *Miller EN. California Computerized Assessment Battery (CalCAP) Manual*. Los Angeles: Norland Software, 1990.
4. Heilman KM, Valenstein E (Eds.), *Clinical Neuropsychology*, 4th ed. New York: Oxford University Press, 2003.
5. Lezak MD, Howieson DB, Loring DW, Hannay J, Fischer JS. *Neuropsychological Assessment*, 4th ed. New York: Oxford University Press, 2004.
6. Reichenberg A, Dahlman KL, Mosovich S, Silverstein JH. Neuropsychiatric consequences of coronary artery bypass grafting and noncardiovascular surgery. *Dial Clin Neurosci*. 2007;9:85–91.
7. Selnes OA, McKhann GM, Borowicz LM Jr, Grega MA. Cognitive and neurobehavioral dysfunction after cardiac bypass procedures. *Neurol Clin*. 2006;24:133–45.

8. Randolph C. *RBANS manual: Repeatable Battery for the Assessment of Neuropsychological Status*. San Antonio, TX: The Psychological Corporation, 1998.
9. Loponen P, Luther M, Wistbacka JO, et al. Postoperative delirium and health-related quality of life after coronary artery bypass grafting. *Scand Cardiovasc J*. 2008;42:337–44.
10. Mattis S. Mental status examination for organic mental syndrome in the elderly patient. In Bellak L, Karasu TB (Eds.), *Geriatric psychiatry*. New York: Grune & Stratton, 1976.
11. Mattis S. *Dementia Rating Scale (DRS)*. Odessa, FL: Psychological Assessment Resources, 1988.
12. Psychological Corporation, The. *Wechsler Abbreviated Scale of Intelligence (WASI)*. San Antonio, TX: The Psychological Corporation, 1999.
13. Wechsler D. *Wechsler Adult Intelligence Scale–III*. San Antonio, TX: The Psychological Corporation, 1997.
14. Delis DC, Kramer JH, Kaplan E, Ober BA. *California Verbal Learning Test—Second Edition (CVLT-II)*. San Antonio, TX: Psychological Corporation, 2000.
15. Benedict R. *Brief Visual Memory Test—Revised*. Odessa, FL: Psychological Assessment Resources, 1997.
16. Brandt J. The Hopkins Verbal Learning Test: Development of a new verbal memory test with six equivalent forms. *Clin Neuropsychol*. 1985;5:125–142.
17. Kaplan E, Goodglass H, Weintraub S. *Boston naming test*. Philadelphia: Lea and Febiger, 1983.
18. Benton AL, Hamsher KdeS. *Multilingual aphasia examination*. Iowa City: AJA Associates, 1989.
19. Spreen O, Strauss E. *A compendium of neuropsychological tests*, 2nd ed. New York: Oxford University Press, 1998.
20. Klove H. Clinical neuropsychology. In: Forster FM (Ed.), *The medical clinics of North America*. New York: Saunders, 1963.
21. Reitan R. Validity of the Trail Making Test as an indicator of organic brain damage. *Percept Mot Skills*. 1958;8:271–276.
22. Stroop JR. Studies of interference in serial verbal reactions. *J Exp Psychol*. 1935;18: 643–662.
23. Jensen AR, Rohwer WD. The Stroop Color-Word Test: a review. *Acta Psychologica*. 1966;25:36–93.
24. Berg EA. A simple objective treatment for measuring flexibility in thinking. *J Gen Psychol*. 1948;39:15–22.
25. Grant DA, Berg EA. A behavioral analysis of the degree of reinforcement and ease of shifting to new responses in a Weigl-type card sorting problem. *J Exp Psychol*. 1948;38:404–411.
26. Goel V, Grafman J. Are the frontal lobes implicated in "planning" functions? Interpreting data from the Tower of Hanoi. *Neuropsychologia*. 1995;33:623–642.
27. Cohen RA. *Neuropsychology of attention*. New York: Plenum Publishing, 1993.
28. Cohen RA, Moser DJ, Clark MM, et al. Neurocognitive functioning and improvement in quality of life following participation in cardiac rehabilitation. *Am J Cardiol*. 1999;83: 1374–1378.
29. Han L, McCusker J, Cole M, Abrahamowicz M, Capek R. 12-month cognitive outcomes of major and minor depression in older medical patients. *American J Geriatr Psychiatry*. 2008;16:742–51.
30. Beck AT, Steer RA, Brown GK. *Beck Depression Inventory–II. Manual*. San Antonio, TX: Psychological Corporation, 1996.
31. Brink TL, Yesavage JA, Lum O, et al. Screening tests for geriatric depression. *Clin Gerontologist*. 1982;37–44.

32. Yesavage JA, Brink TL, Rose TL, et al. Development and validation of a geriatric depression screening scale: A preliminary report. *J Psychiatry Res*, 1982;17:37–49.
33. McHorney CA, Ware JE Jr, Raczek AE. The MOS 36-Item Short-Form Health Survey (SF-36): II. Psychometric and clinical tests of validity in measuring physical and mental health constructs. *Med Care*. 1993;31:247–263.
34. Grace J, Malloy P. *Frontal Systems Behavior Scale (FrSBe): Professional manual*. Lutz, Florida: Psychological Assessment Resources, 2001.
35. Cummings JL, Mega MS, Gray K, Rosemberg-Thompson S, Gornbein T. The neuropsychiatric inventory: Comprehensive assessment of psychopathology in dementia. *Neurology*. 1994;44:2308–2314.
36. Marin RS, Biedrzycki RC, Firinciogullari S. Reliability and validity of the Apathy Evaluation Scale. *Psychiatry Res*. 1991;38:143–62.
37. Krupp LB, LaRocca NG, Muir-Nash J, Steinberg AD. The fatigue severity scale. Application to patients with multiple sclerosis and systemic lupus erythematosus. *Arch Neurol*. 1989;46:1121–3.
38. Gunstad J, Cohen RA, Paul RH, Tate DF, Hoth KF, Poppas A. Understanding reported cognitive dysfunction in older adults with cardiovascular disease. *Neuropsychiatr Dis Treat*. 2006;2:213–218.
39. Clément F, Belleville S, Gauthier S. Cognitive complaint in mild cognitive impairment and Alzheimer's disease. *J Int Neuropsychol Soc*. 2008;14:222–232.
40. Selnes OA, Grega MA, Bailey MM, Pham L, Zeger S, Baumgartner WA, McKhann GM. Neurocognitive outcomes 3 years after coronary artery bypass graft surgery: A controlled study. *Ann Thorac Surg*. 2007;84:1885–1896.

8

BLOOD PRESSURE AND COGNITIVE FUNCTION

John Gunstad, Kelly Stanek, Ashley Szabo, and Lynn Kakos

An extensive literature connects blood pressure to neurocognitive outcome, including links to both cognitive function and neuroimaging findings. Traditionally, people have looked at the adverse effects of high blood pressure on cognitive function or dementia status. However, new lines of programmatic research suggest that the relationship between blood pressure and cognitive function is much more complicated that commonly believed and warrants reexamination. For example, recent studies indicate that:

- Persons who develop Alzheimer's disease show a decline in blood pressure in the years immediately preceding onset.[1, 2]
- Longitudinal studies show that lower cognitive function at age 11 is associated with elevated blood pressure in middle age.[3]
- Subtle cognitive deficits are found in normotensive persons who have hypertensive parents.[4]

Key findings from the quickly growing field of blood pressure and cognitive function are presented below. Particular attention will be given to the evolving understanding of how low blood pressure and variability of blood pressure levels over time predict neurocognitive outcome through the following chapter sections:

1) High blood pressure
2) Anti-hypertensive medications
3) Low blood pressure
4) Blood pressure patterns
5) Family history of hypertension

High Blood Pressure

Blood pressure demonstrates a predictable daily and lifetime pattern. During a normal 24-hour period, blood pressure is highest during waking daytime hours, lowest during the night, and slowly rises just prior to awakening.[5–7] Over the course of an individual's lifetime, systolic blood pressure typically increases from the third to eighth decade of life due to changes in the vascular system, whereas diastolic blood pressure rises until a person reaches 60 years of age, when it begins to decline.[8]

Criteria for normal blood pressure levels are a systolic blood pressure less than 120 mmHg and a diastolic blood pressure less than 80 mmHg. Persons with levels of 120–139 or 80–89 are considered prehypertensive. Two categories of hypertension have been established, with Stage 1 having levels of 140–159 or 90–99, and Stage 2 with 160 or higher and 100 or higher, respectively.[9] Hypertension is one of the most common medical conditions, as nearly one-third of adult Americans meet these criteria—including more than 50% of people over 60 years of age.[10] Hypertension is expected to become even more prevalent in coming years through societal shifts in demographic and medical factors.[11, 12] Hypertension is a known risk factor for many other medical conditions, including end-stage renal disease, atrial fibrillation, and congestive heart failure.[13, 14]

High Blood Pressure and Neurocognitive Outcome

In addition to these conditions, hypertension is also a known contributor to poor neurocognitive outcome. Hypertension is the strongest predictor for stroke after age, with hypertensive persons at three to five times greater risk.[15, 16] It has been estimated that up to 80% of stroke-related events could be reduced by making lifestyle changes, including improved management of blood pressure levels.[17] Given its association with stroke, it is not surprising that hypertension is also an important risk factor for vascular dementia.[18] Less clear is the association between hypertension and Alzheimer's disease, perhaps due to the long interval between onset of these conditions.[19] Although most prospective studies demonstrate an increased risk for Alzheimer's disease in hypertensive patients, this finding is not universal.[18]

Rather than using dementia diagnosis as an outcome, studies more frequently assess the association between high blood pressure levels and cognitive test performance. Most cross-sectional studies suggest that hypertension is associated with poorer neuropsychological function, particularly on tests of attention, learning and memory, executive functioning, and some visuospatial abilities.[20–23] However, an excellent review by Qui et al. (2005)[24] illustrates the many conflicting findings in this literature, as study results range from no association, to poorer cognition with higher blood pressure, poorer cognition with lower blood pressure, and a U-shaped relationship.

Prospective studies linking midlife blood pressure levels to late-life cognitive function more consistently show an adverse effect of hypertension on neurocognitive function. Though findings vary somewhat, higher systolic and diastolic blood pressures are typically associated with lower cognitive function, greater cognitive decline, and higher risk for dementia.[26–27] Longitudinal studies in elderly patients also show an adverse effect from high blood pressure on cognitive function, but they suggest that low blood pressure may be an important contributor as well.[28]

Recent, innovative studies have begun to examine the association between high blood pressure and cognitive function in novel patient and community samples. For example, children with elevated systolic blood pressure have been found to exhibit poorer performance on neuropsychological testing, including tests involving attention and visuospatial skills.[29] Large studies also suggest an adverse effect of higher systolic and diastolic pressures on cognitive function in young and middle-aged adults, including reduced attention, verbal learning, memory, verbal fluency, and inductive reasoning.[30–32]

Taken in sum, these findings suggest that hypertension has adverse neurocognitive effects across the lifespan. However, full determination of the impact of hypertension on the brain is precluded due to the many methodological and statistical differences across studies, including the criteria used to define hypertension, specific cognitive tests used, age of participants, duration of blood pressure levels, treatment effects, and medical comorbidities. Each of these factors has the potential to obscure the true relationship and influence the observed findings. For example, some studies have suggested that high blood pressure may interact with age,[33] have greater effects for women,[31] and interact with conditions like obesity or type 2 diabetes to produce even greater cognitive impairment.[22, 34]

Mechanisms of High Blood Pressure

A growing number of physiological mechanisms have been explored to better understand the association between high blood pressure and poor neurocognitive outcome. A recent review by Hanon and colleagues (2003)[35] connects many of these mechanisms and proposes that hypertension initially causes adverse vascular changes, which ultimately produce interruption in cerebral blood flow and metabolism. Additionally, these pathological vascular changes can also cause stroke and chronic hypoperfusion, thus leading to vascular dementia or an interaction with early stages of Alzheimer's pathology. Substantial support exists for each step of this model, including studies demonstrating that high blood pressure is associated with:

- Development and progression of white matter abnormalities[36–40]
- Atrophy in frontal, temporal, and occipital lobes[36–38, 41]
- Atrophy in specific structures important for cognitive function, including the hippocampus, amygdala, anterior cingulate, and thalamus[42–45]
- Neurofibrillary tangles in the neurocortex and hippocampus.[26]

Recent empirical and theoretical work[35, 46–49] extends this work and proposes a number of additional, complementary mechanisms by which hypertension can adversely impact cognitive function, including:

- Disruption in blood–brain barrier function
- Reduced functional neuroconnectivity
- Vascular remodeling and impaired autoregulation
- Greater oxidative stress and/or systemic inflammation
- Amyloid angiopathy
- Cerebral microbleeds

- Altered evoked response potential indices
- Dysregulation of the hypothalamic-pituitary-adrenal (HPA) axis.

An exciting new line of research has started to determine the acute effects of high blood pressure on cognitive function. Using positronic emission tomography (PET), Jennings and colleagues (2003)[50] found hypertensive persons had reduced overall cerebral blood flow and smaller areas of activation in the posterior parietal regions during completion of a spatial two-back task—a pattern they described as the "vascular hypothesis." Further work to clarify how acute fluctuations in blood pressure impact cognitive function is much needed. The increased availability of beat-to-beat blood pressure monitors may facilitate this key insight.

Antihypertensive Medication

Despite the adverse consequences of hypertension and many available medications, many individuals do not know their blood pressure levels.[51] For example, in a sample of older adults with hypertension, 31% were unaware they had the condition, 12% were aware but were not treating it, 37% were treated but still had uncontrolled blood pressure levels, and just 19% had fully controlled levels.[52] In addition to the many medical complications from uncontrolled hypertension, these patients are not benefiting from the stroke-protective effects of these medications.[53–55]

Several classes of antihypertensive medications exist, including:

- Diuretics
- Beta-blockers
- Angiotensin-converting enzyme (ACE) inhibitors
- Angiotensin-receptor blockers (ARBs)
- Calcium-channel blockers
- Alpha blockers
- Vasodilators.

Each of these medications has been shown to reducing blood pressure levels. However, of particular relevance to the current review, they reduce blood pressure through different physiological mechanisms. At the current time, the literature is not sufficient to determine which class of medications, if any, provides the greatest benefits to cognitive function over time. As a result, findings from this complicated literature will be presented in generalized terms.

Neurocognitive Benefits of Antihypertensive Medication

Many studies suggest that, in addition to reducing the risk of poor medical outcome, blood-pressure-lowering medication may also reduce the risk of poor neurocognitive outcome, including stroke.[56] For example, the Syst-Eur randomized clinical trial followed participants for two years and found lower incidence of both stroke and dementia during that time.[56] However, findings have varied widely across studies, and the many methodological differences make direct comparison difficult. For example, the Systolic Hypertension in the Elderly Program[58] and the Medical Research Council Treatment Trial of Hypertension in Older Adults[58] found antihypertensive medication provided little or no cognitive benefit. The Study on Cognition and Prognosis in the Elderly trial enrolled nearly 5000 hypertensive participants between the ages of 70 and 89 and found add-on treatment for blood pressure reduced cognitive decline and stroke risk, but only in those with slightly impaired cognitive function.[59]

While work from large epidemiological studies generally suggests that persons with untreated hypertension have the poorest neurocognitive outcome, treatment does not ensure good outcome.[25, 26] Consistent with this notion, one large study found that untreated hypertensives had an odds ratio of 4:3 for cognitive decline, whereas treated participants had an odds ratio of 1:9.[60] The Rotterdam study[61] found antihypertensive use was associated with lower risk for vascular dementia—a pattern consistent with the lower prevalence of white matter abnormalities in persons who are on these medications.[62, 56, 39] The Perindopril Protection Against Recurrent Stroke Study (PROGRESS) found no generalized effect of antihypertensive medication on dementia onset, but reduced onset in persons with past history of stroke.[60] In persons with reported memory problems, antihypertensive treatment is associated with better cognitive function and lower prevalence of Alzheimer's disease.[63]

As mentioned above, the many methodological differences across studies makes direct comparison difficult. In addition to the potential for direct effects due to the specific medication employed in each study, many other possible moderator variables exist. For example, it is possible that neurocognitive benefits may differ across racial/ethnic groups.[64] Treatment duration may be important, as persons starting antihypertensive medication use prior to the age of 60 appear to have better cognitive outcomes.[65] Few studies have directly examined adherence to prescribed medication regimens, despite the high rates of noncompliance with prescription regimens in persons with cardiovascular disease.[66]

Another potential moderating variable is the possible acute effects of antihypertensive medication on cognitive function. One study, by Muldoon et al. (2002),[67] examined the potential acute effects of six different antihypertensive medications on cognitive function during a six-week period. All medications adversely impacted finger-tapping speed and performance on Trail Making Test A and B, but improved Digit Symbol Substitution and backward Digit Span performance. No effects on tests of learning and memory were reported.

A final consideration for work in this area involves the optimal level of blood pressure for cognitive function, particularly in older adults. A growing number of studies indicate a U-shaped relationship between blood pressure indices and poor neurocognitive outcome. For example, the Swedish Kungsholmen project found that persons with a systolic blood pressure from 141 mmHg –160 mmHg had the lowest risk of dementia, even lower than persons with a systolic blood pressure lower than 140 mmHg.[68, 69] This finding is consistent with the growing literature on the potential adverse effects of low blood pressure on cognitive function. Findings from this rapidly growing area are presented below.

Low Blood Pressure

Though less frequently examined than high blood pressure, there is growing evidence that low blood pressure is also associated with poor neurocognitive outcome. No universal criteria exist for the diagnosis of hypotension, as it is most often diagnosed on the basis of clinical signs and symptoms. The World Health Organization (1978)[70] proposed diagnosis is warranted when systolic blood pressure is below 110 mmHg in males or 100 mmHg in females, regardless of diastolic blood pressure levels. However, studies have employed a wide range of other criteria. Furthermore, it is important to distinguish chronic hypotension from secondary hypotension and orthostatic blood pressure changes.[71, 72] Secondary hypotension is the result of other medical conditions or medications, whereas orthostatic hypotension is often defined as a reduction by 20 mmHg in systolic blood pressure or 10 mmHg diastolic blood pressure within three minutes after standing.[73]

When considered as a whole, low blood pressure is associated with many adverse outcomes, including increased mortality.[74] It is also linked to the experience of a number of unpleasant symptoms, including fatigue, sleepiness, depressed mood, and reduced goal-directed behavior (as briefly reviewed by Duschek 2007).[75] Consistent with these symptoms, persons with low blood pressure exhibit lower quality of life and poorer subjective well-being.[75] More recent work has also demonstrated that low blood pressure is associated with greater risk of Alzheimer's disease, stroke, and cognitive dysfunction.[26, 74, 76, 77] Interestingly, this association appears to be bidirectional, as dementia following lacunar infarct often reduces blood pressure,[78] and blood pressure levels decline with progression of dementia.[28, 79]

Given the different mechanisms that produce chronic and orthostatic hypotension, these conditions will be presented separately below. In each section, brief information will be provided regarding epidemiology and neurocognitive correlates.

Chronic Hypotension

Few studies have directly examined the prevalence of chronic hypotension. One longitudinal, epidemiological study found approximately 0.2% of men and 1.0% of women had systolic pressure below 100 mmHg for eight or more years.[80] The prevalence can be much higher in some patient samples. For example, approximately 5% to 10% of dialysis patients will show persistent hypotension between treatments, with the risk being particularly high for those on long-term dialysis.[81]

Persons with chronic low blood pressure exhibit low heart rate, body temperature, body mass index, and creatinine.[80] Similar to finding elevations of these indices in persons with hypertension, low levels of these indices in persons with chronic hypotension implicate dysregulation in the sympathetic nervous system as a mechanism for the development and maintenance of low blood pressure.

In terms of neurocognitive outcome, persons with essential hypotension are at elevated risk for Alzheimer's disease, and some patient populations with low blood pressure also exhibit increased risk of stroke.[76, 82] A growing number of studies demonstrate that hypotension is associated with cognitive dysfunction prior to the development of these conditions.[83] Deficits are most commonly found in attention, executive function, and memory, particularly on tasks involving information-processing speed.[84–87]

A series of elegant studies by Duschek and colleagues[75, 88] has started to determine the physiological mechanisms for cognitive impairment in persons with essential hypotension. One such study demonstrated that persons with essential hypotension exhibit smaller blood pressure increases during cognitive test completion; in turn, blood pressure increases were closely correlated with blood flow velocity in the middle cerebral artery (MCA) as measured by transcranial Doppler (TCD).[88] A more recent study demonstrated that pharmacologically induced increases in blood pressure were associated with better performance on cognitive testing and increases in multiple TCD indices of cerebral blood flow.[75] These findings implicate reduced cerebral perfusion as a likely mechanism for the observed cognitive difficulties in persons with low blood pressure, though further work is much needed.

Orthostatic Hypotension

The operational definition of orthostatic hypotension (OH) varies widely across studies. However, larger studies often seek to identify three forms of OH; namely, systolic OH—typically a drop of greater than 20 mmHg in systolic blood pressure during standing; diastolic OH—involving a drop of more than 10 mmHg in diastolic blood pressure during standing; and consensus OH—often defined as the presence of either of these conditions.[73]

Reported prevalence rates for OH vary widely across study populations, including approximately 1% of healthy individuals, 7% to 17% of patients in acute care settings, and up to 25% of medically ill older adults.[73, 89] OH is associated with a number of adverse outcomes, including greater risk of falls, disability, and affective disturbance in older adults.[89, 90]

Evidence for the association between OH and poor neurocognitive outcome comes from a wide range of studies. Patients with OH resulting from pure autonomic failure exhibit deficits in multiple cognitive domains, including attention, executive functioning, psychomotor speed, and memory.[91] Similar findings emerge in middle-aged and older adults with asymptomatic OH.[92] Recent work has extended the observed relationship between orthostatic blood pressure changes and cognitive function to non-patient groups. For example, overtrained athletes often exhibit abnormalities during orthostatic testing, and the severity of these abnormalities is correlated with poorer performance on an executive function test.[93] Another interesting study found that poorer orthostatic blood pressure regulation in seven- to eleven-year-old children was associated with teacher-assessed effort, despite no differences in achieved grades.[94]

However, not all studies show this pattern. A recent study by Kuo and colleagues (2004)[95] assessed cognitive function and blood pressure changes during postural testing in healthy older adults. Although persons who exhibited a significant increase in supine systolic blood pressure were more than twice as likely to be impaired on a test of speeded executive function, no effect on cognitive function was found for decline in systolic blood pressure while standing.[95]

Such findings encourage further work to better clarify the specific, independent effects of OH on cognitive function, particularly studies that directly examine potential mechanisms. One frequently proposed mechanism for neurocognitive impairment is structural brain changes. A recent study demonstrated that persons with OH exhibit frequent silent brain infarct on neuroimaging.[96] Even in persons with preexisting dementia, OH is associated with greater hyperintensities on MRI, particularly in deep white matter and basal ganglia regions.[97] Several other mechanisms have also been proposed, including reduced cerebral perfusion, sympathetic dysregulation (including while completing cognitive testing), and altered neurotransmitter release.[91, 94]

Future studies in this area may benefit from using the innovative methods employed in other projects. For example, use of beat-to-beat blood pressure devices during a wide range of tasks (e.g., orthostatic, cognitive testing, completion of activities of daily living, etc.) may provide insight into the frequency, severity, and functional impact of OH. Similarly, studies that combine beat-to-beat blood pressure indices with measures of cerebral blood flow during cognitive testing will better inform the temporal sequence needed for impaired neuropsychological function.

Blood Pressure Patterns

As mentioned above, blood pressure exhibits a diurnal pattern and is typically highest during waking daytime hours, lowest during the night, and slowly rises just prior to awakening.[5–7] Most persons qualify as "dippers" and exhibit a reduction of 10% to 20% in blood pressure levels at night, whereas "non-dippers" show little or no nocturnal reduction in blood pressure.[5, 6] The specific mechanism(s) for the absence or blunting of nocturnal blood pressure reduction remains poorly understood, though it has been hypothesized to reflect increased sympathetic and decreased parasympathetic activation throughout the night.[98–100]

A non-dipping pattern of blood pressure is associated with many consequences, including increased risk for mortality and end organ damage.[101, 102] Consistent with these findings, there is reason to believe that absent or reduced nocturnal reductions in blood pressure are also associated with adverse neurocognitive outcomes, including stroke and vascular dementia.[103–106]

Non-dipping and Neurocognitive Outcome

There is growing evidence that ambulatory patterns of blood pressure fluctuation are important and independent contributions to poor neurocognitive function. Much like heart rate variability indices capture perturbations in beat-to-beat heart rate, blood pressure variability indices attempt to capture variations in systolic blood pressure, diastolic blood pressure, or some combination of both.

Recent work suggests that blood pressure variability indices are associated with adverse neurocognitive outcomes, particularly in persons that exhibit a disruption in the typical nocturnal reduction in blood pressure. For example, many studies show non-dipping is associated with poorer cognitive function and brain MRI abnormalities, including infarct and white matter hyperintensities.[105–108] Interestingly, there is also evidence that extreme nocturnal blood pressure reductions are also associated with risk for cerebrovascular disease.[109]

Work from both cross-sectional and prospective studies links non-dipping blood pressure and reduced cognitive function. One such study found lower Mini Mental Status Examination scores in elderly hypertensives who were non-dippers.[104] Reduced nocturnal dipping has also been associated with poorer performance on specific neuropsychological functions, including memory and sensorimotor speed.[108] A larger, prospective examination ($n = 999$) showed adult males with no or inverted dipping patterns had poorer cognitive function 20 years later.[25]

Several possible explanations for these findings have been proposed. One explanation comes from Bellelli and colleagues (2004)[104] and focuses on the disruption of autonomic nervous system (ANS) function found in non-dippers.[98–100] In their model, ANS dysfunction leads to reduced baroreflex sensitivity and eventual cerebral ischemia.[110] Support for this notion is found in the growing number of studies demonstrating an independent relationship between autonomic nervous system function and neuropsychological test performance in both patient and healthy samples.[111, 112] Bellelli et al. (2004)[104] also propose the possibility that the blunted nocturnal decline is compensatory and prevents cerebral hypoperfusion due to vascular pathology.[113, 114] In effect, this model suggests that the chronic elevations in blood pressure are protective, minimizing risk of ischemia secondary to atherosclerosis or arteriosclerosis. Another possibility is similar to the explanations offered for hypertension, in that non-dipping exposes cerebral arteries to chronic blood pressure overload, which can eventually result in white matter lesions or infarct.[108] Finally, it is possible that the directionality of the observed correlation between non-dipping and neurocognitive damage goes the other way, and that the structural brain changes produce non-dipping patterns. Preliminary evidence for this possibility can be found in the studies showing that cerebrovascular disease is known to cause dysregulation of cardiac indices, including blood pressure.[115, 116]

However, not all studies demonstrate that blunted or absent nocturnal blood pressure reduction is associated with adverse neurocognitive outcome. A comparison of older adults with newly diagnosed hypertension found no differences in Mini Mental Status Examination scores or event-related potential activity between dippers and non-dippers.[117] A sophisticated project from van Boxtel and colleagues (2006)[118] found no association between blunted nocturnal blood pressure reduction and either structural brain findings or neuropsychological test findings after adjusting for possible confounds. However, this study showed that white matter lesions were associated to pulse pressure, mean arterial pressure, and systolic blood pressure.[118] Such findings suggest that dipping status might be less important than average 24-hour blood pressure levels for ultimate outcome.[119, 120]

Further work is much needed in this area, particularly studies that can help clarify the contribution of factors that are known to influence both blood pressure and neurocognitive outcome, such as:

- Demographic characteristics (e.g., age, gender, race/ethnicity)
- Thresholds in blood pressure levels that clearly predict impairment
- Effects of duration (i.e., new onset vs. chronic)
- Role of anti-hypertensive treatment.

For example, the potential effects of a morning surge in blood pressure levels remain poorly understood. Some studies have linked a morning surge in blood pressure to positive outcomes, whereas others identify it as a risk factor for cardiovascular events and stroke.[121] A recent study showed that a morning surge in blood pressure was associated with greater risk of functional impairment, suggesting a likely connection to reduced cognitive function, though empirical work is needed.[122]

Acute Blood Pressure Variability and Neurocognitive Outcome

The above studies examining the association between blood pressure variability and neurocognitive outcome usually employ ambulatory blood pressure measurement. In such studies, participants typically wear a monitoring device that continuously records blood pressure for 24 to 48 hours. However, recent work suggests that blood pressure variability during a shorter time period may also predict neurocognitive outcome. For example, work from our lab showed that blood pressure fluctuations during a two-hour period were better predictors of white matter hyperintensities than resting blood pressure levels and history of hypertension in a sample of older adults with cardiovascular disease.[123] These findings are consistent with others linking daytime blood pressure variability to outcomes like white matter changes on neuroimaging[124–126] as well as poorer cognitive function and reduced quality of life.[127, 128]

In addition to the mechanisms described in the above subsection, it is possible that acute blood pressure variability may reflect an exaggerated blood pressure reactivity that leads to poor cognitive outcome. The autonomic nervous system mediates blood pressure response to mental and physiological stressors. In turn, recent work indicates that blood pressure reactivity is an independent risk factor for development of cerebrovascular disease and poorer cognitive function, including memory and executive function.[129, 130] Such findings encourage further work to more clearly determine physiological mechanisms for these associations and their possible clinical utility.

Family History of Hypertension

The final topic for review is the interesting association between family history of hypertension and cognitive function. A small literature demonstrates that normotensive persons with hypertensive parents exhibit subtle deficits on neuropsychological testing, particularly on tests of visuospatial and visual attention.[4] These findings and their possible mechanisms are presented below.

McCann and colleagues (1990)[131] administered a neuropsychological test battery to 79 normotensive male and female undergraduates. Half of this sample reported at least one hypertensive parent, while the remaining half reported no parental history of hypertension. They found that individuals with a family history of hypertension produced poorer time judgments than persons without a family history of hypertension, though no differences emerged on other tests, including measures of sensory perception, psychomotor functioning, and visuospatial abilities.

Pierce and Elias (1993)[132] followed with a study focused on short-term memory differences between persons with and without parental history of hypertension. They administered the Sternberg task (measuring reaction time and speed of short-term memory search), in addition to a collection of commonly used neuropsychological tests, to 32 individuals with a reported history of hypertension in at least one parent and 45 individuals with no reported parental history of hypertension. Significant differences emerged between groups on the Sternberg measure of speed of short-term memory search and recall, with the parental-history group performing worse than those with no parental history.

Waldstein and colleagues (1994)[4] studied 105 normotensive white male undergraduates. They sought to improve previous methodology in this area by distinguishing individuals with one hypertensive parent, two hypertensive parents, and no hypertensive parents into three equal groups and confirming their self-reports of parental hypertension with medical record review. Results showed that persons with two hypertensive parents performed significantly worse than those with no parental history on Block Design and Visual Span. Additionally, they found that individuals with any parental history of hypertension had a lower visuoperceptual threshold on the Critical Flicker Fusion task. No between-group differences emerged for attentional, psychomotor, memory, information processing, or executive domains.

Thyrum and colleagues (1995)[133] extended this work by evaluating the influence of family history of hypertension on cognitive function in young to middle-aged adults with established hypertension. They found that hypertensive men and women with at least one parent with a reported history of hypertension performed worse on Trails B, Digit Span, and Sternberg Memory Search reaction time than hypertensives without a family history and normotensive controls, suggesting that the cognitive impairments associated with genetic predisposition to hypertension may be distinct from those associated with elevated blood pressure.

More recently, Ditto and colleagues (2006)[134] studied 88 French-Canadian 14-year-old boys. They found that, after controlling for socioeconomic status, self-reported parental history of hypertension and normatively elevated systolic blood pressure was related to poorer performance on semantic and letter fluency tasks, Paired Associates Learning, and Digit Span than in normotensive boys without genetic risk.

In combination, these findings demonstrate that individuals with genetic risk for hypertension frequently exhibit reduced performance on visuospatial and memory tasks prior to the development of elevated blood pressure. Additionally, individuals with elevated blood pressure and genetic risk demonstrate a different pattern of neurocognitive deficits, performing worse on tasks involving attention, memory, and executive function than hypertensive individuals without a family history.

Together these finding suggest that there may be genetic and environmental mechanisms independent of those associated with elevated blood pressure that contribute to cognitive deficits in offspring of hypertensives, and these may result in impaired neurocognitive performance prior to the onset of hypertension. However, the exact mechanisms for these cognitive deficits are unclear. A recent functional MRI study sought to determine whether patterns of neural activation during task completion would help clarify underlying mechanisms. Even after adjusting for task performance, persons with a family history of hypertension exhibited lower 2-Back-related activation in the right inferior parietal lobule and the right inferior temporal gyrus, as well as greater deactivation in the posterior cingulate cortex.[135] Although this pattern of activation may help explain past findings of reduced visuospatial performance, its etiology remains unclear.

As discussed by previous authors,[4] the pattern of deficits in hypertensive persons (i.e., attention, psychomotor speed, executive function) differs from that of normotensive persons with family history of hypertension (i.e., visuospatial and visual attention). As a result, attempts to explain these findings are largely speculative. One possible explanation involves cardiovascular reactivity to mental stress. A recent study showed persons with a family history of hypertension had greater diastolic blood pressure reactivity and poorer overall blood pressure recovery from stressors.[136] It is possible that this generalized response to stress may acutely impact cognitive function and ultimately predispose an individual to subsequent development of hypertension. Although some early studies did not find an association between cardiovascular reactivity and poorer mental function, recent work has extended previous efforts and demonstrates associations for indices like heart rate variability[137] and blood pressure.[138] Further work is clearly needed in this area, as a better understanding of the link between family history of hypertension and neurocognitive function may provide key insight into the development of both cardiac and neurological conditions.

Summary and Conclusions

A substantial literature demonstrates an association between blood pressure and cognitive function, though recent work demonstrates that the relationship is more complicated than typically believed. Elevated and untreated blood pressure levels are associated with cognitive decline, stroke, and dementia. New research suggests that diurnal blood pressure values and low blood pressure are also important, poorly understood contributors. Parental history of hypertension is linked to reduced cognitive function, raising the possibility of a genetic common cause for both cardiac and neurological function. Prospective studies that examine sophisticated blood pressure indices from beat-to-beat and ambulatory assessment are much needed to better understand the mechanisms that link blood pressure to poor neurocognitive outcome, particularly those that employ a combination of neuroimaging, cerebral perfusion, and cognitive function.

Notes

1. Skoog I, Lernflet B, Landahl S, Palmertz B, Andreasson I, Nilsson L, Persson G, Oden A, Svanborg A. A 15-year longitudinal study of blood pressure and dementia. *Lancet.* 1996;347:1141–1145.
2. Qui C, von Strauss E, Winblad B, Fratigilioni L. Decline in blood pressure over time and risk of dementia: A longitudinal study from the Kungsholmen project. *Stroke.* 2004;35: 1810–1815.
3. Starr JM, Taylor MD, Hart CL, Davey Smith G, Whalley LJ, Hole DJ, Wilson V, Deary IJ. Childhood mental ability and blood pressure at midlife: Linking the Scottish Mental Survey 1932 and the Midspan studies. *J Hypertens.* 2004;22(5):893–897.
4. Waldstein SR, Ryan CM, Polefrone JM, Manuck SB. Neuropsychological performance of young men who vary in familial risk for hypertension. *Psychosom Med.* 1994;56(5): 449–456.
5. O'Brien E, Sheridan J, O'Malley K. Dippers and nondippers. *Lancet.* 1988;13:397.
6. Chobanian AV, Bakris GL, Black HR, Cushman WC, Green LA, Izzo JL Jr, Jones DW, Materson BJ, Oparil S, Wright JT Jr, Roccella EJ. Seventh report of the Joint National Committee on Prevention, Detection, Evaluation, and Treatment of High Blood Pressure. *Hypertension.* 2003;42(6):1206–1252.
7. Ernst ME, Bergus GR. Noninvasive 24-hour ambulatory blood pressure monitoring: Overview of technology and clinical applications. *Pharmacotherapy.* 2002;22:597–612.
8. Franklin SS, Gustin W 4th, Wong ND, Larson MG, Weber MA, Kannel WB, Levy D. Hemodynamic patterns of age related changes in blood pressure. The Framingham Heart Study. *Circulation.* 1997;96:308–315.
9. National Heart, Lung, and Blood Institute. Available at: http://www.nhlbi.nih.gov/health/dci/About/index.html. Accessed December 22, 2008.
10. Thom T, Haase N, Rosamond W, Howard VJ, Rumsfeld J, Manolio T, Zheng ZJ, Flegal K, O'Donnell C, Kittner S, Lloyd-Jones D, Goff DC Jr, Hong Y, Adams R, et al. Heart disease and stroke statistics—2006 update: A report from the American Heart Association Statistics Committee and Stroke Statistics Subcommittee. *Circulation.* 2006;113(6):e85–151.
11. Harris MM, Stevens J, Thomas N, Schreiner P, Folsom AR. Associations of fat distribution and obesity with hypertension in a bi-ethnic population: The ARIC study. Atherosclerosis Risk in Communities Study. *Obes Res.* 2000;8(7):516–524.
12. Centers for Disease Control and Prevention and The Merck Institute of Aging and Health. *The State of Aging and Health in America 2004.* Whitehouse Station, NJ: The Merck Institute of Aging and Health; 2004.
13. Heist EK, Ruskin JN. Atrial fibrillation and congestive heart failure: Risk factors, mechanisms, and treatment. *Prog Cardiovasc Dis.* 2006;48(4):256–269.
14. Zoccali C, Mallamaci F, Tripepi G. Hypertension as a cardiovascular risk factor in end-stage renal failure. *Curr Hypertens Rep.* 2002;4(5):381–386.
15. Gil-Nunez A, Vivancos-Mora J. Blood pressure as a risk factor for stroke and the impact of antihypertensive treatment. *Cerebrovasc Dis.* 2005;20:40–52.
16. Kjeidsen S, Julius S, Hedner T, Hansson L. Stroke is more common than myocardial infarction in hypertension: Analysis based on 11 major randomized trials. *Blood Press.* 2001;10: 190–192.
17. Allen CL, Bayraktutan U. Risk factors for ischaemic stroke. *Int J Stroke.* 2008;3(2):105–116.
18. Yamada M, Kasagi F, Sasaki H, Masunari N, Mimori Y, Suzuki G. Association between dementia and midlife risk factors: The radiation effects research foundation adult health study. *J Am Geriatric Soc.* 2003;51:410–414.

19. Staessen JA, Birkenhäger WH. Cognitive impairment and blood pressure: Quo usque tandem abutere patientia nostra? *Hypertension*. 2004;44;612–613.
20. Brady C, Spito A, Gaziano J. Effects of age and hypertension status on cognition: The Veteran's Affairs Normative Aging Study. *Neuropsychology*. 2005;19:770–777.
21. Madden D, Blumenthal J. Interaction of hypertension and age in visual selective attention performance. *Health Psychol*. 1998;17:76–83.
22. Elias P, Elias M, D'Agostino R, Cupples L. NIDDM and blood pressure as risk factors for poor cognitive performance. *Diabetes Care*. 1997;20:1388–1395.
23. Elias M, Robbins M, Elias P, Streeten D. A longitudinal study of blood pressure in relation to performance on the Wechsler Adult Intelligence Scale. *Health Psychol*. 1998;17:486–493.
24. Qui C, Winblad B, Fratiglioni L. The age-dependent relation of blood pressure cognitive function and dementia. *Lancet Neurol*. 2005;4:487–489.
25. Kilander L, Nyman H, Nyman H, Boberg M, Hansson L, Lithell H. Hypertension is related to cognitive impairment: A 20-year follow-up of 999 men. *Hypertension*. 1998;31:780–786.
26. Launer L, Masaki K, Petrovitch H, Foley D, Havlik R. The association between midlife blood pressure levels and late life cognitive function. The Honolulu Asia aging study. *JAMA*. 1995;274:1846–1851.
27. Launer LJ, Ross GW, Petrovitch H, Masaki K, Foley D, White LR, Havlik RJ. Midlife blood pressure and dementia: The Honolulu-Asia aging study. *Neurobiol Aging*. 2000;21:49–55.
28. Guo Z, Viitanen M, Fratiglioni I, Winblad B. Low blood pressure and dementia in elderly people: The Kungsholmen project. *BMJ*. 1996;312:805–808.
29. Lande MB, Kaczorowski JM, Auinger P, Schwartz GJ, Weitzman M. Elevated blood pressure and decreased cognitive function among school-age children and adolescents in the United States. *J Pediatr*. 2003;143(6):720–724.
30. Suhr JA, Stewart JC, France CR. The relationship between blood pressure and cognitive performance in the Third National Health and Nutrition Examination Survey (NHANES III). *Psychosom Med*. 2004;66(3):291–297.
31. Singh-Manoux A, Marmot M. High blood pressure was associated with cognitive function in middle-age in the Whitehall II study. *J Clin Epidemiol*. 2005;58(12):1308–1315.
32. Elias PK, Elias MF, Robbins MA, Budge MM. Blood-pressure related cognitive decline: Does age make a difference? *Hypertension*. 2004;44:631–636.
33. Waldstein SR, Jennings JR, Ryan CM, Muldoon MF, Shapiro AP, Polefrone JM, Fazzari TV, Manuck SB. Hypertension and neuropsychological performance in men: Interactive effects of age. *Health Psychol*.1996;15(2):102–109.
34. Waldstein SR, Katzel LI. Interactive relations of central versus total obesity and blood pressure to cognitive function. *Int J Obes*. 2006;30(1):201–207.
35. Hanon O, Seux ML, Lenoir H, Rigaud AS, Forette F. Hypertension and dementia. *Curr Cardiol Rep*. 2003;5(6):435–440.
36. Raz N, Rodrigu K, Kennedy K, Dahle C, Head, D., Acker, J. Differential age-related changes in the regional metencephalic volumes in humans: A five-year follow-up. *Neurosci Lett*. 2003;349:163–166.
37. Raz N, Rodrigue K, Acker J. Hypertension and the brain: Vulnerability of the prefrontal regions and executive functions. *Behav Neurosci*. 2003;17:1169–1180.
38. Raz N, Rodrigue K, Kennedy K, Head D, Gunning-Dixon, F, Acker J. Differential aging of the human striatum: Longitudinal evidence. *Am J Neuroradiol*. 2003b;24:1849–1856.
39. Dufouil C, de Kersaint-Gilly A, Besançon V, Levy C, Auffray E, Brunnereau L, Alpérovitch A, Tzourio C. Longitudinal study of blood pressure and white matter hyperintensity: The EVA MRI Cohort. *Neurology*. 2001;56:921–926.

40. Veldnick J, Scheltens P, Jonker C, Launer L. Progression of cerebral white matter hyperintensities on MRI is related to diastolic blood pressure. *Neurology*. 1998;51:319–320.
41. Strassburger TL, Lee HC, Daly EM, Szczepanik J, Krasuski JS, Mentis MJ, Salerno JA, DeCarli C, Schapiro MB, Alexander GE. Interactive effects of age and hypertension on volumes of brain structures. *Stroke*. 1997;28:1410–1417.
42. Raz N, Lindenberger U, Rodrigue KM, Kennedy KM, Head D, Williamson A, Dahle C, Gerstorf D, Acker JD. Regional brain changes in aging healthy adults: General trends, individual differences, and modifiers. *Cereb Cortex*. 2005;15: 1676–1689.
43. Du AT, Schuff N, Chao LL, Kornak J, Jagust WJ, Kramer JH, Reed BR, Miller BL, Norman D, Chui HC, Weiner MW. Age effects on atrophy rates of entorhinal cortex and hippocampus. *Neurobiol Aging*. 2006;27:733–740.
44. den Heijer T, Launer LJ, Prins ND, van Dijk EJ, Vermeer SE, Hofman A, Koudstaal PJ, Breteler MM. Association between blood pressure, white matter lesions, and atrophy of the medial temporal lobe. *Neurology*. 2005;64(2):263–267.
45. Gianaros PJ, Greer PJ, Ryan CM, Jennings JR. Higher blood pressure predicts lower regional grey matter volume: Consequences on short-term information processing. *Neuroimage*. 2006;31(2):754–765.
46. Sierra C, Coca A. White matter lesions and cognitive impairment as silent cerebral disease in hypertension. *Scientific World Journal*. 2006;6:494–501.
47. Hoptman MJ, Gunning-Dixon FM, Murphy CF, Ardekani BA, Hrabe J, Lim KO, Etwaroo GR, Kanellopoulos D, Alexopoulos GS. Blood pressure and white matter integrity in geriatric depression. *J Affect Disord*. 2008 Sep 19. [Epub ahead of print.]
48. Cicconetti P, Priami C, Sagrafoli C, Tafaro L, Ettorre E, Donadio C, Cacciafesta M, Marigliano V. Cognitive function by brain event-related potentials (ERP) in elderly with borderline isolated systolic hypertension (BISH). *Arch Gerontol Geriatr*. 2007;44 Suppl 1:105–111.
49. Gold SM, Dziobek I, Rogers K, Bayoumy A, McHugh PF, Convit A. Hypertension and hypothalamo-pituitary-adrenal axis hyperactivity affect frontal lobe integrity. *J Clin Endocrinol Metab*. 2005;90(6):3262–3267.
50. Jennings JR. Autoregulation of blood pressure and thought: Preliminary results of an application of brain imaging to psychosomatic medicine. *Psychosom Med*. 2003;65(3):384–395.
51. Prince M. The treatment of hypertension in older people and its effect on cognitive function. *Biomed Pharmacother*. 1997;51:208–212.
52. Hyman D, Pavlik V. Characteristics of patients with uncontrolled hypertension in the United States. *N Engl J Med*. 2001;345:479–486.
53. Collins R, Peto R, MacMahon S, Hebert P, Fiebach NH, Eberlein KA, Godwin J, Qizilbash N, Taylor JO, Hennekens CH. Blood pressure, stroke, and coronary heart disease. II. Short-term reductions in blood pressure: Overview of randomized drug trials in their epidemiological context. *Lancet*. 1990;335:827–838.
54. SHEP Cooperative Research Group. Prevention of stroke by antihypertensive drug treatment in older persons with isolated systolic hypertension: Final results of the Systolic Hypertension in the Elderly Program (SHEP). *JAMA*. 1991;265:3255–3264.
55. Staessen JA, Gasowski J, Wang JG, Thijs L, Den Hond E, Boissel JP, Coope J, Ekbom T, Gueyffier F, Liu L, Kerlikowske K, Pocock S, Fagard RH. Risks of untreated and treated isolated systolic hypertension in the elderly: Meta-analysis of outcome trials. *Lancet*. 2000;355:865–872.
56. Forette F, Seux ML, Staessen JA, Thijs L, Babarskiene MR, Babeanu S, Bossini A, Fagard R, Gil-Extremera B, Laks T, Kobalava Z, Sarti C, Tuomilehto J, Vanhanen H, Webster J, Yodfat Y, Birkenhäger WH. The prevention of dementia with antihypertensive

treatment: New evidence from the Systolic Hypertension in Europe (Syst-Eur) study. *Arch Intern Med*. 2002;162:2046–2052.

57. Applegate WB, Pressel S, Wittes J, Luhr J, Shekelle RB, Camel GH, Greenlick MR, Hadley E, Moye L, Perry HM Jr, et al. Impact of the treatment of isolated systolic hypertension on behavioral variables: Results from the Systolic Hypertension in the Elderly Program. *Arch Intern Med*. 1994;154: 2154–2160.
58. Cervilla J, Prince M, Joels S, Lovestone S, Mann A. Long-term predictors of cognitive outcome in a cohort of older people with hypertension. *Br J Psychiatry*. 2000;177:66–71.
59. Zanchetti A, Elmfeldt D. Findings and implications of the Study on Cognition and Prognosis in the Elderly (SCOPE)—a review. *Blood Press*. 2006;15(2):71–79.
60. Tzourio C, Dufouil C, Ducimetiere P, Alperovitch A. Cognitive decline in individuals with high blood pressure: A longitudinal study in the elderly. Epidemiology of Vascular Aging Study Group. *Neurology*. 1999;53:1948–1952.
61. Veld B, Ruitenberg A, Holman A, Stricker B, Breteler M. Antihypertensive drugs and incidence of dementia: The Rotterdam Study. *Neurobiol Aging*. 2001;22:407–412.
62. Liao D, Cooper L, Cai J, Toole JF, Bryan NR, Hutchinson RG, Tyroler HA. Presence and severity of cerebral white matter lesions and hypertension, its treatment, and its control. The Atherosclerosis Risk in Communities Study. *Stroke*. 1996;27(12):2262–2270.
63. Hanon O, Pequignot R, Seux ML, Lenoir H, Bune A, Rigaud AS, Forette F, Girerd X. Relationship between antihypertensive drug therapy and cognitive function in elderly hypertensive patients with memory complaints. *J Hypertens*. 2006;24(10):2101–2107.
64. Izquierdo-Porrera AM, Waldstein SR. Cardiovascular risk factors and cognitive function in African Americans. *J Gerontol B Psychol Sci Soc Sci*. 2002;57(4):P377–380.
65. Knopman D, Boland LL, Mosley T, Howard G, Liao D, Szklo M, McGovern P, Folsom AR. Cardiovascular risk factors and cognitive decline in middle-aged adults. *Neurology*. 2001;56:42–48.
66. Munger MA, Van Tassell BW, LaFleur J. Medication nonadherence: An unrecognized cardiovascular risk factor. *Med Gen Med*. 2007;9(3):58.
67. Muldoon M, Waldstein S, Ryan C, Jennings J, Polefrone J, Shapiro A, Manuck S. Effects of six anti-hypertensive medications on cognitive performance. *J Hypertens*. 2002;20:1643–1652.
68. Guo Z, Fratiglioni L, Zhu L, Fastborn J, Winblad B, Viitanen M. Occurrence and progression of dementia in a community population aged 75 years and older: Relationship of antihypertensive medication use. *Arch Neurol*. 1999;56:991–996.
69. Guo Z, Qiu C, Viitanen M, Fastborn J, Winblad B, Fratiglioni L. Blood pressure and dementia in persons 75+ years old: Three-year follow-up results from the Kungsholmen Project. *J Alzheimers Dis*. 2001;3:585–591.
70. World Health Organization. Arterial hypertension. Technical Report Series No. 628. Geneva: World Health Organization, 1978.
71. Novak V, Novak P, Spies JM, Low PA. Autoregulation of cerebral blood flow in orthostatic hypotension. *Stroke*. 1998;29:104–111.
72. Tonkin A. Low blood pressure and low energy: (How) are they related? *J Hypertens*. 2004;22:671–673.
73. Medow MS, Stewart JM, Sanyal S, Mumtaz A, Sica D, Frishman WH. Pathophysiology, diagnosis, and treatment of orthostatic hypotension and vasovagal syncope. *Cardiol Rev*. 2008;16(1):4–20.
74. Guo Z, Viitanen M, Winblad B. Low blood pressure and five-year mortality in a Stockholm cohort of the very old: Possible confounding by cognitive impairment and other factors. *Am J Public Health*. 1997;87(4):623–628.

75. Duschek S, Hadjamu M, Schandry R. Enhancement of cerebral blood flow and cognitive performance following pharmacological blood pressure elevation in chronic hypotension. *Psychophysiology*. 2007;44(1):145–153.
76. Weiner DE, Tighiouart H, Levey AS, Elsayed E, Griffith JL, Salem DN, Sarnak MJ. Lowest systolic blood pressure is associated with stroke in stages 3 to 4 chronic kidney disease. *J Am Soc Nephrol*. 2007;18(3):960–966.
77. Morris M, Scherr P, Hebert L, Glynn R, Bennett D, Evans D. Association of incident Alzheimer disease and blood pressure measured from 13 years before to 2 years after diagnosis in a large community study. *Arch Neurol*. 2001;12:33–39.
78. Yamamoto Y, Akiguchi I, Oiwa K, Hayashi M, Imai K. Twenty-four-hour blood pressure changes in the course of lacunar disease. *Cerebrovasc Dis*. 2001;11:100–106.
79. Hogan DB, Ebly EM, Rockwood K. Weight, blood pressure, osmolarity, and glucose levels across various stages of Alzheimer's disease and vascular dementia. *Dement Geriatr Cogn Disord*. 1997;8:147–151.
80. Akahoshi M, Hida A, Imaizumi M, Soda M, Maeda R, Ichimaru S, Nakashima E, Seto S, Yano K. Basic characteristics of chronic hypotension cases: A longitudinal follow-up study from 1958 through 1999. *Hypertens Res*. 2006;29(1):1–7.
81. Cases A, Coll E. Chronic hypotension in the dialysis patient. *J Nephrol*. 2002;15:331–335.
82. Miklossy J. Cerebral hypoperfusion induces cortical watershed microinfarcts which may further aggravate cognitive decline in Alzheimer's disease. *Neurol Res*. 2003;25(6):605–610.
83. Nilsson SE, Read S, Berg S, Johansson B, Melander A, Lindblad U. Low systolic blood pressure is associated with impaired cognitive function in the oldest old: Longitudinal observations in a population-based sample 80 years and older. *Aging Clin Exp Res*. 2007;19(1):41–47.
84. Weisz N, Schandry R, Jacobs A, Mialet J, Duschek S. Early contingent negative variation of the EEG and attentional flexibility are reduced in hypotension. *Int J Psychophysiol*. 2002;45(3):253–260.
85. Duschek S, Matthias E, Schandry R. Essential hypotension is accompanied by deficits in attention and working memory. *Behav Med*. 2005;30(4):149–158.
86. Waldstein SR, Giggey PP, Thayer JF, Zonderman AB. Nonlinear relations of blood pressure to cognitive function: The Baltimore Longitudinal Study of Aging. *Hypertension*. 2005;45(3):374–379.
87. Wharton W, Hirshman E, Merritt P, Stangl B, Scanlin K, Krieger L. Lower blood pressure correlates with poorer performance on visuospatial attention tasks in younger individuals. *Biol Psychol*. 2006;73(3):227–234.
88. Duschek S, Schandry R. Deficient adjustment of cerebral blood flow to cognitive activity due to chronically low blood pressure. *Biol Psychol*. 2006;72:311–317.
89. Bendini C, Angelini A, Salsi F, Finelli ME, Martini E, Neviani F, Mussi C, Neri M. Relation of neurocardiovascular instability to cognitive, emotional and functional domains. *Arch Gerontol Geriatr*. 2007;44(1):69–74.
90. Mukai S, Lipsitz LA. Orthostatic hypotension. *Clin Geriatr Med*. 2002;18(2):253–268.
91. Heims HC, Critchley HD, Martin NH, Jäger HR, Mathias CJ, Cipolotti L. Cognitive functioning in orthostatic hypotension due to pure autonomic failure. *Clin Auton Res*. 2006;16(2):86–89.
92. Perlmuter LC, Greenberg JJ. Do you mind standing? Cognitive changes in orthostasis. *Exp Aging Res*. 1996;22(4):325–341.
93. Hynynen E, Uusitalo A, Konttinen N, Rusko H. Cardiac autonomic responses to standing up and cognitive task in overtrained athletes. *Int J Sports Med*. 2008;29(7):552–558.

94. Carapetian S, Siedlarz M, Jackson S, Perlmuter LC. Orthostatic blood pressure regulation predicts classroom effort in children. *Int J Psychophysiol.* 2008;68(1):70–74.
95. Kuo HK, Sorond F, Iloputaife I, Gagnon M, Milberg W, Lipsitz LA. Effect of blood pressure on cognitive functions in elderly persons. *J Gerontol A Biol Sci Med Sci.* 2004;59(11):1191–1194.
96. Eguchi K, Kario K, Hoshide S, Hoshide Y, Ishikawa J, Morinari M, Hashimoto T, Shimada K. Greater change of orthostatic blood pressure is related to silent cerebral infarct and cardiac overload in hypertensive subjects. *Hypertens Res.* 2004;27(4):235–241.
97. Ballard C, O'Brien J, Barber B, Scheltens P, Shaw F, McKeith I, Kenny RA. Neurocardiovascular instability, hypotensive episodes, and MRI lesions in neurodegenerative dementia. *Ann N Y Acad Sci.* 2000;903:442–445.
98. Kohara K, Nishida W, Maguchi M, Hiwada K. Autonomic nervous function in non-dipper essential hypertensive subjects. Evaluation by power spectral analysis of heart rate variability. *Hypertension.* 1995;26:808–814.
99. Sherwood A, Steffen PR, Blumenthal JA, Kuhn C, Hinderliter AL. Nighttime blood pressure dipping: The role of the sympathetic nervous system. *Am J Hypertens.* 2002;15:111–118.
100. Nakano Y, Oshima T, Ozono R, Higashi Y, Sasaki S., Matsumoto T., Matsuura H., Chayama K., Kambe M. Non-dipper phenomenon in essential hypertension is related to blunted nocturnal rise and fall of sympatho-vagal nervous activity and progress in retinopathy. *Auton Neurosci.* 2001;88:181–186.
101. Mancia G, Parati G. The role of blood pressure variability in end-organ damage. *J Hypertens* Suppl. 2003;21(6):S17– S23.
102. Ohkubo T, Imai Y, Tsuji I, Nagai K, Watanabe N, Minami N, Kato J, Kikuchi N, Nishiyama A, Aihara A, Sekino M, Satoh H, Hisamichi S. Relation between nocturnal decline in blood pressure and mortality. The Ohasama Study. *Am J Hypertens.* 1997;10(11):1201–1207.
103. Pickering T, Schwartz J, Verdecchia P, Imai Y, Kario K, Eguchi K, Pierdomenico S, Ohkubo T, Wing L. Prediction of strokes versus cardiac events by ambulatory monitoring of blood pressure: Results from an international database. *Blood Press Monit.* 2007;12(6): 397–399.
104. Bellelli G, Frisoni GB, Lucchi E, Guerini F, Geroldi C, Magnifico F, Bianchetti A, Trabucchi M. Blunted reduction in night-time blood pressure is associated with cognitive deterioration in subjects with long-standing hypertension. *Blood Press Monit.* 2004;9(2);71–76.
105. Yamamoto Y, Akiguchi I, Oiwa K, Hayashi M, Kimura J. Adverse effect of night-time blood pressure on the outcome of lacunar infarct patients. *Stroke.* 1998;29:570–576.
106. Yamamoto Y, Akiguchi I, Oiwa K, Hayashi M, Ohara T, Ozasa K. The relationship between 24-hour blood pressure readings, subcortical ischemic lesions and vascular dementia. *Cerebrovasc Dis.* 2005;19(5):302–308.
107. Ohya Y, Ohtsubo T, Tsuchihashi T, Eto K, Sadanaga T, Nagao T, Abe I, Fujishima M. Altered diurnal variation of blood pressure in elderly subjects with decreased activity of daily living and impaired cognitive functions. *Hypertens Res.* 2001;24:655–661.
108. van Boxtel MP, Gaillard C, Houx PJ, Buntinx F, de Leeuw PW, Jolles J. Is nondipping in 24-hour ambulatory blood pressure related to cognitive dysfunction? *J Hypertens.* 1998;16(10):1425–1432.
109. Kario K, Shimada K, Pickering TG. Abnormal nocturnal blood pressure falls in elderly hypertension: Clinical significance and determinants. *J Cardiovasc Pharmacol.* 2003;41: S61–S66.
110. Birhenhäger WH, Forette F, Seux ML, Wang JG, Staessen JA. Blood pressure, cognitive functions, and prevention of dementias in older patients with hypertension. *Arch Intern Med.* 2001;161:152–156.

111. Keary TA, Gunstad J, Poppas A, Paul RH, Jefferson AL, Hoth KF, Sweet LH, Forman DE, Cohen RA. Blood pressure variability and dementia rating scale performance in older adults with cardiovascular disease. *Cogn Behav Neurol*. 2007;20(1);73–77.
112. Hansen AL, Johnsen BH, Sollers JJ 3rd, Stenvik K, Thayer JF. Heart rate variability and its relation to prefrontal cognitive function: The effects of training and detraining. *Eur J Appl Physiol*. 2004;93(3):263–272.
113. Verdecchia P, Schillaci G, Gatteschi C, Zampi I, Battistelli M, Bartoccini C, Porcellati C. Blunted nocturnal fall in blood pressure in hypertensive women with future cardiovascular morbid events. *Circulation*. 1993;88:986–992.
114. Sander D, Lingelhofer J. Diurnal systolic blood pressure variability is the strongest predictor of early carotid atherosclerosis. *Neurology*. 1996;47:500–507.
115. Pickering TG. The clinical significance of diurnal blood pressure variations. Dippers and nondippers. *Circulation*. 1990;81(2):700–702.
116. O'Brien E, Atkins N, Staessen J. Are overnight dip and end-target-organ damage related? A clinical perspective. *Blood Press Monit*. 1996;1:S41–S46.
117. Cicconetti P, Ciotti V, Monteforte G, Moisè A, Chiarotti F, Piccirillo G, Cacciafesta M. Circadian blood pressure pattern and cognitive function in newly diagnosed older hypertensives. *Blood Press*. 2003;12(3):168–174.
118. van Boxtel MP, Henskens LH, Kroon AA, Hofman PA, Gronenschild EH, Jolles J, de Leeuw PW. Ambulatory blood pressure, asymptomatic cerebrovascular damage and cognitive function in essential hypertension. *J Hum Hypertens*. 2006;20(1):5–13.
119. Mancia G, Parati G. Ambulatory blood pressure monitoring and organ damage. *Hypertension*. 2000; 36:894–900.
120. Sierra C, De la Sierra A, Mercader J, Fgomes-Angelats E, Urbano-Marquez A, Coca A. Silent cerebral white matter lesions in middle-aged essential hypertensive patients. *J Hypertens*. 2002; 20:519–524.
121. Ohkubo T, Metoki H, Imai Y. Prognostic significance of morning surge in blood pressure: Which definition, which outcome? *Blood Press Monit*. 2008;13(3):161–162.
122. Nishinaga M, Takata J, Okumiya K, Matsubayashi K, Ozawa T, Doi Y. High morning home blood pressure is associated with a loss of functional independence in the community-dwelling elderly aged 75 years or older. *Hypertens Res*. 2005;28:657–663.
123. Gunstad J, Cohen RA, Tate DF, Paul RH, Poppas A, Hoth K, Macgregor KL, Jefferson AL. Blood pressure variability and white matter hyperintensities in older adults with cardiovascular disease. *Blood Press*. 2005:14(6):353–358.
124. Puisieux F, Monaca P, Deplanque D, Delmaire C, di Pompeo C, Monaca C, Leys D, Pruvo JP, Dewailly P. Relationship between leuko-araiosis and blood pressure variability in the elderly. *Eur Neurol*. 2001;46:115–120.
125. Marti-Fabregas J, Valencia C, Lopez-Contreras J, Roca-Cusachs A, Sole MJ, Garcia-Sanchez C, Marti-Vilalta JL. Blood pressure variability in Binswanger's disease and isolated lacunar infarction. *Cerebrovasc Dis*. 2001;11:230–234.
126. Tohgi H, Chiba K, Kimura M. Twenty-four-hour variation of blood pressure in vascular dementia of the Binswanger type. *Stroke*. 1991;7:477–483.
127. Sakakura K, Ishikawa J, Okuno M, Shimada K, Kario K. Exaggerated ambulatory blood pressure variability is associated with cognitive dysfunction in the very elderly and quality of life in the younger elderly. *Am J Hypertens*. 2007;20(7):720–727.
128. Kanemaru A, Kanemaru K, Kuwajima I. The effects of short-term blood pressure variability and night-time blood pressure levels on cognitive function. *Hypertens Res*. 2001;24:19–24.

129. Waldstein SR, Katzel LI. Stress-induced blood pressure reactivity and cognitive function. *Neurology*. 2005;64(10);1746–1749.
130. Waldstein SR, Siegel EL, Lefkowitz D, Maier KJ, Brown JR, Obuchowski AM, Katzel LI. Stress-induced blood pressure reactivity and silent cerebrovascular disease. *Stroke*. 2004;35(6);1294–1298.
131. McCann BS, Shapiro AP, Whitley B, Manuck SB, Miller RE. Absence of behavioral differences in young normotensive adults as a function of parental history of hypertension. *Am J Hypertens*. 1990;3(3):225–229.
132. Pierce TW, Elias MF. Cognitive function and cardiovascular responsivity in subjects with a parental history of hypertension. *J Behav Med*. 1993;16(3):277–294.
133. Thyrum ET, Blumenthal JA, Madden DJ, Siegel W. Family history of hypertension influences neurobehavioral function in hypertensive patients. *Psychosom Med*. 1995;57(5): 496–500.
134. Ditto B, Séguin JR, Tremblay RE. Neuropsychological characteristics of adolescent boys differing in risk for high blood pressure. *Ann Behav Med*. 2006;31(3):231–237.
135. Haley A, Sweet L, Gunstad J, Cohen R, Jerskey, & Mulligan, R. (in press). Neural correlates of visuospatial working memory in healthy young adults at risk for hypertension. *Brain Imaging and Behavior*.
136. Wright CE, O'Donnell K, Brydon L, Wardle J, Steptoe A. Family history of cardiovascular disease is associated with cardiovascular responses to stress in healthy young men and women. *Int J Psychophysiol*. 2007:63(3):275–282.
137. Hansen AL, Johnsen BH, Thayer JF. Relationship between heart rate variability and cognitive function during threat of shock. *Anxiety Stress Coping*. 2008:9:1–12.
138. Dimsdale JE. Psychological stress and cardiovascular disease. *J Am Coll Cardiol*. 2008:51(13):1237–1246.

9

NEUROPSYCHOLOGICAL SEQUELAE OF METABOLIC DYSREGULATION

V. H. Taylor and G. M. MacQueen

Cognitive functions are frequently divided into perception, attention, memory, and executive function, with executive function including higher-order planning and decision-making. These general categories include several subtypes of function: memory, for example, is commonly divided into *working memory* (holding information in mind for a short period while it is used), implicit or habit memory (memory for skills) and *declarative memory* (which itself is often further subdivided but includes memory for facts and events). These distinctions are not merely descriptive but reflect distinct neuroanatomical circuits that subsume different aspects of memory and cognition more generally. Associations between neuroendorine dysfunction and poor cognitive performance are commonly recognized. Hyperthyroidism and hypothyroidism, Cushing's disease, Addison's disease, and other endocrinological disturbances routinely result in significant cognitive problems, often in the absence of other frank neurological symptoms such as motor or sensory symptoms. More recently it has been recognized that other, more prevalent forms of neuroendocrine disturbance such as that associated with type 2 diabetes, hypercholesterolemia, and hypertension may also exert a negative effect on cognitive performance.[1] Most striking perhaps, is the correlation between atherosclerosis and an increased risk of Alzheimer's disease (AD) and vascular dementia (VD),[2] but while dementia represents an extreme case of impaired cognitive function, there is emerging evidence for an association between subtle cognitive dysfunction and the endocrine disturbances associated with metabolic syndrome and its constituent features.

Below we review the evidence supporting an association between the various components of metabolic syndrome and cognition, highlighting the proposed mechanisms linking metabolic dysregulation with cognitive dysfunction. It is worth noting that studies differ in the degree of cognitive impairment examined. Some have focused on the association between metabolic function and frank dementia, following standard clinical and research definitions of dementia. Others focus on mild cognitive impairment, which is generally accepted to mean measurable deficits in memory performance but intact performance in other cognitive domains and little impairment in daily function.

Finally, some studies refer to "cognitive dysfunction" when the group of interest has statistically significant deficits in performance compared with healthy controls. Although for most patients the associations between aspects of metabolic syndrome and cognitive changes will not be as striking as in illnesses such as thyroid disease or Cushing's, for people living and working in a highly technological, information-based society, even small declines in cognitive performance may have significant functional implications. Furthermore, on a population-based level, the epidemic increases in rates of obesity and metabolic syndrome (MeS) among young and middle-aged adults means that even relatively subtle consequences of these disorders may exert substantial impact on overall levels of societal health and function.

Metabolic Syndrome

Metabolic syndrome now affects more than 20% of the adult population and has become a significant health concern.[2] A number of differing definitions of the MeS have been put forward by various agencies, but the definition most consistently cited is that of the National Cholesterol Education Program (NCEP) Adult Treatment Panel III introduced in 2001 and subsequently modified in 2004. By definition, MeS requires the presence of any three of the following five criteria: (1) central obesity (waist circumference >102 cm [>40 in] in men, >88 cm [>35 in] in women); (2) elevated triglycerides (>150mg/dL [>1.7 mmol/L] or specific treatment for this lipid abnormality); (3) raised blood pressure (systolic BP >130 or diastolic BP >85 mm Hg, or treatment of previously diagnosed hypertension); (4) raised fasting glucose (>100 mg/dL [>5.6 mmol/L]or treatment for type 2 diabetes); and (5) reduced HDL cholesterol (<40 mg/dL [<1.03mm/L] in males, <50 mg/dL [<1.3 mmol/L] in females or specific treatment for this lipid abnormality).[3,4] People with MeS are twice as likely to die from, and three times as likely to have, a heart attack or stroke and have up to a ninefold greater risk of developing type 2 diabetes, compared with people without the syndrome.[5–7]

Obesity

Obesity has emerged as a common medical illness that confers risk for many other medical conditions,[8,9] and it confers risk for a decline in cognitive performance as well, an association that appears to be independent of other comorbid medical conditions. A prospective analysis of over 10,000 participants in a 27-year longitudinal population-based study concluded that obesity increased the risk of dementia even after adjustment for the prevalen ce of diabetes and cardiovascular disease.[10] Obese people (body mass index [BMI] ~30) had a 74% increased risk of dementia while overweight people (BMI 25–30) had a 35% greater risk of dementia compared with normal-weight individuals.[10] These findings were replicated in a population-based study that determined abdominal obesity was associated with cognitive dysfunction as defined by scores obtained on a mini-mental state exam developed for the assessment of cognitive functioning in individuals over 65 years, even after adjustment for age.[11] A population-based study of women aged 70 to 88 years meeting diagnostic criteria for dementia[12, 13] also yielded similar results. This study followed women over an 18-year time period and found that women who developed dementia had higher BMIs at age 70, 75, and 79 years, compared with non-demented women. The degree of cognitive deficit was age-dependent with cognition declining with increasing age,[14, 15] but it is unknown whether this reflects cognitive changes inherent in the aging process or whether age was a proxy for disease duration.

Adiposity has a direct effect on neuronal degradation.[10] Studies using rodent models of obesity report that obese animals have impaired performance on spatial memory tasks[16] and poor long-term potentiation of neurones in the hippocampus.[17] Obesity is also associated with subclinical inflammatory status, a condition linked to dementia[18] and cognitive decline.[19–24] Although the association between obesity and poor cognitive function is prominent in the elderly, middle-aged obese adults may have a greater degree of brain atrophy compared with age-matched, non-obese people.[25] This finding suggests that non-elderly obese people may experience subtle cognitive dysfunction and may be at greater risk of progression to significant cognitive impairment.[25]

Proposed Mechanisms Mediating the Association Between Cognitive Dysfunction and Obesity

The pathways through which obesity negatively affects cognition are not well-described. Several studies report that change in weight is associated with alterations in cognitive performance,[26–28] but these findings have primarily emerged from studies with dieting subjects, and the results are conflicting. Some report that subjects may have reduced reaction times,[26, 27] poor performance in vigilance tests, or poor immediate recall of words[27] with dieting. Other investigators found that dieters in fact have better word-recall performance[26] or that dieting has nearly no impact on cognition.[28] The discrepancies among reports may reflect differences in the amount of weight lost, the level of dietary restriction, and the subject's weight at baseline. In overweight women, being on a prescribed diet has minimal effect on cognitive performance and may even enhance some aspects of memory.[28] In weight loss studies in which normal-weight women lost further weight, working memory and tests of executive function were negatively affected.[29] Restriction of food or nutrition can affect central nervous system function via reduced glucose levels in the brain[29]; studies report positive effects on cognitive performance with glucose administration,[30] and negative effects of long-term fasting due to eating disorders.[31] There is no relationship, however, between lowered glucose levels as a result of missing a meal and cognitive performance, suggesting that cognitive changes are not simply the result of transient, mild hypoglycemia.[32] There is also evidence from rodent and human studies that adrenaline release and its effect on glucose is an important contributor to the process by which memory formation is regulated.[33] A rise in circulating glucose levels occurs with the release of adrenaline, which in turn contributes to neuronal processes responsible for memory formation. The change in cognitive performance after administration of glucose and other foods may depend on the level of sympathetic activation, glucocorticoid secretion, and pancreatic b-cell function, rather than simple fueling of neural activity.

Central obesity is associated with a variety of endocrine disturbances, and one hormone that is consistently deregulated is cortisol.[34] A number of reports document elevated levels of cortisol impacting hippocampal-dependent learning and memory by disrupting synaptic communication called "long-term potentiation" (LTP) and increasing long-term depression (LTD).[35] Thus, exposure to elevated cortisol concentrations for relatively short periods of time will disrupt hippocampal-dependent cognition and the synaptic phenomenon thought to underlie cognition.[36] Obesity is also associated with elevated levels of leptin, a peptide hormone largely secreted by mature adipocytes that plays a role in body weight and energy homeostasis.[37] Leptin receptors have been found in the neocortex and hippocampus, areas involved in cognition; and leptin-deficient obese mice have impaired ability on behavioral tasks.[38, 39] Hyperleptinemia is associated with enhanced sympathetic nervous activity[34, 40] that may promote structural brain abnormalities and increase the risk of cerebrovascular disease and stroke,[41, 42] increasing the risk of vascular dementia (VaD). It also can result in elevations in amyloid beta (A-beta), the major proteinaceous component of the amyloid plaques found in the brains of AD patients.[43] Obesity has also been associated with elevated levels of proinflammatory cytokines such as C-reactive protein, interleukin–6, and tumor necrosis factor.[44, 45] Such proinflammatory factors, in turn, have negative effects on cognitive function.[24, 46]

Another link between obesity and cognition depends on the "economics of obesity."[47] Environmental influences are major contributors to the obesity epidemic.[48–50] Socioeconomic status (SES) may be an important mediating factor of the relations between glycemic control and cognitive function as SES is a strong correlate of obesity, abnormal glucose tolerance, and cognition, with people from low SES being negatively impacted across all three modalities.[51] Low SES is also associated with low consumption of fruits and vegetables and high consumption of fats.[52] Nutritional status may affect cognitive function, with weight gain acting as a surrogate marker for poor nutritional intake. Cognitive processes may also be affected by vitamin levels and dietary influences on neural membrane fluidity.[53] The best evidence for links between nutrition and cognition are arguably in pediatric studies[54]; and the effect of chronically poor nutrition on cognition in adults is less understood. Diets rich in carbohydrates or fat,[26] eating patterns, additives, and the pharmacological effects of certain foods can affect cognitive function, especially in children. In the Isle of Wight studies, the removal of foods with artificial colorings resulted in a decrease in hyperactivity,[55] and further work is ongoing to assess classroom attention in response to diet.[54] Epidemiological data and animal studies indicate that ingestion of a diet rich in saturated fats may result in deficits in cognitive performance (Fig. 9-1).[56–58]

Glucose Abnormalities and Cognition

Cognitive dysfunction is a complication of diabetes.[59] Prospective studies report that diabetes is associated with low cognitive test scores in middle-aged or older adults,[60–62] and this risk extends to those with type 2 diabetes.[63] Several studies link type 2 diabetes with risk for VaD and AD through a variety of biological mechanisms,[64–68] and there is some evidence that impaired glucose tolerance, a precursor to type 2 diabetes, may also be associated with cognitive deficits.[69] A prospective study of 7000 women with diabetes or impaired fasting glucose found that diabetic and prediabetic woman have impaired cognitive performance and a greater risk of developing cognitive impairment than do normoglycemic subjects.[1] The links between diabetes and cognition are supported by several cross-sectional studies. Among woman enrolled in the Nurses Health Study, those with diabetes scored lower on the Telephone Interview of Cognitive Status and on a composite measure of four cognitive tests, even after multivariate adjustment. In that study, longer duration of diabetes was associated with lower cognition scores.[70] Similarly, both a Finnish study[71] and the Framingham study[72] reported an association between diabetes and impaired cognition. Conversely, prospective studies of diabetes

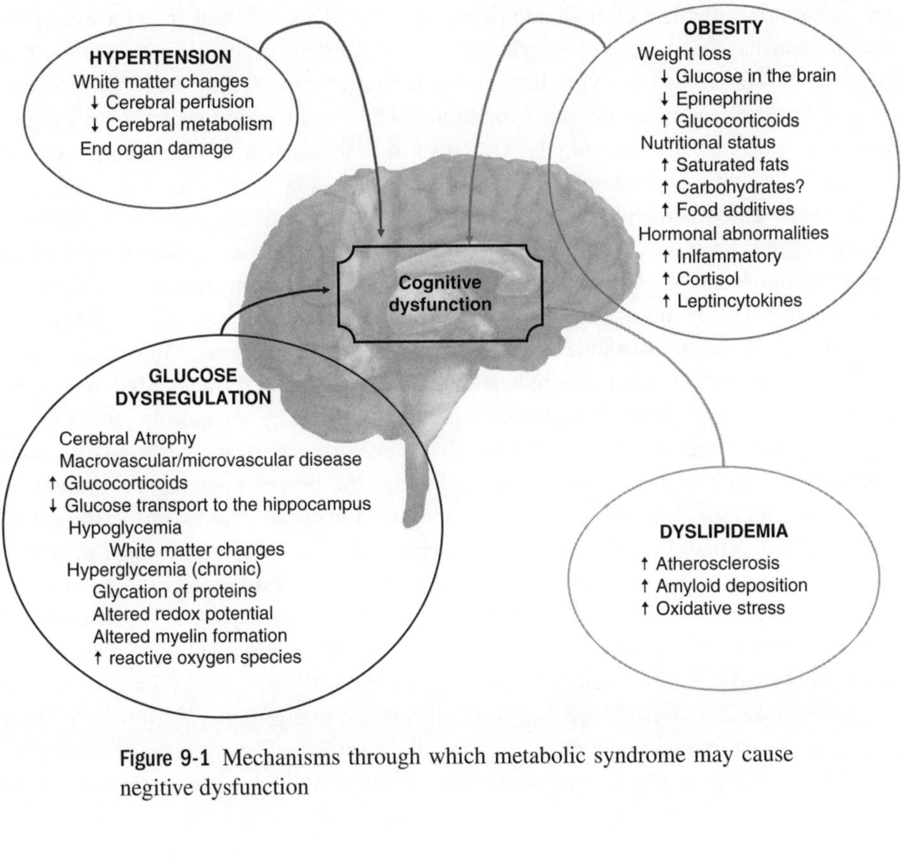

Figure 9-1 Mechanisms through which metabolic syndrome may cause negitive dysfunction

demonstrated that improvement in glucose tolerance is associated with improved cognitive function.[30] The association between glucose regulation and cognition has been consistently replicated, and in some 25 studies, diabetes mellitus has been associated with adverse cognitive changes involving psychomotor efficiency, attention, learning and memory, intelligence, and executive function.[15, 73–76] Furthermore, among the non-diabetic normal middle-aged and elderly population, those with poor glucose regulation have poor memory performance and smaller head size–adjusted hippocampal volumes.[77]

Mediating the Association Between Cognitive Dysfunction and Impaired Glucose Regulation

The cognitive problems associated with diabetes have traditionally been attributed to atherosclerosis,[78] as similar pathological changes are the result of both diseases. Chronic hyperglycemia induces biological toxicity via glycation of proteins, altered redox potential, altered signal transduction, and generation of reactive oxygen species.[79] The resulting oxidative stress contributes to vascular/endothelial dysfunction, and this microvascular damage may be an important determinant of the observed cognitive deficits. The fact that young people with diabetes have cognitive deficits prior to developing comorbid medical complications suggests that diabetes itself may have a direct role in contributing to memory impairment.[77, 80] Proposed mechanisms to explain this include both the effects of hypoglycemia on the developing brain[81] and the effects of chronic hyperglycemia on myelin formation.[82] Deficits in learning and memory also remain in non-diabetic individuals with insulin resistance, after accounting for the possible effects of atherosclerosis.[83]

Elevated glucocorticoid levels are also likely to be a mediating factor in diabetes-related cognitive decline. Cortisol levels and peripheral glucose regulation are linked, and in a longitudinal study, cortisol levels predicted cognitive impairment in older men and women.[84] This is thought to be due in part to the fact that physiological increases in cortisol acutely inhibit insulin release, and pharmacological increases in cortisol cause insulin resistance.[85] Cortisol also reduces the amount of insulin transported across the blood–brain barrier.[86] Not all cognitive functions are equally affected by cortisol and impaired glucose regulation, and it seems that glycemic control most strongly predicts function on cognitive tasks that are dependent on the hippocampus and surrounding structures,[87] regions that are particularly important for declarative memory. In animal studies, glucocorticoid exposure inhibits glucose transport into hippocampal neurones and glia,[88] perhaps because the hippocampus is one of the brain areas with the greatest co-localization of cortisol and insulin receptors.[89] The brain expresses a full range of glucose transporters, including GLUT1, GLUT2, GLUT3, and GLUT4.[90–92] Recent evidence points to the presence and regulation of insulin and/or glucose by a novel glucose transporter, GLUTx1(GLUT8), a receptor that is found in high concentration in the hippocampus.[93] Insulin resistance may potentiate the harmful effects of cortisol elevations on the brain. For example, when diabetic rats are stressed, with a consequent elevation in cortisol levels, they develop extensive hippocampal damage in one-third of the time it takes non-diabetic animals to develop stress-mediated damage.[94] This suggests that the hippocampus is more vulnerable to the deleterious effects of high glucocorticoid levels when glucose regulation is impaired. The hippocampus is very responsive to local tissue glucose levels, and this brain structure also appears to be involved in peripheral glucose regulation. Cognitive tasks activate basal forebrain cholinergic function and concurrently decrease extracellular levels of glucose in the hippocampus.[95, 96] This combination of events appears likely to increase glucose mobilization peripherally, as local stimulation of muscarinic cholinergic receptors in the dentate gyrus[97, 98] increases peripheral glucose levels. When the hippocampus is damaged, as in AD, there is abnormal glucose regulation that is observed in glucose tolerance tests as an abnormal cortisol response.[97] In these patients, the expected decrease in hippocampal glucose utilization and increase in peripheral glucose levels does not occur.[99] These findings suggest that neural circuits involving the hippocampus play some role in sensing glucose levels and regulating the peripheral metabolic response. The hippocampus is affected in type 1 diabetes,[100] and hippocampal neurons have accelerated remodeling in streptozotocin-induced diabetes[94] that can be reversed by insulin replacement.[94] The metabolic alterations in diabetes may also include down-regulation of insulin-like growth factor-1 (IGF-1[101]), which occurs in the early stages of the disease, in rat models at least. IGF-1 deficiency leads to neuroaxonal dystrophy in rats,[18] while direct delivery of IGF-1 in diabetic rats reversed atrophy of myelinated axons in the sural nerve.[102] Global cerebral atrophy has been observed in Laron Syndrome, an illness associated with the inability to generate IGF-1 in humans.[103] Cerebral atrophy has also been identified in diabetic patients. In 1965, Reske-Nielsen described the concept of "diabetic encephalopathy" as a complication of long-term diabetes mellitus.[104] This theory inclusively identified deviations from normoglycemia, macrovascular and microvascular disease, and hormonal and cytokine changes as possible mechanisms of diabetes-associated cerebral atrophy.

Hypoglycemic episodes are associated with cerebral atrophy or white matter lesions in type 1 diabetes.[105] Repeated hypoglycemic episodes are associated with persistent cognitive impairment.[106–108] Cognitive function deteriorates during hypoglycemia if the arterialized venous plasma glucose is reduced below a concentration of 2.7 mmol/L.[109] Severe hypoglycemia may trigger the release of excitatory amino acids such as glutamate and aspartate, which trigger calcium influx, activation of proteases, and structural damage. As hypoglycemia can also occur in type 2 diabetes, these mechanisms may also be relevant for understanding cognitive performance in people with this illness as well[110] (Fig. 9-1).

Hypertension and Cognition

Hypertension is an established risk factor for cerebrovascular illness. Prior to a major cerebrovascular event, however, hypertension exerts a subtle impact on the brain that is revealed by poor performance on tests of attention, learning and memory, executive functions, visuospatial skills, psychomotor abilities and perceptual skills. Hypertension is also predictive of cognitive decline[111–113] although the interval between the respective manifestations of hypertension and cognitive deterioration may vary from a few years to several decades.[114] It is also well know that hypertension or blood pressure elevations are associated with stroke and dementia, and lower levels of performance across a variety of cognitive domains.[115, 116] Anti-hypertensive treatment has a positive effect on cognitive function and quality of life[67, 117] regardless of the duration of illness.

Proposed Mechanisms Mediating the Association Between Cognitive Dysfunction and Hypertension

Several longitudinal studies show an association between middle-age elevations in blood pressure and impaired cognition in later life.[111, 118–121] The mechanisms underlying these associations are unknown, but one association may be between long-standing hypertension and white matter lesions, which are frequently found on cerebral MRI scans of elderly people, particularly those with hypertension.[122] The presence of cerebral white matter lesions is an important prognostic factor for the development of stroke, and also for cognitive impairment and dementia. Correlations between cerebral white matter lesions and elevated blood pressure provide indirect evidence that structural and functional changes in the brain over time may lead to lowered cognitive functioning when blood pressure control is poor or lacking. Subjects with large white matter hyperintensities exhibit disturbed cerebral perfusion, reduced cerebral metabolism,[123–125] abnormalities of cerebral white matter,[126] and cerebral atrophy,[127] all of which are implicated in the pathogenesis of cognitive deficits.[128] Some investigators have even suggested that the presence of white matter lesions in hypertensive patients should be considered an early marker of brain damage[129] (Fig. 9-1).

Dyslipidemia and Cognition

Lipid abnormalities are associated with an increased risk for cardiovascular disease (CVD) and for cognitive impairment. Raised plasma concentrations of cholesterol are implicated as a risk factor for AD,[130–134] and low serum concentrations of high-density lipoprotein (HDL) cholesterol are associated with cognitive impairment and dementia.[135] Elevated total and low-density lipoprotein (LDL) cholesterol levels are reported in very old patients with AD.[136] These findings are supported by a meta-analysis that concluded that patients with probable or possible early-stage AD had elevated total cholesterol values compared with a non-demented population.[133] Subsequent to this meta-analysis, high LDL and total cholesterol levels were statistically linked to lower scores on the most common tests assessing cognitive impairment in a cohort of postmenopausal women. Moreover, a reduction in the LDL cholesterol level during the four-year period of this study was associated with lower odds of cognitive impairment.[137] Although in this study the improved cognitive outcome following statin use further links cognitive deficits to lipid abnormalities, the results of other studies examining the association between statin use and dementia are inconclusive.

Some studies conclude that statin use lowers the risk for dementia,[138] while others suggest that this association is artifactual.[139] Cross-sectional studies of cholesterol-lowering medications report a diminished risk for dementia with medication use, but this relationship may not be robust.[140] A pilot study examined 63 patients who already had a diagnosis of mild to moderate AD and were treated with either placebo or atorvastatin 80 mg day-1. Atorvastatin reduced cholesterol levels as expected, and there was some beneficial reduction in the rate of cognitive and behavioral deterioration, although not all measures achieved statistical significance; again raising the issue of the clinical significance of this effect.[141]

Elevated levels of triglycerides have also been examined for their role in modulating cognitive performance, in part based on case reports that indicate hypertriglyceridemia has led to delirium.[142, 143] In patients with type 2 diabetes, elevated triglycerides have been associated with poor cognitive performance,[144] and in a small study on humans, reducing hypertriglyceridemia with gemfibrozil improved cerebral blood flow and function on the cognitive capacity screening examination.[145] Recent animal work supports these findings, with obese mice that were fed a triglyceride-rich diet showing impaired acquisition in three different cognitive paradigms. These same acquisition problems were noted with injection into the brain of the triglyceride triolein, but not of the free fatty acid palmitate in normal body weight mice. Impaired cognition in obese mice was improved by selectively lowering triglycerides with gemfibrozil.[146]

Mechanisms Mediating the Association Between Cognitive Dysfunction and Dyslipidemia

An association between lipids and cognitive function is usually explained as based on dyslipidemia's being a risk factor for stroke or cerebrovascular hypofunction. Autopsy studies have reported a correlation between elevated levels of cholesterol and amyloid deposition in the brain. A recent study examining autopsy cases of patients over 40 years of age found an association between cholesterolemia and the presence of amyloid deposition (subjects with or without amyloid deposition) as well as cholesterolemia and amyloid load.[147] A study of the circle of Willis in a voluntary brain donation program examined 22 control cases and 18 AD cases, linking circle-of-Willis atherosclerotic lesions with AD lesions and dementia.[148] Women with AD had a higher degree of pathological severity and higher total cholesterol, LDL cholesterol, and triglycerides than controls ($P \sim 0.01$). Among samples from patients with AD, there were positive correlations between brain Abeta n-42 levels and total serum cholesterol, LDL cholesterol, and apolipoprotein B-100, and a negative correlation with HDL cholesterol levels.[149]

The mechanism underlying these post-mortem observations has been pursued in plaque-forming transgenic mouse models, where it has been reported that fat feeding increases brain plaque load, and that hypocholesterolemic agents such as statins lower plaque burden.[150, 151] Sparks and colleagues determined that Watanabe rabbits on a 2% cholesterol diet developed increased levels of beta amyloid immunoreactivity in vesicles inside the neurones of their brains.[152] Cholesterol interacts with Abeta in a reciprocal manner: cellular cholesterol levels modulate Abeta, whereas Abeta alters cholesterol dynamics in neurons, leading to tauopathy.[153] In addition, cholesterol alters the degradation of the amyloid precursor protein (APP), which plays a major role in the pathogenesis of AD.[154] Moreover, vascular disease, which is associated with dyslipidemia, may be related to the risk of cognitive decline and dementia.[155, 156]

A relatively new theory attempting to explain the link between dyslipidemia and cognitive decline comes from animal studies examining the effects of hypertriglyceridemia. The mechanisms via which triglyceride levels impair memory remain unclear, but theories involve linking oxidative stress impacting LTP via alterations in the NMDA-dependent calcium channel.[157, 158] Alternatively, it has been shown that hypertriglyceridemia impairs leptin's ability to cross the blood–brain barrier.[159] Leptin enhances cognition,[160, 161] and leptin-deficient animals have impaired hippocampal LTP and poor spatial memory.[39, 162] Thus triglycerides may impair cognition by preventing leptin from reaching the hippocampal regions important for learning and memory. Triglycerides may also affect cognition via their ability to modify release of peptides involved in feeding behaviors,[163] many of which affect cognition through nitric oxide–dependent pathways.[164, 165]

Simvastatin, atorvastatin, and cyclodextrin, a compound used in the laboratory to deplete cellular cholesterol, lowered Abeta generation while activating the alternate, non-amyloidogenic a-secretase pathway for APP metabolism in cultured neurons.[166, 167] The clinical significance of these preclinical studies is not known, but they support the clinical findings suggesting that there may be an association between cholesterol levels and risk for cognitive deterioration (Fig. 9-1).

Metabolic Syndrome and Cognition

The increased risk of adverse health outcomes associated with metabolic syndrome is related to the concept that the whole is more than simply the sum of its parts; that is, the health risks associated with metabolic syndrome are higher than would be assumed by virtue of combining the risks associated with each component illness required for the diagnosis.[168] It is reasonable to assume that the cognitive risks associated with metabolic syndrome follow a similar exponential increase. Despite many studies examining risk in the individual components of metabolic syndrome, however, few studies have examined this syndrome as a whole. The information that is available does indicate that metabolic syndrome is a risk factor for accelerated cognitive aging. In a study examining 2949 elderly subjects (mean age, 74 years) enrolled in the Health Aging and Body Composition Study, participants with metabolic syndrome were more likely to have cognitive impairment than those without metabolic syndrome (26% vs. 21%).[19] A second study that enrolled 1624 elderly participants of Hispanic descent found a statistically significant decline in cognition amongst patients with metabolic syndrome.[169] Both studies used the modified Mini Mental Status exam (MMSE) to assess cognition. Similar results were obtained from a study based in the Netherlands that evaluated cognitive changes in participants aged 65 to 88 years. This study assessed a variety of cognitive domains including general cognition (the MMSE), memory (verbal learning test), fluid intelligence (Raven's matrices), and information-processing speed (coding task) and found that performance on all cognitive tests was inversely associated with the metabolic syndrome.[170]

Conclusion

People with physical illnesses frequently report problems in multiple cognitive domains. While the mechanisms contributing to cognitive dysfunction in this population remain to be elucidated, the likely combination of neuroanatomical changes and biochemical alterations secondary to dysregulation of various metabolic pathways create a clinically relevant problem. Many patients with one or a combination of obesity, diabetes, hypertension, and dyslipidemia require optimal cognitive function to perform at high levels in their workplaces. While most patients with these illnesses would not meet criteria for dementia or even notable impairment on standard neuropsychological testing, subtle but persistent cognitive dysfunction may contribute to the morbidity experienced by those with metabolic syndrome or its constituent features.

Clinicians must be vigilant to this association and may need to consider a more detailed assessment of patients complaining of impaired cognitive performance and work-related disability. It would be easy to disregard cognitive complaints, but given the mounting evidence supporting a link between cognition and metabolic syndrome, these issues need to be addressed. It is also important to screen for and treat the component illnesses that confer a diagnosis of metabolic syndrome to prevent the detrimental effects these illnesses can have on cognition. The use of statins to control hyperlipidemia and the use of antihypertensive medications may improve cognition. The early diagnosis of diabetes to prevent the effects of chronic hyperglycemia and the consistent regulation of glucose levels to prevent hypoglycemic episodes may minimize the negative impact of diabetes on cognition. Investigators need to consider the inclusion of cognitive measures when examining treatment strategies for metabolic syndrome and related conditions to determine whether treatment of these illnesses has a positive impact on cognitive performance. A better understanding of the mechanisms through which changes in metabolic parameters exert an effect on cognitive performance will improve our understanding of the bidirectional relations between neuronal and somatic systems.

Notes

1. Yaffe K, Clemons TE, McBee WL, Lindblad AS. Impact of antioxidants, zinc, and copper on cognition in the elderly: A randomized, controlled trial. *Neurology*. 2004;63:1705–1707.
2. Ford ES, Giles WH, Dietz WH. Prevalence of the metabolic syndrome among U.S. adults: Findings from the third National Health and Nutrition Examination Survey. *JAMA*. 2002;287: 356–359.
3. Hofman A, Ott A, Breteler MM, Bots ML, Slooter AJ, van Harskamp F, van Duijn CN, Van Broekhoven C, Grobbee DE. Atherosclerosis, apolipoprotein E, and prevalence of dementia and Alzheimer's disease in the Rotterdam Study. *Lancet*. 1997;349:51–154.

4. Grundy SM, Cleeman JI, Daniels SR, Donato KA, Eckel RH, Franklin BA, Gordon DJ, Krauss RM, Savage PJ, Smith Jr SC, Spertus JA, Costa F. Diagnosis and management of the metabolic syndrome. An American Heart Association/National Heart, Lung, and Blood Institute Scientific Statement. Executive summary. *Cardiol Rev*. 2005:322–327.
5. Laaksonen DE, Lakka HM, Niskanen LK, Kaplan GA, Salonen JT, Lakka TA. Metabolic syndrome and development of diabetes mellitus: Application and validation of recently suggested definitions of the metabolic syndrome in a prospective cohort study. *Am J Epidemiol*. 2002;156:1070–1077.
6. Isomaa B, Henricsson M, Almgren P, Tuomi T, Taskinen MR, Groop L. The metabolic syndrome influences the risk of chronic complications in patients with type II diabetes. *Diabetologia*. 2001;44:1148–1154.
7. Lakka HM, Laaksonen DE, Lakka TA, Niskanen LK, Kumpusalo E, Tuomilehto J, Salonen JT. The metabolic syndrome and total and cardiovascular disease mortality in middle-aged men. *JAMA*. 2002;288:2709–2716.
8. Romero-Corral A, Montori VM, Somers VK, Korinek J, Thomas RJ, Allison TG, Mookadam F, Lopez-Jimenez F. Association of bodyweight with total mortality and with cardiovascular events in coronary artery disease: A systematic review of cohort studies. *Lancet*. 2006;368:666–678.
9. Jensen J, Nyberg L, Gustafson Y, Lundin-Olsson L. Fall and injury prevention in residential care—effects in residents with higher and lower levels of cognition. *J Am Geriatr Soc*. 2003;51:627–635.
10. Whitmer RA, Gunderson EP, Barrett-Connor E, Quesenberry CP, Jr., Yaffe K. Obesity in middle age and future risk of dementia: A 27-year longitudinal population based study. *BMJ*. 2005;330:1360.
11. Jeong SK, Nam HS, Son MH, Son EJ, Cho KH. Interactive effect of obesity indexes on cognition. *Dement Geriatr Cogn Disord*. 2005;19:91–96.
12. Gustafson DR, Wen MJ, Koppanati BM. Androgen receptor gene repeats and indices of obesity in older adults. *Int J Obes Relat Metab Disord*. 2003;27:75–81.
13. Gustafson DR, Steen B, Skoog I. Body mass index and white matter lesions in elderly women. An 18-year longitudinal study. *Int Psychogeriatr*. 2004;16:327–336.
14. Messier C. Impact of impaired glucose tolerance and type 2 diabetes on cognitive aging. *Neurobiol Aging*. 2005;26:26–30.
15. Ryan CM. Diabetes, aging, and cognitive decline. *Neurobiol Aging*. 2005;26:21–25.
16. Funahashi H, Yada T, Suzuki R, Shioda S. Distribution, function, and properties of leptin receptors in the brain. *Int Rev Cytol*. 2003;224:1–27.
17. Harvey J. Novel actions of leptin in the hippocampus. *Ann Med*. 2003;35:197–206.
18. Schmidt RE, Dorsey DA, Beaudet LN, Parvin CA, Zhang W, Sima AA. Experimental rat models of types 1 and 2 diabetes differ in sympathetic neuroaxonal dystrophy. *J Neuropathol Exp Neurol*. 2004;63:450–460.
19. Yaffe K, Kanaya A, Lindquist K, Simonsick EM, Harris T, Shorr RI, Tylavsky FA, Newman AB. The metabolic syndrome, inflammation, and risk of cognitive decline. *JAMA*. 2004;292:2237–2242.
20. Bastard JP, Jardel C, Delattre J, Hainque B, Bruckert E, Oberlin F. Evidence for a link between adipose tissue interleukin-6 content and serum C-reactive protein concentrations in obese subjects. *Circulation*. 1999;99:2221–2222.
21. Mohamed-Ali V, Flower L, Sethi J, Hotamisligil G, Gray R, Humphries SE, York DA, Pinkney J. Beta-adrenergic regulation of IL-6 release from adipose tissue: In vivo and in vitro studies. *J Clin Endocrinol Metab*. 2001;86:5864–5869.

22. Schmidt R, Schmidt H, Curb JD, Masaki K, White LR, Launer LJ. Early inflammation and dementia: A 25-year follow-up of the Honolulu-Asia Aging Study. *Ann Neurol.* 2002;52:168–174.
23. Teunissen CE, van Boxtel MP, Bosma H, Bosmans E, Delanghe J, De Bruijn C, Wauters A, Maes M, Jolles J, Steinbusch HW, de Vente J. Inflammation markers in relation to cognition in a healthy aging population. *J Neuroimmunol.* 2003;134:142–150.
24. Yaffe K, Lindquist K, Penninx BW, Simonsick EM, Pahor M, Kritchevsky S, Launer L, Kuller L, Rubin S, Harris T. Inflammatory markers and cognition in well-functioning African-American and white elders. *Neurology.* 2003;61:76–80.
25. Ward MA, Carlsson CM, Trivedi MA, Sager MA, Johnson SC. The effect of body mass index on global brain volume in middle-aged adults: A cross sectional study. *BMC Neurol.* 2005;5:23.
26. Kretsch MJ, Green MW, Fong AK, Elliman NA, Johnson HL. Cognitive effects of a long-term weight reducing diet. *Int J Obes Relat Metab Disord.* 1997;21:14–21.
27. Green MW, Rogers PJ. Impaired cognitive functioning during spontaneous dieting. *Psychol Med.* 1995;25:1003–1010.
28. Bryan J, Tiggemann M. The effect of weight-loss dieting on cognitive performance and psychological well-being in overweight women. *Appetite.* 2001;36:147–156.
29. Benton D, Sargent J. Breakfast, blood glucose and memory. *Biol Psychol.* 1992;33:207–210
30. Korol DL, Gold PE. Glucose, memory, and aging. *Am J Clin Nutr.* 1998;67:764S-771S.
31. Mathias JL, Kent PS. Neuropsychological consequences of extreme weight loss and dietary restriction in patients with anorexia nervosa. *J Clin Exp Neuropsychol.* 1998;20:548–564.
32. Green MW, Elliman NA, Rogers PJ. The effects of food deprivation and incentive motivation on blood glucose levels and cognitive function. *Psychopharmacology (Berl).* 1997;134:88–94.
33. Gold PE. Role of glucose in regulating the brain and cognition. *Am J Clin Nutr.* 1995;61: 987S-995S.
34. Bjorntorp P, Rosmond R. Neuroendocrine abnormalities in visceral obesity. *Int J Obes Relat Metab Disord.* 2000;24:S80-S85.
35. Lupien S, Lecours AR, Lussier I, Schwartz G, Nair NP, Meaney MJ. Basal cortisol levels and cognitive deficits in human aging. *J Neurosci.* 1994;14:2893–2903.
36. McEwen BS, Sapolsky RM. Stress and cognitive function. *Curr Opin Neurobiol.* 1995;5: 205–216.
37. Friedman JM, Halaas JL. Leptin and the regulation of body weight in mammals. *Nature.* 1998;395:763–770.
38. Benoit SC, Clegg DJ, Seeley RJ, Woods SC. Insulin and leptin as adiposity signals. *Recent Prog Horm Res.* 2004;59:267–285.
39. Li XL, Aou S, Oomura Y, Hori N, Fukunaga K, Hori T. Impairment of long-term potentiation and spatial memory in leptin receptor-deficient rodents. *Neuroscience.* 2002;113:607–615.
40. Ren J. Leptin and hyperleptinemia—from friend to foe for cardiovascular function. *J Endocrinol.* 2004;181(1):1–10.
41. Everson SA, Lynch JW, Kaplan GA, Lakka TA, Sivenius J, Salonen JT. Stress-induced blood pressure reactivity and incident stroke in middle-aged men. *Stroke.* 2001;32:1263–1270.
42. Waldstein SR, Siegel EL, Lefkowitz D, Maier KJ, Brown JR, Obuchowski AM, Katzel LI. Stress-induced blood pressure reactivity and silent cerebrovascular disease. *Stroke.* 2004;35:1294–1298.
43. Fewlass DC, Noboa K, Pi-Sunyer FX, Johnston JM, Yan SD, Tezapsidis N. Obesity-related leptin regulates Alzheimer's Abeta. *FASEB J.* 2004;18:1870–1878.
44. Das UN. Metabolic syndrome X: An inflammatory condition? *Curr Hypertens Rep.* 2004;6:66–73.

45. Toni R, Malaguti A, Castorina S, Roti E, Lechan RM. New paradigms in neuroendocrinology: Relationships between obesity, systemic inflammation and the neuroendocrine system. *J Endocrinol Invest*. 2004;27:182–186.
46. Wilson CJ, Finch CE, Cohen HJ. Cytokines and cognition—the case for a head-to-toe inflammatory paradigm. *J Am Geriatr Soc*. 2002;50:2041–2056.
47. Block JP, Scribner RA, DeSalvo KB. Fast food, race/ethnicity, and income: A geographic analysis. *Am J Prev Med*. 2004;27:211–217.
48. Koplan JP, Dietz WH. Caloric imbalance and public health policy. *JAMA*. 1999;282: 1579–1581.
49. Poston WS, Foreyt JP. Obesity is an environmental issue. *Atherosclerosis*. 1999;146: 201–209.
50. Hill JO, Peters JC. Environmental contributions to the obesity epidemic. *Science*. 1998;280:1371–1374.
51. Brunner EJ. Social and biological determinants of cognitive aging. *Neurobiol Aging*. 2005;26:17–20.
52. Townsend MS. Obesity in low-income communities: Prevalence, effects, a place to begin. *J Am Diet Assoc*. 2006;106:34–37.
53. Gibson LE, Green MW. Nutritional influences on cognitive function, mechanisms of susceptibility. *Nutritional Research Reviews*. 2002;15:169–206.
54. Stevenson J. Dietary influences on cognitive development and behaviour in children. *Proc Nutr Soc*. 2006;65:361–365.
55. Bateman B, Warner JO, Hutchinson E, Dean T, Rowlandson P, Gant C, Grundy J, Fitzgerald C, Stevenson J. The effects of a double blind, placebo controlled, artificial food colourings and benzoate preservative challenge on hyperactivity in a general population sample of preschool children. *Arch Dis Child*. 2004;89:506–511.
56. Greenwood CE, Winocur G. High-fat diets, insulin resistance and declining cognitive function. *Neurobiol Aging*. 2005;26:42–45.
57. Winocur G, Greenwood CE. Studies of the effects of high fat diets on cognitive function in a rat model. *Neurobiol Aging*. 2005;26:46–49.
58. Yehuda S, Rabinovitz S, Mostofsky DI. Essential fatty acids and the brain: From infancy to aging. *Neurobiol Aging*. 2005;26:98–102.
59. Cukierman T, Gerstein HC, Williamson JD. Cognitive decline and dementia in diabetes—systematic overview of prospective observational studies. *Diabetologia*. 2005;48:2460–2469.
60. Knopman D, Boland LL, Mosley T, Howard G, Liao D, Szklo M, McGovern P, Folsom AR. Cardiovascular risk factors and cognitive decline in middle-aged adults. *Neurology*. 2001;56:42–48.
61. Haan MN, Shemanski L, Jagust WJ, Manolio TA, Kuller L. The role of APOE epsilon4 in modulating effects of other risk factors for cognitive decline in elderly persons. *JAMA*. 1999;282:40–46.
62. Gregg EW, Yaffe K, Cauley JA, Rolka DB, Blackwell TL, Narayan KM, Cummings SR. Is diabetes associated with cognitive impairment and cognitive decline among older women? Study of Osteoporotic Fractures Research Group. *Arch Intern Med*. 2000;160:174–180.
63. Schnaider BM, Goldbourt U, Silverman JM, Noy S, Schmeidler J, Ravona-Springer R, Sverdlick A, Davidson M. Diabetes mellitus in midlife and the risk of dementia three decades later. *Neurology*. 2004;63:1902–1907.
64. Ott A, Stolk RP, van HF, Pols HA, Hofman A, Breteler MM. Diabetes mellitus and the risk of dementia: The Rotterdam Study. *Neurology*. 1999;53:1937–1942.
65. Peila R, Rodriguez BL, Launer LJ. Type 2 diabetes, APOE gene, and the risk for dementia and related pathologies: The Honolulu-Asia Aging Study. *Diabetes*. 2002;51:256–1262.

66. van den Berg E, Kessels RP, Kappelle LJ, de Haan EH, Biessels GJ. Type 2 diabetes, cognitive function and dementia: Vascular and metabolic determinants. *Drugs Today (Barc).* 2006;42:741–754.
67. Stewart R, Liolitsa D. Type 2 diabetes mellitus, cognitive impairment and dementia. *Diabet Med.* 1999;16:93–112.
68. Farris W, Mansourian S, Chang Y, Lindsley L, Eckman EA, Frosch MP, Eckman CB, Tanzi RE, Selkoe DJ, Guenette S. Insulin-degrading enzyme regulates the levels of insulin, amyloid beta-protein, and the beta-amyloid precursor protein intracellular domain in vivo. *Proc Natl Acad Sci U S A.* 2003;100:4162–4167.
69. Elias MF, Elias PK, Sullivan LM, Wolf PA, D'Agostino RB. Obesity, diabetes and cognitive deficit: The Framingham Heart Study. *Neurobiol Aging.* 2005;26:11–16.
70. Grodstein F, Chen J, Wilson RS, Manson JE. Type 2 diabetes and cognitive function in community-dwelling elderly women. *Diabetes Care.* 2001;24:1060–1065.
71. Hiltunen LA, Keinanen-Kiukaanniemi SM, Laara EM. Glucose tolerance and cognitive impairment in an elderly population. *Public Health.* 2001;115:197–200.
72. Elias PK, Elias MF, D'Agostino RB, Cupples LA, Wilson PW, Silbershatz H, Wolf PA. NIDDM and blood pressure as risk factors for poor cognitive performance. The Framingham Study. *Diabetes Care.* 1997;20:1388–1395.
73. Brands AM, Biessels GJ, de Haan EH, Kappelle LJ, Kessels RP. The effects of type 1 diabetes on cognitive performance: A meta-analysis. *Diabetes Care.* 2005;28:726–735.
74. Lobnig BM, Kromeke O, Optenhostert-Porst C, Wolf OT. Hippocampal volume and cognitive performance in long-standing Type 1 diabetic patients without macrovascular complications. *Diabet Med.* 2006;23:32–39.
75. Strachan MW, Deary IJ, Ewing FM, Frier BM. Is type II diabetes associated with an increased risk of cognitive dysfunction? A critical review of published studies. *Diabetes Care.* 1997;20:438–445.
76. Biessels GT, ter Braak E, Erkelens DW, Hijmna R. Cognitive function in patients with type 2 diabetes mellitus. *Neuroscience Research Communications.* 2006;28:11–22.
77. Bjorgaas M, Gimse R, Vik T, Sand T. Cognitive function in type 1 diabetic children with and without episodes of severe hypoglycaemia. *Acta Paediatr.* 1997;86:148–153.
78. Reaven GM, Thompson LW, Nahum D, Haskins E. Relationship between hyperglycemia and cognitive function in older NIDDM patients. *Diabetes Care.* 1990;13:16–21.
79. McCall AL. Altered glycemia and brain-update and potential relevance to the aging brain. *Neurobiol Aging.* 2005;26:70–75.
80. Northam EA, Anderson PJ, Jacobs R, Hughes M, Warne GL, Werther GA. Neuropsychological profiles of children with type 1 diabetes 6 years after disease onset. *Diabetes Care.* 2001;24:1541–1546.
81. Ryan C, Vega A, Drash A. Cognitive deficits in adolescents who developed diabetes early in life. *Pediatrics.* 1985;75:921–927.
82. Rovet JF, Ehrlich RM, Hoppe M. Intellectual deficits associated with early onset of insulin-dependent diabetes mellitus in children. *Diabetes Care.* 1987;10:510–515.
83. Vanhanen M, Koivisto K, Karjalainen L, Helkala EL, Laakso M, Soininen H, Riekkinen P Sr. Risk for non-insulin-dependent diabetes in the normoglycaemic elderly is associated with impaired cognitive function. *Neuroreport.* 1997;8:1527–1530.
84. Karlamangla AS, Singer BH, Chodosh J, McEwen BS, Seeman TE. Urinary cortisol excretion as a predictor of incident cognitive impairment. *Neurobiol Aging.* 2005;26:80–84.
85. Plat L, Byrne MM, Sturis J, Polonsky KS, Mockel J, Fery F, Van Cauter E. Effects of morning cortisol elevation on insulin secretion and glucose regulation in humans. *Am J Physiol.* 1996;270:E36-E42.

86. Baura GD, Foster DM, Kaiyala K, Porte D, Jr., Kahn SE, Schwartz MW. Insulin transport from plasma into the central nervous system is inhibited by dexamethasone in dogs. *Diabetes*. 1996;45:86–90.
87. Convit A. Links between cognitive impairment in insulin resistance: An explanatory model. *Neurobiol Aging*. 2005;26:31–35.
88. Horner HC, Packan DR, Sapolsky RM. Glucocorticoids inhibit glucose transport in cultured hippocampal neurons and glia. *Neuroendocrinology*. 1990;52:57–64.
89. Jacobson L, Sapolsky R. The role of the hippocampus in feedback regulation of the hypothalamic-pituitary-adrenocortical axis. *Endocr Rev*. 1991;12:118–134.
90. Maher F, Vannucci SJ, Simpson IA. Glucose transporter proteins in brain. *FASEB J*. 1994;8:1003–1011.
91. Reagan LP, Magarinos AM, Yee DK, Swzeda LI, Van Bueren A, McCall AL, McEwen BS. Oxidative stress and HNE conjugation of GLUT3 are increased in the hippocampus of diabetic rats subjected to stress. *Brain Res*. 2000;862:292–300.
92. Cheng CM, Reinhardt RR, Lee WH, Joncas G, Patel SC, Bondy CA. Insulin-like growth factor 1 regulates developing brain glucose metabolism. *Proc Natl Acad Sci U S A*. 2000;97:10236–10241.
93. Reagan LP, Gorovits N, Hoskin EK, Alves SE, Katz EB, Grillo CA, Piroli GG, McEwen BS, Charron MJ. Localization and regulation of GLUTx1 glucose transporter in the hippocampus of streptozotocin diabetic rats. *Proc Natl Acad Sci U S A*. 2001;98:2820–2825.
94. Magarinos AM, McEwen BS. Experimental diabetes in rats causes hippocampal dendritic and synaptic reorganization and increased glucocorticoid reactivity to stress. *Proc Natl Acad Sci U S A*. 2000;97:11056–11061.
95. Ragozzino ME, Pal SN, Unick K, Stefani MR, Gold PE. Modulation of hippocampal acetylcholine release and spontaneous alternation scores by intrahippocampal glucose injections. *J Neurosci*. 1998;18:1595–1601.
96. McNay EC, Fries TM, Gold PE. Decreases in rat extracellular hippocampal glucose concentration associated with cognitive demand during a spatial task. *Proc Natl Acad Sci U S A*. 2000;97:2881–2885.
97. de Leon MJ, McRae T, Tsai JR, George AE, Marcus DL, Freedman M, Wolf AP, McEwen B. Abnormal cortisol response in Alzheimer's disease linked to hippocampal atrophy. *Lancet*. 1988;2:391–392.
98. Iguchi A, Uemura K, Miura H, Ishiguro T, Nonogaki K, Tamagawa T, Goshima K, Sakamoto N. Mechanism of intrahippocampal neostigmine-induced hyperglycemia in fed rats. *Neuroendocrinology*. 1992;55:44–50.
99. de Leon MJ, McRae T, Rusinek H, Convit A, De Santi S, Tarshish C, Golomb J, Volkow N, Daisley K, Orentreich N, McEwen B. Cortisol reduces hippocampal glucose metabolism in normal elderly, but not in Alzheimer's disease. *J Clin Endocrinol Metab*. 1997;82:3251–3259.
100. Gispen WH, Biessels GJ. Cognition and synaptic plasticity in diabetes mellitus. *Trends Neurosci*. 2000;23:542–549.
101. Bereket A, Lang CH, Wilson TA. Alterations in the growth hormone-insulin-like growth factor axis in insulin dependent diabetes mellitus. *Horm Metab Res*. 1999;31:172–181.
102. Brussee V, Cunningham FA, Zochodne DW. Direct insulin signaling of neurons reverses diabetic neuropathy. *Diabetes*. 2004;53:1824–1830.
103. Laron Z. Laron syndrome (primary growth hormone resistance or insensitivity): The personal experience. 1958–2003. *J Clin Endocrinol Metab*. 2004;89:1031–1044.
104. Reske-Nielsen E, Lundbaek K. Pathological changes in the central and peripheral nervous system of young long-term diabetics. II. The spinal cord and peripheral nerves. *Diabetologia*. 1968;4:34–43.

105. Brands AM, Kessels RP, de Haan EH, Kappelle LJ, Biessels GJ. Cerebral dysfunction in type 1 diabetes: Effects of insulin, vascular risk factors and blood-glucose levels. *Eur J Pharmacol.* 2004;490:159–168.
106. Langan SJ, Deary IJ, Hepburn DA, Frier BM. Cumulative cognitive impairment following recurrent severe hypoglycaemia in adult patients with insulin-treated diabetes mellitus. *Diabetologia.* 1991;34:337–344.
107. Lincoln NB, Faleiro RM, Kelly C, Kirk BA, Jeffcoate WJ. Effect of long-term glycemic control on cognitive function. *Diabetes Care.* 1996;19:656–658.
108. Wredling R, Levander S, Adamson U, Lins PE. Permanent neuropsychological impairment after recurrent episodes of severe hypoglycaemia in man. *Diabetologia.* 1990;33:152–157.
109. Mitrakou A, Ryan C, Veneman T, Mokan M, Jenssen T, Kiss I, Durrant J, Cryer P, Gerich J. Hierarchy of glycemic thresholds for counterregulatory hormone secretion, symptoms, and cerebral dysfunction. *Am J Physiol.* 1991;260:E67-E74.
110. de Galan BE, Schouwenberg BJ, Tack CJ, Smits P. Pathophysiology and management of recurrent hypoglycaemia and hypoglycaemia unawareness in diabetes. *Neth J Med.* 2006;64:269–279.
111. Elias MF, D'Agostino RB, Elias PK, Wolf PA. Neuropsychological test performance, cognitive functioning, blood pressure, and age: The Framingham Heart Study. *Exp Aging Res.* 1995;21:369–391.
112. Blumenthal JA, Madden DJ, Pierce TW, Siegel WC, Appelbaum M. Hypertension affects neurobehavioral functioning. *Psychosom Med.* 1993;55:44–50.
113. Waldstein SR, Ryan CM, Manuck SB, Parkinson DK, Bromet EJ. Learning and memory function in men with untreated blood pressure elevation. *J Consult Clin Psychol.* 1991;59: 513–517.
114. Birkenhager WH, Staessen JA. Progress in cardiovascular diseases: Cognitive function in essential hypertension. *Prog Cardiovasc Dis.* 2006;49(1):1–10.
115. Lewington S, Clarke R, Qizilbash N, Peto R, Collins R. Age-specific relevance of usual blood pressure to vascular mortality: A meta-analysis of individual data for one million adults in 61 prospective studies. *Lancet.* 2002;360:1903–1913.
116. Meyer JS, Rauch GM, Rauch RA, Haque A, Crawford K. Cardiovascular and other risk factors for Alzheimer's disease and vascular dementia. *Ann N Y Acad Sci.* 2000;903:411–423.
117. Zanchetti A, Elmfeldt D. Findings and implications of the Study on Cognition and Prognosis in the Elderly (SCOPE)—a review. *Blood Press.* 2006;15:71–79.
118. Elias MF, Wolf PA, D'Agostino RB, Cobb J, White LR. Untreated blood pressure level is inversely related to cognitive functioning: The Framingham Study. *Am J Epidemiol.* 1993;138:353–364.
119. Elias PK, D'Agostino RB, Elias MF, Wolf PA. Blood pressure, hypertension, and age as risk factors for poor cognitive performance. *Exp Aging Res.* 1995;21:393–417.
120. Launer LJ, Masaki K, Petrovitch H, Foley D, Havlik RJ. The association between midlife blood pressure levels and late-life cognitive function. The Honolulu-Asia Aging Study. *JAMA.* 1995;274:1846–1851.
121. Swan GE, Carmelli D, La Rue A. Relationship between blood pressure during middle age and cognitive impairment in old age: The Western Collaborative Group Study. *Aging Neuropsychol Cogn.* 1996;3:241–250.
122. de Leeuw FE, De Groot JC, Oudkerk M, Witteman JC, Hofman A, van Gijn J, Breteler MM. Hypertension and cerebral white matter lesions in a prospective cohort study. *Brain.* 2002;125:765–772.
123. DeCarli C, Murphy DG, Tranh M, Grady CL, Haxby JV, Gillette JA, Salerno JA, Gonzales-Aviles A, Horwitz B, Rapoport SI. The effect of white matter hyperintensity volume on

brain structure, cognitive performance, and cerebral metabolism of glucose in 51 healthy adults. *Neurology*. 1995;45:2077–2084.
124. Mentis MJ, Salerno J, Horwitz B, Grady C, Schapiro MB, Murphy DG, Rapoport SI. Reduction of functional neuronal connectivity in long-term treated hypertension. *Stroke*. 1994;25:601–607.
125. Herholz K, Heindel W, Rackl A, Neubauer I, Steinbrich W, Pietrzyk U, Erasmi-Korber H, Heiss WD. Regional cerebral blood flow in patients with leuko-araiosis and atherosclerotic carotid artery disease. *Arch Neurol*. 1990;47:392–396.
126. Longstreth WT Jr., Manolio TA, Arnold A, Burke GL, Bryan N, Jungreis CA, Enright PL, O'Leary D, Fried L. Clinical correlates of white matter findings on cranial magnetic resonance imaging of 3301 elderly people. The Cardiovascular Health Study. *Stroke*. 1996;27:1274–1282.
127. Salerno JA, Murphy DG, Horwitz B, DeCarli C, Haxby JV, Rapoport SI, Schapiro MB. Brain atrophy in hypertension. A volumetric magnetic resonance imaging study. *Hypertension*. 1992;20:340–348.
128. DeCarli C, Miller BL, Swan GE, Reed T, Wolf PA, Carmelli D. Cerebrovascular and brain morphologic correlates of mild cognitive impairment in the National Heart, Lung, and Blood Institute Twin Study. *Arch Neurol*. 2001;58:643–647.
129. Sierra C, Coca A. White matter lesions and cognitive impairment as silent cerebral disease in hypertension. *Scientific World Journal*. 2006;6:494–501.
130. Jarvik GP, Wijsman EM, Kukull WA, Schellenberg GD, Yu C, Larson EB. Interactions of apolipoprotein E genotype, total cholesterol level, age, and sex in prediction of Alzheimer's disease: A case-control study. *Neurology*. 1995;45:1092–1096.
131. Sparks DL. Coronary artery disease, hypertension, ApoE, and cholesterol: A link to Alzheimer's disease? *Ann N Y Acad Sci*. 1997;826:128–146.
132. Notkola IL, Sulkava R, Pekkanen J, Erkinjuntti T, Ehnholm C, Kivinen P, Tuomilehto J, Nissinen A. Serum total cholesterol, apolipoprotein E epsilon 4 allele, and Alzheimer's disease. *Neuroepidemiology*. 1998;17:14–20.
133. Roher AE, Kuo YM, Kokjohn KM, Emmerling MR, Gracon S. Amyloid and lipids in the pathology of Alzheimer disease. *Amyloid*. 1999;6:136–145.
134. Kivipelto M, Helkala EL, Laakso MP, Hanninen T, Hallikainen M, Alhainen K, Soininen H, Tuomilehto J, Nissinen A. Midlife vascular risk factors and Alzheimer's disease in later life: Longitudinal, population based study. *BMJ*. 2001;322:1447–1451.
135. van Exel E, de Craen AJ, Gussekloo J, Houx P, Bootsma-van der Wiel A, Macfarlane PW, Blauw GJ, Westendorp RG. Association between high-density lipoprotein and cognitive impairment in the oldest old. *Ann Neurol*. 2002;51:716–721.
136. Lesser G, Kandiah K, Libow LS, Likourezos A, Breuer B, Marin D, Mohs R, Haroutunian V, Neufeld R. Elevated serum total and LDL cholesterol in very old patients with Alzheimer's disease. *Dement Geriatr Cogn Disord*. 2001;12:138–145.
137. Yaffe K, Barrett-Connor E, Lin F, Grady D. Serum lipoprotein levels, statin use, and cognitive function in older women. *Arch Neurol*. 2002;59:378–384.
138. Wolozin B, Kellman W, Ruosseau P, Celesia GG, Siegel G. Decreased prevalence of Alzheimer disease associated with 3-hydroxy-3-methyglutaryl coenzyme A reductase inhibitors. *Arch Neurol*. 2000;57:1439–1443.
139. Li G, Higdon R, Kukull WA, Peskind E, Van Valen MK, Tsuang D, van Belle G, McCormick W, Bowen JD, Teri L, Schellenberg GD, Larson EB. Statin therapy and risk of dementia in the elderly: A community-based prospective cohort study. *Neurology*. 2004;63:1624–1628.
140. Nash DT, Fillit H. Cardiovascular disease risk factors and cognitive impairment. *Am J Cardiol*. 2006;97:1262–1265.

141. Sparks DL, Sabbagh MN, Connor DJ, Lopez J, Launer LJ, Browne P, Wasser D, Johnson-Traver S, Lochhead J, Ziolwolski C. Atorvastatin for the treatment of mild to moderate Alzheimer disease: Preliminary results. *Arch Neurol.* 2005;62:753–757.
142. Heilman KM, Fisher WR. Hyperlipidemic dementia. *Arch Neurol.* 1974;31:67–68.
143. Mathew NT, Meyer JS, Achari AN, Dodson RF. Hyperlipidemic neuropathy and dementia. *Eur Neurol.* 1976;14:370–382.
144. Perlmuter LC, Nathan DM, Goldfinger SH, Russo PA, Yates J, Larkin M. Triglyceride levels affect cognitive function in non-insulin-dependent diabetes. *J Diabetes Complications.* 1998;2:210–213.
145. Rogers RL, Meyer JS, McClintic K, Mortel KF. Reducing hypertriglyceridemia in elderly patients with cerebrovascular disease stabilizes or improves cognition and cerebral perfusion. *Angiology.* 1989;40:260–269.
146. Farr SA, Yamada KA, Butterfield DA, Abdul HM, Xu L, Miller NE, Banks WA, Morley JE. Obesity and hypertriglyceridemia produce cognitive impairment. *Endocrinology.* 2008;149:2628–2636.
147. Pappolla MA, Bryant-Thomas TK, Herbert D, Pacheco J, Fabra GM, Manjon M, Girones X, Henry TL, Matsubara E, Zambon D, Wolozin B, Sano M, Cruz-Sanchez FF, Thal LJ, Petanceska SS, Refolo LM. Mild hypercholesterolemia is an early risk factor for the development of Alzheimer amyloid pathology. *Neurology.* 2003;61:199–205.
148. Roher AE, Esh C, Kokjohn TA, Kalback W, Luehrs DC, Seward JD, Sue LI, Beach TG. Circle of Willis atherosclerosis is a risk factor for sporadic Alzheimer's disease. *Arterioscler Thromb Vasc Biol.* 2003;23:2055–2062.
149. Kuo YM, Emmerling MR, Bisgaier CL, Essenburg AD, Lampert HC, Drumm D, Roher AE. Elevated low-density lipoprotein in Alzheimer's disease correlates with brain Abeta 1–42 levels. *Biochem Biophys Res Commun.* 1998;252:711–715.
150. Refolo LM, Malester B, LaFrancois J, Bryant-Thomas T, Wang R, Tint GS, Sambamurti K, Duff K, Pappolla MA. Hypercholesterolemia accelerates the Alzheimer's amyloid pathology in a transgenic mouse model. *Neurobiol Dis.* 2000;7:321–331.
151. Refolo LM, Pappolla MA, LaFrancois J, Malester B, Schmidt SD, Thomas-Bryant T, Tint GS, Wang R, Mercken M, Petanceska SS, Duff KE. A cholesterol-lowering drug reduces beta-amyloid pathology in a transgenic mouse model of Alzheimer's disease. *Neurobiol Dis.* 2001;8:890–899.
152. Sparks DL, Scheff SW, Hunsaker JC, III, Liu H, Landers T, Gross DR. Induction of Alzheimer-like beta-amyloid immunoreactivity in the brains of rabbits with dietary cholesterol. *Exp Neurol.* 1994;126:88–94.
153. Michikawa M. Cholesterol paradox: Is high total or low HDL cholesterol level a risk for Alzheimer's disease? *J Neurosci Res.* 2003;72:141–146.
154. Burns M, Duff K. Cholesterol in Alzheimer's disease and tauopathy. *Ann N Y Acad Sci.* 2002;977:367–375.
155. Breteler MM, Claus JJ, Grobbee DE, Hofman A. Cardiovascular disease and distribution of cognitive function in elderly people: The Rotterdam Study. *BMJ.* 1994;308:1604–1608.
156. Kalmijn S, Feskens EJ, Launer LJ, Kromhout D. Cerebrovascular disease, the apolipoprotein e4 allele, and cognitive decline in a community-based study of elderly men. *Stroke.* 1996;27:2230–2235.
157. Knapp LT, Klann E. Potentiation of hippocampal synaptic transmission by superoxide requires the oxidative activation of protein kinase C. *J Neurosci.* 2002;22:674–683.
158. Knapp LT, Klann E. Role of reactive oxygen species in hippocampal long-term potentiation: Contributory or inhibitory? *J Neurosci Res.* 2002;70(1):1–7.

159. Banks WA, Coon AB, Robinson SM, Moinuddin A, Shultz JM, Nakaoke R, Morley JE. Triglycerides induce leptin resistance at the blood-brain barrier. *Diabetes*. 2004;53: 1253–1260.
160. Farr SA, Banks WA, Morley JE. Effects of leptin on memory processing. *Peptides*. 2006;27:1420–1425.
161. Figlewicz DP, Bennett J, Evans SB, Kaiyala K, Sipols AJ, Benoit SC. Intraventricular insulin and leptin reverse place preference conditioned with high-fat diet in rats. *Behav Neurosci*. 2004;118:479–487.
162. Wayner MJ, Armstrong DL, Phelix CF, Oomura Y. Orexin-A (Hypocretin-1) and leptin enhance LTP in the dentate gyrus of rats in vivo. *Peptides*. 2004;25:991–996.
163. Chang GQ, Karatayev O, Davydova Z, Leibowitz SF. Circulating triglycerides impact on orexigenic peptides and neuronal activity in hypothalamus. *Endocrinology*. 2004;145: 3904–3912.
164. Diano S, Farr SA, Benoit SC, McNay EC, da Silva I, Horvath B, Gaskin FS, Nonaka N, Jaeger LB, Banks WA, Morley JE, Pinto S, Sherwin RS, Xu L, Yamada KA, Sleeman MW, Tschop MH, Horvath TL. Ghrelin controls hippocampal spine synapse density and memory performance. *Nat Neurosci*. 2006;9:381–388.
165. Gaskin FS, Farr SA, Banks WA, Kumar VB, Morley JE. Ghrelin-induced feeding is dependent on nitric oxide. *Peptides*. 2003;24:913–918.
166. Simons M, Keller P, De Strooper B, Beyreuther K, Dotti CG, Simons K. Cholesterol depletion inhibits the generation of beta-amyloid in hippocampal neurons. *Proc Natl Acad Sci U S A*. 1998;95:6460–6464.
167. Kojro E, Gimpl G, Lammich S, Marz W, Fahrenholz F. Low cholesterol stimulates the non-amyloidogenic pathway by its effect on the alpha-secretase ADAM 10. *Proc Natl Acad Sci U S A*. 2001;98:5815–5820.
168. Hu G, Qiao Q, Tuomilehto J. The metabolic syndrome and cardiovascular risk. *Curr Diabetes Rev*. 2005;1:137–143.
169. Yaffe K, Haan M, Blackwell T, Cherkasova E, Whitmer RA, West N. Metabolic syndrome and cognitive decline in elderly Latinos: Findings from the Sacramento Area Latino Study of Aging study. *J Am Geriatr Soc*. 2007;55:758–762.
170. Dik MG, Jonker C, Comijs HC, Deeg DJ, Kok A, Yaffe K, Penninx BW. Contribution of metabolic syndrome components to cognition in older individuals. *Diabetes Care*. 2007;30:2655–2660.

10

NEUROLOGICAL SEQUELAE AND COGNITIVE OUTCOMES FOLLOWING CARDIOSURGICAL INTERVENTION

Jeffrey Browndyke and Patrick Smith

The past three decades have witnessed significant reductions in cardiac morbidity and mortality associated with cardiosurgical interventions, yet central nervous system (CNS) injuries, such as stroke, secondary to these common procedures remain a significant concern.[1–6] A little over a twofold increase in cardiosurgical bypass (CPB) neurological complications was reported for an eight-year period from the late 1970s to the mid-1980s[3, 7]—an increase that sadly has broadened further over the intervening decades. These CNS complication concerns are unfortunately greatest in elderly populations for which cardiac surgery is generally more efficacious than medical therapy alone.[8] Ironically, the general benefits and concerns are born from the same substrate (i.e., greater comorbidities and advanced cardiovascular disease), resulting in a delicate balance between the risk of greater neurological morbidity and mortality versus possible lifespan extension and quality-of-life improvement.[9–13] Additional factors, such as the health economics of cardiosurgical intervention and possible neurological injury, come into play, providing an even greater impetus to tackle the issue of cardiosurgical CNS complications as the sizable "Baby Boom generation" is the next population wave of poor cardiac health risk.[14]

The spectrum of CNS complications ranges in severity from fatal stroke and coma to relatively less severe and often temporary acute conditions, such as encephalopathy and postoperative delirium.[4, 15, 16] While these lesser complications do not carry as high a mortality risk, they may have lasting effects on cognition well beyond acute recovery periods, and they are known to contribute to prolonged health-care utilization and decreased quality of life.[5] Complicated postoperative recovery of independent function and premorbid cognitive abilities may then lead to psychiatric complications, such as depression, which further decrease patient satisfaction.[17, 18]

Acknowledgments: Manuscript preparation and production supported, in part, by National Institute of Health grants NIA P30-AG028377 and L30-AG029001.

The question of cognitive difficulties post-cardiosurgical intervention, for many, is fraught with problems because of the often varying reports regarding the functional significance of any cognitive change, and disagreement regarding the standard by which clinically "meaningful" change is measured.[19, 20] Often because these cognitive changes were perceived in the past as transient, they were just dismissed, but seminal work by Newman and colleagues[15, 21] suggests that the cognitive changes observed early in the recovery process may be important to long-term (five-year) general health outcomes and functional capacities,[22] long after the surgical procedure. This new understanding of possible longitudinal impact[10, 15, 21, 23–29] has underscored the importance of accurately measuring and characterizing iatrogenic neurological injury and any associated cognitive impairment following cardiosurgical intervention; yielding a fresh set of controversies for the growing study of post-interventional cognitive change.

For the convenience of the reader, this chapter is divided into two broad sections. Beginning with the incidence and etiology of various perioperative neurological injuries, chapter discussion then transitions to the incidence and characteristics of cognitive change most often associated with cardiosurgical interventions. After this, the chapter is rounded out by a brief coverage of perioperative genetics and how this growing subfield, in concert with neuropsychological/behavioral and neuroimaging expertise, may be uniquely poised to assist in preoperative risk-identification of possible cardiosurgical injury and associated cognitive decline.

Perioperative Neurological Injury

Incidence

Just behind heart disease and cancer, stroke remains among the top three leading causes of death in the United States. Overall, death rates associated with cerebrovascular disease have declined, but not appreciably enough to remove it from its perch as one of the leading factors in U.S. deaths.[30] Among the causes of iatrogenic stroke, coronary artery bypass graft (CABG) procedures have been consistently reported as being leading contributors, with an average risk rate of 2%.[31, 32]

Care associated with perioperative stroke secondary to CABG also accounts for a significant financial burden to the health-care system and individuals.[33] It has been estimated that approximately 25% of the annual expenditures for stroke treatment in the United States are accounted by perioperative stroke complications.[34] Tuman and colleagues have observed that cardiosurgical CNS complications tended to increase ICU stays from 3 + 3 days to 9 + 11 days, and mortality rates were significantly greater in those with perioperative CNS complications (36%) than in unaffected cardiosurgical patients (4%).[4, 35] More recent data by Stamou and colleagues suggest that prolonged hospital length of stay (11 + 4 day) and ICU utilization (2 + 2 days) is the norm for patients with cardiosurgical CNS complications,[32] and similar to the observations of Tuman and colleagues,[35] in-hospital mortality rates remain relatively high (14.4%) in these patients.

An early study by Roach and colleagues provided an initial glimpse into the incidence of perioperative CNS complications following elective CABG.[5] Among approximately

2100 patients at 24 medical institutions, the incidence rate of adverse outcomes was 6.1%. This incidence rate was split fairly evenly between patients who were noted to have serious perioperative CNS complications (3.1%—fatal/nonfatal stroke, stupor, or coma at discharge) and those with less life-threatening complications (3%—deterioration in intellectual or memory functions, acute seizures, or acute delirium).

When the incidence of perioperative CNS complications is limited to strokes alone, the incidence rate is reduced to 1.6% (based upon a retrospective review of approximately 3000 cardiosurgical patients by Hogue et al.).[36] Of the strokes reported by Hogue and colleagues, 65% occurred during the postoperative recovery period. More recent data from the Society of Thoracic Surgery's National Cardiac Surgery Database appear to support a reduction in the incidence of perioperative CNS complications. Among approximately 400,000 patients from the years 1996 to 1997, the incidence of CNS events was 3.3%.[37] These data reinforce a recent reduction in perioperative CNS complications,[38] which is paradoxically positioned against the rapid increase in perioperative stroke risk factors in the general population. The disparity is most likely due, in part, to improved surgical techniques and better patient-management during the postoperative period.

Among the various cardiosurgical procedures, perioperative CNS complications vary widely. There is a higher risk for adverse outcomes in patients undergoing open-chamber procedures, such as mitral and aortic valve surgeries, which have typically been ascribed to the increased risk for embolization secondary to thrombi or vegetations.[2, 6, 39, 40] Intraoperative entrapment of air within the cardiac chambers presents an additional complication and is thought to contribute to the higher complication risk associated open-chamber procedures.[4] The incidence of CNS complications for patients undergoing intracardiac and coronary artery surgery has been estimated at 16%; this total incidence, again, was fairly evenly divided between serious/fatal complications and lesser CNS events.[6] And, while the overall incidence of perioperative stroke has declined in recent years, the risk for adverse cerebral outcomes in patients undergoing intracardiac and revascularization procedures has been estimated at two to three times that of either procedure alone.[4, 36]

Etiology

Cerebral hypoperfusion Non-pulsatile perfusion and lower pressure during cardiosurgical intervention have been implicated as important conditions for perioperative neurological injury.[41] These factors, when paired with watershed infarcts, appear to be the most plausible mechanism for many of the stroke difficulties observed in older cardiac patients. Supporting this theory is the observation that lower pressure has been associated with reduced washout of watershed emboli,[42] and, as a result, increased probability of cerebral infarction in distal vascular territories. The prospect that higher pressures (mean arterial pressure of 80–100 mm/Hg) may be protective comes from a study by Gold and colleagues, who found that myocardial and neurological positive outcomes post-CABG were associated with pressures in the aforementioned range relative to patients with low perfusion pressures (50–70 mm/Hg).[43] Additionally, higher pressures may prove to be maximally beneficial to neurological outcomes when the level of aortic atherosclerosis is high,[44] reinforcing the theory that the higher pressures may assist in embolic washout.

Cerebral embolization secondary to aortic atherosclerosis Proximal aortic atherosclerosis has long been associated with increased risk for perioperative neurological complications,[44–46] and as noted in the section above, severe atherosclerosis when paired with low perfusion pressure appears to be most detrimental to postsurgical neurological outcomes. Prior to transesophageal echocardiography, common procedures involving surgeon-palpated aortic atherosclerosis were associated with a significant increase in stroke,[5, 47] and the connections between stroke and aortic atherosclerosis were further strengthened by epiaortic ultrasound data noting an increase in stroke risk with atherosclerosis severity in the ascending aorta.[45] Less obtrusive measurement using transcranial Doppler and carotid ultrasound have supported the connection between cerebral emboli risk and atherosclerosis by observing that cannulation, aortic cross-clamp procedures, and partial occlusion side-biting clamps are associated with increased emboli production.[40, 48, 49] However, support for the pairing of emboli magnitude and outcomes has been mixed, with some suggesting that emboli must exceed a critical threshold before any cognitive consequences are observable.[50–53] Additionally, the inability to distinguish air from particulate emboli has hampered the ability to sort out the contribution of atherosclerosis-related damage from other surgical factors. Whether the emboli are air or particulate, it has been demonstrated that approximately 45% of CABG or aortic surgery patients have visible lesions on diffusion-weighted imaging (DWI) brain scans.[54] Enhanced diffusivity, typically in the deep white matter, underscores that, while cognitive consequences secondary to embolic damage may not be observable, there is often objective evidence of neurological injury. Whether these emboli-related diffusivity lesions represent permanent or reversible damage is still debatable, but it is known that the location of any embolic damage will sway whether cognitive consequences are readily observable (e.g., strategic lesion in the medial-dorsal thalamic nucleus vs. lesion in the centrum semiovale).

Cardiac arrhythmia Atrial fibrillation appears to be another notable contributor to negative neurological outcomes following cardiac surgery, with overall incidence rates between 20% and 40%.[55, 56] Advanced age, gender (males), and chronic obstructive pulmonary disease (COPD) are associated with increased incidence.[55–60] The mechanism by which atrial fibrillation may contribute to neurological insult is not well understood, but it is thought that postoperative arrhythmias may increase the likelihood of embolic damage or hypoperfusion due to reduced cardiac output.[4] Regardless of the mechanism, there is some support for the connection between atrial fibrillation and postoperative neurocognitive status change. Stanley and colleagues demonstrated that cardiosurgical patients with postoperative atrial fibrillation experienced greater cognitive decline than those who did not at a six-week cognitive retest interval.[61]

Perioperative Cognitive Change

Incidence

Perioperative cognitive changes have been frequently reported following cardiosurgical interventions,[62, 63] although the incidence of cognitive decline following cardiosurgical intervention varies markedly in relation to the relatively stable incidence reporting for cardiosurgical CNS complications. This disparity is probably the byproduct of widely disparate measurement techniques for cognitive performance, persistent issues surrounding the operational definition of "meaningful clinical change," variability in surgical procedures, and heterogeneity among the inclusion/exclusion criteria of outcome studies.[64] Newman and colleagues report, "Utilization of a standard deviation, a half standard deviation or a percent decline yields early dysfunction rates from 50% to 70% within the first postoperative week, declining to 30% to 50% in six weeks and 20% to 40% at six months and one year,"[4] lending weight to the observation that the incidence of perioperative cognitive decline is guided largely by the metric with which it is measured.

Measurement issues aside, cognitive performance has been identified as a surrogate marker of neurobehavioral risk in other populations, predicting incident cardiovascular events[65] and dementia.[66] Neurocognitive sequelae of cardiosurgical procedures may therefore have prognostic significance and are the focus of increasing research as these procedures have gained wider clinical usage.[67]

Etiology

Coronary artery bypass grafting Cognitive deficits have been reported in 30% to 80% of patients following CABG,[4, 5, 21] with many individuals' experiencing cognitive decline in the immediate postoperative period.[5, 21] Cognitive dysfunction at discharge following CABG, although highly variable between studies, has been shown to predict future cognitive decline in longitudinal studies.[21] Newman and colleagues[4] have reported that observed perioperative neurocognitive changes are highly dependent on a given study's methodology, including variations in measurement techniques and in criteria for patient inclusion and exclusion. Results may also vary by patient characteristics and assessment modality, as previous studies have found that background factors (age, education level) and assessment location (hospital, clinic, or home) may be associated with significant variations in neurocognitive performance.[68]

Transient fluctuations in neurocognitive function may be most apparent in the first weeks postoperatively. Rates of cognitive dysfunction have been reported between 50%–70% within the first postoperative week, falling to 30%–50% after six weeks and continuing to decline to 20%–40% at six months and one year.[4, 64] In a sample of 261 patients undergoing CABG, Newman and colleagues [21] found that 53% of participants exhibited cognitive dysfunction at discharge. Six weeks postoperatively, however, only 36% of patients showed cognitive decrements; and performance continued to improve, with only 24% of participants demonstrating cognitive dysfunction at a six-month follow-up. Consistent with other findings,[69] however, the authors noted a decrease in cognitive function five years postoperatively, with 42% of patients exhibiting cognitive decrements. This finding may have reflected the additional influence of normal aging processes following CABG, although discrepant findings have also been reported.[70]

Valve replacement Neurobehavioral changes have also been observed following cardiac valve replacement procedures. Valve replacement is particularly common among individuals with aortic stenosis and may improve left ventricular ejection fraction (LVEF) and cardiac survival. Although fewer studies have examined this relationship, rates of cognitive dysfunction appear comparable to those following CABG,[71] possibly with greater severity of deficits.[62] Ebert and colleagues[62] have demonstrated that cognitive deficits associated with valve replacement may be more severe than those exhibited following CABG, with a greater severity of dysfunction in fluency, arithmetic, and working memory. Zimpfer and colleagues[71] have reported neurocognitive decline in 52% of individuals receiving biological valve and 45% receiving mechanical valve replacement one week postoperatively. Cognitive dysfunction may continue decline following hospital discharge, although few studies have examined the stability of cognitive function over extensive postoperative time periods. Grimm and colleagues[72] found that cognitive performance continuously worsened during the initial four months postoperatively among individuals receiving mechanical valve replacement, although individuals receiving mitral valve repair did not experience comparable decline in this study.

Neurological insult Recent studies utilizing magnetic resonance imaging (MRI) and diffusion-weighted imaging techniques have reported that clinically undetected ischemic lesions may occur in up to 45% of patients who have undergone cardiac surgery,[73, 74] and that subclinical ischemic damage may only be observable using high-resolution imaging techniques.[75] Brain swelling, reduced regional blood flow, and neuronal death have all been reported following CABG[76–78] and may be associated with cognitive dysfunction.[19, 79]

Retrospective studies among individuals exhibiting cognitive dysfunction postoperatively have generally found poorer cognition to be associated with new ischemic lesions following CABG.[75] Prospective studies have extended these findings, demonstrating that occult neurological damage following CABG may not manifest in reduced cognitive performance.[80, 81] Floyd and colleagues[82] examined this relationship by conducting diffusion-weighted imaging assessments in 34 patients undergoing various cardiosurgical procedures. Imaging was obtained before and after surgical intervention to assess for the presence of new cerebral infarctions. New infarctions occurred in 18% of patients and, of those, 67% were clinically silent. The patients undergoing procedures involving aortic valve replacement were most likely to experience new infarctions, and baseline white matter lesions tended to predict new postoperative infarctions. Similarly, Bendszus and colleagues[81] found that 26% of CABG patients assessed using diffusion-weighted MRI exhibited new ischemic lesions postoperatively, but the presence of new lesions was not associated with reduced neuropsychological performance.

Decreased cognitive performance may result from neuronal damage following cerebral hypoperfusion or microembolic showers. Cerebral hypoperfusion may also impact neuronal function indirectly by reducing washout of small emboli, resulting in greater neuronal injury.[42, 43] Studies utilizing Doppler imaging have demonstrated that microemboli showers are common during cardiac surgery, particularly during the cannulation and clamping/unclamping.[40] Djaiani and colleagues[83] recently found that new ischemic lesions following CABG were associated with greater embolic count, and that greater cerebral emboli were associated with greater confusion postoperatively. Furthermore, post-mortem examinations of post-CABG patients have reported higher numbers of small-capillary cerebral arteriolar dilatations, which occur in large number as a result of microembolization.[4, 84]

Anesthesia The use of general anesthesia in both cardiac[24, 85] and non-cardiac procedures has been associated with postoperative cognitive decline, particularly among older patients.[23, 86] Many of the cognitive deficits observed in the immediate postoperative period have been attributed to insufficient drug clearance and/or postoperative pain,[19] and are not hypothesized to reflect neuronal damage. In animal models, however, anesthesia administration has been associated with changes in gene expression, cerebral protein synthesis, and cognitive dysfunction.[87–89] Despite plausible mechanisms underlying the relationship between cardiosurgery and cognition,[4] few clinical investigations have examined this relationship.[90] Williams-Russo and colleagues,[90] in the largest trial to date, examined the cognitive sequelae following random assignment to epidural or general anesthesia in a sample of 262 patients. Assessments were conducted one week and six months postoperatively using ten cognitive tests assessing performance in multiple cognitive domains, including memory, psychomotor speed, and language skills. Few participants experienced cognitive dysfunction, and rates did not differ between groups.

Personality and affective change Personality and emotional changes are commonly reported following CABG surgery. Although depression has been most often examined,[91] anxiety, stress,[92] and quality of life[18] changes have also been observed. As with cognitive changes, alterations in mood may be most apparent during the acute postoperative period. Rothenhausler and colleagues,[18] for example, reported that adjustment disorder, post-traumatic stress disorder, and major depression are all relatively common immediately following CABG, but that the prevalence of psychological dysfunction returned to preoperative levels 12 months postoperatively. Studies that have investigated personality characteristics prospectively have generally reported weaker findings, with preoperative mood state consistently predicting postoperative mood.[91]

Psychological functioning may influence cognitive test performance during the postoperative period. Andrew and colleagues[92] found that preoperative depression was associated with postoperative deficits on cognitive measures of attention and memory, but that changes in depression, anxiety, and stress from preoperative levels were unrelated to cognitive performance. Despite studies demonstrating a relationship between postoperative depression and cognition, findings have generally found little evidence that depression affects postoperative cognitive function.[17, 93] Nevertheless, moderate-to-severe depression following CABG has been prospectively shown to double the risk of mortality.[94] Moreover, mild-to-moderate depression levels that persisted up to six months were associated with comparable mortality rates, indicating that depression status may have important implications for the clinical management of CABG patients, regardless of its association with cognitive function.

Impact of preexisting CVD Although the impact of postoperative CVD has been studied extensively,[61] an emerging body of evidence suggests that preexisting differences in CVD may be associated with differential cognitive performance following CABG. Individual differences in CVD have been hypothesized to influence the variation in rates of cognitive dysfunction observed in the extant literature. Baumgartner and colleagues,[95] for example, have hypothesized that preexisting variations in CVD comorbidities may explain the discrepant findings in cognitive dysfunction observed in studies utilizing longer follow-up periods.

Several studies have demonstrated that preoperative CVD may be associated with greater detriments following surgery. Boodhwani and colleagues[96] have shown that impaired left ventricular ejection fraction, a marker of cardiovascular risk, is associated with elevated risk for postoperative cognitive dysfunction. Peripheral indices of CVD have also been shown to predict poorer cognition during the postoperative period. Goto and colleagues[97] found that severity of aortic arteriosclerosis assessed preoperatively was associated with postoperative cognitive decrements in a graded fashion, with increasing severity predicting poorer cognitive function. Similarly, Collison and colleagues[98] reported that peripheral vascular disease was associated with greater postoperative neurological complications in a prospective study of 11,398 CABG patients.

Preexisting CVD may impair cognitive performance by increasing the operative embolic load. Djaiani and colleagues[83] examined this relationship by studying the association between aortic atherosclerosis, diffusion-weighted ischemic lesions, operative embolic load, and postoperative mental status in a group of 110 older adults scheduled for CABG surgery. Atherosclerosis in the ascending aorta and aortic arch predicted postoperative ischemic lesions and greater embolic count during the procedure. Furthermore, greater preoperative atherosclerosis was associated with postoperative mental status changes.

Several studies utilizing imaging data have identified presurgical white matter disease as a predictor of postoperative cognitive dysfunction. In a prospective study of 421 Japanese patients aged 60 years and older, Goto and colleagues[99] found that postoperative cognitive dysfunction varied systematically by degree of white matter damage at baseline. Among individuals with greater white matter disease at baseline (i.e., multiple cerebral infarctions), 20% demonstrated postoperative cognitive dysfunction. In comparison, only 7% of those with minimal white matter damage exhibited comparable deficits. Goto and colleagues[100] conducted a similar study in which a total atherosclerotic score was derived by combining risk-assessment measures from the carotid arteries, ascending aorta, and cerebral white matter from MRI. Participants were classified into low-, intermediate-, and high-risk groups based on their total atherosclerotic burden. Neuropsychological dysfunction was present in 25%, 33%, and 79% of participants in the low-, intermediate-, and high-risk groups, respectively.

Longitudinal Cognitive Outcomes

CABG outcomes Several studies have examined long-term cognitive changes following CABG. Longitudinal assessment of cognition is particularly important following CABG, as population-based data from the Cache County Study have demonstrated CABG patients may show a steeper rate of cognitive decline compared with healthy control participants.[69]

In a longitudinal examination, Selnes and colleagues[25] found that CABG patients exhibited comparable improvement in the first year postoperatively compared with nonsurgical controls. Similarly, a nonsignificant decline in overall cognitive function was observed between postoperative testing and a three year follow-up, similar to the decline observed in nonsurgical controls. In a separate study, Selnes and colleagues[26] investigated the cognitive performance of 102 patients approximately five years following CABG. The authors found that patients experienced declines in visuoconstruction and psychomotor speed during the five-year follow-up, but exhibited improvements in executive function.

Newman and colleagues[21] examined this association in 261 patients undergoing CABG. Although only 24% of these patients exhibited cognitive dysfunction six months postoperatively, there was a marked increase during the five-year follow-up, with 42% of patients demonstrating cognitive dysfunction. Interestingly, cognitive dysfunction at discharge was a significant predictor of subsequent cognitive decline, regardless of small improvements during intermediate follow-up assessments.

Valve replacement outcomes Several studies have examined longitudinal changes in cognitive function following valve replacement. Zimpfer and colleagues[29] examined the long-term changes in electroencephalogram (EEG) P300 evoked potential following aortic valve replacement, finding that P300 latency had increased approximately seven days postoperatively. When patients were assessed again four months following surgery, P300 latencies had returned to presurgical levels and remained normal up to 3 years postoperatively. Sotaniemi and colleagues[27] examined the cognitive sequelae of valve replacement surgery in a sample of 44 patients, finding that five-year cognitive performance varied by cognitive performance immediately following discharge. Specifically, patients exhibiting cognitive gains during their two-month assessment continued to improve at a one-year follow-up, with only a marginal decline in performance thereafter. In contrast, patients exhibiting cognitive deficits two months following surgery continued to experience relative deficits at their five-year assessment.

Controversies, Cutting Edge, and Conclusions

CABG: On-pump vs. Off-pump

In recent years, the effects of on-pump and off-pump CABG procedures have been investigated. Off-pump CABG may be associated with the production of fewer microemboli,[101] which have been associated with acute cognitive decrements in some studies.[51] Bucerius and colleagues[102] found a lower incidence of perioperative stroke in off-pump CABG patients. Among the 16,000 adult cardiosurgical patients they studied, the overall incidence of stroke was 4.6%, but incidence varied as a function of the cardiosurgical procedure, with off-pump CABG showing the lowest (1.9%), and double- or triple-valve surgery, the highest (9.7%). On-pump CABG stroke incidence was 3.8% in this large surgical cohort. Despite the apparent disparity in stroke incidence between off- and on-pump CABG, controlled trials have generally found little or no difference between patients randomly assigned to receive on- or off-pump CABG. Hernandez and colleagues[103] examined differences in cognitive function among 102 patients randomly assigned to receive conventional on-pump CABG compared to 99 individuals undergoing off-pump CABG. Using a comprehensive neuropsychological battery, the authors reported only marginal differences between groups, with off-pump patients demonstrating lower performance on tasks of processing speed and executive function at discharge and marginal differences in spatial attention during a six-month follow-up. In the largest trial to date, van Dijk and colleagues[28] conducted a longitudinal study comparing the cognitive sequelae of on-pump and off-pump CABG, reporting comparable cognitive performance, quality of life, and cardiac event rates during a five-year follow-up assessment. However, despite its size, the trial was underpowered to fully examine cognitive outcomes and was populated by a lower-risk patient population.

Overall, there has been insufficient prospective controlled study of on- or off-pump CABG to firmly establish which procedure may be preferential for reduced perioperative neurological injury and positive cognitive outcomes. However, the limited evidence todate appears to favor off-pump procedures in both reduced stroke incidence and reduced cognitive complications.

Perioperative Genetics of Cardiosurgical Neurological and Cognitive Outcomes

Genetic predisposition to cardiosurgically related cerebral injuries and perioperative cognitive change is an area of recent, but intense, research interest. The subfield of perioperative genetics pairs genetic analyses with neurological outcomes to allow for the modeling of candidate risk genotypes with the likelihood and pattern characteristics of perioperative cognitive decline, as well as larger genome-wide searches for single-nucleotide polymorphisms that may be associated with poor clinical outcomes.

The apolipoprotein E (APOE) hypothesis of cognitive outcome post-CABG serves as the fountainhead for perioperative genetics research. In their seminal study, Tardiff and colleagues[104] discovered that cognitive outcomes were poorer in carriers of the APOE e4 allele. Consistent replication of the APOE finding has been elusive, however, and has led many to question whether APOE e4 allele carrier status confers poor cognitive-outcome risk beyond what might be normally attributable to cardiosurgical iatrogenesis.[105–108] The Tardiff et al. finding, however controversial, opened the door for other researchers to move beyond the candidate gene approach to the characterization of individual genetic variations in single-nucleotide polymorphisms (SNPs).

Mathew and colleagues have conducted a few studies utilizing this broader SNP search approach and have found that stroke complications during cardiosurgical procedures were associated with a combination of interleukin-6 single-nucleotide polymorphisms and two minor C-reactive protein alleles.[4, 109, 110] Additionally, the glycoprotein

(GP) IIIa P1A2 polymorphism, related to platelet integrin receptors, has been associated with poorer cognitive outcomes and is postulated to reflect the likelihood of cerebral insult secondary to increased prothrombotic time in P1A2 carriers.[110] Inflammatory processes, and the genes regulating them, have been posited as increasing the risk for poor cardiosurgical outcome[111] and are likely to be the next logical pathophysiological target for both the candidate gene and genome-wide approaches.

Conclusion

The field of perioperative cognitive decline will continue to be advanced by emerging subfields and diagnostic techniques, such as perioperative genetics and advanced functional imaging technologies (as discussed elsewhere in this book), but it remains incumbent upon researchers to steer these advances properly and to avoid the stumbling blocks of the past. A better understanding of the interaction among surgical technique, pathophysiology, genetics, premorbid personality/mood characteristics, and age-related factors will be key to disentangling the often mixed results found in the literature. However, the task before researchers should not just be description of the problem, though this is a necessary step in scientific discovery, but also the development of better screening techniques to identify cardiosurgical patients at risk for cerebral injury or perioperative cognitive decline. It is here that researchers and clinicians must work in concert, calling upon the intellectual resources of cardiothoracic surgical specialists, anesthesiology, neuroradiology, clinical neuropsychology, and social work, to build and refine the reliable screening tools to characterize perioperative risk profiles. Robust risk identification will then allow clinicians to target the patients most likely to profit from prevention strategies, and move the field that much closer to the ultimate goal of stemming the tide of perioperative neurological injury and cognitive decline.

Notes

1. Boeken U, Litmathe J, Feindt P, Gams E. Neurological complications after cardiac surgery: Risk factors and correlation to the surgical procedure. *Thorac Cardiovasc Surg*. 2005;53:33–36.
2. Cleveland JC, Shroyer LW, Chen A, Peterson E, Grover FL. Off-pump coronary artery bypass grafting significantly decreases risk-adjusted mortality and morbidity. *Ann Thorac Surg*. 2001;72:1282–1288. Discussions 8–9.
3. Mack MJ, Brown PP, Kugelmass AD, et al. Current status and outcomes of coronary revascularization. 1999 to 2002: 148,396 surgical and percutaneous procedures. *Ann Thorac Surg*. 2004;77:761–766.
4. Newman MF, Mathew JP, Grocott HP, et al. Central nervous system injury associated with cardiac surgery. *Lancet*. 2006;368:694–703.
5. Roach GW, Kanchuger M, Mora-Mangano C, et al. Adverse cerebral outcomes after coronary bypass surgery. *N Engl J Med*. 1996;335:1857–1863.
6. Wolman RL, Nussmeier NA, Aggarwal A, et al. Cerebral injury after cardiac surgery: Identification of a group at extraordinary risk. *Stroke*. 1999;30:514–522.
7. Hogue CW, Sundt TM, Goldberg M, et al. Neurological complications of cardiac surgery: The need for new paradigms in prevention and treatment. *Semin Thorac Cardiovasc Surg*. 1999;11:105–15.

8. Ferguson TB, Hammill BG, Peterson ED, DeLong ER, Grover FL. A decade of change—Risk profiles and outcomes for isolated coronary artery bypass grafting procedures, 1990–1999: A report from the STS National Database Committee and the Duke Clinical Research Institute. *Ann Thorac Surg*. 2002;73:480–489.
9. Hammermeister KE, Burchfiel C, Johnson R, Grover FL. Identification of patients at greatest risk for developing major complications at cardiac surgery. *Circulation*. 1990;82:380–389.
10. Hannen EL, Racz MJ, Walford G, et al. Long-term outcomes of coronary-artery bypass grafting versus stent implantation. *N Engl J Med*. 2005;352:2174–2183.
11. Jones EL, Weintraub WS, Carver JM, Guyton RA, Cohen CL. Coronary bypass surgery: Is the operation different today? *J Thorac Cardiovasc Surg*. 1991;101:108–115.
12. Malenka DJ, Leavitt BJ, Hearne MJ, et al. Comparing long-term survival of patients with multivessel coronary disease after CABG or PCI: Analysis of BARI-like patients in northern New England. For the Northern New England Cardiovascular Disease Study Group. *Circulation*. 2005;112:I371–I376.
13. Mohan R, Amsel BJ, Walter PL. Coronary artery bypass grafting in the elderly: A review of studies on patients older than 64, 69, or 74 years. *Cardiology*. 1992;80:215–225.
14. Weinstein MC, Coxson PG, Williams LW, Pass TM, Stason WB, Goldman L. Forecasting coronary heart disease incidence, mortality, and cost: The Coronary Heart Disease Policy Model. *Am J Public Health*. 1987;77:1417–1426.
15. Newman MF, Grocott HP, Mathew JP, et al. Report of the substudy assessing the impact of neurocognitive function on quality of life five years after cardiac surgery. *Stroke*. 2001;32: 2874–2881.
16. Selnes OA, Goldsborough MA, Borowicz LM, McKhann GM. Neurobehavioral sequelae of cardiopulmonary bypass. *Lancet*. 1999;353:1601–1606.
17. McKhann GM, Borowicz LM, Goldsborough MA, Enger C, Selnes OA. Depression and cognitive decline after coronary artery bypass grafting. *Lancet*. 1997;349:1282–1284.
18. Rothenhausler HB, Grieser B, Nollert G, Reichart B, Schelling G, Kapfhammer HP. Psychiatric and psychosocial outcome of cardiac surgery with cardiopulmonary bypass: A prospective 12-month follow-up study. *Gen Hosp Psychiatry*. 2005;27:18–28.
19. Gao L, Taha R, Gauvin D, Othmen LB, Wang Y, Blaise G. Postoperative cognitive dysfunction after cardiac surgery. *Chest*. 2005;128:3664–3670.
20. Murkin JM, Newman SP, Stump DA, Blumenthal JA. Statement of consensus on assessment of neurobehavioral outcomes after cardiac surgery. *Ann Thorac Surg*. 1995;59:1289–1295.
21. Newman MF, Kirchner JL, Phillips-Bute B, et al. Longitudinal assessment of neurocognitive function after coronary-artery bypass surgery. *N Engl J Med*. 2001;344:395–402.
22. Ahlgren E, Lundqvist A, Nordlund A, Aren C, Rutberg H. Neurocognitive impairment and driving performance after coronary artery bypass surgery. *Eur J Cardiothorac Surg*. 2003;23:334–340.
23. Moller JT, Cluitmans P, Rasmussen LS, et al. Long-term postoperative cognitive dysfunction in the elderly ISPOCD1 study. ISPOCD investigators. International Study of Postoperative Cognitive Dysfunction. *Lancet*. 1998;351:857–861.
24. Monk TG, Attix DK. Longitudinal assessment of neurocognitive function: Elderly patients after major noncardiac surgery. *Anesthesiology*. 2004;101:A-62.
25. Selnes OA, Grega MA, Bailey MM, et al. Neurocognitive outcomes three years after coronary artery bypass graft surgery: A controlled study. *Ann Thorac Surg*. 2007;84:1885–1896.
26. Selnes OA, Royall RM, Grega MA, Borowicz LM, Jr., Quaskey S, McKhann GM. Cognitive changes five years after coronary artery bypass grafting: Is there evidence of late decline? *Arch Neurol*. 2001;58:598–604.

27. Sotaniemi KA, Mononen H, Hokkanen TE. Long-term cerebral outcome after open-heart surgery. A five-year neuropsychological follow-up study. *Stroke*. 1986;17:410–416.
28. van DD, Spoor M, Hijman R, et al. Cognitive and cardiac outcomes five years after off-pump vs. on-pump coronary artery bypass graft surgery. *JAMA*. 2007;297:701–708.
29. Zimp fer D, Czerny M, Schuch P, et al. Long-term neurocognitive function after mechanical aortic valve replacement. *Ann Thorac Surg*. 2006;81:29–33.
30. Kung H, Hoyert, D, Xu, J, Murphy, SL Deaths: Final data for 2005. National Vital Statistics Reports. 2008;56:1–121.
31. Naylor AR, Mehta Z, Rothwell PM, Bell PRF. Carotid artery disease and stroke during coronary artery bypass: A critical review of the literature. *Eur J Vasc Endovasc Surg*. 2002;23:283–294.
32. Stamou SC, Hill PC, Dangas G, et al. Stroke after coronary artery bypass: Incidence, predictors, and clinical outcome. *Stroke*. 2001:1508–1513.
33. Andrews RM. The national hospital bill: The most expensive conditions by payer, 2006. In: Heathcare Utilization Project, Statistical Brief. September 2008 ed. Rockville, MD: Agency for Healthcare Research and Quality, 2008.
34. Mangano DT. Perioperative cardiac morbidity. *Anesthesiology*. 1990:153–184.
35. Tuman KJ, McCarthy RJ, March RJ, Najafi H, Ivankovich AD. Morbidity and duration of ICU stay after cardiac surgery. A model for preoperative risk assessment. *Chest*. 1992; 102:36–44.
36. Hogue CW, Jr., Murphy SF, Schechtman KB, Davila Roman VG. Risk factors for early or delayed stroke after cardiac surgery. *Circulation*. 1999:642–647.
37. Hogue CW, Jr., Barzilai B, Pieper KS, et al. Sex differences in neurological outcomes and mortality after cardiac surgery: A Society of Thoracic Surgery national database report. *Circulation*. 2001:2133–2137.
38. Grover FL, Shroyer ALW, Hammermeister KE, et al. A decade's experience with quality improvement in cardiac surgery using the Veterans Affairs' and Society of Thoracic Surgeons' national databases. *Ann Surg*. 2001;234:464–474.
39. Moody DM, Brown WR, Challa VR, Stump DA, Reboussin DM, Legault C. Brain microemboli associated with cardiopulmonary bypass: A histologic and magnetic resonance imaging study. *Ann Thorac Surg*. 1995;59:1304–1307.
40. Mullges W, Franke D, Reents W, Babin-Ebell J. Brain microembolic counts during extracorporeal circulation depend on aortic cannula position. *Ultrasound Med Biol*. 2001;27: 933–936.
41. Gilman S. Cerebral disorders after open heart operations. *N Eng J Med*. 1965;272:489–498.
42. Caplan LR, Hennerici M. Impaired clearance of emboli (washout) is an important link between hypoperfusion, embolism, and ischemic stroke. *Arch Neurol*. 1998:1475–1482.
43. Gold JP, Charlson ME, Williams-Russo P, et al. Improvement of outcomes after coronary artery bypass. A randomized trail comparing intraoperative high versus low mean arterial pressure. *J Thorac Cardiovasc Surg*. 1995;110:1302–1311.
44. Hartman GS, Yao FS, Bruefach M 3rd, et al. Severity of aortic atheromatous disease diagnosed by transesophageal echocardiography predicts stroke and other outcomes associated with coronary artery surgery: A prospective study. *Anesth Analg*. 1996;83:701–708.
45. van der Linden J, Hadjinikolaou L, Bergman P, Lindblom D. Postoperative stroke in cardiac surgery is related to the location and extent of atherosclerotic disease in the ascending aorta. *J Am Coll Cardiol*. 2001;38:131–135.
46. Wareing TH, Davila-Roman VG, Barzilai B, Murphy SF, Kouchoukos NT. Management of the severely atherosclerotic ascending aorta during cardiac operations: A strategy for detection and treatment. *J Thorac Cardiovasc Surg*. 1992;103:453–462.

47. Wareing TH, Davila Roman VG, Daily BB, et al. Strategy for the reduction of stroke incidence in cardiac surgical patients. *Ann Thorac Surg*. 1993;55:1400–1408.
48. Brown WR, Moody DM, Challa VR, Stump DA, Hammon JW. Longer duration of cardiopulmonary bypass is associated with greater numbers of cerebral microemboli. *Stroke*. 2000:707–713.
49. Jones TJ, Deal DD, Vernon JC, Blackburn N, Stump DA. Does vacuum-assisted venous drainage increase gaseous microemboli during cardiopulmonary bypass? *Ann Thorac Surg*. 2002;74:2132–2137.
50. Berman L, Pietrzak RH, Mayes L. Neurocognitive changes after carotid revascularization: A review of the current literature. *J Psychosom Res*. 2007;63:599–612.
51. Browndyke JN, Moser DJ, Cohen RA, et al. Acute neuropsychological functioning following cardiosurgical interventions associated with the production of intraoperative cerebral microemboli. *Clin Neuropsychol*. 2002;16:463–471.
52. Challa VR, Moody DM, Troost BT. Brain embolic phenomena associated with cardiopulmonary bypass. *J Neurol Sci*. 1993;117:224–231.
53. Newman MF, Wolman R, Kanchuger M, et al. Multicenter preoperative stroke risk index for patients undergoing coronary artery bypass graft surgery. *Circulation*. 1996;94:II-74–80.
54. Knipp SC, Matatko N, Wilhelm H, et al. Evaluation of brain injury after coronary artery bypass grafting. A prospective study using neuropsychological assessment and diffusion-weighted magnetic resonance imaging. *Eur J Cardiothorac Surg*. 2004;25:791–800.
55. Creswell LL. Postoperative atrial arrhythmias: Risk factors and associated adverse outcomes. *Semin Thorac Cardiovasc Surg*. 1999;11:303–307.
56. Creswell LL, Schuessler RB, Rosenbloom M, Cox JL. Hazards of postoperative atrial arrhythmias. *Ann Thorac Surg*. 1993;56:539–549.
57. Aranki SF, Shaw DP, Adams DH, et al. Predictors of atrial fibrillation after coronary artery surgery. Current trends and impact on hospital resources. *Circulation*. 1996;94:390–397.
58. Crosby LH, Pifalo WB, Woll KR, Burkholder JA. Risk factors for atrial fibrillation after coronary artery bypass grafting. *Am J Cardiol*. 1990;66:1520–1522.
59. Fuller JA, Adams GG, Buxton B. Atrial fibrillation after coronary artery bypass grafting. Is it a disorder of the elderly? *J Thorac Cardiovasc Surg*. 1989;97:821–825.
60. Mathew JP, Parks R, Savino JS, et al. Atrial fibrillation following coronary artery bypass graft surgery: Predictors, outcomes, and resource utilization. *JAMA*. 1996;276:300–306.
61. Stanley TO, Mackensen GB, Grocott HP, et al. The impact of postoperative atrial fibrillation on neurocognitive outcome after coronary artery bypass graft surgery. *Anesth Analg*. 2002;94:290–295.
62. Ebert AD, Walzer TA, Huth C, Herrmann M. Early neurobehavioral disorders after cardiac surgery: A comparative analysis of coronary artery bypass graft surgery and valve replacement. *J Cardiothorac Vasc Anesth*. 2001;15:15–19.
63. Royter V, Bornstein M, Russell D. Coronary artery bypass grafting (CABG) and cognitive decline: A review. *J Neurol Sci*. 2005;229–230:65–67.
64. Mahanna EP, Blumenthal JA, White WD, et al. Defining neuropsychological dysfunction after coronary artery bypass grafting. *Ann Thorac Surg*. 1996;61:1342–1347.
65. Elkins JS, Knopman DS, Yaffe K, Johnston SC. Cognitive function predicts first-time stroke and heart disease. *Neurology*. 2005;64:1750–1755.
66. Geschwind DH, Robidoux J, Alarcon M, et al. Dementia and neurodevelopmental predisposition: Cognitive dysfunction in presymptomatic subjects precedes dementia by decades in frontotemporal dementia. *Ann Neurol*. 2001;50:741–746.
67. American Heart Association Heart Disease and Stroke Statistics. 2006 Update. Dallas, TX: American Heart Association; 2006.

68. Selnes OA, Grega MA, Borowicz LM, Jr., Royall RM, McKhann GM, Baumgartner WA. Cognitive changes with coronary artery disease: A prospective study of coronary artery bypass graft patients and nonsurgical controls. *Ann Thorac Surg*. 2003;75:1377–1384.
69. Lyketsos CG, Toone L, Tschanz J, et al. A population-based study of the association between coronary artery bypass graft surgery (CABG) and cognitive decline: The Cache County study. *Int J Geriatr Psychiatry*. 2006;21:509–518.
70. Selnes OA, Grega MA, Borowicz LM, et al. Cognitive outcomes three years after coronary artery bypass surgery: A comparison of on-pump coronary artery bypass graft surgery and nonsurgical controls. *Ann Thorac Surg*. 2005;79:1201–1209.
71. Zimpfer D, Kilo J, Czerny M, et al. Neurocognitive deficit following aortic valve replacement with biological/mechanical prosthesis. *Eur J Cardiothorac Surg*. 2003;23:544–551.
72. Grimm M, Zimpfer D, Czerny M, et al. Neurocognitive deficit following mitral valve surgery. *Eur J Cardiothorac Surg*. 2003;23:265–271.
73. Hogue CW Jr., Palin CA, Arrowsmith JE. Cardiopulmonary bypass management and neurological outcomes: An evidence-based appraisal of current practices. *Anesth Analg*. 2006;103:21–37.
74. Leary MC, Caplan LR. Technology insight: Brain MRI and cardiac surgery—detection of postoperative brain ischemia. *Nat Clin Pract Cardiovasc Med*. 2007;4:379–388.
75. Wityk RJ, Goldsborough MA, Hillis A, et al. Diffusion- and perfusion-weighted brain magnetic resonance imaging in patients with neurological complications after cardiac surgery. *Arch Neurol*. 2001;58:571–576.
76. Harris DN, Bailey SM, Smith PL, Taylor KM, Oatridge A, Bydder GM. Brain swelling in first hour after coronary artery bypass surgery. *Lancet*. 1993;342:586–587.
77. Rasmussen LS, Sperling B, Abildstrom HH, Moller JT. Neuron loss after coronary artery bypass detected by SPECT estimation of benzodiazepine receptors. *Ann Thorac Surg*. 2002;74:1576–1580.
78. Schmidt R, Fazekas F, Offenbacher H, et al. Brain magnetic resonance imaging in coronary artery bypass grafts: A pre- and postoperative assessment. *Neurology*. 1993;43:775–778.
79. Santillan GG, Chemnitius JM, Bing RJ. The effect of cardiopulmonary bypass on cerebral blood flow. *Brain Res*. 1985;345:1–9.
80. Bendszus M, Koltzenburg M, Burger R, Warmuth-Metz M, Hofmann E, Solymosi L. Silent embolism in diagnostic cerebral angiography and neurointerventional procedures: A prospective study. *Lancet*. 1999;354:1594–1597.
81. Bendszus M, Reents W, Franke D, et al. Brain damage after coronary artery bypass grafting. *Arch Neurol*. 2002;59:1090–1095.
82. Floyd TF, Shah PN, Price CC, et al. Clinically silent cerebral ischemic events after cardiac surgery: Their incidence, regional vascular occurrence, and procedural dependence. *Ann Thorac Surg*. 2006;81:2160–2166.
83. Djaiani G, Fedorko L, Borger M, et al. Mild to moderate atheromatous disease of the thoracic aorta and new ischemic brain lesions after conventional coronary artery bypass graft surgery. *Stroke*. 2004;35:e356–e358.
84. Challa VR, Lovell MA, Moody DM, Brown WR, Reboussin DM, Markesbery WR. Laser microprobe mass spectrometric study of aluminum and silicon in brain emboli related to cardiac surgery. *J Neuropathol Exp Neurol*. 1998;57:140–147.
85. Bryson GL, Wyand A. Evidence-based clinical update: General anesthesia and the risk of delirium and postoperative cognitive dysfunction. *Can J Anaesth*. 2006;53:669–677.
86. Monk TG, Weldon BC, Garvan CW, et al. Predictors of cognitive dysfunction after major noncardiac surgery. *Anesthesiology*. 2008;108:18–30.

87. Culley DJ, Baxter MG, Yukhananov R, Crosby G. Long-term impairment of acquisition of a spatial memory task following isoflurane-nitrous oxide anesthesia in rats. *Anesthesiology*. 2004;100:309–314.
88. Futterer CD, Maurer MH, Schmitt A, Feldmann RE Jr, Kuschinsky W, Waschke KF. Alterations in rat brain proteins after desflurane anesthesia. *Anesthesiology*. 2004;100:302–308.
89. Mackensen GB, Sato Y, Nellgard B, et al. Cardiopulmonary bypass induces neurological and neurocognitive dysfunction in the rat. *Anesthesiology*. 2001;95:1485–1491.
90. Williams-Russo P, Sharrock NE, Mattis S, Szatrowski TP, Charlson ME. Cognitive effects after epidural vs general anesthesia in older adults. A randomized trial [*see comments*]. *JAMA*. 1995;274:44–50.
91. Oxlad M, Wade TD. Longitudinal risk factors for adverse psychological functioning six months after coronary artery bypass graft surgery. *J Health Psychol*. 2008;13:79–92.
92. Andrew MJ, Baker RA, Kneebone AC, Knight JL. Mood state as a predictor of neuropsychological deficits following cardiac surgery. *J Psychosom Res*. 2000;48:537–546.
93. Tsushima WT, Johnson DB, Lee JD, Matsukawa JM, Fast KM. Depression, anxiety and neuropsychological test scores of candidates for coronary artery bypass graft surgery. *Arch Clin Neuropsychol*. 2005;20:667–673.
94. Blumenthal JA, Lett HS, Babyak MA, et al. Depression as a risk factor for mortality after coronary artery bypass surgery. *Lancet*. 2003;362:604–609.
95. Baumgartner WA. Neurocognitive changes after coronary bypass surgery. *Circulation*. 2007;116:1879–1881.
96. Boodhwani M, Rubens FD, Wozny D, et al. Predictors of early neurocognitive deficits in low-risk patients undergoing on-pump coronary artery bypass surgery. *Circulation*. 2006;114:I461–I466.
97. Goto T, Baba T, Matsuyama K, Honma K, Ura M, Koshiji T. Aortic atherosclerosis and postoperative neurological dysfunction in elderly coronary surgical patients. *Ann Thorac Surg*. 2003;75:1912–1918.
98. Collison T, Smith JM, Engel AM. Peripheral vascular disease and outcomes following coronary artery bypass graft surgery. *Arch Surg*. 2006;141:1214–1218.
99. Goto T, Baba T, Honma K, et al. Magnetic resonance imaging findings and postoperative neurological dysfunction in elderly patients undergoing coronary artery bypass grafting. *Ann Thorac Surg*. 2001;72:137–142.
100. Goto T, Baba T, Yoshitake A, Shibata Y, Ura M, Sakata R. Craniocervical and aortic atherosclerosis as neurological risk factors in coronary surgery. *Ann Thorac Surg*. 2000;69:834–840.
101. Stroobant N, Van NG, Van BY, Vingerhoets G. Relation between neurocognitive impairment, embolic load, and cerebrovascular reactivity following on- and off-pump coronary artery bypass grafting. *Chest*. 2005;127:1967–197 6.
102. Bucerius J, Gummert JF, Borger MA, et al. Stroke after cardiac surgery: A risk factor analysis of 16,184 consecutive adult patients. *Ann Thorac Surg*. 2003;75:472–478.
103. Hernandez F, Jr., Brown JR, Likosky DS, et al. Neurocognitive outcomes of off-pump versus on-pump coronary artery bypass: A prospective randomized controlled trial. *Ann Thorac Surg*. 2007;84:1897–1903.
104. Tardiff BE, Newman MF, Saunders AM, et al. Preliminary report of a genetic basis for cognitive decline after cardiac operations. *Ann Thorac Surg*. 1997;64:715–720.
105. Silbert BS, Evered LA, Scott DA, Cowie TF. The apolipoprotein E epsilon4 allele is not associated with cognitive dysfunction in cardiac surgery. *Ann Thorac Surg*. 2008;86:841–847.

106. Treiber KA, Lyketsos CG, Corcoran C, et al. Vascular factors and risk for neuropsychiatric symptoms in Alzheimer's disease: The Cache County Study. *Int Psychogeriatr.* 2008;20:538–553.
107. Kuukasjarvi P, Tarkka M, Mennander A, et al. Apolipoprotein E polymorphism is not a predictor for repeated coronary artery bypass surgery. *Scand Cardiovasc J.* 2005;39:220–224.
108. Tada H. The E4 allele of apolipoprotein E is associated with increased restenosis after coronary angioplasty. *Tokai J Exp Clin Med.* 2001;26:81–92.
109. Mathew JP, Grocott HP, Podgoreanu MD, White WD, Newman MF. Inflammatory and prothrombotic genetic polymorphisms are associated with cognitive decline after CABG surgery. *Anesthesiology.* 2004:ASA /A-274.
110. Mathew JP, Rinder CS, Howe JG, et al. Platelet PlA2 polymorphism enhances the risk of neurocognitive decline after cardiopulmonary bypass. *Ann Thorac Surg.* 2001;71:663–666.
111. Hineman BJ. Emboli, inflammation, and CNS impairment: An overview. *Heart Surg Forum.* 2002;5:249–53.

11

HEART FAILURE AND COGNITIVE FUNCTION

Karin F. Hoth

The clinical syndrome of heart failure (HF) is an increasingly frequent manifestation of diseases that damage the heart. Heart failure is typically characterized by reduced cardiac output, although the full clinical spectrum of heart failure stems from a complex cascade of physiological changes that result in diminished cardiac, vascular, and renal function. Over five million people living in the United States have heart failure, with 660,000 new patients diagnosed annually.[1] The estimated cost of heart failure in the United States for 2008 is $34.8 billion.[1] The prevalence of heart failure rises with increasing age and represents one of the most significant causes of hospitalization, morbidity and mortality among elderly individuals in the United States.[2, 3] Given the large aging population, the improved prognosis after diagnosis of heart failure, and the high frequency of cardiovascular risk factors (e.g., hypertension, obesity, and diabetes), the prevalence of heart failure is expected to quadruple within the next 30 years.[2]

In addition to symptoms of shortness of breath, edema, exercise intolerance, and fatigue, cognitive complaints are relatively common among patients with heart failure. The reported prevalence of cognitive impairment in heart failure patients ranges from approximately 25% to 75%.[4] Differences in patient samples, including type and severity of heart failure, age of the sample, and inpatient versus outpatient status, probably contribute to this variability. As Heckman and colleagues recently pointed out, distinguishing delirium from long-standing cognitive deficits is important, given the potential for acute symptom exacerbations in patients with heart failure.[5] At present, making direct comparisons of the prevalence of impairment across studies is difficult because of differences in the cognitive measures and cutoffs used to define "impairment."

Cognitive deficits have been shown to negatively impact activities of daily living[6, 7] and to increase risk of mortality above and beyond the presence of HF alone.[8] Examining cognition among patients with heart failure is important both because of the prevalence and functional impact of cognitive impairment for patients, and because heart failure provides a model for improving our understanding of how changes in cardiovascular physiology affect the brain. The goals of the chapter are twofold. First, the chapter will review the literature that has examined cognitive functioning among patients with a clinical diagnosis of HF, including treatment studies. Second, directions for future research will be addressed. The effects of specific physiological mechanisms on cognition are covered in other chapters in this book (Chapters 12–13); thus, the focus of the current chapter will be on the clinical syndrome of heart failure, including an overview of the range of physiological factors that may be relevant as the field moves toward more comprehensive models of cognitive impairment in heart failure.

The Syndrome of Heart Failure

"Heart failure" refers to a clinical syndrome where the heart is unable to pump enough blood to meet the body's metabolic needs.[9] Heart failure typically involves abnormalities of ventricular functioning, including either problems with ventricular filling (diastole) and/or ventricular contraction and emptying (systole).[10] Ventricular dysfunction may involve the left or right ventricle, or both. Although patients can have heart failure with normal cardiac output, as when the diastolic relaxation properties of the left ventricle are impaired, most studies examining cognition in heart failure have focused on patients with reduced cardiac output.

Heart failure typically evolves over time from predisposing conditions that affect the heart, although in some cases it can develop rapidly (e.g., exposure to toxins or viral etiology). The most common risk factors for heart failure are hypertension, diabetes, and coronary artery disease.[1] Data from the Framingham Heart Study indicate that 75% of cases of heart failure have antecedent hypertension.[11] Heart failure is progressive and evolves through a dynamic process as the body attempts to compensate for cardiac damage or strain[10] (see Table 11-1). The pathophysiology of heart failure from predisposing conditions such as hypertension or coronary artery disease involves physical forces and neuroendocrine activation that change the structure and function of the ventricle (i.e., *ventricular remodeling*). Changes that are initially adaptive are ultimately

Table 11-1 Compensatory mechanisms in heart failure

Autonomic nervous system activation
Increased heart rate
Arterial and venous vasoconstriction
Increased cardiac relaxation
Renin-Angiotensin-Aldosterone System
Arterial and venous vasoconstriction
Sodium and water retention
Redistribution of cardiac output
Altered peripheral oxygen delivery
Altered oxygen-hemoglobin dissociation
Increased oxygen extraction by tissues
Ventricular remodeling
Hypertrophy
Myocyte elongation

insufficient to compensate for cardiac damage and result in fluid congestion, inadequate blood flow to tissues, and impaired endothelial and vascular function.[12–14] In some cases, ventricular dysfunction causes blood to back up in the pulmonary circulation, resulting in pulmonary edema, shortness of breath, and altered oxygen and gas exchange with the blood. Given the dynamic evolution of heart failure, a comprehensive model of cognitive impairment must ultimately consider the effects of cardiac and systemic changes (i.e., neuroendocrine, renal, and pulmonary) on the brain.

Pattern of Cognitive Impairment in Heart Failure

The term *cardiogenic dementia* was introduced in 1977 to describe a link between cardiac disease and cognitive impairment.[15] The concept of vascular cognitive impairment has evolved considerably since that time,[16, 17] and an increasing number of studies have focused specifically on cognition in patients with a clinical diagnosis of heart failure. Many studies of cognition in heart failure have been limited by small sample sizes, lack of matched control samples, use of relatively few cognitive measures, and/or lack of longitudinal data.[18] However, several large population-based studies and recent systematic reviews of the literature provide convincing evidence that patients with heart failure are at an increased risk for cognitive impairment compared to their age-matched peers and patients with other types of cardiovascular disease.[4, 5, 18, 19]

Previous large-scale clinical trials of heart failure have included brief global cognitive-screening measures. The CHF Italian Study I, a multicenter study of elderly inpatients with heart failure, included the MMSE. The average MMSE score, after adjusting for age, education, blood pressure, and history of cerebrovascular accidents, was approximately one point lower in patients with heart failure than in patients with other types of cardiovascular disease and no heart failure.[20] The Helsinki Aging Study assessed 650 community-dwelling 75-, 80-, and 85-year-olds at baseline and after one, five, and ten years.[21] Heart failure was a predictor of five-year cognitive decline, but not ten-year decline. In a study of 1075 Italian citizens, Cacciatore and colleagues examined history of heart failure and risk of cognitive impairment (defined as MMSE <24).[21] The authors found that the risk of cognitive impairment was 1.96 times greater in participants with a history of heart failure than for those without.

Several reviews of the literature on cognition in heart failure have identified impairments in more specific cognitive domains, including learning, recall, attention, problem solving, and reaction time/psychomotor speed.[4, 5, 18, 19, 22] In 2007, Vogels and colleagues conducted a systematic search of medical databases (i.e., MEDLINE, Ovid, Cochrane Controlled Trials Register of the Cochrane Library) to identify randomized clinical trials or case-control surveys that investigated cognitive impairment in heart failure. The authors required that the studies had used validated cognitive measures with age- and/or education-corrected normative data. Twenty-two studies published between 1966 and 2006 met their inclusion criteria. Due to heterogeneity among the neuropsychological tests that were used, the authors focused on the measures that were most commonly included to describe impairment: the MMSE, memory measures, and Trial Making

Test Part A. The authors examined standardized mean differences using the Mantel-Haenszel method. The pooled analysis included 2937 heart failure patients and 14,848 control subjects, with a resulting odds ratio for cognitive impairment of 1.62 among participants with heart failure. Significant differences were observed for all primary measures (i.e., MMSE, a pooled memory domain, and psychomotor speed assessed using Trail Making Test Part A). The authors pointed out that while the pooled analysis confirms an association between heart failure and cognitive impairment, it also highlights the need for systemic neuropsychological data across multiple cognitive domains.

Clinical Factors Associated with Cognitive Impairment in Heart Failure

In general, greater heart failure severity has been associated with more severe cognitive deficits.[19] Several studies examining New York Heart Association functional lower class suggest that the severity of memory deficits progressively increases across classes.[23, 24] Duration of heart failure, measured by years of illness, has also been associated with more severe cognitive deficits, presumably due to sustained reduction of systemic and cerebral perfusion over time.[19] Given the heterogeneity of risk factors that underlie heart failure, global severity ratings are limited in addressing the etiology of cognitive impairment. The pathophysiology of cognitive deficits in heart failure is multifactorial, including both predisposing risk factors and physiological changes that are more specific to the progression of cardiac dysfunction. Circulatory insufficiency and cardiogenic thromboemboli have historically received the most attention in the literature; however, in the last decade, conceptual models have begun to reflect a broader range of physiological changes (e.g., reduced oxygen saturation) that extend beyond the primary effects of reduced circulatory insufficiency.[19, 25]

Risk Factors for Cognitive Decline and Clinical History

The cumulative effects of risk factors for cognitive decline, such as older age, hypertension, and diabetes, contribute to the development of heart failure and are independently associated with cognitive impairment. Comorbid medical conditions (e.g., renal insufficiency, COPD) may have additive effects or interact with cardiac dysfunction to compound cognitive impairment. A population-based study in Italy examined sociodemographic characteristics and cardiovascular diseases as predictors of global cognitive impairment (defined with a score of <24 on the MMSE).[26] Among 1075 participants, cognitive impairment was associated with sex, age, education, depressive symptoms, diabetes, hypertension, alcohol consumption, smoking, atrial fibrillation, systolic and diastolic blood pressure, and heart rate. The risk of cognitive impairment was 1.96-fold greater in participants with heart failure. Another large (n = 14,089) population-based study in the United States examined demographic, socioeconomic, health-behavior, and medical comorbidity as risk factors for global cognitive impairment among participants with and without probable heart failure.[27] The authors found that a history of stroke and/or TIA, depression, and lower hemoglobin level were all associated with global cognitive impairment among those with probable heart failure. Several clinical studies in patients with heart failure have observed that patients with greater depressive symptoms have worse cognitive function.[24, 28] Metabolic abnormalities including low serum albumin, sodium, and potassium levels, hyperglycemia and anemia were associated with a global cognitive rating score in another study of individuals with heart failure admitted for inpatient hospitalization.[29] In addition to metabolic abnormalities, systolic blood pressure and a cumulative "comorbidity score" reflecting number of comorbid medical conditions were associated with cognitive impairment. Mauro and colleagues (2007) found that high plasma brain natriuretic peptide was associated with lower MMSE scores.[30] At least one study has found that the presence of the apolipoprotein (Apo) ε4 allele is an independent predictor of cognitive impairment in stable outpatients with heart failure.[31] Taken together, this range of risk factors for cognitive decline underscores the importance of carefully describing the population being studied and including specific physiological measures to clarify underlying mechanisms.

Decreased Ejection Fraction/Cardiac Output

Research on the etiology of cognitive impairment in heart failure has focused on a model of circulatory insufficiency. Diminished cardiac pumping efficiency may lead to reduced systemic circulation and, ultimately, cerebral hypoperfusion.[19, 32–34] Cardiac disease has been implicated in transient severe reductions in cardiac output that result in watershed infarcts.[35] Typically, autoregulatory mechanisms maintain cerebral blood flow during brief fluctuations in systemic blood flow; however, cerebrovascular autoregulatory mechanisms may be less effective in older adults, particularly those with chronic heart failure. Modest reductions in perfusion of blood to the brain over a prolonged period can also result in ischemic damage, particularly in regions of the brain that are vulnerable to oxygen deprivation.[36] Indeed, research suggests that reduced cardiac pumping efficiency may decrease both systemic and cerebral perfusion, altering the oxygen and nutrient supply to the brain.[37]

Several studies have suggested that impaired ventricular ejection fraction (EF) and depressed cardiac output, both measures of forward blood flow out of the heart, are associated with diminished cognition among patients with cardiovascular disease.[34, 38, 39] There is some evidence that reduced cardiac output is associated with specific deficits in executive functioning among stable geriatric outpatients with a range of cardiovascular diseases.[38] This suggests that the typical profile of executive dysfunction observed among patients with cardiovascular disease may be associated, at least in part, with reduced blood flow to vulnerable subcortical structures in the brain. Among patients with more advanced heart failure, reduced ejection fraction has been associated with a wider range of cognitive deficits, including global cognition, attention, working memory, fluency, and delayed memory.[39] Bennett and colleagues[18] have suggested that inconsistent findings regarding the relationship between left ventricular ejection fraction and cognition could be due to a nonlinear association, with most pronounced and global effects for patients with severely impaired cardiac function. A comprehensive discussion of reduced cardiac function and cognition is provided in Chapter 13.

Cardiogenic Thromboemboli

Heart failure ranks second to atrial fibrillation in cardiogenic stroke risk.[40] Congestive heart failure conveys a two- to threefold increase in relative risk, and cardiac failure is associated with increased mortality following cardiogenic stroke.[40] Heart failure, particularly with left ventricular dysfunction, involves endothelial dysfunction, rheological abnormalities, and altered cardiac blood flow, which promote platelet adhesion and thrombus formation.[14] While it is clear that patients with heart failure are at an increased risk for cardiogenic thromboembolic stroke, the extent to which this is a primary mechanism of cognitive decline in heart failure has been debated.[20] For some individuals, thromboemboli may be a significant cause of cognitive impairment, but given the prevalence of cognitive impairment among heart failure patients in the absence of stroke, other mechanisms are also important.

Neuroimaging Findings

Heart failure has long been known as a risk factor for adverse brain changes, including stroke and small vessel ischemic disease.[19, 41–44] Heart failure patients show brain abnormalities on neuroimaging prior to stroke or dementia, which may adversely impact cognitive function. Older adults with heart failure exhibit significant white matter hyperintensities on MRI, pointing to vascular- and myelin-related pathology.[45] Low forward flow (cardiac output) and low perfusion pressure (systolic blood pressure) have been associated with alterations in white matter observed on neuroimaging.[33, 46–48] There is some evidence that decreased cardiac output is most strongly related to the presence of white matter hyperintensities contiguous to the subcortical nuclei, an area that may be particularly susceptible to decreases in blood flow.[48] Reduced gray matter volume is also common, including in multiple regions important for cognitive function such as the frontal cortex, parahippocampus, and cingulate.[49]

Functional neuroimaging studies have documented altered cerebrovascular hemodynamics[50, 51] and cerebral metabolism[52, 53] in heart failure patients. Reduced resting global cerebral blood flow has been found among patients with heart failure, and there is evidence that certain cortical regions may be differentially affected, including the precuneus and cuneus, the right lateral temporoparietal cortex, and posterior cingulate.[54] Patients with heart failure show reduced middle-cerebral-artery blood-flow velocity compared to healthy controls and patients with other types of cardiovascular disease.[50] Importantly, reduced middle-cerebral-artery blood-flow velocity has been related to both neuropsychological deficits and white matter hyperintensities.[50]

Cerebrovascular reactivity is reduced in heart failure patients.[55] Georgiadis and colleagues[55] examined changes in middle-cerebral-artery blood flow in response to hypercapnia among 50 patients with NYHA class II–IV heart failure. Compared to 20 age-matched and 20 younger comparison participants, patients with heart failure had impaired reactivity. There was a linear relationship between left ventricular ejection fraction and cerebrovascular reactivity. The authors suggested that patients whose brain resistance vessels are impaired may be unable to compensate for the effects of reduced systemic blood flow. No studies in heart failure have combined measures of vascular reactivity and cognition, although there is evidence of a link between peripheral vascular reactivity and cognition in patients with other cardiovascular diseases such as atherosclerosis[56–58] (see Chapter 14).

Proton magnetic resonance spectroscopy studies have documented cerebral metabolic abnormalities in patients with heart failure, including decreased creatine level in the parietal white matter and decreased N-acetylaspartate, creatine, choline, and myoinositol in the occipital gray matter.[52] Occipital N-acetylaspartate level was an independent predictor of mortality in advanced HF, suggesting that cerebral metabolic abnormalities may be a useful prognostic marker.[53]

Despite these findings, relatively few studies have directly examined the relationship between structural and functional brain changes and cognitive function in heart failure patients, and no study has conducted longitudinal analyses combining these measures. Vogels and colleagues[59] did examine cross-sectional correlations between white matter hyperintensities, lacunar and cortical infarcts, global and medial temporal-lobe atrophy, and several cognitive measures in nondemented patients with heart failure. The authors found that medial temporal lobe atrophy was related to cognitive dysfunction involving memory and executive dysfunction, whereas white matter hyperintensities were related to symptoms of depression and anxiety. The authors had anticipated a relationship between white matter hyperintensities and cognition, and commented that the relationship may not have been apparent yet, given the relatively mild severity of heart failure in their sample.

Effects of Treatments for Heart Failure

Treatment studies that include cognitive measures provide important information about patient outcomes and underlying mechanisms of cognitive impairment in heart failure. To date, research has examined medication treatment, cardiac rehabilitation, heart transplantation, and cardiac-assist devices.

Research on potential medication effects has focused on ACE inhibitors. In a multicenter observational study, Zuccala and colleagues[60] found that use of ACE inhibitors during inpatient hospitalization was associated with improved performance on a global cognitive measure (i.e., Hodkinson Abbreviated Mental Test). Among patients with heart failure, cognition improved in 30% of patients who started ACE inhibitors during their hospitalization, and in 22% of the remaining patients. Although this was not a randomized controlled trial, it is notable that the association between use of ACE inhibitors and improved cognition was not accounted for by systolic blood pressure levels either before or during treatment. Several small studies suggest that treatment with

ACE inhibitors is associated with improved cerebral blood flow.[61, 62] For example, in 11 patients with NYHA Class II or III heart failure, four weeks of daily enalapril administration was associated with an increase in cerebral blood flow measured using radionuclide angiography.[62] The increased cerebral blood flow was not related to increased cardiac output in this sample. Future studies incorporating both cognitive and cerebral blood-flow measures will be important to strengthen the implied mechanistic link.

Alves and colleagues examined the possibility that effective treatment for symptoms of depression could have a positive impact on the cognitive function of patients with heart failure.[63] The authors focused on NYHA class II–III heart failure and compared the cognitive performance of 20 patients with major depressive disorder (HF-depressed) to 23 nondepressed patients (HF-nondepressed) and 18 healthy controls. Baseline cognitive performance on the CAMCOG (i.e., Cambridge Mental Disorders of the Elderly Examination Battery) was lower in both heart failure groups compared to the control participants. The heart failure group with major depressive disorder scored lower than the nondepressed heart failure patients. In the heart failure group with depression, there was significant improvement in cognitive scores following an eight-week trial with SSRIs, bringing their average performance to a level that was comparable to the nondepressed heart failure group. These findings reinforce the clinical significance of depressive symptoms in heart failure and the importance of treatment.

There is some evidence that electrolyte imbalance contributes to cognitive impairment, at least among patients being admitted to the hospital for heart failure. Using data from a hospital-based multi-site study (i.e., Gruppo Italiano di Farmacoepidemiologia nell Anziano [GIFA]), Zuccala and colleagues found that among patients admitted to the hospital with abnormal lab values, normalization of glucose and potassium during their hospital stay improved their performance on a brief cognitive screening measure.[29] It will be important to determine whether the findings can be replicated in an outpatient setting as well.

There is considerable support for the idea that exercise can improve cognitive status in general.[64, 65] A few small studies of consecutively referred patients with heart failure suggest that cognitive function may improve following exercise training.[66, 67] One study found that undergoing an 18-week exercise training program was associated with improvement on general attention and psychomotor speed but not other cognitive measures.[67] Larger clinical trials will be necessary to determine if this effect can be replicated.

Several studies have reported improved cognitive performance among patients following heart transplantation.[28, 68] In a small sample of 17 transplant candidates, memory recall was impaired during the pre-transplant evaluation.[68] An average of 36 months following cardiac transplant, memory function significantly improved to normal levels. No associations with changes in cardiovascular function were examined because of the small sample size. Grimm and colleagues[69] examined the effect of using cyclosporine following heart transplantation on brain function (i.e., P300 evoked potentials on EEG, the MMSE and Trail Making Test A). The study included 55 patients (mean age = 54.8) and 55 matched controls. At baseline, P300 evoked potentials and performance on Trail Making A were impaired in the transplant candidates. After heart transplantation, P300 measures normalized at four months, but declined again at 12 months, and Trail Making A performance continued to improve across the follow-up period. Cumulative cyclosporine dosage was the only predictor of P300 potential at four months and 12 months after transplantation. The authors concluded that improved cognitive brain function may be subclinically affected by long-term cyclosporine immunosuppressive treatment. Longer follow-up studies will be important to better understand the role of cyclosporine treatment on cognitive function.

Due to limited organ availability for heart transplantation, use of mechanical cardiac-assist devices for heart failure is sometimes necessary until a definitive treatment is available. In one study of 29 patients with severe heart failure, successful ventricular-assist device implantation was associated with improved P300 evoked potentials captured on EEG at up to a 12-week follow-up.[70] Interestingly, the change in P300 duration was associated with improvement in cardiac index, suggesting that increased cardiac output may have been an important underlying mechanism.

Implantation of traditional cardiac pacemakers for bradycardia has also been associated with improved cognition in small studies.[71, 72] These studies were not specific to heart failure alone, and included a wider range of patients (e.g., atrial fibrillation). Cardiac resynchronization therapy is a pacemaker/defibrillator treatment for heart failure with ventricular dyssynchrony. In a small pilot study, Conti and Sears examined neuropsychological function among 10 patients undergoing cardiac resynchronization therapy prior to and three months after implantation.[73] The mean cognitive performance of the group improved on two measures of attention and information processing (i.e., Digit Span and Symbol Digit) but not delayed memory (i.e., Hopkins Verbal Learning Test). The authors did not examine change in cardiac function following implantation; thus, these data do not address the underlying mechanism of improvement. The finding does underscore the idea that cognitive deficits in heart failure may be attenuated by treatment and suggests that more data are needed on cardiac resynchronization therapy specifically.

Summary and Future Directions for Research

There is increasing evidence that heart failure confers an independent risk for cognitive impairment above and beyond the presence of cardiovascular risk factors alone. Cerebral hypoperfusion is the leading model, with several studies demonstrating that diminished cardiac output is associated with greater white matter hyperintensity volume on MRI of the brain and cognitive deficits, particularly in the domains of attention, executive functioning, information processing speed, and memory retrieval.

There is a call for and need to move toward more comprehensive models of cognitive impairment in heart failure rather than focusing on individual medical variables in relation to cognition.[19, 25] Bennett and colleagues recently proposed a conceptual model of cognitive impairment in heart failure including background contributing factors (e.g., age), covariates (e.g., medications), and several aspects of heart failure (i.e., severity [NYHA class, ejection fraction], duration of circulatory insufficiency, and decreased oxygen saturation).[19] Clark and colleagues identified an expanded list of additional potentially relevant mechanisms that have been examined in the larger literature on cardiovascular disease and cognition (e.g., electrolyte and sleep disturbances, hormone changes). Pulmonary dysfunction and sympathetic nervous system activation may prove to be important for cognitive function in heart failure as well. Figure 11-1 represents a proposed model of cognitive impairment including many of the factors identified in the past literature, such as individual history variables, physiological changes associated with heart failure, comorbid medical conditions, and treatment effects. This model reflects a range of potential etiologies and contributing factors that will need to be revised over time.

In addition to expanding the range of underlying mechanisms that are examined, researchers need to carefully define the cardiovascular characteristics of each sample to promote comparison across studies. Differences in the etiology of heart failure—including systolic versus diastolic dysfunction, ischemic vs. nonischemic heart failure, chronicity of ventricular dysfunction, comorbid medical conditions, and inpatient vs. outpatient status—are potentially important characteristics. Longitudinal studies may be helpful in differentiating between the course of acute cognitive disturbances from transient events (e.g., delirium) and stable and lasting cognitive impairments.

Finally, additional studies are needed that include comprehensive neuropsychological assessments, which allow us to fully characterize the pattern of relative cognitive

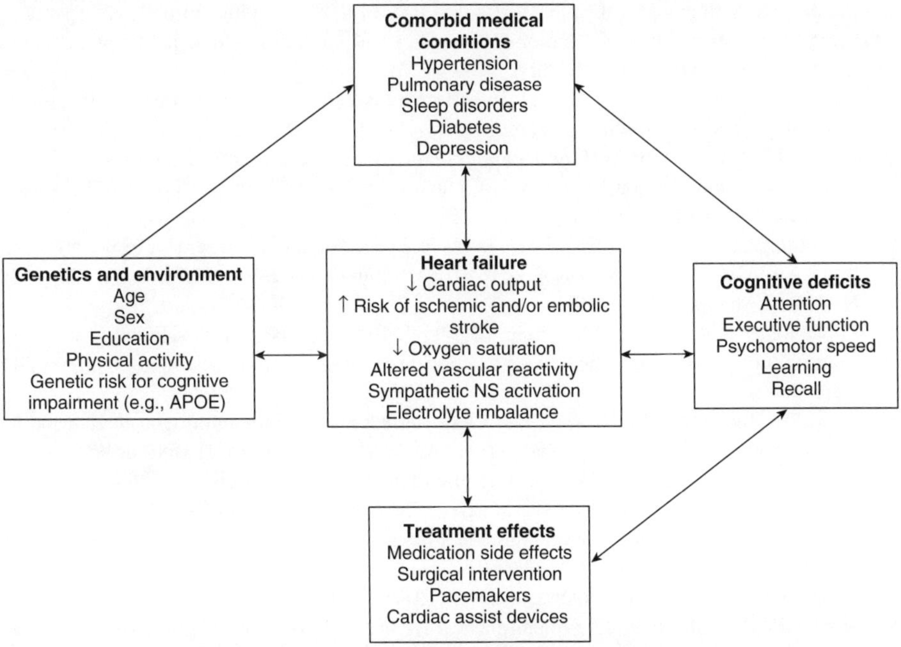

Figure 11-1 Model of cognitive impairment in heart failure.

strengths and weaknesses. This is particularly important given that some of the deficits hypothesized to be most affected by heart failure (i.e., executive dysfunction, speed of processing) are not typically covered by brief cognitive screening measures such as the MMSE. Ultimately, studies that include neuroimaging and neuropsychological measures in the same patients will be most helpful in clarifying the underlying mechanisms of cognitive impairment in heart failure.

Notes

1. Rosamond W, Flegal K, Furie K, et al. Heart disease and stroke statistics—2008 update: A report from the American Heart Association Statistics Committee and Stroke Statistics Subcommittee. *Circulation*. 29 2008;117(4):e25–146.
2. Rich MW. Heart failure in the 21st century: A cardiogeriatric syndrome. *J Gerontol A Biol Sci Med Sci*. 2001;56(2):M88–96.
3. Berry C, Murdoch DR, McMurray JJ. Economics of chronic heart failure. *Eur J Heart Fail*. 2001;3(3):283–291.
4. Vogels RL, Scheltens P, Schroeder-Tanka JM, et al. Cognitive impairment in heart failure: A systematic review of the literature. *Eur J Heart Fail*. 2007;9(5):440–449.
5. Heckman GA, Patterson CJ, Demers C, et al. Heart failure and cognitive impairment: Challenges and opportunities. *Clin Interv Aging*. 2007;2(2):209–218.
6. Zuccala G, Onder G, Pedone C, et al. Cognitive dysfunction as a major determinant of disability in patients with heart failure: Results from a multicentre survey. On behalf of the GIFA (SIGG-ONLUS) Investigators. *J Neurol Neurosurg Psychiatry*. 2001;70(1):109–112.
7. Putzke JD, Williams MA, Daniel FJ, Bourge RC, Boll TJ. Activities of daily living among heart transplant candidates: Neuropsychological and cardiac function predictors. *J Heart Lung Transp*. 2000;19(10):995–1006.
8. Zuccala G, Pedone C, Cesari M, et al. The effects of cognitive impairment on mortality among hospitalized patients with heart failure [*see comment*]. *Am J Med*. 2003;115(2):97–103.
9. Francis FS, Wilson Tang WH, Sonnenblick EH. Pathophysiology of heart failure. In Furster V, Alexander RW, O'Rourke RA (Eds.), Hurst's *The Heart*, 11th ed. (pp. 697–722). New York: McGraw-Hill, 2004.
10. Lejermtel TH, Sonnenblick EH, Frishman WH. Diagnosis and management of heart failure. In: Fuster V, Alexander RW, O'Rourke RA (Eds.), Hurst's *The Heart*, 11th ed. (pp. 723–762). New York: McGraw-Hill, 2004.
11. Lloyd-Jones DM, Larson MG, Leip EP, et al. Lifetime risk for developing congestive heart failure: The Framingham Heart Study [*see comment*]. *Circulation*. 2002;106(24): 3068–3072.
12. Kubo SH, Rector TS, Bank AJ, Williams RE, Heifetz SM. Endothelium-dependent vasodilation is attenuated in patients with heart failure. *Circulation*. 1991;84(4):1589–1596.
13. Treasure CB, Vita JA, Cox DA, et al. Endothelium-dependent dilation of the coronary microvasculature is impaired in dilated cardiomyopathy. *Circulation*. 1990;81(3):772–779.
14. Lip GY, Gibbs CR. Does heart failure confer a hypercoagulable state? Virchow's triad revisited. *J Am Coll Cardiol*. 1999;33(5):1424–1426.
15. Anonymous. Cardiogenic Dementia. *Lancet*. 1977;1(8001):27–28.
16. Bowler JV. Vascular cognitive impairment. *J Neurol Neurosurg Psychiatry*. 2005;76 Suppl 5:v35–44.

17. Gorelick PB, Bowler JV. Advances in vascular cognitive impairment 2007. *Stroke.* 2008;39(2):279–282.
18. Bennett S, Sauve M. Cognitive deficits in patients with heart failure: A review of the literature. *J Cardiovasc Nurs.* 2003;18(3):219–242.
19. Bennett S, Sauve M, Shaw R. A conceptual model of cognitive deficits in chronic heart failure. *J Nurs Scholarsh.* 2005;37(3):222–228.
20. Acanfora D, Trojano L, Iannuzzi GI, et al. The brain in congestive heart failure. *Arch Gerontol Geriatr.* 1996;23:247–256.
21. Tilvis RS, Kahonen-Vare MH, Jolkkonen J, et al. Predictors of cognitive decline and mortality of aged people over a 10-year period. *J Gerontol A Biol Sci Med Sci.* 2004;59(3):268–274.
22. Almeida OP, Flicker L. The mind of a failing heart: A systematic review of the association between congestive heart failure and cognitive functioning. *Int Med J.* 2001;31(5):290–295.
23. Gorkin L, Norvell NK, Rosen RC, et al. Assessment of quality of life as observed from the baseline data of the Studies of Left Ventricular Dysfunction (SOLVD) trial quality-of-life substudy. *Am J Cardiol.* 1993;71(12):1069–1073.
24. Trojano L, Incalzi R, Acanfora D, et al. Cognitive impairment: A key feature of congestive heart failure in the elderly. *J Neurol.* 2003;250:1456–1463.
25. Clark AP, McDougall G. Cognitive impairment in heart failure. *DCCN—Dimensions of Critical Care Nursing.* May-Jun 2006;25(3):93–100; quizzes 101–102.
26. Cacciatore F, Abete P, Ferrara N, et al. Congestive heart failure and cognitive impairment in an older population. Osservatorio Geriatrico Campano Study Group. *J Am Geriatr Soc.* 1998;46(11):1343–1348.
27. Pullicino PM, Wadley VG, McClure LA, et al. Factors contributing to global cognitive impairment in heart failure: Results from a population-based cohort. *J Card Fail.* May 2008;14(4):290–295.
28. Bornstein RA, Starling RC, Myerowitz PD, Haas GJ. Neuropsychological function in patients with end-stage heart failure before and after cardiac transplantation. *Acta Neurol Scand.* Apr 1995;91(4):260–265.
29. Zuccala G, Marzetti E, Cesari M, et al. Correlates of cognitive impairment among patients with heart failure: Results of a multicenter survey [*see comment*]. *Am J Med.* 2005;118(5): 496–502.
30. Feola M, Rosso GL, Peano M, et al. Correlation between cognitive impairment and prognostic parameters in patients with congestive heart failure. (Erratum appears in *Arch Med Res.* 2007;38(5):590, Note: Mauro, Feola [*corrected to Feola, Mauro*].) *Arch Med Res.* 2007;38(2):234–239.
31. Vogels RL, Oosterman JM, van Harten B, et al. Profile of cognitive impairment in chronic heart failure. *J Am Geriatr Soc.* 2007;55(11):1764–1770.
32. Sulkava R, Erkinjuntti T. Vascular dementia due to cardiac arrhythmia and systemic hypotension. *Acta Neurol Scand* 1987;76(2):123–128.
33. Zuccala G, Onder G, Pedone C, et al. Hypotension and cognitive impairment: Selective association in patients with heart failure. *Neurology.* 2001;57(11):1986–1992.
34. Zuccala G, Cattel C, Gravina-Manes E, DiNiro M, Cocchi A, Bernabei R. Left ventricular dysfunction: A clue to cognitive impairment in older patients with heart failure. *J Neurol Neurosurg Psychiatry.* 1997;63:509–512.
35. Bladin CF, Chambers BR. Clinical features, pathogenesis, and computed tomographic characteristics of internal watershed infarction. *Stroke.* 1993;24(12):1925–1932.
36. Moody D, Bell M, Challa V. Features of the cerebral vascular pattern that predict vulnerability to perfusion or oxygenation deficiency: An anatomic study. *Am J Neuroradiol.* 1990;11:431.

37. Saxena P, Schoemaker R. Organ blood flow protection in hypertension and congestive heart failure. *Am J Med*. 1993;94:4S-12S.
38. Jefferson A, Poppas A, Paul R, Cohen R. Systemic hypoperfusion is associated with executive dysfunction in geriatric cardiac patients. *Neurobiol Aging*. 2007;28:477–483.
39. Hoth KF, Poppas A, Moser DJ, et al. Cardiac dysfunction and cognition in older adults with heart failure. *Cogn Behav Neurol*. 2008;21(2):65–72.
40. Wolf PA, Abbott RD, Kannel WB. Atrial fibrillation: A major contributor to stroke in the elderly. The Framingham Study. *Arch Int Med*. 1987;147(9):1561–1564.
41. Roman GC. Vascular dementia prevention: A risk factor analysis. *Cerebrovasc Dis*. 2005;20 Suppl 2:91–100.
42. Wang TJ, Massaro JM, Levy D, et al. A risk score for predicting stroke or death in individuals with new-onset atrial fibrillation in the community: The Framingham Heart Study [*see comment*]. *JAMA*. 27 2003;290(8):1049–1056.
43. Schmidt R, Fazekas F, Offenbacher H, Dusleag J, Lechner H. Brain magnetic resonance imaging and neuropsychologic evaluation of patients with idiopathic dilated cardiomyopathy. *Stroke*. 1991;22(2):195–199.
44. Siachos T, Vanbakel A, Feldman DS, et al. Silent strokes in patients with heart failure [*see comment*]. *J Card Fail*. 2005;11(7):485–489.
45. Almeida JR, Alves TC, Wajngarten M, et al. Late-life depression, heart failure and frontal white matter hyperintensity: A structural magnetic resonance imaging study. *Braz J Med Biol Res*. 2005;38(3):431–436.
46. Raiha I, Tarvonen S, Kurki T, Rajala T, Sourander L. Relationship between vascular factors and white matter low attenuation of the brain. *Acta Neurol Scand*. 1993;87(4):286–289.
47. Travonen-Schroder S, Roytta M, Raiha I, Kurki T, Rajala T, Sourander L. Clinical features of leuko-araiosis. *J Neurol Neurosurg Psychiatry*. 1996;60(4):431–436.
48. Jefferson A, Tate D, Poppas A, et al. Lower cardiac output is associated with greater white matter hyperintensites in older adults with cardiovascular disease. *J Am Geriatr Soc*. 2007;55:1044–1048.
49. Woo MA, Macey PM, Fonarow GC, et al. Regional brain gray matter loss in heart failure. *J Appl Physiol*. 2003;95(2):677–684.
50. Vogels RL, Oosterman JM, Laman DM, et al. Transcranial Doppler blood flow assessment in patients with mild heart failure: Correlates with neuroimaging and cognitive performance. *Congest Heart Fail*. 2008;14(2):61–65.
51. Jesus PA, Vieira-de-Melo RM, Reis FJ, et al. Cognitive dysfunction in congestive heart failure: Transcranial Doppler evidence of microembolic etiology. *Arquivos de Neuro-Psiquiatria*. 2006;64(2A):207–210.
52. Lee CW, Lee JH, Kim JJ, et al. Cerebral metabolic abnormalities in congestive heart failure detected by proton magnetic resonance spectroscopy. *J Am Coll Cardiol*. 1999;33(5): 1196–1202.
53. Lee CW, Lee JH, Lim TH, et al. Prognostic significance of cerebral metabolic abnormalities in patients with congestive heart failure [see comment]. *Circulation*. 2001;103(23): 2784–2787.
54. Alves TC, Rays J, Fraguas R, Jr., et al. Localized cerebral blood flow reductions in patients with heart failure: A study using 99mTc-HMPAO SPECT. *J Neuroimaging*. 2005;15(2): 150–156.
55. Georgiadis D, Sievert M, Cencetti S, et al. Cerebrovascular reactivity is impaired in patients with cardiac failure [*see comment*]. *Eur Heart J*. 2000;21(5):407–413.
56. Moser D, Cohen R, Clark M, et al. Neuropsychological functioning among cardiac rehabilitation patients. *J Cardiopulm Rehabil*. 1999;19(2).

57. Moser DJ, Hoth KF, Robinson RG, et al. Blood vessel function and cognition in elderly patients with atherosclerosis. *Stroke*. 2004;35(11):e369–372.
58. Moser DJ, Miller IN, Hoth KF, et al. Vascular smooth muscle function is associated with initiation and processing speed in patients with atherosclerotic vascular disease. *J Int Neuropsychol Soc*. 2008;14(4):535–541.
59. Vogels RL, Oosterman JM, van Harten B, et al. Neuroimaging and correlates of cognitive function among patients with heart failure. *Dement Geriatr Cogn Dis*. 2007;24(6):418–423.
60. Zuccala G, Onder G, Marzetti E, et al. Use of angiotensin-converting enzyme inhibitors and variations in cognitive performance among patients with heart failure. *Eur Heart J*. 2005;26:226–233.
61. Paulson OB, Jarden JO, Godtfredsen J, Vorstrup S. Cerebral blood flow in patients with congestive heart failure treated with captopril. *Am J Med*. 1984;76(5B):91–95.
62. Kamishirado H, Inoue T, Fujito T, et al. Effect of enalapril maleate on cerebral blood flow in patients with chronic heart failure. *Angiology*. 1997;48(8):707–713.
63. Alves TC, Rays J, Telles RM, et al. Effects of antidepressant treatment on cognitive performance in elderly subjects with heart failure and comorbid major depression: An exploratory study. *Psychosomatics*. 2007;48(1):22–30.
64. Lautenschlager NT, Cox KL, Flicker L, et al. Effect of physical activity on cognitive function in older adults at risk for Alzheimer disease: A randomized trial. *JAMA*. 2008;300(9): 1027–1037.
65. Angevaren M, Aufdemkampe G, Verhaar HJ, et al. Physical activity and enhanced fitness to improve cognitive function in older people without known cognitive impairment. *Cochrane Database Syst Rev*. 2008(3):CD005381.
66. Carles S, Jr., Curnier D, Pathak A, et al. Effects of short-term exercise and exercise training on cognitive function among patients with cardiac disease. *J Cardiopulm Rehabil Prev*. 2007;27(6):395–399.
67. Tanne D, Freimark D, Poreh A, et al. Cognitive functions in severe congestive heart failure before and after an exercise training program. *Int J Cardiol*. 2005;103:145–149.
68. Roman DD, Kubo SH, Ormaza S, Francis GS, Bank AJ, Shumway SJ. Memory improvement following cardiac transplantation. *J Clin Exp Neuropsychol*. 1997;19(5):692–697.
69. Grimm M, Yeganehfar W, Laufer G, et al. Cyclosporine may affect improvement of cognitive brain function after successful cardiac transplantation [*see comment*]. *Circulation*. 1996;94(6):1339–1345.
70. Zimpfer D, Wieselthaler G, Czerny M, et al. Neurocognitive function in patients with ventricular assist devices: A comparison of pulsatile and continuous blood flow devices. *ASAIO Journal*. 2006;52(1):24–27.
71. Barbe C, Puisieux F, Jansen I, et al. Improvement of cognitive function after pacemaker implantation in very old persons with bradycardia. *J Am Geriatr Soc*. 2002;50(4):778–780.
72. Koide H, Kobayashi S, Kitani M, Tsunematsu T, Nakazawa Y. Improvement of cerebral blood flow and cognitive function following pacemaker implantation in patients with bradycardia. *Gerontology*. 1994;40(5):279–285.
73. Conti JB, Sears SF. Cardiac resynchronization therapy: Can we make our heart failure patients smarter? Transactions of the American Clinical and Climatological Association. 2007;118:153–164.

Part III

SYSTEMIC AND CEREBROVASCULAR MECHANISMS UNDERLYING VCI

12

CARDIOEMBOLIC STROKE

E. Jesus Duffis and Marc Fisher

There are approximately 780,000 strokes in the United States every year.[1] Cardioembolic stroke has been reported to account for roughly 20% to 30% of ischemic strokes.[2, 3] However, the true incidence of cardioembolic stroke may be higher, as some strokes classified as having undetermined etiology have features suggestive of cardioembolism.[4] Across races, the proportion of cardioembolic strokes may be greater in Caucasians when compared to blacks and Hispanics.[5] In the young, cardioembolic stroke is among the most common causes of stroke, accounting for up 30% of ischemic strokes.[6]

Clinical Features

It is often difficult to distinguish cardioembolic stroke from other ishcemic stroke subtypes based on clinical presentation alone. Cardioembolic stroke has classically been described as presenting with sudden and maximal deficits at onset.[7] Transient ischemic attack (TIA) and stuttering symptoms are thus less likely to represent cardioembolism. However, sudden symptom onset is not specific for cardioembolic strokes. Large-artery atherosclerosis causing arterial embolism can present in this fashion. Conversely, cardioembolic stroke may at times present with stuttering symptoms as the embolic material may dislodge from a more proximal location into distal branches.[8] Depressed level of consciousness at presentation has also been described as being seen more frequently in cardioembolic stroke.[9] Other reported historical features include onset during valsalva-type maneuvers, suggesting paradoxical embolism.

Hemorrhagic transformation has been reported to occur in 40% to 70% of cardioembolic strokes.[10–11] This is perhaps related to delayed spontaneous recanalization leading to reperfusion-induced hemorrhagic transformation.[12] Despite this classical teaching, a recent systematic review did not identify cardioembolism as a risk for hemorrhagic transformation of ischemic stroke.[13]

High-Risk Sources of Embolism

Atrial Fibrillation

Atrial fibrillation is the most common cause of cardioembolism. It accounts for approximately 25% to 30% of all cardioembolic strokes.[14] The incidence of atrial fibrillation increases with age and thus is an important risk factor for stroke in the elderly.[15] Formation of thrombus within the left atrial appendage as a result of stasis of blood within the atrium appears to be the principal mechanism of embolism.

The risk of stroke is similar for persistent atrial fibrillation and paroxysmal atrial fibrillation. Management strategies aimed at maintaining sinus rhythm have not shown a reduction in thromboembolism.[16] Stroke risk in atrial fibrillation varies with the presence of coexisting cardiovascular risk factors. It increases with advanced age as well as with the presence of hypertension, congestive heart failure, and diabetes. The increased risk of stroke with advanced age is independent of the presence of additional risk factors.[17] Prior history of stroke or TIA is the most important risk factor, with an 11% per year risk of recurrent stroke.[18] Additional risk factors include spontaneous echo contrast[19] and the presence of rheumatic valve disease, which confers a 17-fold increase of stroke compared to controls with neither.[20]

The CHADS2 score, derived from two of the randomized controlled trials of stroke prevention in atrial fibrillation, is a useful tool to quantify the annual risk of stroke in atrial fibrillation. Furthermore, it has been validated in a large population.[21] One point each is assigned to the presence of CHF, hypertension, diabetes, or age greater than 75. Prior stroke or TIA adds two points to the score. Higher scores are associated with a higher annual risk of stroke. In the absence of any of these risk factors, so-called lone atrial fibrillation, the annual risk of stroke is as low as 0.5% to 1% per year.[17, 21]

The effectiveness of anticoagulation over aspirin has been established in five major randomized trials of stroke prevention in atrial fibrillation[22–26] A combined total of 4000 patients were randomized. The overall relative risk reduction of stroke with coumadin was found to be 66% compared to a 16% reduction with aspirin, both compared to placebo.[21] Given these data, patients with one or more additional risk factors are generally treated with anticoagulation drugs unless there is a strong contraindication. Aspirin may be used in low-risk patients or those not eligible for anticoagulation therapy.

Cardiomyopathy

Like atrial fibrillation, dilated cardiomyopathy is associated with stasis of blood and thrombus formation. The annual rate of stroke has been reported to be approximately 1.5% to 3.5% in dilated cardiomyopathy.[27, 28] The risk of stroke increases with decrease in ejection fraction. Retrospective analysis from the studies of left ventricular dysfunction data SOLVD, demonstrated a 54% increase in the risk of thromboembolism for every 10% decrease in ejection fraction in women.[29] A similar increase risk of 18% for every 5% decrease in EF was seen in SAVE.[30] It is unclear if the coexistence of atrial fibrillation confers an increased risk of thromboembolism.[31]

There is uncertainty about the benefits of anticoagulation drugs in prevention of embolic events in dilated cardiomyopathy. Some benefit was suggested by earlier retrospective studies.[27] However, this was not confirmed in subsequent analysis.[29, 31] Two randomized trials have compared the efficacy of coumadin to aspirin in reducing death and cardiovascular events and found no difference in a composite outcome of death MI, and stroke between these treatments.[32, 33] Given the lack of clear evidence in favor of anticoagulation, aspirin or coumadin may be used in stroke prevention.

Acute Myocardial Infarction (MI)

The overall incidence of stroke is in the range of 2% during the first 30 days following MI. Acute MI, especially anterior MI with apical akinesis, may lead to the formation of thrombus within the ventricle and a source of potential embolism. Most thrombi arise within the first two weeks after MI.[34] In the era of PCI and thrombolytic therapy for MI, the incidence of left ventricular thrombus has been reported to be approximately 5%.[35, 36] The presence of mobile thrombus component as well as protrusion into the left ventricular cavity has been associated with increased risk of embolism from intracardiac thrombus.[37]

Anticoagulation may be of benefit in acute MI when a mural thrombus has formed. However, there are no randomized prospective data to support this. Meta-analysis of observational studies suggests a benefit of anticoagulation over antiplatelet therapy in this setting.[38] The duration of treatment is controversial, but generally three to 12 months of anticoagulation has been advocated.

Valvular Heart Disease

Rheumatic heart disease, particularly mitral stenosis, increases the risk of embolization. The vast majority of these emboli involve the cerebral vasculature. Mitral stenosis is often complicated by atrial fibrillation, which occurs in 30% to 40% of symptomatic patients.[39] As mentioned, the two conditions confer a 17-fold increase in the risk of stroke compared to patients with neither. Even in the absence of atrial fibrillation, embolism may be present in 20% of cases.[40] Anticoagulation is recommended in the presence of atrial fibrillation or prior embolic event for mitral stenosis resulting from rheumatic fever.[39] Prophylaxis for endocarditis is also suggested.

Both mechanical and bio-prosthetic valves are also associated with increased risk of stroke, but it is greater with mechanical valves. The annual risk of stroke is estimated to be 1% to 4% after valve replacement.[41, 42] The risk of stroke appears to be greatest for mitral valve replacement compared to aortic valve replacement. As in rheumatic valvular disease, the risk is further increased by the presence of atrial fibrillation.[42] Anticoagulation is recommended for patients with mechanical prosthetic valves, while aspirin may suffice for those with bio-prosthetics and no risk factors for stroke.[39]

Valvular involvement may occur in the setting of bacterial infection or systemic malignancy or connective tissue disease. Both bacterial and non-infective (marantic) endocarditis can be complicated by stroke. In infective endocarditis, the incidence of ischemic stroke is 15% to 20%. The risk of stroke is highest within the first two weeks of presentation. Risk is greatly diminished after initiation of appropriate antibiotic therapy, falling to approximately 3% after one week of treatment.[43] The risk of stroke in bacterial endocarditis is higher with involvement of the mitral valve compared to the aortic valve.[44] Additional risk factors may be ascertained by echocardiography and include size of vegetation and mobility.[44, 45]

Anticoagulation therapy is considered to be contraindicated in infective endocarditis because of an increased risk of cerebral hemorrhage. Treatment is centered around an appropriate antibiotic regimen and valve replacement if indicated. Anticoagulation therapy has been suggested in the treatment of marantic endocarditis.[42]

Sources with Medium or Uncertain Risk

Aortic Arch Atheroma

The annual risk of stroke for patients with severe plaque in the aortic arch has been reported to be 10% to 12%.[46–48] These figures, however, were obtained from selected patient populations at high risk for ischemic event. A recent prospective population-based study failed to show an independent association between aortic atheroma and stroke.[49]

The prevalence of aortic atheroma in stroke patients is about 14% to 21% and is on the same order as the prevalence of atrial fibrillation and carotid artery disease.[50] For rather obvious reasons, only atheromatous plaques involving the ascending aorta and arch should confer an increased risk of cerebral embolism. Increasing plaque size confers an additional risk. The French Aortic Plaque in Stroke study group found a recurrence rate of 11.9% per year for plaques greater than or equal to 4mm, compared to only 3.5% for atheroma of a size less than 4 mm.[47] Similarly mobile and ulcerated plaque components also appear to increase the risk of embolism.[48, 51]

The optimal treatment of aortic atheroma remains unclear. A potential benefit of anticoagulation was suggested in some observational studies with a limited number of patients.[52, 53] A larger retrospective examination of 519 patients with complex aortic plaque greater than 4 mm found no statistically significant benefit to anticoagulation therapy.[54] In this same series, statins were associated with an absolute risk reduction of 17%. Given the lack of convincing data to support anticoagulation therapy in the treatment of aortic arch atheroma, a reasonable strategy may be risk-factor reduction, including aggressive cholesterol-lowering and antiplatelet therapy.

Patent Foramen Ovale

Patent foramen ovale (PFO) represents a remnant of fetal circulation. It is present in approximately 25% of the population. The association of PFO with stroke has been suggested in several case-control studies.[55] The relationship is stronger for patients younger than 55 and in those with cryptogenic stroke. In the general population, however, the risk of stroke in the presence of PFO is extremely low, and no independent association between the two has been found.[56, 57] Furthermore, in patients younger than 55 treated with aspirin, the recurrent rate of stroke is only 1% to 2% per year.[58, 59]

Additional risk factors besides the presence of PFO may be important in predicting the occurrence of stroke. For example, the size of right-to-left shunting as measured by microbubbles seen on echocardiogram may increase the likelihood of paradoxical embolism.[60] The size of the PFO may also be associated with the recurrence of stroke, however, the evidence for this is conflicting.[61, 62]

Atrial Septal Aneurysm

Atrial septal aneurysm (ASA) is defined as an excursion of atrial septum into the atrial chambers. It occurs in 1% of patients at autopsy.[63] ASA is found more frequently in patients with prior ischemic stroke than in the general population. Several reports have suggested a link between ASA and an increase risk of embolic events.[64–66] Several potential mechanisms for thromboembolism have been suggested, including local thrombus formation within the aneurysm, as well as predisposition to cardiac arrhythmias. The great frequency with which coexisting right-to-left shunt is seen makes paradoxical embolism a likely possibility.

PFO with ASA

PFO is present in combination with ASA in approximately 4% of patients.[57] There is conflicting evidence about whether the presence of both defects increases the risk of recurrent stroke. Two studies suggested a fourfold increase in the annual risk of recurrence.[59, 61] In contrast, the PFO in Cryptogenic Stroke Study (PICSS) found no difference in the event rate between patients with PFO alone and those with PFO in association with ASA.[67] Other studies have also failed to show an increased risk of recurrent stroke with the combination of PFO and ASA.[68, 69]

There is no evidence of benefit of anticoagulation drugs over aspirin for secondary stroke prevention in patients with either isolated PFO or in combination with ASA.[67] Treatment with aspirin may suffice in most patients. An exception may be patients with documented venous thrombosis or evidence of hypercoagulability, in which paradoxical embolism is suspected. Surgical or percutaneous closure may be another option; however, these procedures carry risks of complications. Furthermore, as of yet, results of prospective trials comparing closure with medical management have not been reported.

Mitral Valve Prolapse

Mitral valve prolapse (MVP) is present in approximately 2.4% to 4% of the population.[71, 72] In early studies MVP was reported in up to 30% of patients with ischemic stroke under the age of 45.[70] After revision of the echocardiographic criteria for the diagnosis of MVP, recent studies have failed to show an association between MVP and first or recurrent stroke, even in young patients.[73, 74] As with PFO, additional risk factors for stroke in MVP may be important. These may include the presence of arrhythmias, age, and presence of valve thickening.[75] In the absence of strong indication for coumadin such as coexisting atrial fibrillation, antiplatelet therapy seems reasonable for secondary stroke prevention.

Valvular Calcification

Mitral annular calcification (MAC) refers to the degenerative deposition of calcium within the fibrous supportive structure of the mitral valve. MAC is associated with the presence of cardiovascular risk factors and with vascular atherosclerosis.[76] The presence of MAC increases with age. It is seen in approximately 8% of patients younger than 60 and 47% of those older than 80.[76, 77] The association of MAC with stroke was suggested in an analysis of the Framingham Heart Study, which showed that MAC doubles the risk of stroke. The increased risk was independent of the presence of traditional stroke risk factors.[78] Increased risk of stroke with MAC has been subsequently confirmed in other reports, however, no increased risk has been seen with aortic calcification.[79] Now there is no widely accepted mechanism of embolism in MAC. It remains unclear if MAC is itself directly a cause of stroke or merely a marker for other precursors of stroke.[80] Here again, initial antiplatelet treatment for secondary prevention is acceptable.

Diagnosis

The diagnosis of cardioembolic stroke relies on detection of a high-risk source of embolism and exclusion of other causes of stroke. As mentioned previously, features of the history and neurological exam may be highly suggestive of embolism. In addition, neuroimaging may show distinct patterns, which may further suggest the diagnosis. These patterns include the involvement of multiple vascular territories, as well proximal occlusion of vessels, particularly the posterior cerebral artery.[81]

Echocardiography should be performed in patients with suspected cardioembolic stroke, however, its routine use in the evaluation of stroke is not likely to be cost-effective. The yield of transthoracic echocardiography in identifying a potential source of embolism is higher in the presence of clinical features of cardiac disease. In the absence of cardiac disease, however, the diagnostic yield is less than 5%.[82, 83] Transesophageal echocardiogram (TEE) allows for improved visualization of the aortic arch and the left atrium as well as the atrial septum, and thus improves the detection of potential sources of cardiac embolism. The overall yield of TEE in identifying a potential cardiac source of embolism is 43% compared with 14% for TTE.[84] Despite improved detection of cardiac sources with TEE, the information obtained from TEE may not impact management, because no change of medication may be made.[85]

Identification of atrial fibrillation is easily accomplished with ECG monitoring. Serial ECG examination may increase the detection of atrial fibrillation almost threefold.[86] Identification of paroxysmal atrial fibrillation may be somewhat harder and may require holter monitoring. A recent study reported that up to 5% of patients with unexplained stroke show evidence of paroxysmal atrial fibrillation on holter monitoring in the first 24 hours, and an additional 5% may be detected after one week of monitoring.[87] Event-loop recorders may have a similar rate of detection.[88]

Treatment

The role of heparin in the treatment of acute cardioembolic stroke remains controversial. On one hand, the potential for early recurrence of embolic stroke may necessitate immediate anticoagulation therapy. However, the risk of bleeding while on heparin may offset any potential gains in preventing recurrent events. As an example, a recent meta-analysis of randomized controlled trials showed no significant reduction in the number of early recurrent ischemic strokes in patients treated with heparin, while demonstrating a statistically significant increase in the number of symptomatic intracranial bleeding.[89] Despite these findings, heparin may still benefit selected patients, including those with high-risk embolic sources such as those with intracardiac thrombus, in which the risk of recurrent embolism may outweigh the risk of hemorrhage. In addition, early anticoagulation within the first six hours has only been addressed in a limited number of trials, which have shown that anticoagulation can be accomplished safely and may be of some benefit.[90–92] Management strategies for specific sources of embolism have been discussed previously. In many centers, oral anticoagulation is initiated within one to two days after stroke onset, if the patient can swallow safely.

Prognosis

The overall mortality appears to be higher in cardioembolic stroke than in other stroke subtypes. Mortality may be close to 25% within the first 30 days.[93] Even at two years, the mortality rate has been reported to be three times that of strokes due to small-vessel occlusion.[2] Based on prospective data, the early risk of recurrence within the first 14 days may be as high as 5%.[94]

Notes

1. Rosamond W, Flegal K, Furie K, et al. Heart disease and stroke statistics—2008 update: A report from the American Heart Association Statistics Committee and Stroke Statistics Subcommittee. *Circulation*. 2008;117:e25–146.
2. Sandercock PA, Warlow CP, Jones LN, Starkey IR. Predisposing factors for cerebral infarction: The Oxfordshire Community Stroke Project. *BMJ*. 1989;298:75–80.
3. Klominsky-Rabas PL, Weber M, Gefeller O Neundoerfer B, Heuschmann PU. Epidemiology of ischemic stroke subtypes according to TOAST criteria: Incidence, recurrence, and long-term survival in ischemic stroke subtypes: A population-based study. *Stroke*. 2001;32(12): 2735–2740.
4. Sacco RL, Ellenberg JH, Mohr JP, et al. Infarcts of undetermined cause: The NINCDS Stroke Data Bank. *Ann Neurol*. 1989;25:382–390.

5. White H, Boden-Albala B, Wang C, et al. Ischemic stroke subtype incidence among whites, blacks, and Hispanics: The Northern Manhattan Study. *Circulation*. 2005;111(10): 1327–1331.
6. Kittner SJ, Stern BJ, Wozniak M, et al. Cerebral infarction in young adults: The Baltimore-Washington Cooperative Young Stroke Study. *Neurology*. 1998;50(4):890–894.
7. Arboix A, Oliveres M, Massons J, Pujades R, Garcia-Eroles J. Early differentiation of cardioembolic from atherothrombotic cerebral infarction: A multivariate analysis. *Eur J Neurol*.1999;6(6):677–683.
8. Minematsu K, Yamaguchi T, Omae T. "Spectacular shrinking deficit": Rapid recovery from a major hemispheric syndrome by migration of an embolus. *Neurology*.1992;42(1): 157–162.
9. Timsit SG, Sacco RL, Mohr JP, et al. Brain infarction severity differs according to cardiac or arterial embolic source. *Neurology*. 1993;43(4):728–733.
10. Okada Y, Yamaguchi T, Minematsu K, et al. Hemorrhagic transformation in cerebral embolism. *Stroke*. 1989;20(5):598–603.
11. Hornig CR, Bauer T, Simon C, Trittmacher S, Dorndorf W. Hemorrhagic transformation in cardioembolic cerebral infarction. *Stroke*. 1993;24(3):465–468.
12. Molina CA, Montaner J, Abilleira S, et al. Timing of spontaneous recanalization and risk of hemorrhagic transformation in acute cardioembolic stroke. *Stroke*. 2001;32:1079–1084.
13. Lindley RI, Wardlaw JM, Sandercock PA, et al. Frequency and risk factors for spontaneous hemorrhagic transformation of cerebral infarction. *J Stroke Cerebrovasc Dis*. 2004;13(6): 235–246.
14. Cardiogenic brain embolism. Cerebral Embolism Task force. *Arch Neurol*. 1986;43(1): 71–84.
15. Wolf PA, Abbott RD, Kannel WB. Atrial fibrillation: A major contributor to stroke in the elderly. The Framingham Study. *Arch Intern Med*. 1987;147(9):1561–1564.
16. Wyse DG, Waldo AL, DiMarco JP, et al. A comparison of rate control and rhythm control in patients with atrial fibrillation. *N Engl J Med*. 2002;347(23):1825–1833.
17. Risk factors for stroke and efficacy of antithrombotic therapy in atrial fibrillation. Analysis of pooled data from five randomized controlled trials. *Arch Intern Med*. 1994;154(13): 1449–1457.
18. Gage BF, van Walraven C, Pearce L, et al. Selecting patients with atrial fibrillation for anticoagulation. Stroke risk stratification in patients taking aspirin. *Circulation*. 20004; 110:2287–2292.
19. Zabalgoitia M, Halperin JL, Pearce LA, Blackshear JL, Asinger RW, Hart RG. Transesophageal echocardiographic correlates of clinical risk of thromboembolism in nonvalvular atrial fibrillation. Stroke Prevention in Atrial Fibrillation III Investigators. *J Am Coll Cardiol*. 1998;31:1622–1626.
20. Wolf PA, Dawber TR, Thomas HE Jr, Kannel B. Epidemiologic assessment of chronic atrial fibrillation and risk of stroke: The Framingham Study. *Neurology*. 1978;28:973–977.
21. Albers GW, Amarenco P, Easton JD, Sacco RL, Teal P. Antithrombotic and thrombolytic therapy for ischemic stroke: American College of Chest Physicians Evidence-Based Clinical Practice Guidelines (8th ed.). *Chest*. 2008;133:630–669.
22. The effect of low-dose warfarin on the risk of stroke in patients with nonrheumatic atrial fibrillation. The Boston Area Anticoagulation Trial for Atrial Fibrillation Investigators. *N Engl J Med*. 1990;323:1505–1511.
23. Ezekowitz MD, Bridgers SL, James KE, et al. Warfarin in the prevention of stroke associated with nonrheumatic atrial fibrillation. Veterans Affairs Stroke Prevention in Nonrheumatic Atrial Fibrillation Investigators. *N Engl J Med*. 1992;327(20):1406–1412.

24. Petersen P, Boysen G, Godtfredsen J, Andersen ED, Andersen B. Placebo-controlled, randomised trial of warfarin and aspirin for prevention of thromboembolic complications in chronic atrial fibrillation. The Copenhagen AFASAK study. *Lancet.* 1989;1:175–179.
25. Connolly SJ, Laupacis A, Gent M, Roberts RS, Cairns JA, Joyner C. Canadian Atrial Fibrillation Anticoagulation (CAFA) Study. *J Am Coll Cardiol.* 1991;18:349–355.
26. *Stroke.* Prevention in Atrial Fibrillation Study. Final results. Circulation 1991;84(2):527–539.
27. Fuster V, Gersh BJ, Giuliani ER, et al. The natural history of idiopathic dilated cardiomyopathy. *Am J Cardiol.* 1981, 47:525.
28. Freudenberger RS, Hellkamp AS, Halperin JL, et al. Risk of thromboembolism in heart failure: An analysis from the Sudden Cardiac Death in Heart Failure Trial (SCD-HeFT). *Circulation.* 2007;115:2637.
29. Dries DL, Rosenberg YD, Waclawiw MA, Domanski MJ. Ejection fraction and risk of thromboembolic events in patients with systolic dysfunction and sinus rhythm: Evidence for gender differences in the studies of left ventricular dysfunction trials. *J Am Coll Cardiol.* 1997;29(5):1074–1080.
30. Loh E, St. John Sutton M, Wun CC, et al. Ventricular dysfunction and the risk of stroke after myocardial infarction. *N Engl J Med.* 1997;336:251.
31. Dunkman WB, Johnson GR, Carson PE, et al. Incidence of thromboembolic events in congestive heart failure. The V-HeFT VA Cooperative Studies Group. *Circulation.* 1993; 87(6 Suppl):VI94–101.
32. Cleland JGF, Findlay I, Jafri S, et al. The Warfarin/Aspirin Study in Heart failure (WASH), a randomized trial comparing antithrombotic strategies for patients with heart failure. *Am Heart J.* 2004;148:157–64.
33. Cokkinos DV, Haralabopoulos GC, Kostis JB, et al. Efficacy of antithrombotic therapy in chronic heart failure: The HELAS study. *Eur J Heart Fail.* 2006;8:428–432.
34. Asinger RW, Mikell FL, Elsperger J, Hodges, M. Incidence of left-ventricular thrombosis after acute transmural myocardial infarction. Serial evaluation by two-dimensional echocardiography. *N Engl J Med.* 1981;305:297.
35. Rehan A, Kanwar M, Rosman H, et al. Incidence of post-myocardial infarction left ventricular thrombus formation in the era of primary percutaneous intervention and glycoprotein IIb/IIIa inhibitors. A prospective observational study. *Cardiovasc Ultrasound.* 2006;4:20.
36. Chiarella F, Santora E, Domenicucci S, et al., on behalf of the GISSI-3 Investigators. Predischarge two-dimensional echocardiographic evaluation of left ventricular thrombosis after acute myocardial infarction in the GISSI-3 study. *Am J Cardiol.* 1998;81:822.
37. Visser CA, Kan G, Meltzer RS, et al. Embolic potential of left ventricular thrombus after myocardial infarction: A two-dimensional echocardiographic study of 119 patients. *J Am Coll Cardiol.* 1985;5:1.
38. Vaitkus PT, Barnathan ES. Embolic potential, prevention and management of mural thrombus complicating anterior myocardial infarction: A meta-analysis. *J Am Coll Cardiol.* 1993;22:1004–1009.
39. Bonow RO, Blasé AC, Kanu C, et al. ACC?AHA. 2006 guidelines for the management of patients with valvular heart disease. A report of the American College of Cardiology/American Heart Association Task Force on Practice Guidelines (writing committee to revise the 1998 guidelines for the management of patients with valvular heart disease). *J Am Coll Cardiol.* 2006;48:e1–148.
40. Szekely P. Systemic embolism and anticoagulant prophylaxis in rheumatic heart disease. *BMJ.* 1964;1:209–212.
41. Israel DH, Sharma Sk, Fuster V. Antithrombotic therapy in prosthetic heart valve replacement. *Am Heart J.* 1994:127:400–411.

42. Salem DN, Stein PD, Al-Ahmad A, et al. Antithrombotic therapy in valvular heart disease-native and prosthetic. *Chest.* 2004;126:457S-8S.
43. Dickerman SA, Abrutyn E, Barsic B, et al. The relationship between the initiation of antimicrobial therapy and the incidence of stroke in infective endocarditis: An analysis from the ICE Prospective Cohort Study (ICE-PCS). *Am Heart J.* 2007;154:1086–1094.
44. Cabell CH, Pond KK, Peterson GE, et al. The risk of stroke and death in patients with aortic and mitral valve endocarditis. *Am Heart J.* 2001;142:75–80.
45. Di Salvo G, Habib G, Pergola V, et al. Echocardiography predicts embolic events in infective endocarditis. *J Am Coll Cardiol.* 2001;37:1069–1076.
46. Tunick PA, Katz ES, Freedberg RS, Rosenzweig BP, Perez JL, Kronzon I. High risk for vascular events in patients with protruding aortic atheromas: A prospective study. *J Am Coll Cardiol* 1994;23:1085–1090.
47. Atherosclerotic disease of the aortic arch as a risk factor for recurrent ischemic stroke: The French Study of Aortic Plaques in Stroke Group. *N Engl J Med.* 1996;334:1216–1221.
48. Transesophageal echocardiographic correlates of thromboembolism in high-risk patients with nonvalvular atrial fibrillation: The Stroke Prevention in Atrial Fibrillation Investigators Committee on Echocardiography. *Ann Intern Med.* 1998;128:639–647.
49. Meissner I, Khandheria BK, Sheps SG, et al. Atherosclerosis of the aorta: Risk factor, risk marker, or innocent bystander? A prospective population-based transesophageal echocardiography study. *J Am Coll Cardiol.* 2004, 44:1018.
50. Kronzon I, Tunick PA. Aortic atherosclerotic disease and stroke. *Circulation.* 2006; 114:63–75.
51. Karalis DG, Chanddrasekaran K, Victor MF, et al. Recognition and embolic potential of intra-aortic atherosclerotic debris. *J Am Coll Cardiol.* 1991;17:73–78.
52. Dressler FA, Craig WR, Castello R, Labovitz AJ. Mobile aortic atheroma and systemic emboli: Efficacy of anticoagulation and influence of plaque morphology on recurrent stroke. *J Am Coll Cardiol.* 1998;31:134–138.
53. Ferrari E, Vidal R, Chevallier T, Baudouy M. Atherosclerosis of the thoracic aorta and aortic debris as a marker of poor prognosis: Benefit of oral anticoagulants. *J Am Coll Cardiol.* 1999;33:1317–1322.
54. Tunick PA, Nayar AC, Goodkin GM, et al. Effect of treatment on the incidence of stroke and other emboli in 519 patients with severe thoracic aortic plaque. *Am J Cardiol.* 2002;90: 1320–1325.
55. Overell JR, Bone I, Less KR. Interarterial septal abnormalities and stroke. A meta-analysis of case-control studies. *Neurology.* 2000;55:1172–1179.
56. Di Tullio MR, Sacco RL, Sciacca RR, Jin Z, Homma S. Patent foramen ovale and the risk of ischemic stroke in a multiethnic population. *J Am Coll Cardiol.* 2007;49:797–802.
57. Meissner I, Khandheria BK, Heit JA, et al. patent foramen ovale: Innocent or guilty? Evidence from a prospective population-based study. *J Am Coll Cardiol.* 2006;47:440–445.
58. Homma S, Di Tullio MR, Sacco RL, et al. Age as a determinant of adverse events in medically treated crytogenic stroke patients with patent foramen ovale. *Stroke.* 2004;35:2145–2149.
59. Mas JL, Zuber M. Recurrent cerebrovascular events in patients with patent foramen ovale, atrial septal aneurysm, or both and cryptogenic stroke or transient ischemic attack. French Study Group on Patent Foramen Ovale and Atrial Septal Aneurysm. *Am Heart J.* 1995;130:1083–1088.
60. Serena J, Segura T, Perez-Ayuso MJ, Bassaganyas J, Molins A. The need to quantify right-to-left shunt in acute ischemic stroke: A case control study. *Stroke.* 1998;29:1322–1328.
61. Mas JL, Arquizan C, Lamy C, et al. Recurrent cerebrovascular events associated with patent foramen ovale, atrial septal aneurysm, or both. *N Engl J Med.* 2001;345(24):1740–1746.

62. Schuchlenz HW, Weihs W, Horner S, Quehenberger F. The association between the diameter of a patent foramen ovale and the risk of embolic cerebrovascular events. *Am J Med.* 2000;109:456–462.
63. Belkin RN, Kisslo J. Atrial septal aneurysm: Recognition and clinical relevance. *Am Heart J.* 1990;120:948–957.
64. Schneider B, Hanrath P, Vogel P, Meinertz T. Improved morphologic characterization of atrial septal aneurysm by transesophageal echocardiography: Relation to cerebrovascular events. *J Am Coll Cardiol.* 1990;16(4):1000–1009.
65. Belkin RN, Hurwitz BJ, Kisslo J. Atrial septal aneurysm: Association with cerebrovascular and peripheral embolic events. *Stroke.*1987;18:856–862.
66. Pearson AC, Nagelhout D, Castello R, Gomez CR, Labovitz AJ. Atrial septal aneurysm and stroke: A transesophageal echocardiographic study. *J Am Coll Cardiol.* 1991;18: 1223–1229.
67. Homma S, Sacco RL, Di Tullio MR, et al. Effect of medical treatment in stroke patients with patent foramen ovale. Patent Foramen Ovale in Cryptogenic Stroke Study. *Circulation.* 2002;105:2625–2631.
68. Bogousslavsky J, Garazi S, Jeanrenaud X, et al. Stroke recurrence in patients with patent foramen ovale: The Lausanne Study. Lausanne Stroke with Paradoxal Embolism study group. *Neurology.* 1996;46:1301–1305.
69. Cerrato P, Priano L, Imperiale D, et al. Recurrent cerebrovascular ischaemic events in patients with interatrial septal abnormalities: A follow up study. *Neurol Sci.* 2006;26:411–418.
70. Barnett HJM, Boughner DR, Taylor DW, Cooper PE, Kostuk WJ, Nichol PM. Further evidence relating mitral-valve prolapse to cerebral ischemic events. *N Engl J Med.* 1980;302: 139–144.
71. Freed LA, Levy D, Levine RA, et al. Prevalence and clinical outcome of mitral-valve prolapse. *N Engl J Med.* 1999;341:1741–1742.
72. Levine RA, Stathogianni E, Newell JB, et al. Reconsideration of echocardiographic standards for mitral valve prolapse: Lack of association between leaflet displacement isolated to the apical four chamber view and independent echocardiographic evidence of abnormality. *J Am Coll Cardiol.* 1988;11:1010–1015.
73. Orencia AJ, Petty GW, Khandheria BK, et al. Risk of stroke with mitral valve prolapse in population-based cohort study. *Stroke.* 1995;26:7–13.
74. Gilon D, Buonannd FS, Joffe MM, et al. Lack of association between mitral-valve prolapse and stroke in young patients. *N Engl J Med.* 1999;341:8–13.
75. Avierinos JF, Brown RD, Foley DA, et al. Cerebral ischemic events after diagnosis of mitral valve prolapse: A community-based study of incidence and predictive factors. *Stroke.* 2003;34(6):1339–1344.
76. Allison MA, Cheung P, Criqui MH, Langer RD, Wright CM. Mitral and aortic annular calcification are highly associated with systemic calcified atherosclerosis. *Circulation.* 2006;113(6):861–866.
77. Aronow WS, Ahn C, Kronzon I, Gutstein H. Association of mitral annular calcium with new thromboembolic stroke at 44-month follow-up of 2,148 persons, mean age 81 years. *Am J Cardiol.* 1998;81(1):105–106.
78. Benjamin EJ, Plehn JF, D'Agostino RB, et al. Mitral annular calcification and the risk of stroke in an elderly cohort. *N Engl J Med.* 1992 6;327(6):374–379.
79. Kizer JR, Wiebers DO, Whisnant JP, et al. Mitral annular calcification, aortic valve sclerosis, and incident stroke in adults free of clinical cardiovascular disease: The Strong Heart Study. *Stroke.* 2005;36:2533–2537.

80. Boon A, Lodder J, Cheriex E, Kessels F. Mitral annulus calcification is not an independent risk factor for stroke: A cohort study of 657 patients. *J Neurol.* 1997;244(9):535–541.
81. Yamamoto Y, Georgiadis AL, Chang HM, Caplan LR. Posterior cerebral artery territory infarcts in the New England Medical Center Posterior Circulation Registry. *Arch Neurol.* 1999;56(7):824–832.
82. Wolber T, Maeder M, Atefy R, Bluzaite I, Blank R, Rickli H, Ammann P. Should routine echocardiography be performed in all patients with stroke? *J Stroke Cerebrovasc Dis.* 2007;16:1–7.
83. Sansoy V, Abbott RD, Jayaweera AR, Kaul S. Low yield of transthoracic echocardiography for cardiac source of embolism. *Am J Cardiol.* 1995;75:166–169.
84. Pearson AC. Transthoracic echocardiography versus transesophageal echocardiography in detecting cardiac sources of embolism. *Echocardiography.* 1993;10:397–403.
85. Hata JS, Ayres RW, Biller J, et al. Impact of transesophageal echocardiography on the anticoagulation management of patients admitted with focal cerebral ischemia. *Am J Cardiol.* 1993;72:707–710.
86. Douen AG, Pageau N, Medic S. Serial electrocardiographic assessments significantly improve detection of atrial fibrillation 2.6-fold in patients with acute stroke. *Stroke.* 2008, 39: 480–482.
87. Jabaudon D, Sztajzel J, Sievert K, Landis T, Sztajzel R. Usefulness of ambulatory 7-day ECG monitoring for the detection of atrial fibrillation and flutter after acute stroke and transient ischemic attack. *Stroke.* 2004;35:1647–1651.
88. Liao J, Khalid Z, Scallan C, Morillo C, O'Donnell M. Noninvasive cardiac monitoring for detecting paroxysmal atrial fibrillation or flutter after acute ischemic stroke: A systematic review. *Stroke.* 2007;38(11):2935–2940.
89. Paciaroni M, Agnelli G, Micheli S, Caso V. Efficacy and safety of anticoagulant treatment in acute cardioembolic stroke: A meta-analysis of randomized controlled trials. *Stroke.* 2007;38:423–430.
90. Chamorro A, Vila N, Saiz A, Alday M, Tolosa E. Early anticoagulation after large cerebral embolic infarction: A safety study. *Neurology.* 1995;45:861–865.
91. Immediate anticoagulation of embolic stroke: A randomized trial. Cerebral Embolism Study Group. *Stroke.* 1983;14:668–676.
92. Chamorro A, Vila N, Ascaso C, Blanc R. Heparin in acute stroke with atrial fibrillation: Clinical relevance of very early treatment. *Arch Neurol.* 1999;56:1098–1102.
93. de Jong G, van Raak L, Kessels F, Lodder J. Stroke subtype and mortality: A follow-up study in 998 patients with a first cerebral infarct. *J Clin Epidemiol.* 2003;56(3):262–268.
94. Saxena R, Lewis S, Berge E, Sandercock PA, Koudstaal PJ. Risk of early death and recurrent stroke and effect of heparin in 3,169 patients with acute ischemic stroke and atrial fibrillation in the International Stroke Trial. *Stroke.* 2001;32(10):2333–2337.

13

CARDIAC OUTPUT AND EJECTION FRACTION

IMPACT ON BRAIN STRUCTURE AND FUNCTION

Farzin Irani

Cardiovascular disease (CVD) is an umbrella term for various conditions, including coronary artery disease, myocardial infarction, heart failure, and hypertension. It is a leading cause of death and morbidity in Western society and a major health concern. CVD has been associated with a wide range of cognitive deficits even in the absence of clinically identified stroke.[1–4] Recent interest in these "vascular cognitive impairments" (VCI) that are evident early in the disease process has led to efforts to preemptively identify risk factors prior to deterioration.[5–7] The underlying pathophysiological mechanism for vascular cognitive impairments remains an area of rigorous study, but a complex interaction of impaired cardiac and cerebral hemodynamic factors is likely to be involved.[8] Towards this end, a variety of cardiac and systemic risk vascular factors have been investigated and shown to impact cognitive performance, structural integrity, and brain response to cognitive challenges.[2, 9–22]

Of the etiological factors implicated in VCI, the role of cerebral hypoperfusion has garnered recent interest. Reductions in cardiac performance can alter blood flow through the body (systemic perfusion), which then impacts blood flow to the brain (cerebral perfusion). Specifically, reduced cardiac performance based on aging, hypertension, atherosclerosis, or a number of CVD risk factors can have a significant impact on brain microcirculation that then influences both systemic and cerebral perfusion via changes to the oxygen and nutrient supply of the brain.[23] When hypoperfusion is chronic, there can be a decrease in the effectiveness of autoregulatory mechanisms that augment blood flow to the brain.[24] This is particularly relevant for elderly individuals in whom CVD-associated brain dysfunction is significant.[3, 4] Thus, in addition to mechanisms involving single strategic infarcts, multiple infarcts, and leukoaraiosis, chronic hypoperfusion is an important factor in the pattern of cognitive deficits associated with vascular degeneration.[25] Consistently with this, several studies have shown that cerebral hypoperfusion is a primary alternative mechanism for developing VCI and vascular dementia, independent of cerebral infarcts in small and large vessels.

This chapter will focus on describing the studies conducted to date on two indices of cerebral perfusion and cardiac performance. These indices are ventricular ejection fraction (EF) and cardiac output (CO), both of which are predictors of chronic hypoperfusion. This is a growing line of investigation, and the few studies conducted to date using neuropsychological and neuroimaging methodologies will be reviewed here in an attempt to summarize what has been gleaned thus far about the relationship between cardiac performance, hypoperfusion, and brain structure and function.

Description of Cardiac Output and Ejection Fraction

CO and EF are both widely used echocardiogram measures that reflect heart output and subsequent cerebral perfusion. Both these measures have been shown to load heavily as "cardiac factors" as compared to "systemic vascular factors such as brachial artery distensibility, intima-media-thickening and diastolic variability."[8] CO measures the absolute volume of blood leaving the heart into systemic circulation per minute. It is measured by the amount of blood in liters per minute (L/min) that is pumped from the heart to perfuse the systemic circulation. Because the flow is pulsatile, CO is a function of stroke volume (SV) and heart rate (HR). SV is a function of mean velocity of blood flow from the left ventricle multiplied by the area of left-ventricular-outflow tract measured from the 2D echo image (CO = [TVI x CSA] x HR, where TVI = time velocity integral, CSA = cross-sectional area, and HR = heart rate). It can be recorded with noninvasive Doppler echocardiography methods, which are strongly correlated with more invasive measures of CO.[26] CO for an average individual at rest is usually 4.9 1/minute.

EF is more often used as a clinical indicator of heart health and is a strong prognostic indicator of morbidity and mortality. It refers to the fraction of blood ejected by the left ventricle during the contraction (ejection phase) of the cardiac cycle. It is calculated by dividing SV by the end-diastolic volume. EF dysfunction has been characterized as being mild in the 41% to 49% range, moderate in the 35% to 40% range, and greater than 35% as severe.[27] EF may decrease when the heart muscle has been damaged, such as due to myocardial infarction, heartmuscle disease (cardiomyopathy), or heart valve problems.

Neuropsychological Studies

A few studies have evaluated the relationship between reduced cardiac performance as measured by CO and/or EF and neuropsychological test performance. One recent study examined these relationships using a variety of neuropsychological tests in a geriatric cohort of patients with CVD without clinically identified stroke and globally intact cognition.[21] They estimated cardiac performance using CO and found that patients with low CO performed significantly worse than those with normal CO on tests of sequencing and planning. Since tests of sequencing and planning are most sensitive to executive dysfunction, this study provided initial support for the hypothesis that frontal-subcortical circuitry involved in executive control may be impacted in patients with reduced cardiac performance. This is particularly relevant for elderly individuals in whom age-associated breakdown of the cerebrovasculature along with chronic hypoperfusion could exacerbate susceptibility towards alterations in heart efficiency.

Another recent study extended these findings by examining the relationship between cognition and more pronounced reductions in cardiac performance in a cohort of elderly patients with New York Heart Association class II–IV heart failure.[28] Using EF as a proxy measure for cardiac performance, Hoth et al. (2008) showed below-expected levels of cognitive performance in domains associated with executive function. In particular, they found a significant association between decreased EF and weaker performance on tests of attention, working memory, and fluency, despite adjustments for age, education, and systolic blood pressure. Lower EF was also associated with global cognition and marginally associated with delayed memory. They also examined the overall cardiac index, which was found to be associated with poorer immediate memory and global cognition. Thus, consistently with Jefferson et al. (2007) this study also indicated the presence of executive dysfunction in a population at particularly high risk for the negative effects of reduced systemic perfusion.

Similarly, lower EF has recently also been shown to be specifically associated with decrements in sustained attention and vigilance in older CVD patients.[29] In particular, performance on tests of continuous vigilance and discriminability were lower for patients with lower EF in this study, supporting the hypothesis that a decrease in cardiac performance leads to decrements in some aspects of attention.

Overall, the handful of studies conducted so far has suggested that the typical profile of attentional and executive dysfunction observed among patients with CVD may be associated, at least in part, with hypoperfusion secondary to inefficiencies in heart performance.

Structural Neuroimaging

Findings of attentional-executive dysfunction in older CVD patients without clinically identified stroke and intact global cognition have led to suggestions of subtle impairment in frontal-subcortical circuitry in these patients. To investigate this further, the potential impact of structural brain abnormalities and its relationship with cardiac pumping efficiency has been examined more closely.[21] Jefferson et al. (2007) used magnetic resonance imaging indices of white matter hyperintensities (WMHs) to more closely examine a common finding on brain magnetic resonance images that becomes increasingly prevalent with age.[30] Results indicated that, independently of age and history of hypertension, WMHs next to subcortical nuclei were inversely related to CO. Thus, as CO decreased, subcortical WMHs increased significantly. This indicated that cerebrovascular degeneration and chronicity of hypoperfusion may exacerbate the susceptibility of white matter integrity to alterations in blood flow in older adults. Given reciprocal white matter pathways connecting frontal and subcortical structures, subcortical white matter damage could in fact be a mediating factor between the hypoperfusion and executive dysfunction associations observed in this population.

Functional Neuroimaging

The presence of associations between subcortical white matter integrity, executive dysfunction, and reduced cardiac performance suggests that inefficiencies in brain function could also be detected in this population. We recently applied functional magnetic resonance imaging (fMRI) methods to further characterize any brain inefficiencies secondary to decreased cardiac performance.[31] We recruited a small cohort of CVD patients from those participating in an ongoing prospective study examining the effects of CVD on brain function in the elderly. We chose a 2-back verbal working-memory task to assess relationships between executive function, and with task-related activation based on *a priori* regions of interest (dorsolateral prefrontal, posterior parietal, supplemental motor area, medial prefrontal gyrus, insula, and posterior cingulated gyrus: see Fig. 13-1). Based on the aforementioned literature, we hypothesized that reduced cardiac performance, as reflected by reductions in CO and EF, would be associated with decreased brain activation in regions of interest previously shown to respond to the verbal working memory challenge.

Our findings supported the previously discussed line of work by demonstrating that in elderly CVD patients with intact global cognition, poorer EF was associated with less brain activity in a task-related region (i.e., insula) and tended to be associated with slower reaction times and poorer verbal working-memory accuracy. We also found that CO was associated with insula activation as well as activation in the supplemental motor area and the dorsolateral prefrontal cortex. These are regions previously shown to be reliably associated with activity on this task,[19, 32, 33] indicating that EF is tightly coupled with performance during cognitive challenges, and CO is related to dysfunction in brain areas responsible for articulatory rehearsal and executive processes crucial for successful verbal working-memory function. In addition, our findings also indicate that some

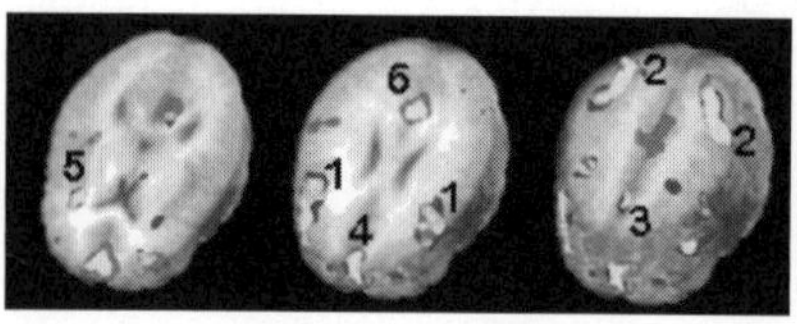

Bilateral ROIs*	Center Coordinates		
	x	y	z
1) Dorsolateral prefrontal	±40	16	31
2) Posterior parietal	±35	–47	44
3) Supplementary motor area	±02	18	47
4) Medial prefrontal gyrus	±04	56	07
5) Insula	±34	0	13
6) Posterior cingulate gyrus	±05	–49	19

z = 10 z = 25

z = 45

*ROIs based on[32]

Figure 13-1 *A priori* regions of interest related to verbal working memory.

brain areas and their functions appear to be differentially affected by intermittent cardiac changes, as reflected by CO, while others might be more affected by chronic changes in cardiac performance, as measured by EF.

Conclusions

The observed associations discussed here lend some support for the value of using neuroimaging and neuropsychological methods to detect perfusion-related changes in brain function early in the disease process and while cognitive functioning is globally intact. The studies reviewed here indicate that cardiac performance indices could be valuable proxy measures for examining mechanisms of cerebrovascular dysfunction in elderly populations at increased risk for hypoperfusion and vascular cognitive degeneration. This line of work supports the hypothesis that low heart performance, as indicated by decreases in CO and/or EF, impacts cerebral perfusion, which is reflected in observable attentional and executive dysfunction and alterations in frontal-subcortical white matter circuitry. This dysfunction is further apparent during cognitive challenges, as detected using functional neuroimaging methods. More studies, however, are required to more directly examine concomitant relationships between cardiac performance and cerebral perfusion using longitudinal designs. This could aid in improving our understanding of the underlying mechanisms of CVD dysfunction in elderly patients particularly vulnerable to the negative effects of chronic or intermittent cerebral hypoperfusion and may aid in prospective efforts geared towards minimizing the effects of these cardiac and systemic abnormalities on vascular degeneration. Longitudinal studies will also clarify whether there is an underlying causal relationship linking systemic hypoperfusion to cerebral hypoperfusion and decreased cognition and neuroimaging abnormalities. More treatment-focused studies that examine any changes in cognitive and functional performance following treatment of CVD risk factors would also be valuable in further clarifying the underlying mechanisms of cognitive decline in patients with cardiovascular disease.

Notes

1. Moser DJ, Cohen RA, Clark MM, et al. Neuropsychological functioning among cardiac rehabilitation patients. *J Cardiopulm Rehabil.* 1999;19(2):91–97.
2. Paul RH, Gunstad J, Poppas A, et al. Neuroimaging and cardiac correlates of cognitive function among patients with cardiac disease. *Cerebrovasc Dis.* 2005;20(2):129–133.
3. Verhaegen P, Borchelt M, Smith J. Relation between cardiovascular and metabolic disease and cognition in very old age: Cross-sectional and longitudinal findings from the Berlin Aging Study. *Health Psychol.* 2003;22(6):559–569.
4. Rastas S, Pirttila T, Viramo P, et al. Association between blood pressure and survival over 9 years in a general population aged 85 and older. *J Am Geriatr Soc.* 2006;54(6):912–918.
5. Bowler JV, Steenhuis R, Hachinski V. Conceptual background to vascular cognitive impairment. *Alzheimer Dis Assoc Disord.* 1999;13(Suppl 3):S30–S37.
6. Rockwood K. Vascular cognitive impairment and vascular dementia. *J Neurol Sci.* 2002; 203–204:23–27.

7. Roman GC, Erkinjuntti T, Wallin A, Pantoni L, Chui HC. Subcortical ischaemic vascular dementia. *Lancet Neurol.* 2002;1(7):426–436.
8. Cohen RA, Poppas A, Forman D, et al. Vascular and cognitive functions associated with cardiovascular disease in the elderly. *J Clin Exp Neuropsychol.* 2009, 31(1) 96–110.
9. de Leeuw FE, Richard F, de Groot JC, et al. Interaction between hypertension, apoE, and cerebral white matter lesions. *Stroke.* 2004;35(5):1057–1060.
10. DeCarli C, Miller BL, Swan GE, et al. Predictors of brain morphology for the men of the NHLBI twin study. *Stroke.* 1999;30(3):529–536.
11. Claus JJ, Breteler MM, Hasan D, et al. Vascular risk factors, atherosclerosis, cerebral white matter lesions and cerebral perfusion in a population-based study. *Eur J Nucl Med.* 1996;23(6):675–682.
12. Vermeer SE, Hollander M, van Dijk EJ, Hofman A, Koudstaal PJ, Breteler MM. Silent brain infarcts and white matter lesions increase stroke risk in the general population: The Rotterdam Scan Study. *Stroke.* 2003;34(5):1126–1129.
13. den Heijer T, Launer LJ, Prins ND, et al. Association between blood pressure, white matter lesions, and atrophy of the medial temporal lobe. *Neurology.* 25 2005;64(2):263–267.
14. Vermeer SE, Koudstaal PJ, Oudkerk M, Hofman A, Breteler MM. Prevalence and risk factors of silent brain infarcts in the population-based Rotterdam Scan Study. *Stroke.* 2002; 33(1):21–25.
15. Birkenhager WH, Forette F, Seux ML, Wang JG, Staessen JA. Blood pressure, cognitive functions, and prevention of dementias in older patients with hypertension. *Arch Intern Med.* 2001;161(2):152–156.
16. Jefferson AL, Poppas A, Paul RH, Cohen RA. Systemic hypoperfusion is associated with executive dysfunction in geriatric cardiac patients. *Neurobiol Aging.* 2007;28(3):477–483.
17. Haley AP, Forman DE, Poppas A, et al. Carotid artery intima-media thickness and cognition in cardiovascular disease. *Int J Cardiol.* 2006; 121(2),148–54.
18. Gunstad J, Cohen RA, Tate DF, et al. Blood pressure variability and white matter hyperintensities in older adults with cardiovascular disease. *Blood Press.* 2005;14(6):353–358.
19. Haley AP, Sweet LH, Gunstad J, et al. Verbal working memory and atherosclerosis in patients with cardiovascular disease: An fMRI study. *J Neuroimaging.* 2007;17(3):227–233.
20. Hoth KF, Tate DF, Poppas A, et al. Endothelial function and white matter hyperintensities in older adults with cardiovascular disease. *Stroke.* 2007;38(2):308–312.
21. Jefferson AL, Tate DF, Poppas A, et al. Lower cardiac output is associated with greater white matter hyperintensities in older adults with cardiovascular disease. *J Am Geriatr Soc.* 2007;55(7):1044–1048.
22. Mulligan RC, Haley AP, Jerskey BA, et al. Endothelial function predicts fMRI activity in the medial prefrontal cortex [poster]. *J Int Neuropsychol Soc.* 2008;15(51):48.
23. Moody DM, Bell MA, Challa VR. Features of the cerebral vascular pattern that predict vulnerability to perfusion or oxygenation deficiency: An anatomic study. *AJNR Am J Neuroradiol.* 1990;11(3):431–439.
24. Saxena PR, Schoemaker RG. Organ blood flow protection in hypertension and congestive heart failure. *Am J Med.* 1993;94(4A):4S-12S.
25. Moorhouse P, Rockwood K. Vascular cognitive impairment: Current concepts and clinical developments. *Lancet Neurol.* 2008;7(3):246–255.
26. Moulinier L, Venet T, Schiller NB, Kurtz TW, Morris RC, Jr., Sebastian A. Measurement of aortic blood flow by Doppler echocardiography: Day to day variability in normal subjects and applicability in clinical research. *J Am Coll Cardiol.* 1991;17(6):1326–1333.

27. Mahadevan G, Davis RC, Frenneaux MP, et al. Left ventricular ejection fraction: Are the revised cut-off points for defining systolic dysfunction sufficiently evidence based? 2008; 94:426–428.
28. Hoth KF, Poppas A, Moser DJ, Paul RH, Cohen RA. Cardiac dysfunction and cognition in older adults with heart failure. *Cogn Behav Neurol*. 2008;21(2):65–72.
29. Jerskey BA, Cohen RA, Jefferson AL, et al. Sustained attention is associated with left ventricular ejection fraction in older adults with heart disease. *J Int Neuropsychol Soc*. 2009; 15(1):137–141.
30. Gunning-Dixon FM, Raz N. The cognitive correlates of white matter abnormalities in normal aging: A quantitative review. *Neuropsychology*. 2000;14(2):224–232.
31. Irani F, Sweet LH, Haley AP, et al. A fMRI study of verbal working memory, cardiac output, and ejection fraction in elderly patients with cardiovascular disease. *Brain Imaging and Behavior*, in press.
32. Sweet LH, Paskavitz JF, Haley AP, et al. Imaging phonological similarity effects on verbal working memory. *Neuropsychologia*. 2008;46(4):1114–1123.
33. Braver TS, Cohen JD, Nystrom LE, Jonides J, Smith EE, Noll DC. A parametric study of prefrontal cortex involvement in human working memory. *Neuroimage*. 1997;5(1):49–62.

14

SYSTEMIC VASCULAR FUNCTION AND COGNITIVE FUNCTION

Ivy N. Miller, William G. Haynes, and David J. Moser

It is known that vascular disease is a significant contributor to more than 50% of cases of dementia, regardless of specific dementia subtype.[1] Given that vascular disease is prevalent around the world, and is potentially modifiable,[2] developing a better understanding of the pathophysiological mechanisms of this association is important for both research and clinical purposes. For the purposes of this chapter, *vascular disease* will be defined as changes in blood vessel structure and function that range from modest impairment of blood flow regulation to atherosclerotic occlusion of a blood vessel. Thus, vascular disease represents the blood vessel effects of single or multiple cardiovascular risk factors, such as hypertension, diabetes, smoking, aging, and hyperlipidemia, as well as atherosclerosis itself.

A necessary prerequisite of this type of research is the accurate assessment of vascular disease severity, a process that can be quite challenging, given that vascular disease patients typically represent a very heterogeneous group with regard to the presence and severity of myriad vascular risk factors. Further study is needed to elucidate the mechanism by which vascular disease affects cognition. There is not yet a safe and practical way to directly study the early pathology of vascular cognitive impairment in the brain in the same way it can be studied in the peripheral vasculature. Because vascular disease is known to be a generalized condition, it is plausible that the relationship between systemic vascular function and cognition reflects compromised cerebrovascular function. Therefore, the study of systemic vascular function has been a growing area of research. This chapter attempts to outline the current research in this field as well as implications for future study of vascular disease.

Why Study Systemic Vascular Function?

For the purposes of this chapter, *vascular function* will be defined as the ability of blood vessels to dilate, which can provide a valid and reliable index of overall vascular health. A 2000 study by Suwaidi et al. showed that coronary vascular-flow dysfunction was strongly predictive of the occurrence of cardiac events during a 28-month follow-up.[3]

It is important to note that vascular dysfunction was predictive of cardiac events independently of conventional risk factors and baseline degree of atherosclerosis, suggesting that it provides unique and additional information to that provided by conventional cardiovascular risk factor assessment. This relationship has been well supported in the literature.[4–6]

Vascular function declines very early in the development of atherosclerotic vascular disease (AVD), prior to the appearance of atherosclerotic plaques.[7] This chapter focuses on the effects of AVD, as atherosclerosis is the underlying cause of many cardiovascular events and complications. All known risk-factors for AVD (hypertension, hyperlipidemia, obesity, etc.) are also associated with impaired vascular function.[8] Additionally, assessment of vascular function takes account of emerging and unknown risk factors (i.e., visceral obesity, inflammation, renal disease, genetic predisposition) that are not included in standard algorithms (such as the Framingham equation). Therefore, assessment of vascular function may serve as an integrated measure of total atherosclerotic risk factor burden, or a physiological proxy measure for overall vascular health.

Much of the research on vascular disease and cognition has focused on individuals who have already developed severe cognitive impairment and vascular dementia, for which there is now no effective treatment. Therefore, the current challenge is to identify specific patterns of vascular risk factors and/or mechanisms that will allow for the earlier identification of individuals at high risk for future cognitive decline.

Endothelium and Vascular Smooth Muscle

The study of systemic vascular flow function is largely focused on the endothelium and vascular smooth muscle layers of blood vessels. The endothelium is the single layer of cells that makes up the innermost lining of all the body's blood vessels. It is the body's largest endocrine organ, with an approximate total weight of 1.5 kg and a surface area that is equivalent to that of two tennis courts.[8] Although initially thought to be a simple semipermeable membrane, the endothelium is now known to be a physiologically active organ that carries out a number of vital functions. These functions include regulation of vascular tone, platelet adhesion and aggregation, lipid transport, macrophage migration, vascular smooth-muscle proliferation, thrombosis, and fibrinolysis.[8] Most *in vivo* assessments of endothelial function focus on the degree to which an individual's blood vessels can dilate or constrict when necessary to deliver blood in appropriate proportions to various parts of the body, including the brain. Changes in endothelial regulation of blood flow correlate with changes in endothelial regulation of other functions, such as fibrinolysis. Recent studies have shown that endothelial dysfunction contributes both to the pathogenesis and to the subsequent complications of atherosclerosis.[9] It has been shown to be strongly associated with atherosclerosis in both human[10, 11] and animal[12, 13] studies, and there is clear evidence that changes in endothelial function *precede* development of atherosclerotic lesions in non-human primates.[7] Additional evidence that endothelial function is an early and central process in the development of atherosclerotic vascular disease is provided by the fact that every known risk factor for atherosclerosis impairs endothelial function. These risk factors include advancing age, male sex, family history of coronary artery disease, smoking, increased cholesterol, low HDL cholesterol, hypertension, diabetes, obesity, high fat diet, and increased homocysteine.[14] Aging is particularly strongly associated with both endothelial dysfunction and atherosclerosis,[15, 16] because endothelial cells typically die after approximately 30 years and the new endothelial cells that replace them do not function as effectively as their precursors. Therefore, as men and women approach the age of 40 or 50, endothelial function begins to decline progressively,[17] placing them at increasing risk for atherosclerotic vascular disease.

Immediately outside the layer of endothelial cells lies a layer of vascular smooth muscle, which is responsible for controlling peripheral resistance, arterial and venous tone, and the distribution of blood throughout the body. Contraction of vascular smooth muscle narrows the vessel lumen, while relaxation dilates the vessel.[18] Endothelial cells interact with vascular smooth muscle by, among other means, releasing nitric oxide, which causes smooth muscle relaxation and, subsequently, vasodilation. Therefore, any impairment of vascular smooth muscle and/or endothelial cell function will impair vascular dilator function.

Often discussed in the study of vascular function are the roles of endothelium-dependent and -independent vascular function. Vasodilation that occurs due to direct involvement of the endothelial cells or due to nitric oxide release is classified as endothelium-dependent vascular function. Vasodilation mediated only by actions within vascular smooth muscle cells is classified as endothelium-independent vascular function. A better understanding of the mechanisms involved in both types of vasodilation is discussed later in the chapter and provides another necessary component in the study of the effects of vascular function on cognition.

How Is Systemic Vascular Function Assessed?

There are several methodologies now used to study vascular function both centrally and in the periphery. In this chapter, the peripheral methods of venous occlusion plethysmography (VOP), flow-mediated dilatation (FMD), and pulse wave velocity (PWV) are discussed, and PET and MRI methodology are briefly reviewed. While this is not a comprehensive list, these represent a variety of ways to study vascular disease systemically.

VOP assesses vascular function in resistance (small) vessels using a plethysmograph, a device that is used to measure volume in a variety of organs, while FMD is conducted using Doppler techniques to assess conduit (large) vessels through ultrasound. Results from each method are correlated with risk for cardiovascular disease.[19] Pulse wave analysis and pulse wave velocity provide measurements of arterial stiffness. While this chapter focuses mainly on assessments conducted in the forearms, the study of systemic vascular disease also includes the lower limbs[20–22] and the abdomen and gluteal areas.[23–26]

Venous Occlusion Plethysmography to Assess Resistance Vessel Function

The study of forearm vascular function has been accomplished using venous occlusion plethysmography for almost 100 years. This method of studying human vascular physiology *in vivo* measures forearm blood flow, which is regulated by small (10 μm –100 μm) resistance vessels. When conducted alone, VOP can be used to crudely assess endothelial function of the resistance arteries through the measurement of reactive hyperemia, the increase in blood flow that occurs in response to ischemia and reperfusion of the forearm.[27] For more accurate assessment, VOP is combined with brachial artery infusion of vasoactive drugs to assess vascular health.[28–31] This combination of techniques permits multiple measures of forearm resistance vessel function to be obtained.[29, 30] The ability of the blood vessels to respond (dilate) in response to vasoactive agents provides a valuable physiological marker of vascular disease severity.

During venous occlusion plethysmography of the forearm, the patient lies with both arms supported above the normal level of the central venous pressure and with venous emptying unimpeded. VOP combined with intra-arterial infusions is usually conducted bilaterally, as the non-infused arm is often used as a control for the infused arm,[32] which provides more reproducible results than assessing just the manipulated arm alone.[33] A ratio of flows in the two arms at each time-point is calculated using this control. The primary measure in this procedure is the percentage of change from baseline in the ratio of blood flow between the infused and non-infused arms.

Forearm blood flow is then measured using strain gauges applied to the widest part of each forearm and attached to a plethysmography unit. Upper-arm cuffs are intermittently inflated to temporarily prevent venous outflow from the forearm and thus obtain plethysmographic recordings. It is important to make sure that hand circulation is occluded by inflation of a wrist cuff during VOP measurements[29] because, unlike forearm blood flow, which comes mostly from skeletal muscle, most of the blood flow to the hands comes from the skin and can be affected by cutaneous variables unrelated to VOP methods. The addition of the wrist cuff can also reduce intraindividual variability, allowing for more reproducible results.[34] However, some authors have found that the use of a cuff does not significantly alter the VOP results.[35]

Vasoactive Agents

In brachial artery drug infusion, the patient's forearm length is measured and the non-dominant forearm is cannulated under local anesthesia. Drugs administered are chosen for their actions on the endothelium and vascular smooth muscle, as described in the previous section. In this case, drugs are given in doses that act locally only. Because the reaction to some drugs (e.g., acetylcholine) depends on circulation time it is necessary to measure forearm length prior to drug infusion.[36] The total rate of intra-arterial infusion is maintained at a constant level throughout the VOP procedure to prevent confounded interpretation of the results by alterations in the flow rate, causing changes in blood flow.

Previous studies have introduced a variety of vasoactive drugs to the brachial artery. Acetylcholine[16, 19, 20, 37–42] and methacholine[43–47] are often used, both of which cause vasodilation through the endothelial-cell muscarinic receptors, thereby activating endothelial nitric oxide synthase and increasing nitric oxide production, which then relaxes underlying vascular smooth muscle, resulting in resistance vessel dilatation. Sodium nitroprusside[16, 19, 20, 39, 40, 42–47] is a direct nitric oxide donor, causing vascular smooth-muscle relaxation without involvement of endothelial cells. Verapamil[39, 40, 44, 47] acts directly on vascular smooth muscle cells, causing relaxation without altering endothelial cell function or generation of nitric oxide. For these reasons, vasodilation that occurs as the result of acetylcholine administration is often referred to as "endothelium-dependent," and that which occurs in response to nitroprusside and verapamil is described as "endothelium-independent." The effects of a number of other vasoactive medications have also been examined (bradykinin,[20] phenylephrine,[43] L-NMMA, glibenclamide, indomethacin, and miconazol[37]).

It should be noted, however, that examining the response to a vasoactive drug that acts directly on the endothelial cells such as acetylcholine alone does not yield a truly specific index of endothelium-dependent vasodilation. For example, if a disease caused only vascular smooth-muscle dysfunction, vasodilation in response to acetylcholine would still be impaired, although endothelial function would be normal. Therefore, the most robust parameter for endothelium-dependent vasodilation is obtained by assessing vascular response to an endothelium-dependent vasodilator and correcting that for dilatation that occurs in response to a vascular smooth-muscle-specific dilator. In the example of acetylcholine, this can be accomplished by using simple ratios between acetylcholine response/nitroprusside response and acetylcholine response/verapamil response.

Strengths and Weaknesses of VOP Measurement

The combination of venous occlusion plethysmography and brachial-artery drug infusion is strong in many respects. There is debate in the literature over labeling this technique a "gold standard" in the study of endothelial function.[28, 37, 41, 48] This method is generally considered safe in that the drug infusion acts locally and does not carry the risk factors of a systemic administration.[29] Another benefit is that computerization of the procedure allows for immediate and detailed data collection without operator subjectivity. However, VOP is not without limitations. One study suggests that venous occlusion plethysmography underestimates blood flow.[49] Motion artifact during VOP is also a common methodological problem.[50] Also, due to the potential discomfort to the patient during the process of cannulation and the time commitment required, repeated studies of venous occlusion plethysmography are not often practical.[29, 30, 41] In our experience, discomfort can be mitigated by use of a very-fine-gauge catheter (27 SWG).[39, 40, 51] These fine-bore catheters cause less discomfort than standard venepuncture, but have a diameter sufficient for drug infusion, though not arterial pressure measurement or blood sampling.

Flow-Mediated Dilation to Assess Conduit Vessel Function

Vascular ultrasound can be used to assess conduit endothelial function by measuring flow-mediated dilatation, thereby studying endothelial function in a different blood vessel type than venous occlusion plethysmography.[52] Conduit vessels are the larger arteries typically affected by occlusive atherosclerosis, such as occurs in the carotid or coronary circulations. Dilatation of vessels in response to an increase in blood flow is a fundamental physiological response that is mediated by endothelial cell mechanosensors. While FMD can be studied in the axillary, radial, and superficial femoral arteries,[53] the brachial artery is the most practical location, and has been widely used.[52] The primary measure of endothelial function in this procedure is the total change in vessel diameter from resting to one minute after onset of a hyperemic response to distal forearm ischemia and, as such, is an accurate index of conduit (large) vessel endothelial function.

During FMD measurement of the brachial artery, the patient lies supine, and a length of the brachial artery is imaged while the image depth and gain settings are adjusted to optimally define the vessel wall–lumen interface. Since FMD is sensitive to a number of stimuli, including temperature and sympathetic stimuli, these parameters and other environmental stimuli are kept constant during the procedure.[53] Baseline images of brachial artery diameter and Doppler velocities from the center of the vessel are recorded. An occluding forearm cuff is then placed just below the elbow and is inflated to above systolic pressure and then deflated to induce reactive hyperemia. Some groups have used an upper-arm cuff to induce a more robust hyperemic response; this approach has the disadvantage that the brachial artery itself is rendered ischemic, sometimes leading to poorly reproducible responses. Brachial artery diameter and velocity are then continuously measured during cuff inflation and after deflation. The forearm cuff causes vasodilation through the release of nitric oxide,[54] providing a measure of endothelium-dependent function.[6, 52] This relies upon the fact that increases in flow through a vessel stimulate shear–stress-sensitive endothelial mechanosensors that then stimulate release of nitric oxide and cause endothelial-dependent dilatation.

Just as with forearm resistance-vessel testing with VOP, it is necessary to record endothelium-independent responses to ascertain whether dysfunction occurs at endothelial or vascular smooth-muscle cell layers. Administration of vascular smooth muscle dilators during Doppler ultrasound provides a measurement of endothelium-*independent* vasodilation: the percentage of change between the diameter of the vessel after drug administration as compared to the baseline diameter.[6, 52] A dilator that has an endothelium-independent effect, usually nitroglycerin,[20, 25, 26, 46, 50, 55, 56] is administered sublingually after basal diameter and flow have been fully restored to baseline after the initial FMD procedure. Brachial artery diameter and Doppler velocity are then recorded after the drug administration. Arterial pressure is measured throughout the study: at baseline, at the end of ischemia, after cuff release, and after nitroglycerine administration. Nitroglycerin is used because changes in responses to increased flow can also be due to vascular smooth-muscle-cell insensitivity to dilators (e.g., nitric oxide) released by the endothelium. Thus, if flow-dependent vasodilatation without nitroglycerin and nitroglycerin-induced dilatation are both abnormal, this suggests smooth muscle dysfunction rather than endothelial dysfunction.

To analyze FMD data, videotapes of brachial artery images are transferred to computer. Brachial artery diameter measurements are made manually, and mean Doppler flow velocity is calculated and averaged over consecutive cardiac cycles. Percentage change in diameter and velocity is calculated for the interventions of distal ischemia, reactive hyperemia, and sublingual nitroglycerine. Velocity measures are used to check that the intensity of the stimulus (increase in velocity elicited by ischemia-reperfusion) is similar between subjects/groups.

Strengths and Weaknesses of Doppler Ultrasound Techniques

The Doppler ultrasound method of evaluating endothelial function is popular because of its brevity and noninvasive nature. For these reasons, studies can be repeated without undue stress on the patient. A potential disadvantage is the fact that the stimulus (hyperemia following ischemia) cannot be standardized in the same way that a dose of a drug can, and the standard approach to FMD does not permit assessment of a stimulus-response association. In addition, flow-mediated dilatation is sensitive to a variety of stimuli such as diet, temperature, and sympathetic stimuli,[53] and keeping all these conditions constant is difficult. Perhaps more important, obtaining and measuring a consistent image is heavily observer-dependent, and small movements of the ultrasound probe can invalidate an assessment where the typical difference between groups is on the order of 5% of brachial artery diameter. The rather lengthy post-procedure analysis required for Doppler ultrasound is also a limitation of the technique. Brachial artery diameter and blood velocity measurements must be formally analyzed by a blinded observer who does not know the identity of the subject and who has demonstrated the ability to reproducibly analyze records. Training and the processing are heavily time-intensive and require frequent analyses to maintain technique.

Pulse Wave Analysis and Velocity

Pulse wave analysis and pulse wave velocity are measures of arterial stiffness. Arterial stiffness is difficult to study because of the complex structure of the vasculature and the dynamic nature of the circulation.[57] Arterial stiffness has been associated with cardiovascular risk factors,[58] and PWV in particular has been associated with cardiovascular events[58–60] and death.[61] PWA is a measure of the form of the pulse wave, while PWV is a measure of the speed of the pressure pulse as it travels through the vasculature.

For PWA, a peripheral artery (commonly the radial artery) waveform is imaged, often either by ultrasound or with an applanation tonometer.[62] Combined with noninvasive limb blood pressure, measures of central blood pressure can be derived from the radial pulse wave form. The radial pulse waveform is a complex pressure variation that includes pressure changes due to systolic ejection of blood from the left ventricle, as well as waves reflected back from resistance vessels. From this radial waveform, various validated equations are used to derive a corresponding central aortic pressure waveform.

The importance of this measure is that it directly links peripheral vascular structure and function to adverse cardiac hemodynamics. As atherosclerosis develops and the arteries stiffen, blood velocity increases and reflected waves return to the heart more quickly than in healthy vessels, creating an altered central-aortic-pressure waveform. This waveform tends to have elevated systolic pressure and reduced diastolic pressure, as a result of the reflected wave's arriving earlier in the cardiac cycle.[63] These changes will lead to increased left-ventricular afterload (wall stress), predisposing to left-ventricular hypertrophy, and reduced diastolic coronary perfusion, predisposing to myocardial ischemia. Increased arterial stiffness will also cause higher systolic pressure in large arteries near to the heart, including the carotid vessels, which may accentuate atherosclerosis in those arteries. PWA has been found to be correlated with endothelial function as measured by FMD, suggesting that endothelial function and arterial stiffness are related in the development of atherosclerosis.[64]

PWV is an alternative and more direct method of gauging arterial stiffness. It is calculated by first measuring the external distance between the skin sites of two arteries, most commonly the carotid and femoral arteries. These vessels are readily available for imaging because of their proximity to the surface of the skin.[58] PWV has also been measured between the brachial artery and the ankle.[65] A pressure-sensitive transducer is used in conjunction with an electrocardiogram to calculate the time necessary for the cardiac systolic impulse to reach each vessel. When combined with the distance from the heart to the respective vessels, the speed that the arterial systolic wave travels in large arteries can be calculated. Higher PWV is associated with increased age as well as high blood pressure.[57]

Several different devices have been developed for PWA and PWV measurements, including Sphygmocor, Complior, Doppler ultrasound systems, and WallTrack.[58, 59, 62] Because these measurements can be affected by a number of environmental stimuli, it is important that the patient lie supine in a temperature-controlled room, as in VOP and FMD measurement procedures.

Strengths and Weaknesses of PWA and PWV Measurement

PWA and PWV measurements are useful in that they are noninvasive, brief, and therefore well tolerated by patients.[45] Information such as blood pressure, wave form, and pressure speed can be gathered in a short time, and the expense of conducting these measurements is low. Criticisms of these methods include questions of validity, particularly for PWA, as each method relies on theoretical calculations.[59] Just as in FMD measurement, PWA and PWV can be greatly influenced by a number of confounds, such as room temperature, caffeine, alcohol and food intake, vasoactive medications, and time of day,[59, 62] perhaps to a greater extent than in other methods of vascular function assessment. PWA and PWV can be very difficult to assess in obese patients as excess adipose tissue can make it difficult to make accurate external measurements.[66, 67] Finally, unlike stimulated measures of resistance (dilatation to drug infusion) and conduit vessel function (dilatation to shear stress), PWV and PWA are usually performed as resting measures, and so do not indicate vascular "reserve" in the systemic circulation.

Positron Emission Tomography

Studies using positron emission tomography (PET), which allows for imaging of brain activity through the use of nuclear medicine, have been conducted to assess vascular flow function[68] and have been used in studies of vascular disease as well as cognitive impairment for a number of years. When combined with structural imaging techniques in a process known as *co-registration*, PET imaging provides a wealth of information on brain structure and function not previously available.

PET studies typically use radioactive tracers such as [^{18}F]-fluorodeoxyglucose (FDG) or^{15}O-water to trace metabolism and blood flow, respectively. PET studies using FDG have been the more popular type of PET studies conducted and provide clearer lesion images,[69] while^{15}O-water studies better measure the distribution of tumor volume and require less time to trace.[70, 71] However, these two tracers show similar distributions, as cerebral blood flow and metabolism are closely related in the brain,[72] especially in relation to vascular dementia and Alzheimer's disease.

One aspect of brain physiology that PET examines is the level of cerebral blood flow (CBF), both globally and region-specific. Global CBF is known as a strong predictor of cognitive and synaptic function.[73] In an elderly sample, it has been shown to be reduced when difficult cognitive tasks are performed[71] and in brains with vascular lesions. PET can also be used to measure the degree of cerebrovascular reserve (CVR), a measure of the ability of the vasculature in the brain to respond (dilate) to the need for oxygen and nutrients.[74] Levels of CBF and CVR can vary based on the patient's physiological and cognitive status at a particular time.[71] Low levels of CBF can be compensated by better CVR, so it is important to examine the relationship between the two entities as well as the basic levels of CBF and CVR.[74]

PET imaging studies of CVR in vascular disease often use acetazolamide, a carbonic anhydrase inhibitor, allowing for assessment of the brain's CVR by causing a maximal vasodilatory state.[75–78] In a healthy brain, the introduction of acetazolamide causes an increase in global CBF.[79] Because people with vascular lesions in the brain often have low CBF, the amount of increase in CBF after acetazolamide administration provides a measurement of CVR. Patients with high CVR show enhanced cognitive performance, while impaired CVR is associated with poorer cognitive performance.[74] Indeed, CVR is compromised in patients with vascular dementia.[80]

Strengths and Weaknesses of PET

PET studies provide detailed information on both cerebral blood flow and cerebrovascular reserve in regions of interest as well as for the whole brain. When co-registered with structural magnetic resonance imaging scans, a much clearer picture of the brain is possible than with either technique alone. However, PET scans are expensive, as the radioactive tracers need to be created at the scan location immediately before the study begins, and PET scanners are not as widely available as MRI scanners. PET scanning is also more invasive than some of the other imaging techniques.

Arterial Spin Labeling

In recent years, a new MRI technique that directly measures cerebral blood flow similarly to PET imaging has been developed. Arterial spin labeling (ASL) uses an inversion pulse to tag arterial water before it flows into a region of interest in the brain. After a time delay to allow the labeled water to enter the specified region, images are obtained and then compared to a control image. The control image is taken of the same region, but without the tagged blood. The image with labeled water is then subtracted from the control image and a measure of cerebral blood flow (CBF) is obtained. Generally, ASL images of CBF are consistent with PET CBF images.[81–83]

There are two types of ASL typically conducted: continuous ASL (CASL), imaged over several seconds, and pulsed ASL (PASL), in which the image is obtained with a single pulse. CASL has a higher signal-to-noise ratio than PASL,[84] but the technique is more challenging than PASL.[82] Though PET imaging is still more widely used in clinical populations than ASL, recent studies have shown that ASL is a valuable tool in distinguishing CBF in various types of dementia,[85, 86] and in the future, ASL MRI techniques are likely to become more widespread in clinical application as further validation studies are conducted.

Strengths and Weaknesses of ASL

ASL has several advantages over PET studies. Where PET uses radioactive tracers, ASL uses magnets, which do not require injections. The absence of radioactivity allows for repeated studies as there is no concern about subject radiation-dose levels. A type of MRI, the scanners used in ASL are more widely available than PET scanners. The resolution of ASL images is also much better than that of PET scans.[81, 87] However, ASL cannot directly assess cerebral blood volume[88] and has a relatively low signal-to-noise ratio.[81] ASL imaging sessions also tend to be longer than PET's, and PET images also provide more sensitive information regarding specifics of the labeled blood movement.[81]

How Is Vascular Function Related to Cognition?

Many large epidemiological studies of vascular disease and cognition have been conducted in the central and peripheral vascular systems. Much research has also been conducted with atherosclerotic vascular-disease patients who have already developed severe cognitive impairments. Studies of this nature have often focused on the cognitive effects of open-heart surgeries,[89] stroke,[90] and the placement of cardiac stents.[91] Another theme in the research on cerebrovascular disease and cognition is that of distinguishing

Alzheimer's disease from vascular dementia. This distinction is quite often muddled, as it is known that patients with AD often show vascular pathology, and patients diagnosed with vascular disease are at risk for developing AD.[92]

Several studies have focused on the conventional risk factors of vascular disease and often include brief neurocognitive assessments.[93–101] Data from the Kuopio Heart Disease Risk Factor Study, a cross-sectional epidemiological study of more than 500 men, clearly indicated an association between atherosclerosis and cognitive dysfunction. Specifically, the degree of atherosclerotic disease in the internal carotid arteries was found to be significantly associated with performance on tests of global mental status, nonverbal memory, verbal memory, verbal fluency, and cognitive speed and flexibility.[102] Another report from a large investigation, the Atherosclerosis Risk in Communities (ARIC) study, revealed significant associations between the degree of carotid artery atherosclerosis and performance on tests of psychomotor processing speed and memory.[103] A study conducted in France by Auperin and co-investigators yielded very similar findings, showing impaired performance on a test of global cognition and psychomotor processing speed in subjects with carotid atherosclerosis.[104]

Peripheral Vascular Disease and Cognition

In addition to studies that have focused primarily on carotid atherosclerotic disease, several studies have also demonstrated cognitive dysfunction in peripheral vascular disease (PVD), which involves atherosclerotic claudication of the peripheral arteries.[105] Though atherosclerosis is known to be a generalized process, it had previously been thought that patients with PVD were cognitively intact.[106]

In the first of three studies by Phillips et al., neuropsychological performance of patients who had undergone extremity amputations due to PVD, but had no history of stroke, was compared to that of age- and education-matched controls. The patient group performed significantly more poorly on a test of psychomotor processing speed and also on a measure of higher-level executive functioning.[107] Deficits attributed to executive dysfunction are widely described in patients with vascular cognitive decline. Executive function, though not singularly defined, is the set of abilities that allows for complex, higher-order functioning: planning, organizing, and managing finances are examples. Some have suggested that executive deficits are the primary characteristic of patients with vascular cognitive decline[108] and vascular dementia.[109–113] Executive abilities tend to decline before memory loss and other cognitive changes associated with dementia,[108, 114] and patients with executive deficits often perform poorly on tests of processing speed, initiation, and psychomotor speed, all of which are necessary for the completion of daily life tasks.[111]

In a subsequent study, Phillips and co-investigators compared subjects who had PVD with subjects who had suffered strokes and with healthy controls. Results showed that the PVD group performed significantly worse than controls on a range of commonly used tests that assess attention, psychomotor processing speed, higher-level executive function, visuospatial/constructional skills, and nonverbal memory. Furthermore, on the vast majority of these tests, the PVD group did not perform significantly better than the stroke group.[115] A small one-year follow-up study that included some of the PVD subjects from this study revealed that baseline performance on tests of attention, memory, and visuospatial functioning significantly predicted level of daily functioning as measured by the Functional Activities Questionnaire.[116, 117] This means that even the initial stages of vascular cognitive decline can greatly affect an individual's ability to carry out daily activities, which has serious implications for the prevention and treatment of vascular disease.

Pulse Wave Velocity and Cognition

Studies of arterial stiffness and cognition have focused on pulse wave velocity measurement. There is debate over whether PWV should be labeled an independent marker for cognitive decline, as studies on this theme have shown conflicting results.[118–120] Some authors have used a global measure of cognition such as the MMSE,[119, 121] while others have examined more specific aspects of cognition in relation to PWV such as verbal and nonverbal learning and memory[118, 122] and the Cognitive Efficiency Profile.[118] For example, Hanon et al. in 2005 found a significant relationship between measures of PWV and tests of global cognition (MMSE and the Cognitive Efficiency Profile, or CEP), independent of traditional risk factors for cardiovascular disease such as age, gender, systolic blood pressure, and cardiovascular disease status.[118] This study, as well as similar findings in others listed above (see Scuteria et al., 2007,[121] for another example), supports the idea of an independent association between PWV and cognition after controlling for well-known cardiovascular risk factors. In other studies of pulse wave velocity, the strength of the association between PWV and cognition was greatly attenuated after controlling for cardiovascular risk factors. For example, a study conducted by Poels et al. in 2007 showed that decreased scores on an abbreviated version of the Stroop Test, a test of executive abilities, were associated with higher PWV, though this relationship did not exist with other tests of executive skills and global cognition.[120] Though the Poels group initially found associations between PWV and all cognitive tests administered (MMSE, Letter-Digit Substitution Task, Word Fluency Test, and an abbreviated Stroop Test), after controlling for cardiovascular risk factors the Stroop Test was the only cognitive measure that remained statistically significant.

More specifically, pulse wave velocity has also been associated, though somewhat weakly, with decreased executive function and processing capacity in recent years, outside of the Poels study previously discussed. Muller et al. (2007) studied middle-aged and elderly men and found that those with higher PWV (i.e., more arterial stiffness) were more likely to have deficits in these areas of cognitive function, though not at a significant level.[123] A pilot study by Scuteri et al. (2005) found an association between increased PWV and scales of activities of daily living (ADLs),[124] examples of a person's functional skills that are considered indicative of executive abilities. While more attention has been drawn to studies of this nature in recent years, much remains to be explored.

Resistance Vessel Function and Cognition

In the resistance-vessel function literature, a small 2004 study by our group (Moser et al.) produced the first published evidence of a significant association between forearm resistance-vessel function (using VOP with brachial artery drug infusion) and neuropsychological performance.[39] Indeed, the association between vascular function and cognition in that study was stronger than the relationship between cognition and individual conventional vascular-related variables such as blood pressure, glucose level, lipid levels, etc. These findings supported the concept that forearm resistance-vessel function might be used as an integrated measure of total atherosclerotic risk-factor burden—in effect, an index of a given patient's general vascular health—regardless of that particular patient's pattern of risk factors, and that this measure could then be examined in relation to cognition. A follow-up study, on a much larger non-overlapping sample, confirmed a significant cross-sectional relation between forearm vascular function and cognition in a larger sample.[40] Intriguingly, vascular smooth muscle (endothelium-independent) function appeared to be more strongly associated with cognition than did endothelium-dependent function.

A subsequent 2008 study from our group suggested that vascular smooth-muscle function of forearm resistance vessels, defined once again by VOP, is significantly associated with performance on tests of initiation and processing speed, whereas endothelium-dependent vascular function was not associated with these measures.[125]

Flow-Mediated Dilatation and Cognition

In some contrast to the Moser et al. resistance-vessel findings, in an FMD study of the brachial conduit vessel, Hoth et al. (2007) found an inverse association between endothelial-*dependent* forearm vasodilation and white matter hyperintensity volume in patients with cardiovascular disease,[56] suggesting that the poor vascular health is reflected in the brain with a greater degree of white matter lesions. These divergent findings on the role of the endothelium raise the possibility that resistance and conduit vessels have different roles in the cerebrovascular contribution to cognitive decline.

Several other recent studies have examined conduit vessel function (by FMD) in relation to cognition. One study, by Dede et al., in examining the possibility of vascular etiology for Alzheimer's disease (AD), measured FMD in patients with Alzheimer's disease and in healthy elderly controls. The authors found, after adjusting for age, that a significant association exists between endothelial function as measured by FMD and the stage of (severity of) AD. That is, subjects in the more advanced stages of AD showed poorer endothelial function (FMD).[126] Smith et al. looked at cerebrovascular risk factors, FMD, and neuropsychological functioning in adults with major depressive disorder (MDD). Results from this study indicated an association between poor FMD and neuropsychological factors such as executive function and working memory. These results were significant even after the authors controlled for cerebrovascular risk factors.[127] Another study, in a healthy elderly population, found that high levels of trait anxiety were accompanied by greater sympathetic activation and were also associated with decreased FMD.[128] In a study of elderly participants with cardiovascular disease diagnoses, Cohen et al. measured brachial artery FMD along with other measures of vascular function and neuropsychological function and found that FMD was significantly related to results on tests of attention, executive function, and psychomotor speed. The FMD data in this study were also strongly associated with total WMH volume.[129]

Positron Emission Tomography and Cognition

In the PET literature, the concept of cognitive reserve has recently become a focus in the interests of accounting for the difference between poor anatomical brain health and intact cognitive function. A review by Stern (2002) proposed that cognitive reserve either signifies that such a patient has a greater number of neurons, leaving enough intact even after disease for greater-than-expected cognitive function, or that the patient's neurons are simply more efficient than someone without this level of cognitive reserve.[73] Cognitive reserve has often been studied in the aging population. In this population, *cognitive reserve* is defined as the brain's reorganization as a coping mechanism for changes associated with aging.[130] Similar to the risk factors for vascular disease, it has been suggested that a person's cognitive reserve is a modifiable entity. Higher levels of leisure activity and intellectual stimulation are associated with greater cognitive reserve and less risk of developing dementia.[131–133]

In patients with cerebrovascular disease, PET scans have been used to describe functional versus structural changes in the brain. In a study of the effects of both Alzheimer's disease and subcortical ischemic vascular disease (SIVD), Tullberg et al. (2004) found that frontal regional PET glucose metabolism (rCMRglc) was related to executive function in all patients, including control subjects: increases in glucose metabolism were associated with higher scores of executive function as described by executive neuropsychological tests such as the Dementia Rating Scale Initiation-Perseveration subscale, Wechsler Memory Scale—Revised backwards visual and digit spans, and a controlled oral word-fluency test. These authors also examined status of memory function in the same group and found that while rCMRglc was not significantly associated with memory function, frontal cortical gray matter voxel levels were positively associated with scores of memory on neuropsychological tests in all subjects.[134]

Also in 2004, Sturm et al. found that an alertness training program increased PET activation and neuropsychological function in three out of four patients who showed deficits in alertness in the post-acute phase of right-hemisphere stroke. Of the patients who showed improvement, PET scans revealed reactivation in the superior, middle, and/or inferior right frontal lobe, with some variation. Patients who improved also showed improvement in an alertness task as well as a visual vigilance task after training. These effects were not seen in a control group who completed a general memory training program. The authors posited that reactivation as revealed by PET is necessary for behavioral changes to be seen.[135]

In another study of neuropsychological function as compared to PET imaging, Jacobs et al. studied cerebrovascular patients who had undergone coronary artery bypass grafting (CABG), after which many patients suffer from some level of neuropsychological decline. Results from this study suggest that the degree of functional decline does not always correspond with the degree of structural damage, and that imaging techniques such as PET, in combination with neuropsychological testing, are valuable in determining the extent and location of injury in postoperative cardiac patients.[136] These studies suggest that PET (along with other types of functional imaging) now has, and will continue to play, an important role in the evaluation of vascular disease in a variety of patients.

Arterial Spin Labeling and Cognition

A handful of studies have been conducted that examine CBF as measured by ASL during cognitive tasks. Most have compared blood-oxygen-level-dependent (BOLD) imaging, a functional MRI technique often used in the study of CBF, to ASL during various tasks. For example, in 2007, Bangen et al. used a picture-encoding task during the scan to compare the CBF of older and younger adults. The authors found that the CBF in older adults was reduced during a resting state, which is consistent with previous literature. Also, CBF in older, but not younger, adults changed significantly during the cognitive task according to ASL, though no such change in BOLD signal was detected.[137] A study by Kim et al. used a visual sustained-attention task as well as a working memory task in continuous ASL (CASL). Results showed activation in similar regions as detected by PET and BOLD fMRI studies, and the authors predict that ASL will soon become a more popular method of measuring CBF.[138]

In the future, ASL may become more widely used in clinical practice. Xu and coauthors, in 2007, used ASL to compare participants with amnestic mild cognitive impairment (aMCI) with cognitively normal adults. Participants completed neuropsychological testing and ASL MRI with a memory-encoding photograph task. As in the elderly participants from the Bangen study, participants with aMCI showed reduced CBF in the regions of interest at resting state. During the memory-encoding task, cognitively normal participants were able to increase CBF as expected, while the aMCI group did not.[139] Using ASL MRI, Du et al. found hypoperfusion in the right frontal regions of patients with frontotemporal dementia (FTD) as compared to cognitively normal participants. These authors note the differences in regions affected by FTD as compared to Alzheimer's disease and suggest that ASL could become an important tool in distinguishing between the two.[86] Strouse et al. looked at CASL imaging as compared to IQ in children with sickle-cell anemia and found a strong inverse relationship between performance IQ and CBF. Strouse and coauthors suggest that CASL may be useful to detect early neurocognitive impairment in children with sickle-cell anemia.[140]

Limitations and Future Direction of the Field

One of the major challenges in any type of vascular research is the heterogeneity of participants. For example, a population selected on the basis of having atherosclerosis will undoubtedly vary with regard to age, weight, and family history of vascular disease, among other risk factors. Such variable risk-factor profiles are difficult to characterize and/or statistically control. Additionally, there are almost certainly risk factors for, and contributors to, cerebrovascular disease that are yet unknown. Nonetheless, it is likely that such factors would contribute to reduced vascular function and, therefore, be measurable. It is precisely this research problem that makes vascular function such a promising variable to be studied in relation to cognition. Another limitation of vascular research, as in all biomedical research, is that often, subjects take a variety of medications to manage their risk factors and other health problems. As it is not practical or ethical to take subjects off of medications for extended periods of time, results obtained may reflect a vascular profile that is biased toward a healthy state. Again, this is an interesting limitation in that an ideal treatment is lacking for vascular cognitive decline and for all types of dementia; therefore studying medicated patients may lead to preventions and treatments supplemental to current therapy for the cognitive effects of vascular disease.

In the future, research that is focused on the understanding of the mechanisms by which cerebrovascular disease affects cognition is likely to provide insight into the detection of the disease. A clearer picture of how resistance- and conduit-vessel health and function are related to the effects of cerebrovascular disease on the brain is necessary for understanding these mechanisms. The potential differing impact of endothelial and vascular smooth-muscle-cell regulation of blood flow on cognition is intriguing and deserves further attention. More detailed and specific cognitive testing in relation to systemic vascular function should also be a focus in determining the overall burden of vascular disease on the brain. Clarifying the involvement of vascular function in Alzheimer's disease and other dementia types will be useful in determining which aspects of preventive health individuals predisposed to such dementias should follow. Further imaging studies like PET, MRI, and functional MRI should be analyzed to develop a better picture of vascular pathology in the brain. Because vascular disease is a generalized condition, continued studies in the peripheral circulation as described in this chapter will provide a better understanding of the development of cerebrovascular disease and better enable us to determine who is at greatest risk for vascular decline. Ultimately, these studies may lead to identification of novel therapeutic options that could reverse cerebrovascular impairment and cognitive decline.

Notes

1. Breteler MM, Claus JJ, Grobbee DE, Hofman A. Cardiovascular disease and distribution of cognitive function in elderly people: The Rotterdam Study. *BMJ*. 1994;308(6944): 1604–1608.

2. Bowler JV, Steenhuis R, Hachinski V. Conceptual background to vascular cognitive impairment. *Alzheimer Dis Assoc Disord.* 1999;13(Suppl 3):S30–37.
3. Suwaidi JA, Hamasaki S, Higano ST, Nishimura RA, Holmes DR, Jr., Lerman A. Long-term follow-up of patients with mild coronary artery disease and endothelial dysfunction. *Circulation.* 2000;101(9):948–954.
4. Schachinger V, Britten MB, Zeiher AM. Prognostic impact of coronary vasodilator dysfunction on adverse long-term outcome of coronary heart disease. *Circulation.* 2000;101(16): 1899–1906.
5. Fichtlscherer S, Breuer S, Zeiher AM. Prognostic value of systemic endothelial dysfunction in patients with acute coronary syndromes: Further evidence for the existence of the "vulnerable" patient. *Circulation.* 2004;110(14):1926–1932.
6. Campuzano R, Moya JL, Garcia-Lledo A, et al. Endothelial dysfunction, intima-media thickness and coronary reserve in relation to risk factors and Framingham score in patients without clinical atherosclerosis. *J Hypertens.* 2006;24(8):1581–1588.
7. Lopez JA, Armstrong ML, Piegors DJ, Heistad DD. Effect of early and advanced atherosclerosis on vascular responses to serotonin, thromboxane A2, and ADP. *Circulation.* 1989;79(3):698–705.
8. Vogel RA. Brachial artery ultrasound: A noninvasive tool in the assessment of triglyceride-rich lipoproteins. *Clin Cardiol.* 1999;22(Suppl 6):II34–39.
9. Heistad DD, Armstrong ML. Sick vessel syndrome. Can atherosclerotic arteries recover? *Circulation.* 1994;89(5):2447–2450.
10. Corretti MC, Plotnick GD, Vogel RA. Technical aspects of evaluating brachial artery vasodilatation using high-frequency ultrasound. *Am J Physiol.* 1995;268(4 Pt 2):H1397–1404.
11. Hirooka Y, Egashira K, Imaizumi T, et al. Effect of L-arginine on acetylcholine-induced endothelium-dependent vasodilation differs between the coronary and forearm vasculatures in humans. *J Am Coll Cardiol.* 1994;24(4):948–955.
12. Bossaller C, Habib GB, Yamamoto H, Williams C, Wells S, Henry PD. Impaired muscarinic endothelium-dependent relaxation and cyclic guanosine 5'-monophosphate formation in atherosclerotic human coronary artery and rabbit aorta. *J Clin Invest.* 1987;79(1):170–174.
13. Freiman PC, Mitchell GG, Heistad DD, Armstrong ML, Harrison DG. Atherosclerosis impairs endothelium-dependent vascular relaxation to acetylcholine and thrombin in primates. *Circ Res.* 1986;58(6):783–789.
14. Vogel RA, Corretti MC. Estrogens, progestins, and heart disease: Can endothelial function divine the benefit? *Circulation.* 1998;97(13):1223–1226.
15. Yildiz O. Vascular smooth muscle and endothelial functions in aging. *Ann N Y Acad Sci.* 2007;1100:353–360.
16. Al-Shaer MH, Choueiri NE, Correia ML, Sinkey CA, Barenz TA, Haynes WG. Effects of aging and atherosclerosis on endothelial and vascular smooth muscle function in humans. *Int J Cardiol.* 2006;109(2):201–206.
17. Celermajer DS, Sorensen KE, Spiegelhalter DJ, Georgakopoulos D, Robinson J, Deanfield JE. Aging is associated with endothelial dysfunction in healthy men years before the age-related decline in women. *J Am Coll Cardiol.* 1994;24(2):471–476.
18. Berne R, Levy M. *Cardiovascular Physiology.* St. Louis, MO: Mosby, 2001.
19. Lind L, Fors N, Hall J, Marttala K, Stenborg A. A comparison of three different methods to evaluate endothelium-dependent vasodilation in the elderly: The Prospective Investigation of the Vasculature in Uppsala Seniors (PIVUS) study. *Arterioscler Thromb Vasc Biol.* 2005;25(11):2368–2375.
20. Arcaro G, Solini A, Monauni T, et al. ACE genotype and endothelium-dependent vasodilation of conduit arteries and forearm microcirculation in humans. *Arterioscler Thromb Vasc Biol.* 2001;21(8):1313–1319.

21. Kramer CM. Peripheral arterial disease assessment: Wall, perfusion, and spectroscopy. *Top Magn Reson Imaging*. 2007;18(5):357–369.
22. Kooijman M, Poelkens F, Rongen GA, Smits P, Hopman MT. Leg blood flow measurements using venous occlusion plethysmography during head-up tilt. *Clin Auton Res*. 2007;17(2):106–111.
23. Aalkjaer C, Heagerty AM, Petersen KK, Swales JD, Mulvany MJ. Evidence for increased media thickness, increased neuronal amine uptake, and depressed excitation–contraction coupling in isolated resistance vessels from essential hypertensives. *Circ Res*. 1987;61(2):181–186.
24. Aalkjaer C, Pedersen EB, Danielsen H, et al. Morphological and functional characteristics of isolated resistance vessels in advanced uraemia. *Clin Sci (Lond)*. 1986;71(6):657–663.
25. Buus NH, Jorgensen CG, Mulvany MJ, Sorensen KE. Large and small artery endothelial function in patients with essential hypertension—Effect of ACE inhibition and beta-blockade. *Blood Press*. 2007;16(2):106–113.
26. Park JB, Charbonneau F, Schiffrin EL. Correlation of endothelial function in large and small arteries in human essential hypertension. *J Hypertens*. 2001;19(3):415–420.
27. Higashi Y, Sasaki S, Nakagawa K, Matsuura H, Kajiyama G, Oshima T. A noninvasive measurement of reactive hyperemia that can be used to assess resistance artery endothelial function in humans. *Am J Cardiol*. 2001;87(1):121–125, A129.
28. Leslie SJ, Attina T, Hultsch E, et al. Comparison of two plethysmography systems in assessment of forearm blood flow. *J Appl Physiol*. 2004;96(5):1794–1799.
29. Wilkinson IB, Webb DJ. Venous occlusion plethysmography in cardiovascular research: Methodology and clinical applications. *Br J Clin Pharmacol*. 2001;52(6):631–646.
30. Yvonne-Tee GB, Rasool AH, Halim AS, Rahman AR. Noninvasive assessment of cutaneous vascular function *in vivo* using capillaroscopy, plethysmography and laser-Doppler instruments: Its strengths and weaknesses. *Clin Hemorheol Microcirc*. 2006;34(4):457–473.
31. Joyner MJ, Dietz NM, Shepherd JT. From Belfast to Mayo and beyond: The use and future of plethysmography to study blood flow in human limbs. *J Appl Physiol*. 2001;91(6):2431–2441.
32. Strachan FE, Newby DE, Sciberras DG, McCrea JB, Goldberg MR, Webb DJ. Repeatability of local forearm vasoconstriction to endothelin-1 measured by venous occlusion plethysmography. *Br J Clin Pharmacol*. 2002;54(4):386–394.
33. Petrie JR, Ueda S, Morris AD, Murray LS, Elliott HL, Connell JM. How reproducible is bilateral forearm plethysmography? *Br J Clin Pharmacol*. 1998;45(2):131–139.
34. Burggraaf J, Kemme MJ, Muller LM, Schoemaker RC, Cohen AF. The influence of the hand circulation on the assessment of venous distensibility of the human forearm with venous occlusion plethysmography. *Br J Clin Pharmacol*. 2000;50(6):621–623.
35. Lind L, Sarabi M, Millgard J. Methodological aspects of the evaluation of endothelium-dependent vasodilatation in the human forearm. *Clin Physiol*. 1998;18(2):81–87.
36. Chowienczyk PJ, Cockcroft JR, Ritter JM. Blood flow responses to intra-arterial acetylcholine in man: Effects of basal flow and conduit vessel length. *Clin Sci (Lond)*. 1994;87(1):45–51.
37. Higashi Y, Yoshizumi M. New methods to evaluate endothelial function: Method for assessing endothelial function in humans using a strain-gauge plethysmography: Nitric oxide-dependent and -independent vasodilation. *J Pharmacol Sci*. 2003;93(4):399–404.
38. Duff F, Greenfield AD, Shepherd JT, Thompson ID. A quantitative study of the response to acetylcholine and histamine of the blood vessels of the human hand and forearm. *J Physiol*. 1953;120(1–2):160–170.
39. Moser DJ, Hoth KF, Robinson RG, et al. Blood vessel function and cognition in elderly patients with atherosclerosis. *Stroke*. 2004;35(11):e369–372.

40. Moser DJ, Robinson RG, Hynes SM, et al. Neuropsychological performance is associated with vascular function in patients with atherosclerotic vascular disease. *Arterioscler Thromb Vasc Biol*. 2007;27(1):141–146.
41. Irace C, Ceravolo R, Notarangelo L, et al. Comparison of endothelial function evaluated by strain gauge plethysmography and brachial artery ultrasound. *Atherosclerosis*. 2001;158(1):53–59.
42. Lind L. Endothelium-dependent vasodilation, insulin resistance and the metabolic syndrome in an elderly cohort: The Prospective Investigation of the Vasculature in Uppsala Seniors (PIVUS) study. *Atherosclerosis*. 2008;196(2):795–802.
43. Creager MA, Cooke JP, Mendelsohn ME, et al. Impaired vasodilation of forearm resistance vessels in hypercholesterolemic humans. *J Clin Invest*. 1990;86(1):228–234.
44. Kahn DF, Duffy SJ, Tomasian D, et al. Effects of black race on forearm resistance vessel function. *Hypertension*. 2002;40(2):195–201.
45. Lind L, Hall J, Johansson K. Evaluation of four different methods to measure endothelium-dependent vasodilation in the human peripheral circulation. *Clin Sci (Lond)*. 2002;102(5): 561–567.
46. Lind L, Hall J, Larsson A, Annuk M, Fellstrom B, Lithell H. Evaluation of endothelium-dependent vasodilation in the human peripheral circulation. *Clin Physiol*. 2000;20(6): 440–448.
47. Williams SB, Cusco JA, Roddy MA, Johnstone MT, Creager MA. Impaired nitric oxide–mediated vasodilation in patients with non-insulin-dependent diabetes mellitus. *J Am Coll Cardiol*. 1996;27(3):567–574.
48. Ishibashi Y, Takahashi N, Shimada T, et al. Short duration of reactive hyperemia in the forearm of subjects with multiple cardiovascular risk factors. *Circ J*. 2006;70(1):115–123.
49. Chuah SS, Woolfson PI, Pullan BR, Lewis PS. Plethysmography without venous occlusion for measuring forearm blood flow: Comparison with venous occlusive method. *Clin Physiol Funct Imaging*. 2004;24(5):296–303.
50. Naylor LH, Weisbrod CJ, O'Driscoll G, Green DJ. Measuring peripheral resistance and conduit arterial structure in humans using Doppler ultrasound. *J Appl Physiol*. 2005;98(6):2311–2315.
51. Moser DJ, Miller IN, Hoth KF, Correia M, Arndt S, Haynes WG. Vascular smooth muscle function is associated with initiation and processing speed in patients with atherosclerotic vascular disease. *J Int Neuropsychol Soc*. 2008;14(4):535–541.
52. Celermajer DS, Sorensen KE, Gooch VM, et al. Non-invasive detection of endothelial dysfunction in children and adults at risk of atherosclerosis. *Lancet*. 1992;340(8828): 1111–1115.
53. Corretti MC, Anderson TJ, Benjamin EJ, et al. Guidelines for the ultrasound assessment of endothelial-dependent flow-mediated vasodilation of the brachial artery: A report of the International Brachial Artery Reactivity Task Force. *J Am Coll Cardiol*. 2002;39(2): 257–265.
54. Joannides R, Haefeli WE, Linder L, et al. Nitric oxide is responsible for flow-dependent dilatation of human peripheral conduit arteries *in vivo*. *Circulation*. 1995;91(5):1314–1319.
55. Raitakari OT, Seale JP, Celermajer DS. Impaired vascular responses to nitroglycerin in subjects with coronary atherosclerosis. *Am J Cardiol*. 2001;87(2):217–219, A218.
56. Hoth KF, Tate DF, Poppas A, et al. Endothelial function and white matter hyperintensities in older adults with cardiovascular disease. *Stroke*. 2007;38(2):308–312.
57. As R, Benetos A, Topouchian J, et al. Assessment of arterial distensibility by automatic pulse wave velocity measurement. Validation and clinical application studies. *Hypertension*. 1995;26(3):485–490.

58. Oliver JJ, Webb DJ. Noninvasive assessment of arterial stiffness and risk of atherosclerotic events. *Arterioscler Thromb Vasc Biol.* 2003;23(4):554–566.
59. Laurent S, Cockcroft J, Van Bortel L, et al. Expert consensus document on arterial stiffness: Methodological issues and clinical applications. *Eur Heart J.* 2006;27(21):2588–2605.
60. Lehmann ED, Hopkins KD, Rawesh A, et al. Relation between number of cardiovascular risk factors/events and noninvasive Doppler ultrasound assessments of aortic compliance. *Hypertension.* 1998;32(3):565–569.
61. Matsuoka O, Otsuka K, Murakami S, et al. Arterial stiffness independently predicts cardiovascular events in an elderly community—Longitudinal Investigation for the Longevity and Aging in Hokkaido County (LILAC) study. *Biomed Pharmacother.* 2005;59 (Suppl 1):S40–44.
62. Ter Avest E, Stalenhoef AF, de Graaf J. What is the role of non-invasive measurements of atherosclerosis in individual cardiovascular risk prediction? *Clin Sci (Lond).* 2007;112(10): 507–516.
63. O'Rourke MF, Gallagher DE. Pulse wave analysis. *J Hypertens Suppl.* 1996;14(5): S147–157.
64. Wilson AM, O'Neal D, Nelson CL, Prior DL, Best JD, Jenkins AJ. Comparison of arterial assessments in low and high vascular disease risk groups. *Am J Hypertens.* 2004;17(4): 285–291.
65. Matsumoto C, Tomiyama H, Yamada J, Yoshida M, Shiina K, Yamashina A. Brachial-ankle pulse wave velocity as a marker of subclinical organ damage in middle-aged patients with hypertension. *J Cardiol.* 2008;51(3):163–170.
66. Lehmann ED. Noninvasive measurements of aortic stiffness: Methodological considerations. *Pathol Biol (Paris).* 1999;47(7):716–730.
67. Van Bortel LM, Duprez D, Starmans-Kool MJ, et al. Clinical applications of arterial stiffness, Task Force III: Recommendations for user procedures. *Am J Hypertens.* 2002;15(5): 445–452.
68. Gould KL. Positron emission tomography in coronary artery disease. *Curr Opin Cardiol.* 2007;22(5):422–428.
69. Sinzinger H, Granegger S. Radionuclide vascular imaging and characterization of human metabolic endothelial surface lining. *Q J Nucl Med Mol Imaging.* 2006;50(3):226–235.
70. Macapinlac HA. Positron emission tomography of the brain. *Neuroimaging Clin N Am.* 2006;16(4):591–603, viii.
71. Boles Ponto LL, Schultz SK, Watkins LG, Hichwa RD. Technical issues in the determination of cerebrovascular reserve in elderly subjects using ^{15}O-water PET imaging. *Neuroimage.* 2004;21(1):201–210.
72. Silverman DH, Alavi A. PET imaging in the assessment of normal and impaired cognitive function. *Radiol Clin North Am.* 2005;43(1):67–77, x.
73. Stern Y. What is cognitive reserve? Theory and research application of the reserve concept. *J Int Neuropsychol Soc.* 2002;8(3):448–460.
74. Boles Ponto LL, Magnotta VA, Moser DJ, Duff KM, Schultz SK. Global cerebral blood flow in relation to cognitive performance and reserve in subjects with mild memory deficits. *Mol Imaging Biol.* 2006;8(6):363–372.
75. Yonas H, Pindzola RR, Meltzer CC, Sasser H. Qualitative versus quantitative assessment of cerebrovascular reserves. *Neurosurgery.* 1998;42(5):1005–1010; discussion, 1011–1002.
76. Nariai T, Suzuki R, Hirakawa K, Maehara T, Ishii K, Senda M. Vascular reserve in chronic cerebral ischemia measured by the acetazolamide challenge test: Comparison with positron emission tomography. *AJNR Am J Neuroradiol.* 1995;16(3):563–570.

77. Murakami M, Yonehara T, Takaki A, Fujioka S, Hirano T, Ushio Y. Evaluation of delayed appearance of acetazolamide effect in patients with chronic cerebrovascular ischemic disease: Feasibility and usefulness of SPECT method using triple injection of ECD. *J Nucl Med.* 2002;43(5):577–583.
78. Hirano T, Minematsu K, Hasegawa Y, Tanaka Y, Hayashida K, Yamaguchi T. Acetazolamide reactivity on 123I-IMP single photon emission computed tomography in patients with major cerebral artery occlusive disease: Correlation with positron emission tomography parameters. *J Cereb Blood Flow Metab.* 1994;14(5):763–770.
79. Bonte FJ, Devous MD, Reisch JS. The effect of acetazolamide on regional cerebral blood flow in normal human subjects as measured by single-photon emission computed tomography. *Invest Radiol.* 1988;23(8):564–568.
80. Pavics L, Grunwald F, Reichmann K, et al. Regional cerebral blood flow single-photon emission tomography with 99mTc-HMPAO and the acetazolamide test in the evaluation of vascular and Alzheimer's dementia. *Eur J Nucl Med.* 1999;26(3):239–245.
81. Wong EC, Buxton RB, Frank LR. Quantitative perfusion imaging using arterial spin labeling. *Neuroimaging Clin N Am.* 1999;9(2):333–342.
82. Wolf RL, Detre JA. Clinical neuroimaging using arterial spin-labeled perfusion magnetic resonance imaging. *Neurotherapeutics.* 2007;4(3):346–359.
83. Feng CM, Narayana S, Lancaster JL, et al. CBF changes during brain activation: FMRI vs. PET. *Neuroimage.* 2004;22(1):443–446.
84. Alsop DC, Detre JA. Reduced transit-time sensitivity in noninvasive magnetic resonance imaging of human cerebral blood flow. *J Cereb Blood Flow Metab.* 1996;16(6):1236–1249.
85. Alsop DC, Detre JA, Grossman M. Assessment of cerebral blood flow in Alzheimer's disease by spin-labeled magnetic resonance imaging. *Ann Neurol.* 2000;47(1):93–100.
86. Du AT, Jahng GH, Hayasaka S, et al. Hypoperfusion in frontotemporal dementia and Alzheimer disease by arterial spin labeling MRI. *Neurology.* 10 2006;67(7):1215–1220.
87. Ludemann L, Warmuth C, Plotkin M, et al. Brain tumor perfusion: Comparison of dynamic contrast enhanced magnetic resonance imaging using T(1), T(2), and T(2)(*) contrast, pulsed arterial spin labeling, and H(2)(15)O positron emission tomography. *Eur J Radiol.* 2009;70(3):465-74.
88. Deibler AR, Pollock JM, Kraft RA, Tan H, Burdette JH, Maldjian JA. Arterial spin-labeling in routine clinical practice, Part 2: Hypoperfusion patterns. *AJNR Am J Neuroradiol.* 2008;29(7):1235-41.
89. Knipp SC, Matatko N, Wilhelm H, et al. Cognitive outcomes three years after coronary artery bypass surgery: Relation to diffusion-weighted magnetic resonance imaging. *Ann Thorac Surg.* 2008;85(3):872–879.
90. Jokinen H, Kalska H, Mantyla R, et al. White matter hyperintensities as a predictor of neuropsychological deficits post-stroke. *J Neurol Neurosurg Psychiatry.* 2005;76(9):1229–1233.
91. Grunwald IQ, Supprian T, Politi M, et al. Cognitive changes after carotid artery stenting. *Neuroradiology.* 2006;48(5):319–323.
92. Victoroff J, Mack WJ, Lyness SA, Chui HC. Multicenter clinicopathological correlation in dementia. *Am J Psychiatry.* 1995;152(10):1476–1484.
93. Peila R, White LR, Petrovich H, et al. Joint effect of the APOE gene and midlife systolic blood pressure on late-life cognitive impairment: The Honolulu-Asia Aging Study. *Stroke.* 1 2001;32(12):2882–2889.
94. Elias MF, D'Agostino RB, Elias PK, Wolf PA. Neuropsychological test performance, cognitive functioning, blood pressure, and age: The Framingham Heart Study. *Exp Aging Res.* 1995;21(4):369–391.

95. Elias MF, Robbins MA, Elias PK, Streeten DH. A longitudinal study of blood pressure in relation to performance on the Wechsler Adult Intelligence Scale. *Health Psychol.* 1998;17(6):486–493.
96. Elias MF, Schultz NR, Jr., Robbins MA, Elias PK. A longitudinal study of neuropsychological performance by hypertensives and normotensives: A third measurement point. *J Gerontol.* 1989;44(1):P25–P28.
97. Elias PK, Elias MF, D'Agostino RB, et al. NIDDM and blood pressure as risk factors for poor cognitive performance. The Framingham Study. *Diabetes Care.* 1997;20(9): 1388–1395.
98. DeCarli C, Miller BL, Swan GE, Reed T, Wolf PA, Carmelli D. Cerebrovascular and brain morphological correlates of mild cognitive impairment in the National Heart, Lung, and Blood Institute Twin Study. *Arch Neurol.* 2001;58(4):643–647.
99. Swan GE, Carmelli D, Larue A. Systolic blood pressure tracking over 25 to 30 years and cognitive performance in older adults. *Stroke.* 1998;29(11):2334–2340.
100. Swan GE, DeCarli C, Miller BL, et al. Association of midlife blood pressure to late-life cognitive decline and brain morphology. *Neurology.* 1998;51(4):986–993.
101. Launer LJ, Masaki K, Petrovitch H, Foley D, Havlik RJ. The association between midlife blood pressure levels and late-life cognitive function. The Honolulu-Asia Aging Study. *JAMA.* 1995;274(23):1846–1851.
102. Kaplan GA, Everson SA, Koivisto K, Salonen R, Salonen JT. Cognitive function and carotid atherosclerosis in eastern Finnish men. *Ann Behav Med.* 1996;18(Suppl.):S47.
103. Cerhan JR, Folsom AR, Mortimer JA, et al. Correlates of cognitive function in middle-aged adults. Atherosclerosis Risk in Communities (ARIC) Study Investigators. *Gerontology.* 1998;44(2):95–105.
104. Auperin A, Berr C, Bonithon-Kopp C, et al. Ultrasonographic assessment of carotid wall characteristics and cognitive functions in a community sample of 59- to 71-year-olds. The EVA Study Group. *Stroke.* 1996;27(8):1290–1295.
105. Juergens JL, Bernatz PE. Atherosclerosis of the extremities. In: Juergens JL, Spittel JAJ, Fairbairn JF (Eds.), *Peripheral Vascular Diseases*, 5th ed. (pp. 253–293). Philadelphia: W.B. Saunders, 1980.
106. Everson SA, Helkala E, Kaplan GA, Salonen JT. Atherosclerosis and cognitive functioning. In Waldstein SR, Elias MF (Eds.), *Neuropsychology of Cardiovascular Disease*. Mahway, NJ: Lawrence Erlbaum; 2001.
107. Phillips NA, Mate-Kole CC, Kirby RL. Neuropsychological function in peripheral vascular disease amputee patients. *Arch Phys Med Rehabil.* 1993;74(12):1309–1314.
108. Roman GC, Sachdev P, Royall DR, et al. Vascular cognitive disorder: A new diagnostic category updating vascular cognitive impairment and vascular dementia. *J Neurol Sci.* 15 2004;226(1–2):81–87.
109. Looi JC, Sachdev PS. Differentiation of vascular dementia from AD on neuropsychological tests. *Neurology.* 1999;53(4):670–678.
110. Jefferson AL, Cahn-Weiner D, Boyle P, et al. Cognitive predictors of functional decline in vascular dementia. *Int J Geriatr Psychiatry.* 2006;21(8):752–754.
111. Boyle PA, Cohen RA, Paul R, Moser D, Gordon N. Cognitive and motor impairments predict functional declines in patients with vascular dementia. *Int J Geriatr Psychiatry.* 2002;17(2):164–169.
112. Boyle PA, Paul R, Moser D, Zawacki T, Gordon N, Cohen R. Cognitive and neurological predictors of functional impairment in vascular dementia. *Am J Geriatr Psychiatry.* 2003;11(1):103–106.

113. Kramer JH, Reed BR, Mungas D, Weiner MW, Chui HC. Executive dysfunction in subcortical ischaemic vascular disease. *J Neurol Neurosurg Psychiatry*. 2002;72(2):217–220.
114. Almkvist O. Cognitive syndrome(s) in preclinical and clinical vascular dementia. *Int Psychogeriatr*. 2003;15(Suppl 1):127–131.
115. Phillips NA, Mate-Kole CC. Cognitive deficits in peripheral vascular disease. A comparison of mild stroke patients and normal control subjects. *Stroke*. 1997;28(4):777–784.
116. Pfeffer RI, Kurosaki TT, Harrah CH, Jr., Chance JM, Filos S. Measurement of functional activities in older adults in the community. *J Gerontol*. 1982;37(3):323–329.
117. Phillips NA. Neuropsychological function in patients with peripheral vascular disease [unpublished doctoral dissertation]. Halifax, Nova Scotia: Dalhousie University, 1996.
118. Hanon O, Haulon S, Lenoir H, et al. Relationship between arterial stiffness and cognitive function in elderly subjects with complaints of memory loss. *Stroke*. 2005;36(10): 2193–2197.
119. Fujiwara Y, Chaves PH, Takahashi R, et al. Arterial pulse wave velocity as a marker of poor cognitive function in an elderly community-dwelling population. *J Gerontol A Biol Sci Med Sci*. 2005;60(5):607–612.
120. Poels MM, van Oijen M, Mattace-Raso FU, et al. Arterial stiffness, cognitive decline, and risk of dementia: The Rotterdam study. *Stroke*. 2007;38(3):888–892.
121. Scuteri A, Tesauro M, Appolloni S, Preziosi F, Brancati AM, Volpe M. Arterial stiffness as an independent predictor of longitudinal changes in cognitive function in the older individual. *J Hypertens*. 2007;25(5):1035–1040.
122. Waldstein SR, Rice SC, Thayer JF, Najjar SS, Scuteri A, Zonderman AB. Pulse pressure and pulse wave velocity are related to cognitive decline in the Baltimore Longitudinal Study of Aging. *Hypertension*. 2008;51(1):99–104.
123. Muller M, Grobbee DE, Aleman A, Bots M, van der Schouw YT. Cardiovascular disease and cognitive performance in middle-aged and elderly men. *Atherosclerosis*. 2007;190(1):143–149.
124. Scuteri A, Brancati AM, Gianni W, Assisi A, Volpe M. Arterial stiffness is an independent risk factor for cognitive impairment in the elderly: A pilot study. *J Hypertens*. 2005;23(6):1211–1216.
125. Moser DJ, Miller IN, Hoth KF, Correia ML, Arndt S, Haynes WG. Vascular smooth muscle function is associated with initiation and processing speed in patients with atherosclerotic vascular disease. *J Int Neuropsychol Soc*. 2008;14(4):535–541.
126. Dede DS, Yavuz B, Yavuz BB, et al. Assessment of endothelial function in Alzheimer's disease: Is Alzheimer's disease a vascular disease? *J Am Geriatr Soc*. 2007;55(10): 1613–1617.
127. Smith PJ, Blumenthal JA, Babyak MA, et al. Cerebrovascular risk factors, vascular disease, and neuropsychological outcomes in adults with major depression. *Psychosom Med*. 2007;69(6):578–586.
128. Narita K, Murata T, Hamada T, et al. Interactions among higher trait anxiety, sympathetic activity, and endothelial function in the elderly. *J Psychiatr Res*. 2007;41(5):418–427.
129. Cohen RA, Poppas A, Forman DE, et al. Vascular and cognitive functions associated with cardiovascular disease in the elderly. *J Clin Exp Neuropsychol*. 2009;31(1):96-110.
130. Scarmeas N, Zarahn E, Anderson KE, et al. Cognitive reserve modulates functional brain responses during memory tasks: A PET study in healthy young and elderly subjects. *Neuroimage*. 2003;19(3):1215–1227.
131. Scarmeas N, Zarahn E, Anderson KE, et al. Association of life activities with cerebral blood flow in Alzheimer disease: Implications for the cognitive reserve hypothesis. *Arch Neurol*. 2003;60(3):359–365.

132. Scarmeas N, Stern Y. Cognitive reserve and lifestyle. *J Clin Exp Neuropsychol.* 2003;25(5):625–633.
133. Alexander GE, Furey ML, Grady CL, et al. Association of premorbid intellectual function with cerebral metabolism in Alzheimer's disease: Implications for the cognitive reserve hypothesis. *Am J Psychiatry*. 1997;154(2):165–172.
134. Tullberg M, Fletcher E, DeCarli C, et al. White matter lesions impair frontal lobe function regardless of their location. *Neurology*. 2004;63(2):246–253.
135. Sturm W, Longoni F, Weis S, et al. Functional reorganisation in patients with right hemisphere stroke after training of alertness: A longitudinal PET and fMRI study in eight cases. *Neuropsychologia*. 2004;42(4):434–450.
136. Jacobs A, Neveling M, Horst M, et al. Alterations of neuropsychological function and cerebral glucose metabolism after cardiac surgery are not related only to intraoperative microembolic events. *Stroke*. 1998;29(3):660–667.
137. Bangen KJ, Restom K, Liu TT, et al. Differential age effects on cerebral blood flow and BOLD response to encoding: Associations with cognition and stroke risk. *Neurobiol Aging*. Dec. 19, 2007.
138. Kim J, Whyte J, Wang J, Rao H, Tang KZ, Detre JA. Continuous ASL perfusion fMRI investigation of higher cognition: Quantification of tonic CBF changes during sustained attention and working memory tasks. *Neuroimage*. 2006;31(1):376–385.
139. Xu G, Antuono PG, Jones J, et al. Perfusion fMRI detects deficits in regional CBF during memory-encoding tasks in MCI subjects. *Neurology*. 2007;69(17):1650–1656.
140. Strouse JJ, Cox CS, Melhem ER, et al. Inverse correlation between cerebral blood flow measured by continuous arterial spin-labeling (CASL) MRI and neurocognitive function in children with sickle-cell anemia (SCA). *Blood*. 2006;108(1):379–381.

15

CEREBROVASCULAR HEMODYNAMICS AND CEREBRAL AUTOREGULATION IN THE AGING BRAIN

Jorge M. Serrador and William P. Milberg

Regulation of cerebral blood flow is critical for proper neural function. Therefore, alterations in cerebral blood flow regulation due to aging or age-related disease may have important clinical consequences, including cognitive impairment, gait disorders, falls, and syncope. This chapter will review mechanisms of cerebral blood flow regulation, their changes with hypertension and aging, and their clinical implications, including the frontal subcortical dysfunction in cognition and gait that is commonly observed in elderly people.

The regulation of cerebral blood flow involves several interacting mechanisms.[1, 2] Barcroft in 1914 proposed that cerebral flow was matched to metabolic demands.[1] This has since been validated in both animal and human studies. Cognitive activation in humans increases both global and local blood flow to the brain.[3–5] The ability to augment flow is critical; for example, cognitive deficits with cerebral ischemia are reversed by increases in global cerebral blood flow.[6] Although vasodilation related to neuronal activity increases regional brain blood flow during cognitive activation, this vasodilation may be insufficient if global flow is already limited. To ensure sufficient cerebral blood flow is available, the cerebrovasculature must dilate or constrict in response to prevailing perfusion pressure. The ability to maintain brain blood flow over a wide range of pressures is termed *cerebral autoregulation*.[2] Thus, impairment of either metabolic cerebral vasodilation or cerebral autoregulation could adversely affect cognitive function in the elderly possibly leading to cerebrovascular disease and dementia.

Autoregulation of Cerebral Blood Flow

Cerebral autoregulation maintains blood flow relatively constant across a wide range of cerebral perfusion pressures. Cerebral blood flow (CBF) is determined by cerebral perfusion pressure (CPP) and cerebrovascular resistance (CVR), with CPP being a result of arterial minus intracranial pressure. The relationship between these variables can be defined as

$$CBF = \frac{CPP}{CVR}$$

Thus to maintain constant cerebral blood flow in the face of changing perfusion pressure, the vascular resistance must be adjusted. For example, to maintain flow during increases in pressure, resistance must increase. The pial arteries constrict in response to increased cerebral perfusion pressure, causing an increase in cerebrovascular resistance.[2] Figure 15-1 demonstrates that within a normal pressure range, cerebrovascular resistance adjusts to the prevailing cerebral perfusion pressure to maintain flow relatively constant. When pressure becomes excessively low, resulting in maximal vasodilation, resistance can no longer adjust to decreasing perfusion pressures, and cerebral blood flow will fall. In contrast, when pressures become too high, the pial arterioles will be forced open by the driving pressure, and thus resistance will decrease, resulting in an increase in cerebral blood flow. This condition is termed *autoregulatory breakthrough.*

Previous research has demonstrated that the autoregulatory curve is not static and is affected by a variety of conditions. It is well known that changing arterial carbon dioxide levels will result in changes in cerebral blood flow without affecting cerebral autoregulation (Fig. 15-2).[2] For example, a decrease in arterial CO_2 will cause an overall cerebral vasoconstriction, which will reduce global cerebral blood flow; however, the inherent ability of the cerebrovasculature to respond to pressure changes will remain intact. Thus, cerebral blood flow will now be autoregulated around this new lower level of cerebral blood flow (i.e. this can be described as a downward shift in the curve). Similarly, stimulation of the fastigial nucleus in primates has been found to result in vasodilatation, which increases cerebral blood flow[7, 8] without a loss of autoregulation (i.e. an upward shift in the autoregulation curve).[8] This vasodilatation may be mediated by parasympathetic pathways.[9] Another example of a shift in the curve is the observation that cerebral blood flow is maintained during hypotension in both chronic local cerebral hypoperfusion[1, 10] and orthostatic hypotension.[11, 12] Thus, individuals with these conditions are able to maintain cerebral blood flow at pressures that would be expected to cause maximal vasodilation and thus impair the ability of the cerebral vessels to adjust to perfusion pressure. This increased ability to vasodilate at lower perfusion pressures can be described as a leftward shift in the autoregulation curve.

It is possible that leftward/rightward shifts in the curve are mediated by changes in sympathetic activity. For example, sympathectomized baboons demonstrate a leftward shift in the curve,[8] presumably because the sympathetically mediated vasoconstriction of cerebral vessels is no longer present and thus greater cerebral vasodilation is possible. Although the role of sympathetic tone in humans is still under debate,[2, 13–15] studies have suggested that interruption of cerebral sympathetic pathways through the superior cervical ganglia in spinal cord injured patients may shift autoregulation to a lower pressure zone. Similar to the sympathectomized baboons, a reduction in vasoconstrictive inputs

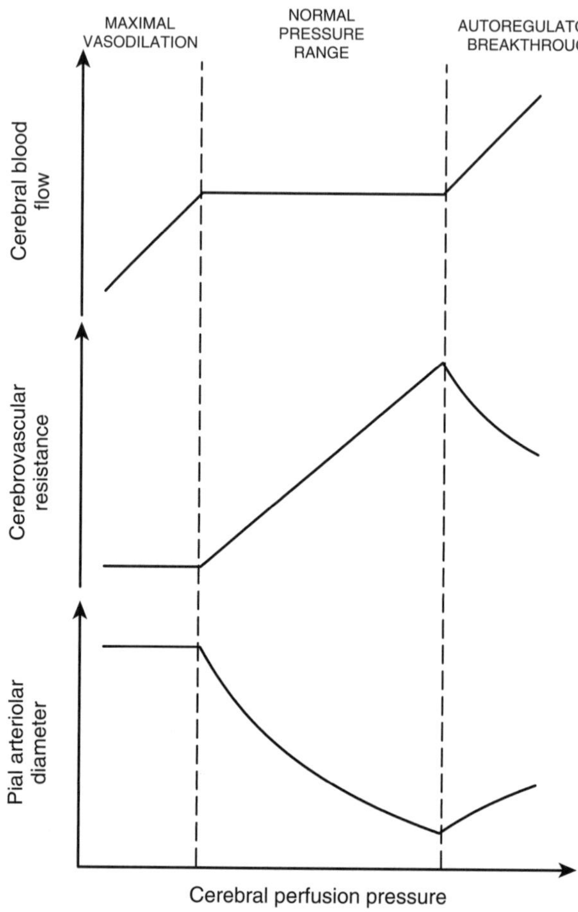

Figure 15-1 Representation of autoregulatory response to changes in cerebral perfusion pressure. Cerebral blood flow is maintained constant over a wide range of perfusion pressures by adjusting cerebrovascular resistance via dilating or constricting pial arterioles. Once pial arterioles are maximally dilated, further reductions in perfusion pressure result in decreases in cerebral blood flow (lower limit of autoregulation). If perfusion pressure is sufficiently high, pial arterioles are forced open, and cerebral blood flow increases with increasing perfusion pressure (autoregulatory breakthrough).

would allow for greater dilation, and thus explain the ability of these patients to tolerate lower cerebral perfusion pressures.[12] However, spinal cord–injured patients with high cervical lesions demonstrate decreases in cerebral blood flow similar to those of controls, suggesting they have not shifted their curve leftward.[16]

There are also data suggesting that acute changes in sympathetic outflow can shift the autoregulation curve. Levine et al.[17] have proposed that a rightward shift of the

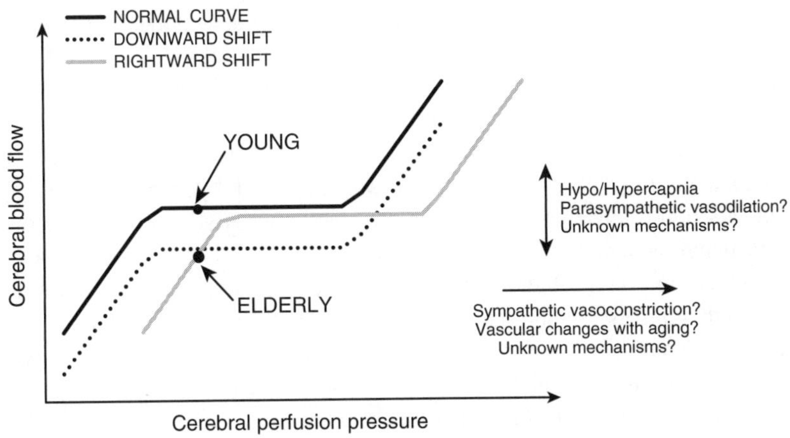

Figure 15-2 Theoretical shifts in the cerebral autoregulation curve associated with changes in arterial carbon dioxide and sympathetic nervous system activity. Elderly subjects are known to have reduced global cerebral blood flow at the same perfusion pressure. One possible explanation is a rightward shift in the curve due to diminished vasodilatory capacity. In this case, elderly subjects are no longer able to autoregulate in response to perfusion pressure, and therefore cerebral blood flow falls. Another explanation is that a downward shift in the curve occurs so that overall cerebrovascular resistance increases, decreasing flow without affecting cerebral autoregulation. The underlying mechanism of this aging-related cerebral hypoperfusion remains unclear.

autoregulation curve during lower-body negative pressure results from sympathetic activation (i.e., increased sympathetic cerebral vasoconstriction). This derives from the finding that decreases in cerebral blood flow occur without any appreciable alteration in arterial pressure.[17, 18] This could occur if there is a rightward shift in the autoregulation curve so that the current cerebral perfusion pressure falls onto the downward slope of the curve, decreasing cerebral blood flow without drops in pressure (Fig. 15-2). Moreover, previous work found evidence of a decreased ability to regulate against fluctuations in pressure during higher levels of lower-body negative pressure[19] or upright tilt.[20] Furthermore, ganglionic blockade using trimethaphan resulted in further impairment of autoregulation during lower-body negative pressure.[21] Since autoregulation works to maintain constant cerebral blood flow in the face of changing perfusion pressure, this decreased ability to regulate against fluctuations in pressure suggests that autoregulation is impaired; thus, these subjects may be on the linear portion of the curve associated with maximal vasodilation.

In contrast, early studies of cats found no effect of acute sympathetic denervation on autoregulatory responses.[22] Consistent with this, animal studies have found no effect on autoregulation of chronic or acute sympathetic denervation, or electrical stimulation if blood pressure is kept stable.[23, 24] In humans, sympathetic activation caused by upright tilt does not impair the ability to regulate against pressure fluctuations,[25, 26] despite having decreases in cerebral flow velocity similar to those of previous studies.[19, 20] These data suggest that sympathetic activation does not impair cerebral autoregulation (i.e., shift the curve right) and thus a downward shift in the curve must have occurred.

One possible explanation for these contradictory results may be provided by the contradictory findings that autoregulation was impaired by ganglionic blockade,[21] which blocks both parasympathetic and sympathetic activity, and improved by pharmacological sympathetic blockade using beta-blockers in stroke patients.[27] Thus, in the study in which only sympathetic activity was blocked, autoregulation was improved, but when both sympathetic and parasympathetic activity were blocked, autoregulation was impaired. Thus, parasympathetic inputs may improve autoregulatory responses. However, these are insufficient data at the moment to determine this.

Thus, while it remains unclear what mechanisms are involved in shifting the autoregulation curve, current data suggest that the curve does shift. Since autoregulation is critical to the maintenance of cerebral blood flow, impaired autoregulation in the elderly could have detrimental effects resulting in impaired cognition, orthostatic intolerance and even permanent neuronal damage.

Cerebral Blood Flow and Hypertension

Hypertension has been shown as a significant modifiable risk factor for stroke, dementia and cerebrovascular diseases.[28] Previous work has suggested that hypertension results in a rightward shift in the curve.[29, 30] While the lower limit of autoregulation may be shifted to the right, regulation of cerebral blood flow in response to spontaneous pressure oscillations remains intact.[31–36] Therefore, while cerebral autoregulation remains intact, the increased lower limit of the curve could result in a greater potential for individuals to fall onto the lower leg of the curve during periods of hypotension, such as during standing.

Recent work examining a sit-to-stand response in normotensive, controlled hypertensive and uncontrolled hypertensive subjects demonstrated that decreases in cerebral blood flow when standing were similar across groups, suggesting that none of the hypertensive patients reached the lower limit of autoregulation (Fig. 15-4).[36] Previous work has found similar intact autoregulatory responses in younger hypertensives (age ~49 ± 14 years), both when moving from a squatting to standing position[35] and during head-up tilt.[37]

Despite this preservation of cerebral autoregulation, hypertension is associated with cerebral remodeling including hypertrophy and stiffening of larger cerebral vessels, and reduced lumen diameter and structural changes in pial vessels.[38, 39] The rightward shift in the autoregulatory curve is related to the increase in myogenic tone induced by an increase in Ca2+ sensitivity of myocytes.[40] In addition reducing vascular lumen size will increase cerebrovascular resistance,[38] maintaining constant cerebral blood flow in the face of increased cerebral perfusion pressure. Surprisingly, small cerebral vessels demonstrate increased distensibility with hypertension.[41] This appears to also

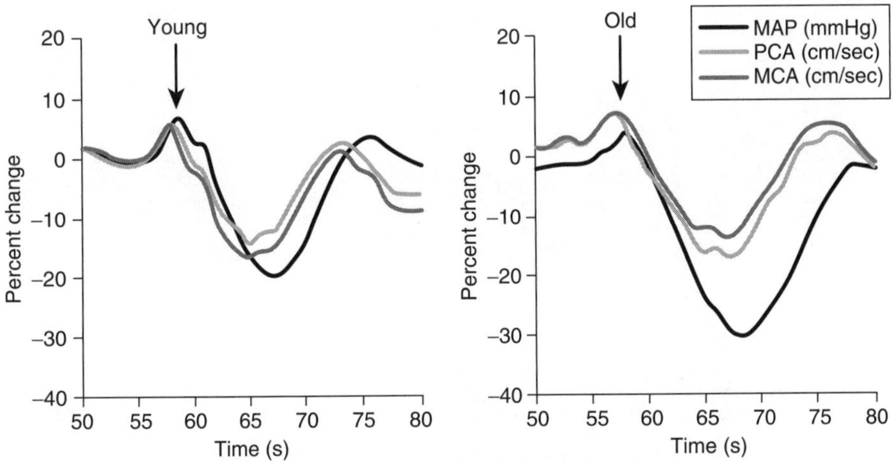

Figure 15-3 Response of a healthy young and an elderly subject to a sit-to-stand maneuver. Arrow indicates initiation of the stand. Both the young and elderly subjects were able to maintain cerebral blood flow velocity in the middle (MCA) and posterior cerebral artery (PCA), despite a decrease in mean arterial pressure (MAP) with standing. But both groups were not able to return cerebral flow back to baseline levels by ~15 seconds. These data indicate that autoregulation remains intact with healthy aging. Adapted from Sorond et al.[105]

be true in humans, since previous work found the transfer of arterial pulse pressure to the pulsatility of cerebral flow velocity was reduced in hypertensive elderly subjects.[36] This suggests that the increased distensibility acted to absorb some of the pulse wave pressure, reducing stress on capillary walls that would be induced by large variations in pressure.

Other effects of hypertensive remodeling include a reduction in cerebrovascular reactivity[36, 42] and impairment of endothelium-dependent relaxation.[39] However, reductions in cerebrovascular reactivity are probably not due to endothelium impairment, since previous work has shown that cerebrovascular reactivity is nitric oxide-independent.[43]

Hypertension has also been found to be associated with decreased global cerebral blood flow[44] and longitudinal reductions in cerebral blood flow.[45] Furthermore, increased blood pressure has been associated with greater brain atrophy and white matter hyperintensities.[46–48] Despite the clear necessity to reduce blood pressure to reduce risk factors for cerebrovascular events, concern has been raised over the possibility that aggressive treatment may cause cerebral hypoperfusion and associated syncope, falls, or cognitive dysfunction.[49] However, recent work has demonstrated that six months of antihypertensive therapy based primarily on an angiotensin-converting enzyme inhibitor regimen improved cerebral blood flow without affecting cerebral autoregulation.[42] In addition, improved carotid distensibility was correlated with increased cerebral blood flow. The increase in distensibility may serve to dampen oscillations in pressure and

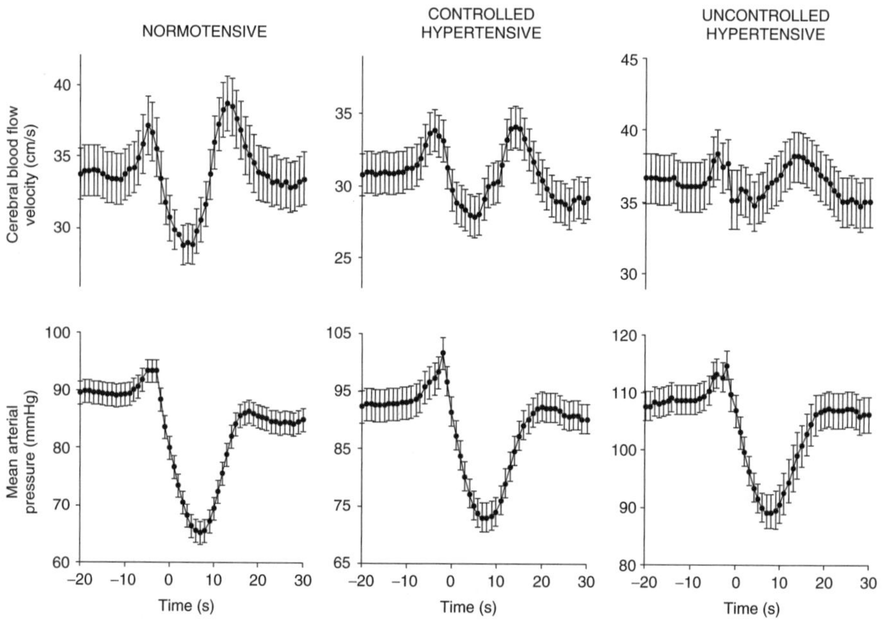

Figure 15-4 Response of elderly normotensive, controlled and uncontrolled hypertensives during a sit-to-stand test. All subjects demonstrated similar decreases in pressure; however, cerebral blood flow was better maintained in the hypertensive groups than in the normotensive subjects, suggesting intact cerebral blood flow regulation. Adapted from Serrador et al.[103]

thereby maintain continuous blood flow through the cerebral circulation, similar to the findings of Serrador et al.[36] Interestingly, a recent review examined the effect of antihypertensive drugs on dementia in randomized, placebo-controlled studies and found that the three studies that used angiotensin-converting enzyme inhibitors were also the only trials to demonstrate a reduction in dementia risk.[28] Since Lipsitz et al.[42] used angiotensin-converting enzyme inhibitors in their study, it is possible the reduction in dementia risk was related to increased cerebral blood flow.

While treatment of hypertension was able to improve cerebral blood flow, it did not change the indirect measures of cerebral distensibility and did not improve cerebrovascular reactivity.[42] In addition, cross-sectional examination of elderly subjects with long-term controlled hypertension also demonstrated increased cerebral distensibility, although arterial pulse pressure was significantly lower than in the uncontrolled hypertensive group.[36] These findings suggest that some aspects of hypertensive remodeling of cerebral vessels may not be reversible.

In summary, these data demonstrate that, despite the fact that hypertension does not impair cerebral autoregulation, it results in reductions in cerebral blood flow, brain atrophy, increased incidence of white matter hyperintensities, vascular remodeling, impaired cerebrovascular reactivity, and rightward shift in the autoregulation curve. Treatment of hypertension improves cerebral blood flow without affecting cerebral autoregulation or cerebral flow response to orthostatic stress.

Effects of Age on Cerebral Blood Flow

Aging is associated with a well-documented decrease in global cerebral blood flow[50–56] and increase in cerebral vascular resistance.[50] One possible cause of this decrease could be a rightward shift in the cerebral autoregulation curve (Fig. 15-2). A chronic rightward shift in the absence of increased perfusion pressure could result in the greatest risk for hypoperfusion, since elderly individuals would now be operating on the linear downward sloping portion of the curve, compromising their ability to defend cerebral blood flow against rises and falls in arterial pressure (i.e., impaired autoregulation). Couple that with impaired blood-pressure regulation in elderly individuals,[57, 58] and one would expect large swings in cerebral blood flow, resulting in repeated bouts of cerebral hypoperfusion.

Since aging is associated with increased sympathetic activity,[59] and increased sympathetic activity has been suggested to cause a rightward shift in the curve,[17] it seems logical that impaired autoregulation be considered as a possible cause of the global reduction in cerebral blood flow with aging (i.e. a rightward shift in the curve). Evidence supporting this hypothesis can be found in previous work demonstrating that older rats are less able to tolerate hypotensive stimuli[60, 61] have reduced cerebrovascular reactivity to CO_2 (often used as an indicator of intact autoregulation), and an increased lower limit of autoregulation.[62–64] These findings suggest a rightward shift in the autoregulation curve.

Studies of cerebral blood flow in elderly humans have produced conflicting results. Examining the response to changes in arterial CO_2 levels, studies have reported that aging has either no effect on cerebrovascular reactivity[65, 66] or is associated with reduced reactivity.[31, 67–70] Myogenic tone in isolated human pial arteries was found to be unaffected by age, suggesting intact autoregulatory capacity.[71] Furthermore, measures of cerebral autoregulation in elderly humans based on the response of cerebral blood flow to spontaneous fluctuations in blood pressure have found that autoregulation remains intact.[31, 33, 36, 72–75]

Examination of the response of elderly individuals to sudden changes in blood pressure has also demonstrated intact autoregulatory responses. During a sit-to-stand maneuver in which subjects experience transient hypotension, elderly subjects are able to maintain cerebral flow velocity effectively despite demonstrating larger decreases in mean arterial pressure[31, 76] (Fig. 15-3). In fact, during standing, elderly subjects demonstrated better attenuation of spontaneous blood pressure oscillations than younger subjects, suggesting *improved* autoregulation.[31] Elderly subjects are either better able to maintain cerebral blood flow[69] or have similar responses to those of young subjects[75] during head-up tilt. These data demonstrate that autoregulation remains intact in healthy elderly individuals.

If impaired autoregulation is not involved in the reduction in cerebral blood flow, could a direct sympathetically mediated vasoconstriction be the cause? Sympathetic innervation of cerebral vessels has been found in animals to originate in the superior cervical ganglion, stellate ganglion, and via several central pathways, including the locus coeruleus, fastigial nucleus, dorsal raphe nucleus, dorsal medullary reticular formation, and rostral ventrolateral medulla.[13] However, the role of sympathetic pathways in humans remains unclear. For example, blockade of sympathetic activity through the stellate ganglion has been found to increase cerebral blood flow, as measured by single photon emission computed tomography (SPECT), presumably through the blockade of a sympathetic vasoconstrictor signal.[77] However, MRI measures of cerebral blood flow using the same blocking technique found no change in internal carotid flow, but did demonstrate an increase in common carotid flow suggesting vasodilatation in the extracerebral beds.[78] Therefore, it is possible that the increase in cerebral blood flow observed with SPECT[77] was partly due to increased scalp and facial blood flow. In contrast, direct stimulation of the cervical ganglia and presumably sympathetic pathways during surgery caused an increase in cerebral blood flow and arterial pressure.[79] However, patients in this study were anesthetised with isoflurane, which has been shown to ablate autoregulation,[80] and nitrous oxide, which is a potent vasodilator, particularly when used in combination with isoflurane.[81] These considerations suggest that the elevated cerebral perfusion was the result of increased arterial pressure augmenting cerebral flow through vessels with pharmacologically impaired autoregulation.

In primates, cerebral vasoconstriction has been found with stimulation of the locus coeruleus.[82] This vasoconstriction was unaffected by sectioning of the vagus nerve or sympathetic trunk, suggesting no peripheral sympathetic role. In humans, direct measures of middle cerebral-artery diameter using MRI during sympathetic activation induced by lower-body negative pressure did not demonstrate a vasoconstriction at the basal artery level, even though flow decreased, suggesting the constriction occurred at the peripheral resistance arteries.[83] Direct intrathecal infusion of the locus coeruleus with clonidine, an α2-agonist which at low doses inhibits central sympathetic activity, resulted in a reduction in cerebral flow velocity in one patient, presumably through a downstream vasoconstriction.[84] In healthy individuals, clonidine has been found to minimize the decrease in cerebral flow velocity during sympathetic activation by the cold pressor test,[84, 85] presumably by reducing sympathetic activation. Furthermore, the use of beta-blockers attenuated the decrease in cerebral blood flow velocity of patients with orthostatic intolerance during head-up tilt testing.[86] In all these studies, it was proposed that the observed changes in cerebral blood flow were due to a decrease in cerebrovascular resistance as a result of reduced cerebral sympathetic activity. However, low-dose clonidine also produced hypotension and caused a reduction in baseline cerebral flow velocity,[84] suggesting a cerebral vasoconstriction. This reduction in flow was present even when the hypotension was eliminated with phenylephrine.[87]

In contrast, increasing peripheral sympathetic activity using cold face stimulation[88] or skin surface cooling[89] did not increase cerebrovascular resistance. Increasing muscle sympathetic nerve activity by ~50% using static handgrip did not cause a reduction in

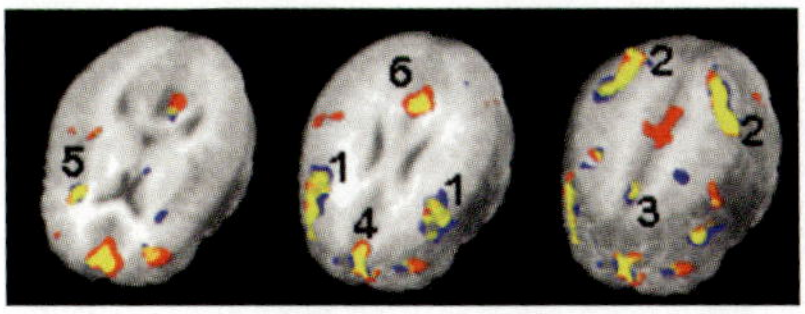

Bilateral ROIs*	Center Coordinates		
	x	y	z
1) Dorsolateral prefrontal	±40	16	31
2) Posterior parietal	±35	–47	44
3) Supplementary motor area	±02	18	47
4) Medial prefrontal gyrus	±04	56	07
5) Insula	±34	0	13
6) Posterior cingulate gyrus	±05	–49	19

*ROIs based on[32]

Figure 13-1 *A priori* regions of interest related to verbal working memory.

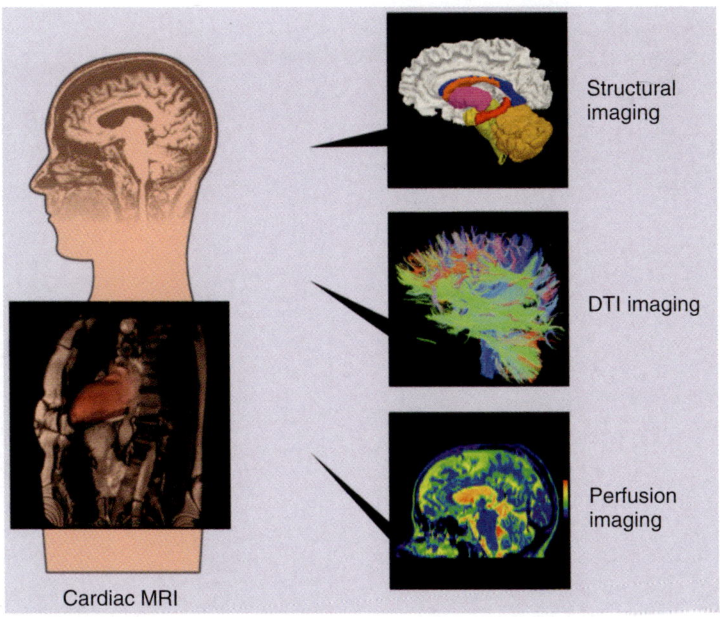

Figure 18-4 The combination of different imaging modalities should greatly enhance pathological specificity.

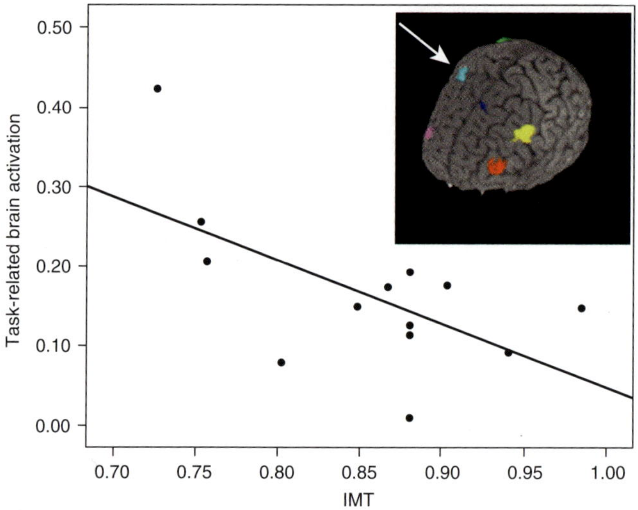

Figure 19-2 BOLD response to a verbal working memory challenge among cardiovascular disease patients as a function of atherosclerosis (inta-media thickness).

cerebral flow velocity,[90] suggesting no sympathetically mediate cerebral vasoconstriction. Similarly ganglionic blockade[91, 92] and sympathoexcitation using lower-body negative pressure[93] did not change the response of subjects to CO_2 or improve their cerebral blood flow response. Interruption of the sympathetic pathway through stellate ganglion block caused a reduction in cerebral flow velocity without a change in pressure, suggesting a cerebral vasoconstriction rather than a vasodilation as would be expected if sympathetic vasoconstriction were interrupted.[94] Similarly, spinal cord–injured patients with cervical lesions that should have had interrupted sympathetic pathways through the stellate ganglia demonstrated similar decreases in cerebral flow velocity to those of controls with intact pathways.[16, 95] Finally, direct infusions of norepinephrine in both anesthetised[96] and conscious patients[97, 98] have not been shown to affect cerebral blood flow or vascular resistance. Therefore, the role of sympathetic activation on cerebrovascular tone is as yet unclear.

If direct sympathetic vasoconstriction is not responsible, other mechanisms may be involved in the age-related decline in cerebral blood flow. In animals, infusion of adenosine, a vasodilator, has been found to produce an attenuated vasodilatory response in aged rats.[99] Similarly, endothelium-dependent vasodilation is attenuated in aged animals.[100–102] In addition, cholinergic vasodilator systems are impaired in older rats.[103, 104] In contrast, application of a high dose of intravascular serotonin, a dose dependent vasoconstrictor, produced augmented vasoconstriction in aged rats.[105] These data suggest that in older animals, vasoconstrictor stimuli may dominate. Extrapolating these mechanisms to aged humans may prove difficult, since there appear to be inherent differences in the cerebrovascular systems of aged animals and humans. For example, as mentioned previously, myogenic tone remains intact with age in isolated human pial arteries,[71] but is reduced in older rat cerebral arteries, reducing their ability to dilate or constrict in response to pressure changes.[100]

Finally, aging is associated with a general cerebral atrophy that includes the loss of gray matter.[54] Thus, reductions in cerebral blood flow may just be the result of reduced metabolic demand due to the reduced volume of neural tissue. Yoshii et al.[106] found that age-related reductions in global cerebral metabolic rate were eliminated when metabolic rate was normalized to brain volume. However, use of advanced imaging techniques over the last decade suggest that reductions in cerebral metabolic rate with aging, especially in the frontal lobes, are independent of brain atrophy.[54]

While current data do not provide a clear mechanism for the reduction in cerebral blood flow with aging, the fact that older individuals have reduced cerebral blood flow but are still able to attenuate fluctuations in pressure (i.e., cerebral autoregulation is intact) suggests that a rightward shift in the cerebral autoregulation curve is not involved. Regardless of the mechanism, it is possible that reductions in cerebral blood flow with aging may result in chronic hypoperfusion and ischemic damage to watershed areas, particularly in frontal subcortical regions. For example, older adults have a high prevalence of orthostatic and postprandial hypotension, which are not only risk factors for falls and syncope, but also threaten cerebral perfusion during everyday activities. In fact, older adults demonstrate a paradoxical cerebral vasoconstriction during postprandial hypotension, which probably threatens cerebral perfusion.[107] With near-infrared spectroscopy, it has been shown that healthy older adults frequently develop decreased cortical oxygenation levels in the frontal lobes when assuming an upright posture.[108, 109] Since humans spend a majority of their time in the upright posture, these data raise the question of what effect repeated bouts of cerebral hypoperfusion have on cerebral function.

Cerebral Hypoperfusion: Cause or Consequence?

The human frontal lobe is necessary to plan and execute goals, coordinate complex motor functions, make decisions, express creativity, and navigate through complex social situations. Aging is associated with loss of frontal lobe volume, changes in frontal subcortical white matter, and the familiar geriatric syndrome of gait impairment, falls, executive cognitive dysfunction, and depression, which are common manifestations of frontal subcortical dysfunction.[110] The pathogenesis of age-related white matter abnormalities, which are seen with increasing frequency as multifocal as well as diffuse areas of white matter hyperintensity on T2-weighted brain MRIs of older people,[111] is still a matter of rigorous investigation. The strong association of these white matter hyperintensities with cardiovascular risk factors[112, 113] supports a vascular basis for the development of white matter abnormalities and age-related frontal lobe dysfunction. These white matter hyperintensities have been related pathologically to cerebral microangiopathy[111, 114, 115] and clinically to hypoperfusion in affected areas.[116, 117] However, it is not known whether hypoperfusion causes damage to subcortical white matter with the subsequent development of symptoms, or whether hypoperfusion is simply due to loss of brain tissue.

Chronic hypoperfusion in animals has been found to be related to reductions in cerebral metabolism,[118] impaired cognitive function,[118, 119] and white matter degeneration.[120] These data suggest that white matter degeneration caused by cerebrovascular dysfunction may constitute a major determinant of common neurological symptoms in older persons with risk factors for cardiovascular disease.[110]

Evidence Linking Hypoperfusion to Frontal Lobe Dysfunction

The notion that hypoperfusion plays a role in the pathogenesis of white matter abnormalities is supported by xenon contrast CT,[121] and MRI[122] studies showing reduced cerebral blood flow in regions with high concentrations of white matter hyperintensities. Using a new quantitative MR perfusion imaging technique, O'Sullivan et al.[117] have shown reduced cerebral blood flow in white matter, but not gray matter, of older adults with white matter abnormalities. This study also demonstrates a reduction of cerebral blood flow in normal-appearing periventricular white matter in patients with white matter hyperintensities compared with controls, providing evidence that hypoperfusion may precede the appearance of new lesions on T2-weighted images.

Further evidence linking hypoperfusion to frontal lobe dysfunction comes from a limited, but emerging, set of data, which shows that abnormalities of blood pressure regulation may lead to perfusion abnormalities in the frontal lobes and contribute to functional frontal-subcortical deficits. With near-infrared spectroscopy, it was shown that healthy elderly persons frequently develop decreased cortical oxygenation levels in the frontal lobes when assuming an upright posture, even in the absence of clinical symptoms of orthostasis.[108] Both orthostatic hypotension and postprandial hypotension are associated with cognitive abnormalities and white matter hyperintensities.[123–125] Since the subcortical white matter is supplied by terminal vessels with scarce anastamoses, it is a "watershed" region in the cerebral circulation, and thus it is particularly vulnerable to ischemic injury during periods of hypotension.[126] Increased blood-pressure variability is also associated with white matter hyperintensities of the brain.[127, 128] In Binswanger's disease patients with diffuse white matter abnormalities, Tohgi et al.[129] reported greater 24-hour systolic blood-pressure standard deviations, and a larger difference between the maximum and minimum systolic blood pressure compared to normal controls. While it is not known whether frequent daily pressure declines in older patients increase the risk of developing white matter abnormalities and their clinical consequences, there is some evidence that lower standing blood pressure increases the risk of falls during one year of follow-up among community-dwelling adults over age 65.[130] In a nursing home population, we have found that increased orthostatic blood pressure variability is a risk factor for stroke.[131]

These data suggest that elderly subjects with white matter abnormalities may have impaired frontal blood flow regulation, resulting in repeated hypoperfusion during periods of hypotension. Previous work demonstrating intact cerebral autoregulation in healthy elderly subjects has examined flow velocity in the middle cerebral artery, which primarily feeds the temporal and parietal cortex.[31, 33] It is possible that abnormal regulation to the frontal lobes was present but undetected. Further work is necessary to examine cerebral autoregulation in the frontal lobes of these individuals.

Summary

Aging is associated with a number of physiological changes that affect cerebral blood flow and possibly cerebrovascular blood flow regulation. These changes may result in both global reductions in cerebral blood flow and regional cerebral hypoperfusion in the frontal lobes. Sustained or intermittent cerebral hypoperfusion could be involved in the development of subcortical and periventricular white matter abnormalities. Atrophy of the frontal lobes may be responsible for impairment of executive function in elderly individuals and may underlie the development of vascular dementia. Future work needs to focus prospectively on age-related structural and functional changes in the brain, and how they may lead to common geriatric symptoms affecting cognition.

Notes

1. Lassen NA. Cerebral blood flow and oxygen consumption in man. *Physiol Rev*. 1959;39(2): 183–238.

2. Paulson OB, Strandgaard S, Edvinsson L. Cerebral autoregulation. *Cerebrovasc Brain Metab Rev*. 1990;2(2):161–192.
3. Gur RC, et al. Effects of memory processing on regional brain activation: Cerebral blood flow in normal subjects. *Int J Neurosci*. 1993;72(1–2):31–44.
4. Perani D, et al. PET studies of cognitive functions: A review. *J Nucl Biol Med*. 1992;36(4): 324–336.
5. Ramsay SC, et al. Regional cerebral blood flow during volitional expiration in man: A comparison with volitional inspiration. 1993;461:101.
6. Nunn J, Hodges H. Cognitive deficits induced by global cerebral ischemia: Relationship to brain damage and reversal by transplants. *Behav Brain Res*. 1994;65(1):1–31.
7. Goadsby PJ, Lambert GA. Electrical stimulation of the fastigial nucleus increases total cerebral blood flow in the monkey. *Neurosci Lett*. 1989;107(1–3):141–144.
8. McKee JC, Denn MJ, Stone HL. Neurogenic cerebral vasodilation from electrical stimulation of the cerebellum in the monkey. *Stroke*. 1976;7(2):179–186.
9. Toda N, et al. Cerebral vasodilatation induced by stimulation of the pterygopalatine ganglion and greater petrosal nerve in anesthetized monkeys. *Neuroscience*. 2000;96(2):393–398.
10. Keunen RW, et al. Chronic cerebral hypotension induces a downward shift of the cerebral autoregulation: A hypothesis based on TCD and OPG-GEE studies in ambulatory patients with occlusive cerebrovascular disease. *Neurol Res*. 1994;16(6):413–416.
11. Novak V, et al. Autoregulation of cerebral blood flow in orthostatic hypotension. *Stroke*. 1998;29(1):104–111.
12. Nanda RN, et al. Cerebral blood flow in paraplegia. *Paraplegia*. 1974;12(3):212–218.
13. Sandor, P. Nervous control of the cerebrovascular system: Doubts and facts. *Neurochem Int*. 1999;35(3):237–259.
14. Strandgaard S, Sigurdsson ST. Point:counterpoint: Sympathetic activity does/does not influence cerebral blood flow. Counterpoint: Sympathetic nerve activity does not influence cerebral blood flow. *J Appl Physiol*. 2008;105(4):1366–1367. discussion, 1367–1368.
15. Levine BD, Zhang R. Comments on Point:counterpoint: Sympathetic activity does/does not influence cerebral blood flow. Autonomic control of the cerebral circulation is most important for dynamic cerebral autoregulation. *J Appl Physiol*. 2008;105(4):1369–1373.
16. Houtman S, et al. Changes in cerebral oxygenation and blood flow during LBNP in spinal cord–injured individuals. *J Appl Physiol*. 2001;91(5):2199–2204.
17. Levine BD, et al. Cerebral versus systemic hemodynamics during graded orthostatic stress in humans. *Circulation*. 1994;90(1):298–306.
18. Bondar RL, et al. Simultaneous cerebrovascular and cardiovascular responses during presyncope. *Stroke*. 1995;26(10):1794–1800.
19. Zhang R, et al. Transfer function analysis of dynamic cerebral autoregulation in humans. *Am J Physiol*. 1998;274(1 Pt 2):H233–H241.
20. Carey BJ, et al. Cerebral autoregulatory responses to head-up tilt in normal subjects and patients with recurrent vasovagal syncope. *Circulation*. 2001;104(8):898–902.
21. Zhang R, et al. Autonomic neural control of dynamic cerebral autoregulation in humans. *Circulation*. 2002;106(14):1814–1820.
22. Fog M. Cerebral circulation. I. Reaction of pial arteries to epinephrine by direct application and intravenous injection. *Arch Neurol Psychiatr*. 1939;41:109–118.
23. Eklof B, et al. Persistence of cerebral blood flow autoregulation following chronic bilateral cervical sympathectomy in the monkey. *Acta Physiol Scand*. 1971;82(2):172–176.
24. Waltz AG, Yamaguchi T, Regli F. Regulatory responses of cerebral vasculature after sympathetic denervation. *Am J Physiol*. 1971;221(1):298–302.

25. Serrador JM, et al. Cerebral vasoconstriction precedes orthostatic intolerance after parabolic flight. *Brain Res Bull.* 2000;53(1):113–120.
26. Diehl RR, et al. Cerebrovascular mechanisms in neurocardiogenic syncope with and without postural tachycardia syndrome. *J Auton Nerv Syst.* 1999;76(2–3):159–166.
27. Meyer JS, et al. Effects of alpha adrenergic blockade on autoregulation and chemical vasomotor control of CBF in stroke. *Stroke.* 1973;4(2):187–200.
28. Veglio F, et al. Hypertension and cerebrovascular damage. *Atherosclerosis.* 2009;205(2): 331–341.
29. Waldemar G, et al. Angiotensin converting enzyme inhibition and cerebral blood flow autoregulation in normotensive and hypertensive man. *J Hypertens.* 1989;7(3):229–235.
30. Strandgaard S. Autoregulation of cerebral blood flow in hypertensive patients. The modifying influence of prolonged antihypertensive treatment on the tolerance to acute, drug-induced hypotension. *Circulation.* 1976;53(4):720–727.
31. Lipsitz LA, et al. Dynamic regulation of middle cerebral artery blood flow velocity in aging and hypertension. *Stroke.* 2000;31(8):1897–1903.
32. Narayanan K, et al. Predicting cerebral blood flow response to orthostatic stress from resting dynamics: Effects of healthy aging. *Am J Physiol Regul Integr Comp Physiol.* 2001; 281(3):R716–22.
33. Carey BJ, et al. Dynamic cerebral autoregulation is unaffected by aging. *Stroke.* 2000;31(12):2895–2900.
34. Eames PJ, et al. Cerebral autoregulation indices are unimpaired by hypertension in middle aged and older people. *Am J Hypertens.* 2003;16(9 Pt 1):746–753.
35. Traon AP, et al. Dynamics of cerebral blood flow autoregulation in hypertensive patients. *J Neurol Sci.* 2002;195(2):139–144.
36. Serrador JM, et al. Cerebral pressure-flow relations in hypertensive elderly humans: Transfer gain in different frequency domains. *J Appl Physiol.* 2005;98(1):151–159.
37. Novak V, et al. Altered cerebral vasoregulation in hypertension and stroke. *Neurology.* 2003;60(10):1657–1663.
38. Baumbach GL, Heistad DD. Cerebral circulation in chronic arterial hypertension. [Review] [68 refs]. *Hypertension.* 1988;12(2):89–95.
39. Iadecola C, Davisson RL. Hypertension and cerebrovascular dysfunction. *Cell Metab.* 2008;7(6):476–484.
40. Chrissobolis S, Sobey CG. Recent evidence for an involvement of rho-kinase in cerebral vascular disease. *Stroke.* 2006;37(8):2174–2180.
41. Baumbach GL, MA Hajdu. Mechanics and composition of cerebral arterioles in renal and spontaneously hypertensive rats. *Hypertension.* 1993;21(6 Pt 1):816–826.
42. Lipsitz LA, et al. Antihypertensive therapy increases cerebral blood flow and carotid distensibility in hypertensive elderly subjects. *Hypertension.* 2005;45(2):216–221.
43. Ide K, et al. Effects of the nitric oxide synthase inhibitor L-NMMA on cerebrovascular and cardiovascular responses to hypoxia and hypercapnia in humans. *J Physiol.* 2007; 584(Pt 1):321–332.
44. Dai W, et al. Abnormal regional cerebral blood flow in cognitively normal elderly subjects with hypertension. *Stroke.* 2008;39(2):349–354.
45. Beason-Held LL, et al. Longitudinal changes in cerebral blood flow in the older hypertensive brain. *Stroke.* 2007;38(6):1766–1773.
46. Firbank MJ, et al. Brain atrophy and white matter hyperintensity change in older adults and relationship to blood pressure. Brain atrophy, WMH change and blood pressure. *J Neurol.* 2007;254(6):713–721.

47. Enzinger C, et al. Risk factors for progression of brain atrophy in aging: Six-year follow-up of normal subjects. *Neurology*. 2005;64(10):1704–1711.
48. Goldstein FC, et al. Hypertension and cognitive performance in African Americans with Alzheimer disease. *Neurology*. 2005;64(5):899–901.
49. Rigaud AS, et al. Hypertension and dementia. *Curr Hypertens Rep*. 2001;3(6):454–457.
50. Krejza J, et al. Transcranial color Doppler sonography of basal cerebral arteries in 182 healthy subjects: Age and sex variability and normal reference values for blood flow parameters. *Am J Roentgenol*. 1999;172(1):213–218.
51. Marchal G, et al. Regional cerebral oxygen consumption, blood flow, and blood volume in healthy human aging. *Arch Neurol*. 1992;49(10):1013–1020.
52. Catafau AM, et al. Regional cerebral blood flow pattern in normal young and aged volunteers: A 99mTc-HMPAO SPET study. *Eur J Nucl Med*. 1996;23(10):1329–1337.
53. Krausz Y, et al. Age-related changes in brain perfusion of normal subjects detected by 99mTc-HMPAO SPECT. *Neuroradiology*. 1998;40(7):428–434.
54. Nobler MS, Mann JJ, Sackeim HA. Serotonin, cerebral blood flow, and cerebral metabolic rate in geriatric major depression and normal aging. *Brain Res Rev*. 1999;30(3):250–263.
55. Schultz SK, et al. Age-related changes in regional cerebral blood flow among young to mid-life adults. *Neuroreport*. 1999;10(12):2493–2496.
56. Stoquart-ElSankari S, et al. Aging effects on cerebral blood and cerebrospinal fluid flows. *J Cereb Blood Flow Metab*. 2007;27(9):1563–1572.
57. Lipsitz LA. Orthostatic hypotension in the elderly. *N Engl J Med*. 1989;321(14):952–957.
58. Lipsitz LA, et al. Reduced susceptibility to syncope during postural tilt in old age. Is beta-blockade protective? 1989;149(12):2709–2712.
59. Seals DR, Esler MD. Human aging and the sympathoadrenal system. *J Physiol*. 2000; 528(Pt 3):407–417.
60. Larsen FS, et al. Transcranial Doppler is valid for determination of the lower limit of cerebral blood flow autoregulation. *Stroke*. 1994;25(10):1985–1988.
61. Hoffman WE, Miletich DJ, Albrecht RF. The influence of antihypertensive therapy on cerebral autoregulation in aged hypertensive rats. *Stroke*. 1982;13(5):701–704.
62. Hoffman WE, Albrecht RF, Miletich DJ, The influence of aging and hypertension on cerebral autoregulation. *Brain Res*. 1981;214(1):196–199.
63. Fujishima M, et al. Autoregulation of cerebral blood flow in young and aged spontaneously hypertensive rats (SHR). *Gerontology*. 1984;30(1):30–36.
64. Toyoda K, et al. Effect of aging on regulation of brain stem circulation during hypotension. *J Cereb Blood Flow Metab*. 1997;17(6):680–685.
65. Kastrup A, et al. Changes of cerebrovascular C02 reactivity during normal aging. *Stroke*. 1998;29(7):1311–1314.
66. Ito H, et al. Effect of aging on cerebral vascular response to Pac02 changes in humans as measured by positron emission tomography. *J Cereb Blood Flow Metab*. 2002;22(8): 997–1003.
67. Lartaud I, et al. *In vivo* cerebrovascular reactivity in Wistar and Fischer 344 rat strains during aging. *Am J Physiol*. 1993;264(3 Pt 2):H851–H858.
68. Matteis M, et al. Age and sex differences in cerebral hemodynamics: A transcranial Doppler study. *Stroke*. 1998;29(5):963–967.
69. Oblak JP, et al. The effect of age on cerebrovascular reactivity to cold pressor test and head-up tilt. *Acta Neurol Scand*. 2002;106(1):30–33.
70. Bakker SL, et al. Cerebral hemodynamics in the elderly: The Rotterdam Study. *Neuroepidemiology*. 2004;23(4):178–184.

71. Thorin-Trescases N, et al. Diameter dependence of myogenic tone of human pial arteries. Possible relation to distensibility. *Stroke*. 1997;28(12):2486–2492.
72. Fisher JP, et al. Regulation of middle cerebral artery blood velocity during dynamic exercise in humans: Influence of aging. *J Appl Physiol*. 2008;105(1):266–273.
73. Lewis PM, et al. Slow oscillations in middle cerebral artery cerebral blood flow velocity and aging. *Neurol Res*. 2007;29(3):260–263.
74. Yam AT, et al. Cerebral autoregulation and aging. *J Clin Neurosci*. 2005;12(6):643–646.
75. Carey BJ, Panerai RB, Potter JF, Effect of aging on dynamic cerebral autoregulation during head-up tilt. *Stroke*. 2003;34(8):1871–1875.
76. Sorond FA, et al. Regional cerebral autoregulation during orthostatic stress: Age-related differences. *J Gerontol A Biol Sci Med Sci*. 2005;60(11):1484–1487.
77. Umeyama T, et al. Changes in cerebral blood flow estimated after stellate ganglion block by single photon emission computed tomography. *J Auton Nerv Syst*. 1995;50(3):339–346.
78. Nitahara K, Dan K. Blood flow velocity changes in carotid and vertebral arteries with stellate ganglion block: Measurement by magnetic resonance imaging using a direct bolus tracking method. *Reg Anesth Pain Med*. 1998;23(6):600–604.
79. Wahlgren NG, et al. Sympathetic nerve stimulation in humans increases middle cerebral artery blood flow velocity. *Cerebrovasc Dis*. 1992;2(6):359–364.
80. Strebel S, et al. Dynamic and static cerebral autoregulation during isoflurane, desflurane, and propofol anesthesia. *Anesthesiology*. 1995;83(1):66–76.
81. Strebel S, et al. Nitrous oxide is a potent cerebrovasodilator in humans when added to isoflurane. A transcranial Doppler study. *Acta Anaesthesiol Scand*. 1995;39(5):653–658.
82. Goadsby PJ, Duckworth JW. Low frequency stimulation of the locus coeruleus reduces regional cerebral blood flow in the spinalized cat. *Brain Res*. 1989;476(1):71–77.
83. Serrador JM, et al. MRI measures of middle cerebral artery diameter in conscious humans during simulated orthostasis. *Stroke*. 2000;31(7):1672–1678.
84. Bramanti P, et al. The first in vivo experience of the effects of the continuous intrathecal infusion of clonidine on the locus coeruleus in the regulation of cerebral blood flow: A TCD study. *Ital J Neurol Sci*. 1997;18(3):139–144.
85. Micieli G, et al. Intracerebral vascular changes induced by cold pressor test: A model of sympathetic activation. *Neurol Res*. 1994;16(3):163–167.
86. Jordan J, et al. Raised cerebrovascular resistance in idiopathic orthostatic intolerance: Evidence for sympathetic vasoconstriction. *Hypertension*. 1998;32(4):699–704.
87. Lee HW, et al. The effect of clonidine on cerebral blood flow velocity, carbon dioxide cerebral vasoreactivity, and response to increased arterial pressure in human volunteers. *Anesthesiology*. 1997;87(3):553–558.
88. Brown CM, Sanya EO, Hilz MJ. Effect of cold face stimulation on cerebral blood flow in humans. *Brain Res Bull*. 2003;61(1):81–86.
89. Durand S, et al. Skin surface cooling improves orthostatic tolerance in normothermic individuals. *Am J Physiol Regul Integr Comp Physiol*. 2004;286(1):R199–205.
90. Ainslie PN, et al. Differential responses to C02 and sympathetic stimulation in the cerebral and femoral circulations in humans. *J Physiol*. 2005;566(Pt 2):613–624.
91. Przybylowski T, et al. Mechanisms of the cerebrovascular response to apnea in humans. *J Physiol*. 2003;548(Pt 1):323–332.
92. Zhang R, Levine BD. Autonomic ganglionic blockade does not prevent reduction in cerebral blood flow velocity during orthostasis in humans. *Stroke*. 2007;38(4):1238–1244.
93. LeMarbre G, et al. Baroreflex-induced sympathetic activation does not alter cerebrovascular CO_2 responsiveness in humans. *J Physiol*. 2003;551(Pt 2):609–616.

94. Gupta MM, et al. Effects of stellate ganglion block on cerebral haemodynamics as assessed by transcranial Doppler ultrasonography. *Br J Anaesth*. 2005;95(5):669–673.
95. Handrakis JP, et al. Effect of hypotensive challenge on systemic hemodynamics and cerebral blood flow in persons with tetraplegia. *Clin Auton Res*. 2009;19(1):39–45.
96. Strebel SP, et al. The impact of systemic vasoconstrictors on the cerebral circulation of anesthetized patients. *Anesthesiology*. 1998;89(1):67–72.
97. Olesen J. The effect of intracarotid epinephrine, norepinephrine, and angiotensin on the regional cerebral blood flow in man. *Neurology*. 1972;22(9):978–987.
98. Kimmerly DS, et al, Circulating norepinephrine and cerebrovascular control in conscious humans. *Clin Physiol Funct Imaging*. 2003;23(6):314–319.
99. Jiang HX, et al. Age related alterations in the response of the pial arterioles to adenosine in the rat. *Mech Aging Dev*. 1992;65(2–3):257–276.
100. Geary GG, Buchholz JN. Selected contribution: Effects of aging on cerebrovascular tone and[Ca2+]i. *J Appl Physiol*. 2003;95(4):1746–1754.
101. Geary GG, Buchholz JN, Pearce WJ. Maturation depresses mouse cerebrovascular tone through endothelium-dependent mechanisms. *Am J Physiol Regul Integr Comp Physiol*. 2003;284(3):R734–41.
102. Mayhan WG, et al., Age-related alterations in reactivity of cerebral arterioles: Role of oxidative stress. *Microcirculation*. 2008;15(3):225–236.
103. Sato A, Sato Y, Uchida S. Regulation of cerebral cortical blood flow by the basal forebrain cholinergic fibers and aging. *Auton Neurosci*. 2002;96(1):13–19.
104. Uchida S, et al. Effects of age on cholinergic vasodilation of cortical cerebral blood vessels in rats. *Neurosci Lett*. 2000;294(2):109–112.
105. Hajdu MA, et al. Effects of aging on cerebral vascular responses to serotonin in rats. *Am J Physiol*. 1993;264(6 Pt 2):H2136–H2140.
106. Yoshii F, et al. Sensitivity of cerebral glucose metabolism to age, gender, brain volume, brain atrophy, and cerebrovascular risk factors. *J Cereb Blood Flow Metab*. 1988;8(5): 654–661.
107. Krajewski A, et al. Transcranial Doppler assessment of the cerebral circulation during postprandial hypotension in the elderly. *J Am Geriatr Soc*. 1993;41(1):19–24.
108. Mehagnoul-Schipper DJ, et al. Cerebral oxygenation declines in healthy elderly subjects in response to assuming the upright position. *Stroke*. 2000;31(7):1615–1620.
109. Mehagnoul-Schipper DJ, Colier WN, and Jansen RW. Reproducibility of orthostatic changes in cerebral oxygenation in healthy subjects aged 70 years or older. *Clin Physiol*. 2001;21(1):77–84.
110. Geroldi C, et al. Mild cognitive deterioration with subcortical features: prevalence, clinical characteristics, and association with cardiovascular risk factors in community-dwelling older persons (The InCHIANTI Study). *J Am Geriatr Soc*. 2003;51(8):1064–1071.
111. van Swieten JC, et al., Periventricular lesions in the white matter on magnetic resonance imaging in the elderly. A morphometric correlation with arteriolosclerosis and dilated perivascular spaces. *Brain*. 1991;114 (Pt 2):761–774.
112. Pantoni L, Garcia JH. Cognitive impairment and cellular/vascular changes in the cerebral white matter. *Ann N Y Acad Sci*. 1997;826:92–102.
113. Yamauchi H, et al. Brain arteriolosclerosis and hemodynamic disturbance may induce leukoaraiosis. *Neurology*. 1999;53(8):1833–1838.
114. Takao M, et al. Pathologic findings of silent hyperintense white matter lesions on MRI. *J Neurol Sci*. 1999;167(2):127–131.
115. Fazekas F, Schmidt R, Scheltens P. Pathophysiologic mechanisms in the development of age-related white matter changes of the brain. *Dement Geriatr Cogn Disord*. 1998;9 (Suppl 1):2–5.

116. Meyer JS, et al. Risk factors for cerebral hypoperfusion, mild cognitive impairment, and dementia. *Neurobiol Aging*. 2000;21(2):161–169.
117. O'Sullivan M, et al. Patterns of cerebral blood flow reduction in patients with ischemic leukoaraiosis. *Neurology*. 2002;59(3):321–326.
118. Cada A, de la Torre JC, Gonzalez-Lima F. Chronic cerebrovascular ischemia in aged rats: Effects on brain metabolic capacity and behavior. *Neurobiol Aging*. 2000;21(2):225–233.
119. Sopala M, Danysz W. Chronic cerebral hypoperfusion in the rat enhances age-related deficits in spatial memory. *J Neural Transm*. 2001;108(12):1445–1456.
120. Tomimoto H, et al. Chronic cerebral hypoperfusion induces white matter lesions and loss of oligodendroglia with DNA fragmentation in the rat. *Acta Neuropathol* (Berl). 2003;106(6):527–534.
121. Miyazawa N, et al. Xenon contrast CT-CBF measurements in high-intensity foci on T2-weighted MR images in centrum semiovale of asymptomatic individuals. *Stroke*. 1997; 28(5):984–987.
122. Hatazawa J, et al. Subcortical hypoperfusion associated with asymptomatic white matter lesions on magnetic resonance imaging. *Stroke*. 1997;28(10):1944–1947.
123. Perlmuter LC, Greenberg JJ. Do you mind standing? Cognitive changes in orthostasis. *Exp Aging Res*. 1996;22(4):325–341.
124. Matsubayashi K, et al. Postural dysregulation in systolic blood pressure is associated with worsened scoring on neurobehavioral function tests and leukoaraiosis in the older elderly living in a community. *Stroke*. 1997;28(11):2169–2173.
125. Kohara K, et al. Postprandial hypotension is associated with asymptomatic cerebrovascular damage in essential hypertensive patients. *Hypertension*. 1999;33(1 Pt 2):565–568.
126. De Reuck J. The human periventricular arterial blood supply and the anatomy of cerebral infarctions. *Eur Neurol*. 1971;5(6):321–334.
127. Raiha I, et al. Relationship between vascular factors and white matter low attenuation of the brain. *Acta Neurol Scand*. 1993;87(4):286–289.
128. Puisieux F, et al. Relationship between leuko-araiosis and blood pressure variability in the elderly. *Eur Neurol*. 2001;46(3):115–120.
129. Tohgi H, Chiba K, Kimura M. Twenty-four-hour variation of blood pressure in vascular dementia of the Binswanger type. *Stroke*. 1991;22(5):603–608.
130. Kario K, et al. Lower standing systolic blood pressure as a predictor of falls in the elderly: A community-based prospective study. *J Am Coll Cardiol*. 2001;38(1):246–252.
131. Hossain M, Ooi WL, Lipsitz LA. Intra-individual postural blood pressure variability and stroke in elderly nursing home residents. *J Clin Epidemiol*. 2001;54(5):488–494.

16

MEASUREMENT OF ARTERIAL FUNCTION AND REACTIVITY

Brian E. Hunt

Vascular dementia (VaD) occurs as a consequence of cerebrovascular disease resulting in hemorrhage and hypoperfusion, ultimately leading to neurodegeneration.[1] It's not surprising that the modifiable risk factors for VaD closely parallel those for cardiovascular disease: hypertension, type 2 diabetes, hyperlipidemia, smoking, ischemic heart disease, peripheral vascular disease, and white matter lesions.[2–4] As these risk factors are not isolated to the cerebral vasculature, it is reasonable to presume the vascular dysfunction seen in VaD is not isolated to the cerebral vasculature. Therefore, measurements of peripheral vascular function can provide insight into the etiology of, and vascular mechanisms underlying, VaD. Numerous techniques and indices have been developed to characterize the mechanical properties of the arterial tree (Table 16-1). This chapter will discuss the methodology, advantages, issues, and recommendations for many of the most common approaches available to the physician and physiologist when characterizing arterial function in humans.

Table 16-1

Index (international units)	Equation
Arterial Compliance (cm^2/dyne)	(Ds – Dd)/(Ps – Pd)
Arterial Distensibility (cm^3/dyne)	(Ds – Dd)/(Ps – Pd)Dd
B-Stiffness Index (non-dimensional)	(Dd ln(Ps/Pd))/(Ds – Dd)
Peterson's E lastic Modulus (dyne/cm^2)	((Ps – Pd)Dd)/(Ds – Dd)
Young's Elastic Modulus (dyne/cm)	((Ps – Pd)Dd)/(Ds – Dd)h
Pulse Wave Velocity (cm/sec)	(z1 – z2)/(t1 – t2)

Ds (systolic diameter), Dd (diastolic diameter), Ps (systolic blood pressure), Pd (diastolic blood pressure), z1 – z2 (distance between measurement sites), t1 – t2 (difference in time betwe en arrival of pressure wave at different measurement sites)

Arterial Compliance and Distensibility

The most basic index of arterial wall function is that of arterial compliance. *Compliance* is defined as the change in arterial volume for a given change in arterial pressure. In practice, changes in diameter are used rather than those of volume because the volume of a cylinder is proportional to its diameter. In humans, vessel diameters are determined using ultrasonography, while arterial pressures are often measured in the brachial[5–7] or radial artery,[8] or the finger.[6, 9] The advantage of arterial compliance is that it is relatively simple to measure. However, there are several issues that must be considered when using this index of arterial mechanical function.

The arterial wall is composed of both elastin and collagen fibers. At lower arterial pressures and diameters, the resistance to stretch is provided primarily by elastin, whereas at higher pressures collagen begins to bear some of the load.[10] Because elastin is less resistant to stretch than collagen, the pressure–diameter relation is curvilinear. Therefore, if one were to compare arterial compliance between normotensive and hypertensive adults, the lower arterial compliance in the hypertensive individuals may be due in large part to differences in arterial distending pressure rather than inherent differences in arterial wall function. *Arterial distensibility* attempts to account for this fact by normalizing compliance to the initial diameter of the vessel. This has little impact on the non-linearity of the relationship. Therefore, if one uses compliance or distensibility to characterize arterial wall function, comparisons should be made at similar arterial pressures.

The resolution of the ultrasound images should also be considered. For example, the B-mode ultrasound image of the brachial artery shown in Fig. 16-1 has 480 vertical pixels/cm. Thus, the smallest measurement error (± 1 pixel) is equal to 50 μm. As a result, one could have confidence if the change in brachial diameter exceeded 1.7%. For the radial artery, one would have to see a change in diameter of at least 3.1%. As the pulsatile changes in diameter of larger arteries (aorta, carotid, brachial, femoral) typically exceed the maximum resolution of the ultrasound images, this is of minor concern. However, for smaller arteries such as the radial artery, image resolution can introduce significant error into the calculation of compliance or distensibility. Automated software for diameter estimation has been shown to improve the reproducibility of diameter measurements, presumably due to a reduction in measurement error.[11, 12]

When estimating arterial compliance, blood pressure is often measured at a site distal to the measurement of arterial diameters.[6, 9] This may create a problem, because systolic and mean arterial pressure increase as the pressure wave moves from the aorta to the periphery,[13] and compliance or distensibility may be underestimated when using pressure measured in the finger and diameter changes measured in the carotid artery. To complicate matters further, this pulse wave amplification does not occur in older adults,[14] making aging comparisons suspect when compliance or distensibility is estimated in this manner. However, in practice, the use of peripheral pressures may have little impact on compliance estimates. For example, Kevin Monahan and colleagues estimated carotid compliance from changes in carotid diameter and concurrent changes

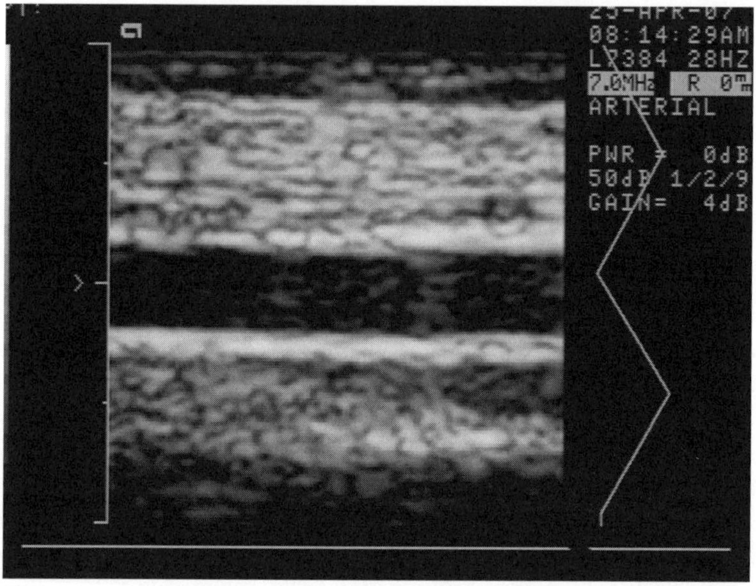

Figure 16-1 Ultrasound (Acuson 128XP) image of the left brachial artery of a 24-year-old male. Arterial diameter is 2.94 mm.

in arterial pressure measured in the contralateral carotid artery using applanation tonometry. These researchers also estimated carotid compliance using concurrent changes in arterial pressure measured in the finger by photoplethysmography (Finapres). When carotid compliance estimates were compared, there were no differences between estimates derived from carotid or finger blood pressures.[15] As a result of the divergent findings regarding the use of peripheral pressures for the estimation of arterial compliance, the best practice is to measure pressure and diameter at the same site. However, when differences in compliance between two groups or conditions exceed what can be explained by pulse wave amplification, peripheral pressures may be of some utility.

Not only is compliance and distensibility non-linear, it differs from vessel to vessel. This is demonstrated in Table 16-2. Therefore, any association between arterial compliance in a single artery and cognitive function does not imply that vascular dysfunction underlies the cognitive decline.

Arterial Stiffness

Arterial stiffness is the inverse of arterial compliance and distensibility. There are several indices of arterial stiffness: the β-stiffness index, Young's and Petersen's elastic modulus, pulse wave velocity, and augmentation index. The β-stiffness index has been proposed to characterize the stiffness of arteries independent of distending pressure,

Table 16-2

Study	Artery	Distensibility (1/mmHg × 10^{-3})
Resnick 1997[48]	Ascending Aorta	7.0
	Descending Aorta	5.1
Laurent 1994[49]	Common Carotid	11.7
	Radial	1.4
Jondeau 1999[50]	Abdominal Aorta	27.7
	Common Carotid	6.9
	Femoral	5.3

thereby eliminating the need to characterize arterial wall function at the same distending pressures. The elastic modulus is another expression of arterial stiffness. The greater the elastic modulus, the stiffer the vessel. Two commonly used expressions are Peterson's elastic modulus and Young's elastic modulus (Table 16-1). The circumferential stress of blood pressure is related to wall thickness. Therefore, Young's modulus may be preferential to other indices of arterial stiffness. As an example, when pressure and arterial dimension data were collected from the same site in the aortas of a four-month-old puppy and a very old dog, the compliance was identical. However, when wall thickness was taken into account, the old dog's artery was revealed to be much stiffer than the puppy's.[16]

All the issues related to the estimation of arterial compliance and distensibility also apply to the measurement of β-stiffness and the elastic modulus. While the β-stiffness index is reported to be linear across a large range of blood pressures, the elastic modulus is curvalinear.[14] Therefore, the elastic modulus should be compared at the same distending pressure. Because β-stiffness index and elastic modulus rely on diameter measurement, the resolution of these measures should be considered. This may be of particular importance when intima-media thickness (IMT) is used as a surrogate for total wall thickness. This is done because the outer boundary of the adventitia can be difficult to discern, whereas the intima-media boundaries can be more easily identified. However, as one can imagine, not only is IMT quite small relative to lumen diameter, but differences between groups are even smaller, often within measurement error bounds. As with compliance and distensibility, the use of blood pressure measured at sites distal to the diameter measurement may confound these estimates of arterial stiffness. Finally, measurements of stiffness can vary substantially from artery to artery within an individual or population.[17]

The mechanical properties of the arterial wall play a central role in determining the rate at which the pulse wave is propagated along the arterial tree. That is, the stiffer the vessel wall, the faster the pressure wave will move through the vessel. In fact, pulse wave velocity (PWV) is directly related to Young's elastic modulus,

$$PWV = \text{sqrt } Ey \,.\, h/2r \,.\, \rho$$

where Ey is Young's modulus, h is arterial wall thickness, r is the lumen radius, and ρ is the density of the blood.[18] Therefore, the greater the PWV, the greater the arterial stiffness. Pulse wave velocity can be calculated by measuring the time delay between the arrival of a pressure wave at two different sites along the arterial tree or by measuring the time of wave propagation at a single point along the arterial tree. The two-site method is the most common. Applanation tonometry can be used to simultaneously measure the arrival of the same pulse wave at two different sites. For example, Fig. 16-2 depicts the pressure wave in the common carotid artery and femoral artery. The foot of the pressure wave is identified at each site, and the time difference is calculated. The distance that the pulse wave traveled is estimated by measuring the linear distance between measurement sites using a simple measuring tape. Pulse wave velocity is simply derived from the distance and time.

To eliminate some of the problems with the two-site method (inaccurate estimation of distance), the PWV can be estimated from the characteristics of a single pulse wave

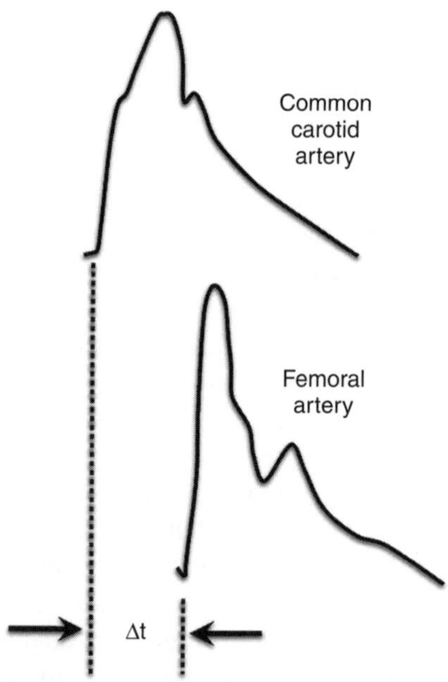

Figure 16-2 Schematic diagram of pressure waveforms from the carotid and femoral arteries. Waveforms can be obtained simultaneously by using two applanation tonometers, or sequentially by using a single tonometer and gating to the ECG. Pulse wave velocity is determined by dividing the distance traveled (estimated as the linear distance between the carotid and femoral arteries) by ΔT.

at a specific site.[19–21] This approach simply estimates the time it takes for the pulse wave to travel past a single point, eliminating the need to estimate the distance the pulse wave travels. As shown in Fig. 16-3, pulse wave velocity, or more accurately, pulse wave transit time, can be estimated as the time difference between the foot of the pressure wave and the reflected wave or dichrotic notch. While the measurement of PWV is non-invasive, relatively simple to perform, and eliminates many of the issues related to other methods discussed above, there are a few issues that must be considered when using this approach.

Pulse wave velocity is affected by any factor that can influence blood pressure. like the elastic modulus, PWV is dependent on distending pressure. Therefore, PWV should be given for a specific mean arterial pressure and diameter.[18] When this is done, apparent differences can disappear.[22] Also, heart rate may affect PWV, though this is greatly debated.[23–26] Another issue is that of the identification of the pressure wave-front or "foot" of the pressure wave. The foot of the pressure wave is defined as the point at the end of diastole when the steep rise of the wave-front begins.[14] While the foot of the pressure wave is rather easily identified visually, reproducible identification is important, given that the delay time between the aorta and carotid artery may be only a few milliseconds. Several approaches have been used. Extrapolating the early portion of the

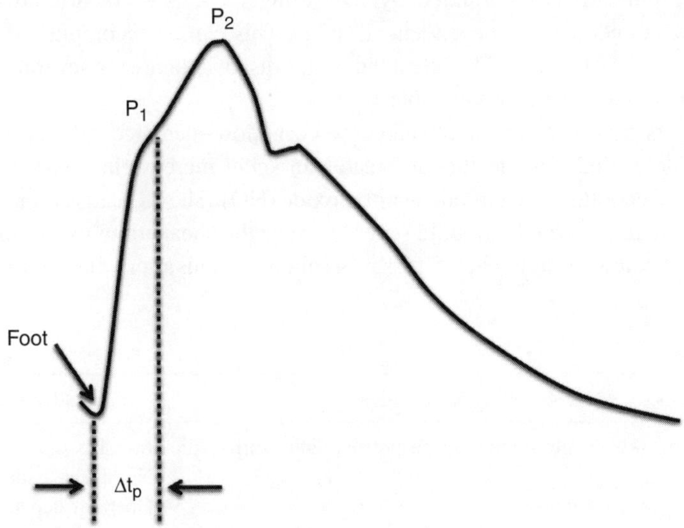

Figure 16-3 Schematic diagram of a pressure waveform from the common carotid artery. P_1 is the inflection point that indicates the beginning of the reflected pressure wave. P_2 is peak systolic pressure. Δt_p represents the time it takes the pressure wave to travel through the periphery and return from major reflecting sites.

pressure wave-front downward and the later portion of the diastolic curve rightward, one can use the intersection of these lines as an estimate of the position of the foot of the wavefront.[27] More recently, the first zero-crossing of the fourth derivative of the pulse wave has been used to identify the foot of the pressure wave.[28] Another method is the use of the time derivative of the pressure wave. The point of maximum rate of rise in pressure occurs in the first half of the wave-front. This portion of the pressure wave is unaffected by distal wave reflection. As such, this point can be used as a reliable reference point on the pulse wave.[29]

There are several commercial devices that can be used to derive PWV. These include the Compilor and SphygmoCor. Each of these devices uses a proprietary algorithm (transfer function) to derive an aortic pulse wave from which one can estimate aortic or "systemic" PWV. However, while the manufacturers claim that the devices have been validated, no such data exist.[30] Thus, any use of these derived aortic waveforms to estimate PWV is suspect.

Endothelial Function

The vascular endothelium is a paracrine organ that produces various molecules that determine vascular tone. Specifically, it has been found that the ability of the endothelium to produce nitric oxide is vital in the modulation of vascular tone.[31] Therefore, vascular endothelial function plays a pivotal role in determining arterial stiffness.[32–37] Endothelial function is determined by measuring the degree of arterial dilation in response to an endothelium-dependent stimulus. This can be accomplished in humans using numerous techniques. The advantages and disadvantages for several of the most common approaches are listed in Table 16-3.

Due to its non-invasive nature and low cost, flow-mediated dilation (FMD) has become widely used. This technique creates an acute increase in shear stress, which stimulates the endothelium to produce nitric oxide (NO). The NO causes smooth-muscle relaxation leading to vasodilation. In order to create the shear stimulus, an inflation cuff is placed just below the ante-cubital fossa. Baseline brachial artery diameter is measured

Table 16-3

Technique	Advantages	Disadvantages
ACh Infusion	– Can determine dose–response relationship	– Invasive – Not nitric-oxide specific
FMD	– Non-invasive – Uses physiological stimulus (shear stress) – Can be specific for endothelial nitric oxide	– Operator-dependent – Possible resolution issues
PWA	– Non-invasive – Can use physiological stimulus (shear stress)	– Not nitric-oxide specific

ACh (acetylcholine), FMD (flow-mediated dilation), PWA (pulse wave analysis: can include changes in pulse wave velocity or changes in wave form morphology–augmentation index)

using ultrasonography, and blood flow velocity is measured using Doppler flowmetry. The cuff is inflated to supra-systolic pressure, typically for five minutes. The resulting ischemia causes dilation of the resistance vessels in the forearm. The cuff is then rapidly deflated, resulting is a brief but profound increase in blood flow. This increased shear stress induces NO production, resulting in vasodilation (Fig. 16-4). Although it is non-invasive and relatively simple, several issues must be considered when using this technique.

Most investigators wish to use FMD in order to selectively assess the ability of the endothelium to produce nitric oxide. Whether the dilation is solely mediated by nitric oxide is a highly debated issue.[38, 39] Several technical aspects appear to be important. First, the position of the inflation cuff is critical. When the cuff is placed distal to the site of diameter measurement and the NO synthase is inhibited, the FMD response is abolished. However, when the cuff is placed proximal to the site of diameter measurement, FMD is reduced only ~33%.[40] Second, the duration of occlusion also determines the mechanisms of the response. When occlusion is limited to five minutes, the FMD response is abolished with NO synthase inhibition. When occlusion time is extended to15 minutes, the FMD is unaffected by NO synthase inhibition.[41] These findings indicate that the FMD response to prolonged shear stress is not NO mediated. Thus, if one wishes to use FMD as a tool to

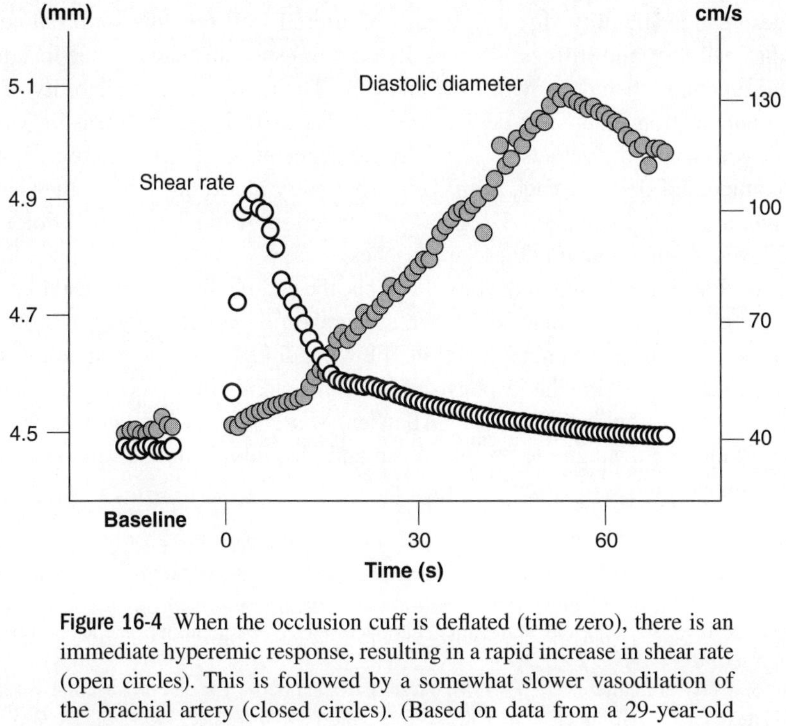

Figure 16-4 When the occlusion cuff is deflated (time zero), there is an immediate hyperemic response, resulting in a rapid increase in shear rate (open circles). This is followed by a somewhat slower vasodilation of the brachial artery (closed circles). (Based on data from a 29-year-old male.)

investigate NO-mediated vasolidation, occlusion should be limited to five minutes. Third, in FMD the dilation must be normalized to the stimulus, the shear stress. Normalization is typically done by dividing the dilation, relative to baseline diameter, by the peak shear rate. It is interesting to note that peak shear stress occurs within the first several seconds, whereas peak dilation occurs one to two minutes after cuff release. Recently, it has been demonstrated that the total shear stress during dilation accounts for the degree of dilation, rather than peak shear stress.[42] Therefore, one should either divide the relative dilation by total shear during dilation or statistically adjust for differences in total shear through use of Analysis of Covariance.[42,43] Lastly, while FMD may vary from vessel to vessel, peripheral endothelial function correlates with endothelial function in the coronary arteries.[44–46] This indicates that endothelial dysfunction is systemic, and that brachial artery FMD may be indicative of endothelial function in other arteries, such as the carotid, and perhaps the cerebral vasculature.

Summary

In humans it is difficult to assess the nature of the cerebral vascular dysfunction that underlies VaD. However, as the vascular impairment leading to VaD is probably not limited to the cerebral vasculature, one can gain insight into the vascular mechanisms by assessing peripheral vascular function. With the advent of vascular ultrasound and its widespread availability, direct measures of arterial wall function—arterial compliance, distensibility, and stiffness—are easily accomplished and can provide insight into vascular function when done with rigor and care. The more recent availability of commercial applanation tonometry devices now allows us to indirectly measure vascular stiffness within specific vessels or across longer segments of the vasculature. However, these commercial devices, each with their proprietary algorithms, are somewhat of a black-box approach in characterizing vascular function. A modicum of caution should be employed when employing these approaches.

Lastly, that simple lining of the blood vessels, the endothelium, is neither simple, nor does it merely line the vasculature. Rather, as a powerful paracrine organ, it profoundly influences vascular mechanical function. Flow-mediated dilation is a non-invasive approach to characterizing the responsiveness of the endothelium. As this methodology is rather new (first used in the 1980s by Allen and Mark[47]) it is continuously developing. All these tools are available to the physician and physiologist to gain insight into the vascular underpinnings of vascular dementia.

Notes

1. Baskys A, Hou AC. Vascular dementia: Pharmacological treatment approaches and perspectives. *Clin Interv Aging*. 2007;2(3):327–335.
2. Desmond DW, Tatemichi TK, Paik M, Stern Y. Risk factors for cerebrovascular disease as correlates of cognitive function in a stroke-free cohort. *Arch Neurol*. 1993;50(2):162–166.

3. Kalaria RN, Maestre GE, Arizaga R, et al. Alzheimer's disease and vascular dementia in developing countries: Prevalence, management, and risk factors. *Lancet Neurol.* 2008;7(9):812–826.
4. Rockwood K, Ebly E, Hachinski V, Hogan D. Presence and treatment of vascular risk factors in patients with vascular cognitive impairment. *Arch Neurol.* 1997;54(1):33–39.
5. Dijk JM, Algra A, van der Graaf Y, Grobbee DE, Bots ML. Carotid stiffness and the risk of new vascular events in patients with manifest cardiovascular disease. The SMART study. *Eur Heart J.* 2005;26(12):1213–1220.
6. Giannattasio C, Achilli F, Failla M, et al. Radial, carotid and aortic distensibility in congestive heart failure: Effects of high-dose angiotensin-converting enzyme inhibitor or low-dose association with angiotensin type 1 receptor blockade. *J Am Coll Cardiol.* 2002;39(8):1275–1282.
7. Rakobowchuk M, McGowan CL, de Groot PC, et al. Effect of whole body resistance training on arterial compliance in young men. *Exp Physiol.* 2005;90(4):645–651.
8. Haluska BA, Fathi R, Jeffriess L, Leano R, Carlier SG, Marwick TH. Noninvasive tests for arterial structure, function, and compliance: Do they identify risk or diagnose disease? *J Am Soc Echocardiogr.* 2004;17(2):195–202; quiz, 203–194.
9. Myers CW, Farquhar WB, Forman DE, Williams TD, Dierks DL, Taylor JA. Carotid distensibility characterized via the isometric exercise pressor response. *Am J Physiol Heart Circ Physiol.* 2002;283(6):H2592–2598.
10. Roach MR, Burton AC. The reason for the shape of the distensibility curves of arteries. *Can J Biochem Physiol.* 1957;35(8):681–690.
11. Stadler RW, Karl WC, Lees RS. New methods for arterial diameter measurement from B-mode images. *Ultrasound Med Biol.* 1996;22(1):25–34.
12. Woodman RJ, Playford DA, Watts GF, et al. Improved analysis of brachial artery ultrasound using a novel edge-detection software system. *J Appl Physiol.* 2001;91(2):929–937.
13. O'Rourke MF, Blazek JV, Morreels CL, Jr., Krovetz LJ. Pressure wave transmission along the human aorta. Changes with age and in arterial degenerative disease. *Circ Res.* 1968;23(4):567–579.
14. Nichols WW, O'Rourke MF, McDonald DA. *McDonald's blood flow in arteries: Theoretic, experimental, and clinical principles*, 5th ed. London/New York: Hodder Arnold; distributed in the U.S.A. by Oxford University Press, 2005.
15. Monahan KD, Tanaka H, Dinenno FA, Seals DR. Central arterial compliance is associated with age- and habitual-exercise-related differences in cardiovagal baroreflex sensitivity. *Circulation.* 2001;104(14):1627–1632.
16. Peterson LH, Jensen RE, Parnell J. Mechanical properties of arteries in vivo. *Circ Res.* 1960;8:17.
17. O'Rourke MF, Staessen JA, Vlachopoulos C, Duprez D, Plante GE. Clinical applications of arterial stiffness; Definitions and reference values. *Am J Hypertens.* 2002;15(5):426–444.
18. O'Rourke M. Arterial stiffness, systolic blood pressure, and logical treatment of arterial hypertension. *Hypertension.* 1990;15(4):339–347.
19. Harada A, Okada T, Niki K, Chang D, Sugawara M. On-line noninvasive one-point measurements of pulse wave velocity. *Heart Vessels.* 2002;17(2):61–68.
20. Marchais SJ, Guerin AP, Pannier BM, Levy BI, Safar ME, London GM. Wave reflections and cardiac hypertrophy in chronic uremia. Influence of body size. *Hypertension.* 1993;22(6):876–883.
21. Murgo JP, Westerhof N, Giolma JP, Altobelli SA. Aortic input impedance in normal man: Relationship to pressure wave forms. *Circulation.* 1980;62(1):105–116.

22. Gribbin B, Pickering TG, Sleight P. Arterial distensibility in normal and hypertensive man. *Clin Sci (Lond)*. 1979;56(5):413–417.
23. Albaladejo P, Copie X, Boutouyrie P, et al. Heart rate, arterial stiffness, and wave reflections in paced patients. *Hypertension*. 2001;38(4):949–952.
24. Haesler E, Lyon X, Pruvot E, Kappenberger L, Hayoz D. Confounding effects of heart rate on pulse wave velocity in paced patients with a low degree of atherosclerosis. *J Hypertens*. 2004;22(7):1317–1322.
25. Liang YL, Gatzka CD, Du XJ, Cameron JD, Kingwell BA, Dart AM. Effects of heart rate on arterial compliance in men. *Clin Exp Pharmacol Physiol*. 1999;26(4):342–346.
26. O'Rourke MF, Hayward CS. Arterial stiffness, gender and heart rate. *J Hypertens*. 2003;21(3):487–490.
27. Laszt L, Muller A. [Comparison of pressure-relationship of blood vessels of the neck and upper extremities with the pressure of aorta ascendens.]. *Helv Physiol Pharmacol Acta*. 1952;10(4):469–481.
28. Kelly R, Hayward C, Avolio A, O'Rourke M. Noninvasive determination of age-related changes in the human arterial pulse. *Circulation*. 1989;80(6):1652–1659.
29. Patel DJ, Janicki JS, Carew TE. Static anisotropic elastic properties of the aorta in living dogs. *Circ Res*. 1969;25(6):765–779.
30. Lehmann ED. Citation of "validation" references for sphygmocor-based estimates of central aortic blood pressure. *J Clin Endocrinol Metab*. 2001;86(4):1844–1845.
31. Furchgott RF, Zawadzki JV. The obligatory role of endothelial cells in the relaxation of arterial smooth muscle by acetylcholine. *Nature*. 1980;288(5789):373–376.
32. Boutouyrie P, Bezie Y, Lacolley P, et al. In vivo/in vitro comparison of rat abdominal aorta wall viscosity. Influence of endothelial function. *Arterioscler Thromb Vasc Biol*. 1997;17(7):1346–1355.
33. Ceravolo R, Maio R, Pujia A, et al. Pulse pressure and endothelial dysfunction in never-treated hypertensive patients. *J Am Coll Cardiol*. 2003;41(10):1753–1758.
34. Ichigi Y, Takano H, Umetani K, et al. Increased ambulatory pulse pressure is a strong risk factor for coronary endothelial vasomotor dysfunction. *J Am Coll Cardiol*. 2005;45(9):1461–1466.
35. McEniery CM, Wallace S, Mackenzie IS, et al. Endothelial function is associated with pulse pressure, pulse wave velocity, and augmentation index in healthy humans. *Hypertension*. 2006;48(4):602–608.
36. Schmitt M, Avolio A, Qasem A, et al. Basal NO locally modulates human iliac artery function in vivo. *Hypertension*. 2005;46(1):227–231.
37. Wilkinson IB, Qasem A, McEniery CM, Webb DJ, Avolio AP, Cockcroft JR. Nitric oxide regulates local arterial distensibility in vivo. *Circulation*. 2002;105(2):213–217.
38. Green D. Point: Flow-mediated dilation does reflect nitric oxide-mediated endothelial function. *J Appl Physiol*. 2005;99(3):1233–1234; discussion, 1237–1238.
39. Tschakovsky ME, Pyke KE. Counterpoint: Flow-mediated dilation does not reflect nitric oxide-mediated endothelial function. *J Appl Physiol*. Sep 2005;99(3):1235–1237; discussion, 1237–1238.
40. Doshi SN, Naka KK, Payne N, et al. Flow-mediated dilatation following wrist and upper arm occlusion in humans: The contribution of nitric oxide. *Clin Sci (Lond)*. 2001;101(6): 629–635.
41. Mullen MJ, Kharbanda RK, Cross J, et al. Heterogenous nature of flow-mediated dilatation in human conduit arteries in vivo: Relevance to endothelial dysfunction in hypercholesterolemia. *Circ Res*. 2001;88(2):145–151.

42. Pyke KE, Tschakovsky ME. Peak vs. total reactive hyperemia: Which determines the magnitude of flow-mediated dilation? *J Appl Physiol.* 2007;102(4):1510–1519.
43. Harris RA, Padilla J. Proper "normalization" of flow-mediated dilation for shear. *J Appl Physiol.* 2007;102(4).
44. Anderson TJ, Uehata A, Gerhard MD, et al. Close relation of endothelial function in the human coronary and peripheral circulations. *J Am Coll Cardiol.* 1995;26(5):1235–1241.
45. Kaku B, Mizuno S, Ohsato K, et al. The correlation between coronary stenosis index and flow-mediated dilation of the brachial artery. *Jpn Circ J.* 1998;62(6):425–430.
46. Neunteufl T, Katzenschlager R, Hassan A, et al. Systemic endothelial dysfunction is related to the extent and severity of coronary artery disease. *Atherosclerosis.* 1997;129(1):111–118.
47. Anderson EA, Mark AL. Flow-mediated and reflex changes in large peripheral artery tone in humans. *Circulation.* 1989;79(1):93–100.
48. Resnick LM, Miltitiau D, Cunnings AJ, et al. Direct magnetic resonance determination of aortic distensibility in essential hypertension: Relation to age, abdominal visceral fat, and in situ intracellular free magnesium. *Hypertension.* 1997;30(pt. 2):654–659.
49. Laurent S, Caviezel B, Beck L, et al. Carotid artery distensibility and distending pressure in humans. *Hypertension.* 1994;23(pt 2):878–883.
50. Jondeau G, Boutouyrie P, Lacolley P, et al. Central pulse pressure is a major determinant of ascending aorta dilatation in Marfan syndrom. *Circulation.* 1999;99:2677–2681.

17

THE AUTONOMIC NERVOUS SYSTEM IN PERSONS WITH NEUROLOGICAL CONDITIONS

Louise Allan

The autonomic nervous system (ANS) is primarily responsible for the short-term cardiovascular control (including heart rate and blood pressure), and many other important homeostatic systems (body temperature, saliva and tear production, pupil size, gut motility, and sphincter control). The ANS innervates every organ in the body via the peripheral NS, which has three divisions: the sympathetic nervous system, the parasympathetic nervous system, and the enteric nervous system (see Fig. 17-1). The sympathetic and parasympathetic systems carry the efferent limbs of the autonomic reflexes and are under central nervous control by descending pathways from the hypothalamus via the brainstem nuclei.[1]

The arterial baroreflexes play a critical physiological role in the homeostasis of arterial blood pressure.[2] Baroreceptors are found in the arch of the aorta, the carotid sinus, and other arteries such as the innominate, common carotid, and subclavian arteries.[3] Baroreceptor activation modifies the heart rate, stroke volume, cardiac contractility, total systemic vascular resistance, and venous capacitance in response to intraluminal or extraluminal pressure changes, thus maintaining relatively constant blood pressure despite complex postural changes during daily activities.[4] There are multiple causes of baroreflex dysfunction, including autonomic failure,[5] polypharmacy,[6] cardiovascular disease,[7] aging, and hypertension.[8, 9]

Autonomic Nervous System Dysfunction

The importance of the ANS is often only appreciated when it is not functioning adequately. Patients with generalized autonomic failure have a recognizable pattern of symptoms and aggravating factors that relate to the severity of autonomic failure.[11] Symptoms include postural dizziness, syncope, fatigue, constipation, and incontinence (see Table 17-1). The most disabling symptoms, postural dizziness and syncope, are due to failure of the arterial baroreflexes, resulting in orthostatic hypotension (a fall in blood pressure when adopting the standing position) or postprandial hypotension (a fall

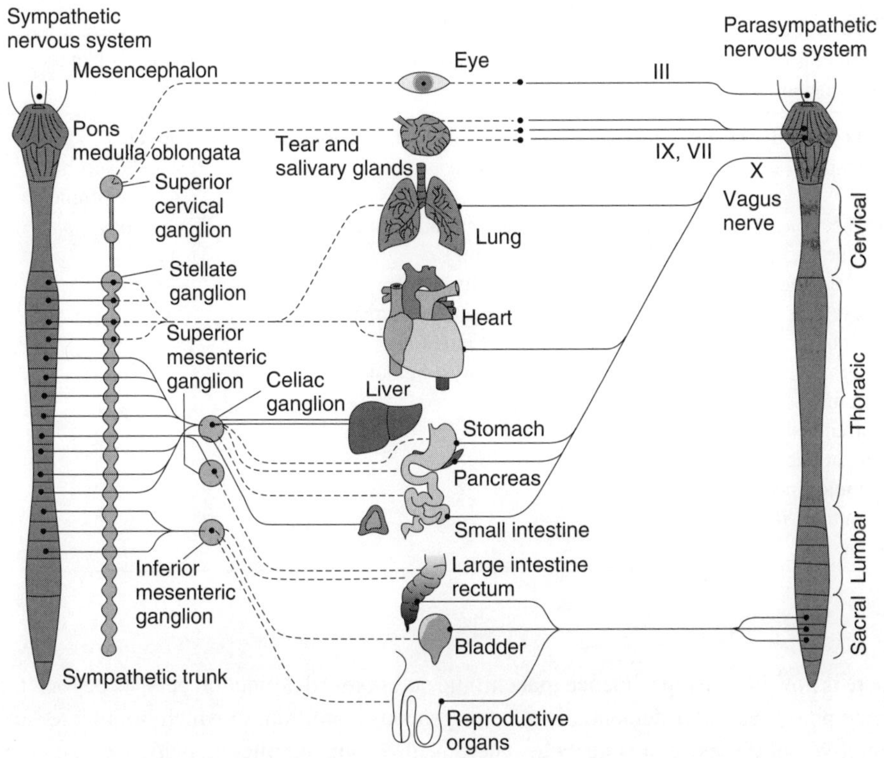

Figure 17-1 Diagrammatic representation of the sympathetic and parasympathetic nervous systems.

in blood pressure following a meal). Syncope can also be neurally mediated, as occurs in vasovagal syncope and carotid sinus syncope.

Autonomic Nervous System Disease in Persons with Neurological Conditions

Autonomic dysfunction is associated with a number of neurological conditions, including both neurodegenerative disorders and cerebrovascular disease. It is a cardinal feature of the alpha-synucleinopathies: multiple system atrophy and pure autonomic failure, and a well recognized feature of Parkinson's disease (PD)[12] and dementia with Lewy bodies (DLB).[13] Autonomic dysfunction has also been reported in the tauopathies: progressive supranuclear palsy (PSP), frontotemporal dementia (FTD), and Alzheimer's disease (AD), although the evidence is less certain in these conditions, as there have been several conflicting research reports. With respect to cerebrovascular disease, acute stroke is known to cause acute disturbance of autonomic function, and

Table 17-1 Symptoms of autonomic failure

Symptoms of orthostatic hypotension	Other autonomic symptoms	Provoking factors
Light-headedness or dizziness	Bloating, nausea, and vomiting	Standing
Syncope	Dry mouth	Physical exertion
Falls	Dry eyes	Warm environment
Weakness	Loss of sweating or excessive sweating	Time of day
Fatigue	Sensitivity to glare	Meals
Head and neck pain (coat-hanger pain)	Diarrea and constipation	
Vertigo	Urinary retention	
Pallor	Erectile dysfunction	
Clamminess		
Blurred vision		
Palpitations		
Tremulousness		
Cognitive difficulties		
Anxiety		

there is now increasing evidence that chronic autonomic dysfunction persists beyond the acute phase. Vascular dementia is a heterogeneous condition, to which both large- and small-vessel disease can contribute. There is also some conflicting evidence that autonomic dysfunction may be a feature of vascular dementia (VaD).

This chapter will review current evidence regarding the presence of autonomic dysfunction in these neurological conditions, with a particular focus on the conditions that are associated with dementia.

Methods of Assessment of Autonomic Nervous System Function in Neurological Conditions

Clinical autonomic function testing usually focuses on the neurocardiovascular system as this can be investigated noninvasively.[14] The most commonly used methods are discussed below and summarized in Table 17-2.

Orthostatic Hypotension

The measurement of postural change in blood pressure is the most easily available investigation in the clinical setting. However, various definitions of orthostatic hypotension (OH) have been used in both clinical settings and research studies, leading to a wide variation in estimates of the prevalence of orthostatic hypotension. The prevalence of OH in any population depends on the methodology employed to determine whether

OH is present, the age and comorbidities of the participants, and the number and type of medications they are taking. There is a consensus definition in which orthostatic hypotension has been defined arbitrarily as a fall in systolic blood pressure of 20 mmHg or to a level below 90 mm Hg, or a fall in diastolic blood pressure of 10 mmHg, within three minutes of standing.[15] Studies that have used this definition or a similar one have found a prevalence of OH in elderly community-dwelling participants varying from 13% to 30%, depending on the age, gender, setting, method of blood pressure measurement, and definition of OH.[16]

It should be remembered that the presence of OH does not confirm autonomic failure, as OH has many causes, including low intravascular volume (e.g., hemorrhage, burns, vomiting, diarrhea and hemodialysis), vasodilatation (e.g., due to glyceryl trinitrate, alcohol or other drugs, pyrexia), and structural heart disease (e.g., constrictive pericarditis, aortic stenosis).

Bedside Testing (Ewing Battery)

Ewing et al.[17] developed a more sensitive and specific battery of bedside tests to detect autonomic dysfunction in the clinical setting, initially described in diabetics. This battery (components marked [E] in Table 17-2) includes three sympathetic and three parasympathetic tests in which the cardiovascular responses to hemodynamic challenges are recorded. Abnormalities in three or more of these tests are usually taken as an indication of clinically significant autonomic failure.[17] Alternatively, a composite scoring system may be used, which has been shown to correlate with severity of disease and prognosis in other common causes of autonomic neuropathy.[18] In addition, various other bedside tests have been devised; for example, assessment of cardiovascular responses to physical or emotional stress, or to body movements during sleep, or arithmetical tasks.[19] These tests are less reproducible, as the degree of stress experienced by each participant depends on their perception of the difficulty of each task.

Some studies have included biochemical measures as well as physical stimuli; for example, change in plasma catecholamine levels during standing. Such studies were only included if they examined an autonomic stimulus such as change in posture. Studies of cerebral spinal fluid (CSF) and plasma catecholamines alone were not included, as these are more likely to reflect the overall status of the neurotransmitter systems producing such amines, rather than autonomic activity.

Neurally Mediated Syncope

Autonomic dysregulation can also cause the neurally mediated syncope syndromes, which include vasovagal syncope and carotid sinus syndrome. Both disorders cause hypotension and/or bradycardia sufficiently profound to produce cerebral ischemia and loss of neural function, due to abnormal vasodilatation and/or abnormal activation of the arterial baroreflexes.[12]

Vasovagal syncope (the common faint) presents with a typical clinical history: often, prodromal symptoms of light-headedness, pallor, weakness, yawning, blurred vision, impaired hearing, and derealization are followed by syncope. Provoking factors include prolonged standing, heat, postprandial state, straining, sudden emotional stress or pain, surgical procedures, or phlebotomy.

Carotid sinus syndrome is diagnosed in subjects with otherwise unexplained recurrent syncope who have carotid sinus hypersensitivity (abnormal response to carotid sinus massage). The syndrome is an important but frequently overlooked cause of syncope and presyncope in older subjects. The symptoms are usually precipitated by mechanical stimulation of the carotid sinus, i.e., by head turning, tight neckwear, and neck pathology, and by vagal stimuli such as prolonged standing. Other recognized triggers for symptoms are postprandial state, straining, looking or stretching upwards, exertion, defecation, and micturition.[20]

Heart Rate Variability

Heart rate variability (HRV) is a noninvasive method of assessing autonomic function, which has been used extensively as a research tool, although it is less suitable for clinical use.[21, 22] It requires less cooperation from the subject than other autonomic function tests and is suitable for use in patients with dementia. Power spectral analysis of heart rate variability produces power bands, or spectra (as shown in Fig. 17-2), which vary according to the tone of modulating autonomic activity.[23] High-frequency changes in heart rate are abolished by atropine and are thus thought to represent the rapid activity of the parasympathetic nervous system, whereas low-frequency variation in heart rate is thought to reflect both sympathetic and parasympathetic activity. Very-low-frequency variability is thought to be due to a combination of factors, including thermoregulation. The ratio of low-frequency to high-frequency bands is taken to represent sympathovagal balance. However, the sympathovagal balance can depend on non-autonomic factors such as the response of the patient to the stress of the test. It is therefore more appropriate to consider absolute rather than relative changes in HRV. The technique is sensitive for the detection of early autonomic neuropathy, as shown in diabetic patients.[24]

Cardiac^{123}I-Meta-iodobenzylguanidine scintigraphy

Meta-iodobenzylguanidine (MIBG) is a physiological analogue of norepinephrine, which has previously been used as a noninvasive method of screening for local myocardial sympathetic-nerve damage in various cardiac and neurological diseases. The test provides evidence of cardiac sympathetic denervation, but is not a measure of autonomic function. There are several studies confirming that cardiac uptake of^{123} I MIBG is reduced in idiopathic Parkinson's disease both with and without autonomic failure.[25–27]

Table 17-2 Clinical autonomic function tests

Sympathetic tests	Blood pressure response
Orthostasis (E)	Active standing for 3 minutes or passive head up tilt to at least 60 degrees: maximum drop in systolic blood pressure
Valsalva maneuver (E)	Expiration against a closed glottis to maintain a pressure of 40 mmHg for 15 sec: maximum rise in systolic blood pressure during phase IV
Isometric exercise (E)	Isometric exercise e.g., handgrip for 3 min: maximum increase in diastolic blood pressure
Emotional stimulus	Cognitive task e.g. mental arithmetic: maximum increase in systolic blood pressure
Physical stimulus	Hand placed in cold water (4°C) for 1 min: maximum increase in diastolic blood pressure
Parasympathetic tests	**Heart rate responses**
Orthostasis (E)	Absolute change in heart rate on orthostasis or ratio of maximum to minimum R-R interval following orthostasis
Respiratory sinus arrhythmia (E)	Mean change in heart rate or ratio of maximum to minimum R-R intervals during 6 cycles of deep breathing at 0.1 Hz
Valsalva maneuver (E)	Ratio of maximum R-R interval immediately following maneuver to minimum R-R interval during maneuver
Oculocardiac reflex (Aschner's test)	Bradycardic response to eyeball compression
Neurally mediated syncope	
Vasovagal syncope[211]	Fall in blood pressure and syncope induced by head up tilt at ≥60 degrees Type 1: Mixed; heart rate falls at the time of syncope, but the ventricular rate does not fall to < 40 beats/min or falls to < 40 beats/min for < 10 sec with or without asystole of < 3 sec. Type 2A: Cardioinhibition without asystole; heart rate falls to a ventricular rate < 40 beats/min for > 10 sec but asystole of > 3 sec does not occur. Type 2B: Cardioinhibition with asystole; asystole occurs for > 3 sec. Heart rate fall coincides with or precedes blood pressure fall. Type 3: Vasodepressor; heart rate does not fall >10%, from its peak, at the time of syncope.
Carotid sinus hypersensitivity[212]	Cardioinhibitory and/or vasodepressor response to 5 to 10 seconds of carotid sinus massage: Cardioinhibitory: asystole exceeding 3 seconds Vasodepressor: fall in systolic blood pressure exceeding 50 mmHg in the absence of cardioinhibition Mixed: combination of the two

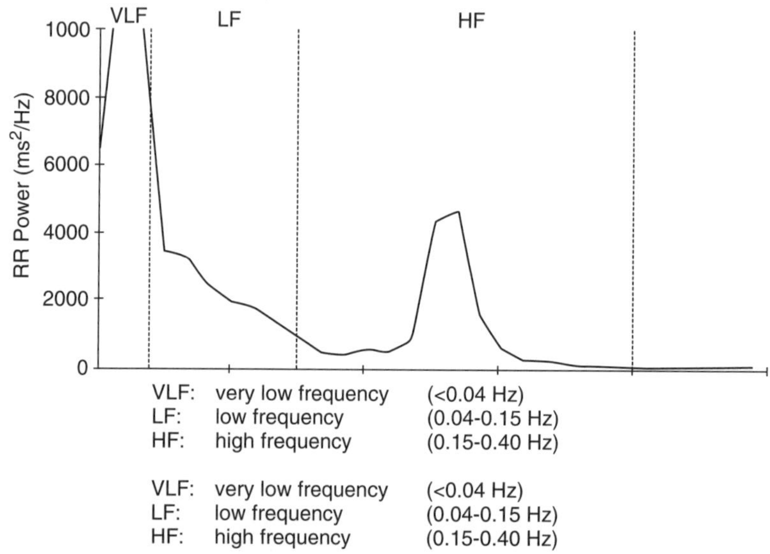

Figure 17-2 Example graph of power spectral analysis of heart rate variability in a healthy elderly control.

Non-cardiovascular Autonomic Function Tests

Other methods of evaluating autonomic function include pupillography; measurement of tear production; quantitative sudomotor axon testing; thermoregulatory sweat testing; sweat imprint testing; electrophysiological assessments, including sympathetic microneurography and sympathetic skin response; studies of gastric motility; urodynamics; penile plethysmography; and sphincter electromyography.[12]

Autonomic Dysfunction in Dementia: Current Evidence

The common dementias, including Alzheimer's disease (AD), vascular dementia (VaD) and dementia with Lewy bodies (DLB), have all been associated with underactivity of the cholinergic nervous systems.[28, 29] A generalized deficit in cholinergic function would be expected to lead to autonomic dysfunction, as acetylcholine is essential for parasympathetic and preganglionic sympathetic neurotransmission. Previous investigators have speculated, on the basis of cholinergic underactivity, that autonomic dysfunction would occur in Alzheimer's disease.[30–32] AD-related cytoskeletal pathology can be found in the brainstem autonomic nuclei at autopsy even in the early Braak stages of AD.[33] There is also evidence that neurofibrillary tangles can occur in the sympathetic and spinal ganglia in older people, but these are not necessarily related to neuropathology in the central nervous system.[34] Moreover, the finding of neuropathology does not necessarily imply clinically significant neuronal dysfunction.

The clinical manifestations of autonomic failure have long been associated with Parkinson's disease (PD).[35–37] Many investigators now believe DLB to be part of a spectrum of Lewy body disorders, including PD, Parkinson's disease dementia (PDD), and pure autonomic failure[38]; it is therefore to be expected that DLB would also be associated with autonomic failure. The Braak staging of PD[39] emphasises early involvement of the brainstem, including the dorsal vagal nucleus. It has been suggested that in PD, Lewy body pathology begins in the brainstem and progresses to the neocortex.[40] However, there may be a different pattern of evolution in DLB, with some studies suggesting that cerebrocortical pathology predominates in DLB,[41, 42] although prominent Lewy body pathology is still evident in the brain stem, including the dorsal vagal nucleus.[43]

Autonomic Symptoms

There are few studies of the prevalence of autonomic symptoms in dementia. Orthostatic dizziness has been reported as an early symptom of DLB in three cases in a series of eight patients,[44] and syncope has been reported as the initial symptom of DLB in two cases of a series of eleven DLB patients.[45] In a retrospective examination for autonomic symptoms in the case notes of a series of cases of DLB, urinary incontinence and constipation were the most commonly documented autonomic symptoms, occurring in 97% and 83%, respectively, whereas syncope occurred in 28%.[46, 47] Prospective studies have suggested that urinary incontinence occurs earlier in DLB than in AD.[48, 49] Falls are a particularly common feature of DLB, and underlying autonomic dysfunction could be a significant contributory cause of such falls.[50–53] Both syncope and falls are included as supporting features in the diagnostic criteria for DLB.[54, 55]

Resting Hypotension

Three studies have examined resting hypotension in dementia. One study[56] found lower resting systolic blood pressure in 38 AD cases (133 mmHg), in comparison with 14 VaD cases (160 mmHg) and 19 cases of other dementias (146 mmHg). A larger community study found similar results, with resting systolic blood pressure lower in AD than in VaD, and also lower than in non-demented controls.[57] However, as there were no direct tests of autonomic function in either of these papers, few conclusions regarding autonomic dysfunction can be drawn from these studies. In a large dementia case series in which diagnoses of DLB or AD were retrospectively applied, Londos et al.[58] found that BP did decline with advancing dementia in both diagnoses, but significant hypotension (systolic BP <120 mmHg) was more prevalent in late DLB than in late AD (40% vs. 31%). This effect was independent of age. In this paper, the orthostatic fall in blood pressure was found to be greater in DLB than AD, but the prevalence of OH was not determined.

Orthostatic Hypotension

Although most studies of autonomic function tests in dementia have included measurements of orthostatic blood pressure responses, very few studies have assessed the prevalence of orthostatic hypotension. Of the ten studies identified for this review, only five papers compared the prevalence of OH with a healthy control group[59–63] and five did not.[45, 64–67] The findings of all these studies are summarized in Table 17-3.

The definition of OH and methods of blood pressure assessment varied widely between studies. Unfortunately, the earliest studies of OH in dementia all had significant problems, being small and/or with methodological difficulties. None used the consensus definition of OH,[15] although most approximated to it, requiring a fall of at least 20 mmHg–30 mmHg in systolic blood pressure.[45, 60, 64–67] Two studies did not give details of the definition of OH that they used.[59, 66] Two studies reported the use of a digital sphygmomanometer,[59, 64] and one used a photoplethysmographic device.[65] The remaining studies did not give any details regarding the method of blood pressure assessment. One study included assessment of post-prandial hypotension (PPH) as well as orthostatic hypotension.[59] Although this study did not find any OH in the AD cases, a high prevalence of PPH was found in AD (70%), in comparison with controls (26%), leading the authors to suggest that abnormalities in cardiac vasomotor regulation or gut hormone secretion might be present in AD.

More recently there have been two studies[61, 62] of OH in dementia without the methodological problems described in the earlier studies. Both included healthy older control groups and did use the consensus definition of OH: the former using a photoplethysmographic device for a period of three minutes standing, and the latter a validated digital sphygmomanometer to record the blood pressure at one, three, five, and ten minutes. Both of these reports compared AD and DLB with control groups, and found a higher prevalence of OH in AD and DLB than in controls. Both found that the drop in blood

Table 17-3 Comparative table of studies examining the prevalence of orthostatic hypotension in dementia

Paper	Healthy controls	AD	VaD	FTD	DLB	PDD	PD without dementia	Length of stand
59	9%	0%						5 min
60	60%	33%						Not stated
64		39%	52%	46%				10 min
66		41%						Not stated
65		32%			40%			2 min
67		29%			93%			10 min
45					63%			Not stated
61	13%	34%	34%		52%	49%		3 min
62	13%	42%			69%			10 min

pressure on orthostasis was substantially more prolonged in DLB, and in the latter, OH was more common in DLB. This is supported by another study, which found a higher prevalence of OH at 10 minutes of standing in DLB than in AD.[67] Only one study has compared the prevalence of OH in VaD with that in healthy controls, AD and DLB,[61] finding that OH in VaD was also higher than in controls.

In conclusion, although there is some conflicting evidence, it does seem that the prevalence of orthostatic hypotension in dementia is higher than in healthy older people. It is likely that the prevalence is even higher in DLB than in the other dementias, but given that OH is common in all dementias, the presence of OH cannot be used to reliably distinguish between dementia subtypes. Despite the clinical relevance of OH in dementia, studies of its prevalence do not allow firm conclusions to be drawn about autonomic dysfunction in dementia, as there are multiple possible causes of OH. It is necessary, therefore, to consider more detailed studies of clinical autonomic function.

Clinical Autonomic Function Tests

For the purposes of this review, 26 studies of bedside clinical autonomic tests in dementia were identified.[19, 30–32, 58, 60–62, 68–85] Most of these included patients with AD only, although three included patients with multi-infarct dementia or Binswanger's encephalopathy,[70, 75, 79] and there was one prospective study of bedside clinical tests in DLB.[61]

The first study to attempt a complete Ewing battery in people with dementia[68] investigated a relatively young group of moderately to severely demented Alzheimer's patients (mean age 62.2 ± 4.1 years) and healthy controls (mean age 59.6 ± 2.5 years). Three of the patients had a family history of dementia. It was reported that they were unable to perform the Ewing battery. In contrast, the same group reported that a group of AD patients was able to perform the Ewing battery and stated that all had normal results.[19] This is a discrepancy, as this study appears to report results on the same cohort of patients as in their previous work. Severity of dementia was not given in the latter paper, but demographic characteristics and other autonomic indices were identical. The outcome of Ewing testing in these two papers is therefore difficult to comment upon.

Sympathetic Function Tests

Thirteen studies included measurements of orthostatic blood pressure responses in patients with dementia in comparison with healthy controls (that is, a quantitative measurement of the fall in BP on standing rather than a categorical description of whether OH is present).[30, 31, 61, 62, 69, 70, 72, 73, 76–79, 84] The results are summarized in Table 17-4. A total of six studies found no differences in postural blood pressure responses in AD in comparison with controls.[30, 69, 70, 73, 77, 78, 84] In one study, the fall in blood pressure on standing was actually smaller in AD than in controls.[76] These studies suggest that sympathetic responses to standing are normal in AD. However, four studies did find evidence of abnormal postural changes in blood pressure in AD.[31, 62, 72, 86] The evidence regarding the degree of orthostatic blood pressure responses in AD in comparison with healthy controls is conflicting, and the results are probably highly dependent on methodology and case selection.

Seven studies reported upon measurements of blood pressure responses to sympathetic stimuli other than orthostasis in AD and healthy controls.[19, 32, 61, 69, 70, 81, 82] The first study of responses to Valsalva maneuver and isometric exercise reported "normal responses," although detailed comparisons were not given, and concerns about this paper have been previously discussed.[19] One study showed a reduction of sympathetic responses in AD to both Valsalva maneuver and isometric exercise.[32] This study included a reasonably elderly group with an age-matched control group. However, eight out of 14 AD patients had a positive family history of dementia, so these patients may not have been typical of most elderly patients. In a more representative study of AD cases, neither responses to Valsalva maneuver nor isometric exercise were impaired in comparison with controls. In addition, the reports of responses to the cold pressor test in AD have been conflicting.[70, 82] Two studies used cognitive and emotional sympathetic stimuli. The first examined studied heart rate, blood pressure, and catecholamine responses to cognitive challenge as well as postural testing.[69] Responses to cognitive effort were blunted, which was taken to indicate impaired sympathetic response. However, the main disadvantage of using a cognitive stimulus is that the effort required is extremely variable, so this result is of limited value in determining whether AD patients do have sympathetic impairment. The second examined studied blood pressure and heart-rate responses to painful electrical stimuli, in a study that was primarily designed to evaluate pain perception in AD patients rather than autonomic responses.[81] They found an increased threshold for autonomic activation in AD, but again it is difficult to control for variation between patients and controls in the cognitive aspects of the stimulus.

There have been fewer studies of sympathetic function in VaD. One study found a greater blood pressure decrease on passive tilt in patients with Binswanger's disease compared with healthy controls,[79] but another study of multi-infarct dementia found no differences in postural blood pressure responses in comparison with controls.[70] One study showed a greater blood pressure decrease in response to active orthostasis in VaD than in controls, but other sympathetic function tests were not impaired.

There have been two studies that have compared sympathetic clinical autonomic function tests in DLB with both controls and AD. As previously noted, both found that the drop in blood pressure on orthostasis was substantially more prolonged in DLB than in controls,[61, 62] and in the latter the response was also more prolonged than in AD. In the former, response to Valsalva also appeared impaired in DLB in comparison with controls and AD, although the difference only reached significance when comparing AD and DLB. A further study compared DLB with controls and also found greater fall in BP on passive tilt in DLB, and significant impairment of responses to the Valsalva maneuver.[63]

Parasympathetic Function Tests

In AD, most studies have found no difference in the absolute change in heart rate, which is a test of parasympathetic function, on either standing,[69, 70, 72, 73, 78, 80] or on passive tilt,[30, 76, 77] in comparison with controls (see Table 17-5).

Table 17-4 Summary of studies examining sympathetic tests in dementia

AD vs. healthy controls		
Orthostasis–Active	Greater blood pressure fall in AD	3 studies[61, 62, 72]
	No differences	5 studies[69, 70, 73, 78, 84]
Orthostasis–Passive	Greater blood pressure fall in AD	1 study[31]
	No differences	2 studies[30, 77]
	Reduced fall in blood pressure	1 study[76]
Valsalva maneuver	Reduced pulse pressure	1 study[32]
	No differences	1 study[61]
	All normal responses	1 study[19]
Isometric exercise	Reduced response	1 study[32]
	No differences	1 study[61]
	All normal responses	1 study[19]
Cold pressor test	No difference	1 study[70]
	Increased response	1 study[82]
Cognitive challenge	Reduced response	1 study[69]
Painful stimulus	Reduced response	1 study[81]
VaD, Multi infarct dementia or Binswanger's disease vs. healthy controls		
Orthostasis–Active	No difference between multi infarct dementia and controls	1 study[70]
	Greater blood pressure fall in VaD	1 study[61]
Orthostasis–Passive	Greater blood pressure fall in Binswanger's disease	1 study[79]
Valsalva maneuver	No differences	1 study[61]
Isometric exercise	No differences	1 study[61]
DLB vs. healthy controls		
Orthostasis–Active	Greater blood pressure fall in DLB	2 studies[61, 62]
	No differences	5 studies[69, 70, 73, 78, 84]
Orthostasis–Passive	Greater blood pressure fall in AD	1 study[63]
Valsalva maneuver	Reduced responses	1 study[63]
	No differences	1 study[61]
Isometric exercise	No differences	1 study[61]

Two studies found a reduction in the ratio of maximal to minimal heart rate on standing (30:15 ratio), one using a passive stand[32] and one using an active stand.[80] However, both of these studies were small, with the former being the study with a significant number of patients having a positive family history. One study found a greater increase in absolute heart rate in AD patients, and this would be expected to reduce the 30:15 ratio. A reduction in 30:15 ratio suggests parasympathetic dysfunction, but can depend on non-parasympathetic factors, including the initial increase in heart rate on standing, which is partly sympathetically mediated, and the time and effort required to achieve the standing position, which may depend on cognition and mobility. This study also used two alternative autonomic markers of heart rate response to passive standing rather than

Table 17-5 Summary of studies examining parasympathetic tests in Alzheimer's disease and vascular dementia

AD vs. healthy controls		
Orthostasis–Active	Reduced 30:15 ratio in AD	2 studies[80]
	No difference in 30:15 ratio	1 study[61]
	No difference in absolute change in heart rate	7 studies[62, 69, 70, 72, 73, 78, 80]
Orthostasis–Passive	Reduced 30:15 ratio in AD	1 study[32]
	No difference in absolute change in heart rate	3 studies[30, 76, 77]
	Greater increase in absolute change in heart rate	1 study[31]
Respiratory sinus arrhythmia	Reduced response	1 study[73]
	No difference	4 studies[31, 32, 61, 80]
Valsalva maneuver	Reduced Valsalva ratio	1 study[32]
	No difference in Valsalva ratio	1 study[61]
	All normal responses	1 study[19]
VaD or Multi infarct dementia vs. healthy controls		
Orthostasis–Active	No difference in 30:15 ratio in VaD	1 study[61]
Valsalva maneuver	Reduced Valsalva ratio in VaD	1 study[61]
Respiratory sinus arrhythmia	Reduced 30:15 ratio	1 study[61]
Oculocardiac reflex	Reduced response in multi-infarct dementia	1 study[70]
DLB vs. healthy controls		
Orthostasis–Active	Reduced 30:15 ratio	1 study[61]
Respiratory sinus arrhythmia	Reduced response	1 study[61]
Valsalva maneuver	Reduced response	1 study[61]
	Reduced baroreflex sensitivity calculated from Valsalva phase IV	1 study[63]

the usual 30:15 ratio. They found greater acceleration followed by reduced deceleration of heart rate in response to an eight-minute tilt. The results were taken to indicate autonomic imbalance. The final study that has examined 30:15 ratio did not find significant differences between AD patients and controls.[61]

Seven studies reported upon measurements of blood pressure responses to parasympathetic stimuli other than orthostasis,[19, 31, 32, 61, 70, 73, 80] and in the majority, no differences in parasympathetic function have been shown between AD patients and controls. In one study that did show a difference, Wang et al.[73] measured R-R interval variation during normal and deep breathing, defined as the difference between longest and shortest R-R interval in 20 successive beats, expressed as percent of mean R-R interval. This index was found to be reduced in a group of elderly AD patients at rest and during deep breathing and was taken as evidence of parasympathetic dysfunction. However, as mean MMSE score was only 10 in this group, they were more severely demented than in other studies. Poor compliance may have reduced the depth of breathing and consequent autonomic stimulus.

In VaD, there is much less evidence regarding parasympathetic function, but two studies have shown evidence of some impairment. Yamamoto did find impaired parasympathetic response to ocular compression in multi-infarct dementia (MID) patients, in comparison with both AD patients and healthy controls,[70] and Allan et al. found reduced Valsalva ratio and 30:15 ratio in VaD compared with controls.[61] In this study, Valsalva ratio, 30:15 ratio, and respiratory sinus arrhythmia were all found to be impaired in DLB patients. Similarly, one study showed impaired baroreflex sensitivity (calculated from phase IV of the Valsalva maneuver) in DLB patients compared with controls.[63]

Heart Rate Variability

Heart rate variability techniques are more sensitive than standard bedside clinical autonomic function tests and therefore might be expected to resolve some of the inconsistencies in the evidence regarding autonomic dysfunction in dementia. There have been six studies of HRV in AD (see Table 17-6).

Two of these used autoregressive models, which can result in spectral smoothing or possibly erroneous frequency peak insertion. The first study[30] did not report any absolute reduction in spectral power or any of its components. They did find changes in the fractions of HRV in different frequency bands and interpreted this as evidence of a relatively hypersympathetic, hypoparasympathetic state in AD patients. It should be remembered that the sympathovagal balance could depend on non-autonomic factors such as the response of the patient to the stress of the test. In addition, the length of the supine recording was not standardized in this study and could vary from five to ten minutes. Manual verification of QRS classification was not recorded, and the control group appeared to be younger than the patient group. The second study[77] found an absolute reduction in total spectral power and each frequency band in the AD patients, which suggested generalized autonomic dysfunction. Few details about the control group were given, but it appears to have been younger than the patient group (AD patients' mean age was 65.7, ± 6.2 years, versus control age 62.5 ± 5.1 years). No details of drug history other than dementia treatment were given. Manual verification of QRS classification and exclusion of arrhythmias were not recorded.

Four studies used a Fast Fourier transformation–based signal processing method, which makes use of all the available data and is more suitable for measurement of HRV over short periods of time.[61, 76, 87, 88] The first of these[76] used HRV as part of a detailed study of the effects of central muscarinic-1 receptor stimulation in a small number of patients with AD compared with healthy age-matched controls. Although significant differences in response to tilt testing were described (see above), few results were given

Table 17-6 Summary of studies examining heart rate variability in dementia

AD vs. healthy controls		
Autoregressive model	Hypersympathetic, Hypoparasympathetic state	1 study[30, 77]
	Absolute reduction in HRV	1 study[77]
Fast Fourier transformation	Decreased HRV in response to xanomeline in AD but not controls	1 study[76]
	No difference in resting HRV in AD compared with controls	2 studies[61,87]
	Altered sympathovagal balance	1 study[88]
VaD or Binswanger's encephalopathy vs. healthy controls		
Fast Fourier transformation	No difference in resting HRV in VaD compared with controls	2 studies[61, 87]
Method of power spectral analysis not known	Reduction in high frequency power in Binswanger's encephalopathy	1 study[83]
DLB vs. healthy controls		
Fast Fourier transformation	Reduced total spectral power and low frequency power	1 study[61]

about the heart rate variability data acquired. Xanomeline (a muscarinic agonist) was found to decrease HRV in AD patients but not significantly in controls. Allan et al. did not find any reduction in HRV in AD compared with either healthy volunteer controls[61] or a community-based sample of controls.[87]

Three studies have examined HRV in the vascular dementias.[61, 83, 87] Watanabe et al. used power spectral analysis to study heart rate variability in patients with Binswanger's encephalopathy. High-frequency power was reduced in comparison with healthy controls and patients with lacunar stroke. In severe cases, the change in sympathovagal balance in response to standing was also impaired. The authors suggested that parasympathetic dysfunction is an early feature of Binswanger's encephalopathy, with progression to include sympathetic dysfunction in the later stages. Unfortunately, the method of power spectral analysis was not given. Again, using Fast Fourier transformation, Allan et al. did not find any reduction in HRV in VaD compared with either healthy volunteer controls[61] or a community-based sample of controls.[87] In DLB, the evidence is consistent with studies of bedside clinical autonomic function tests in finding that autonomic dysfunction is present, with reduced total spectral power and low-frequency power, although an apparent reduction in high-frequency power did not reach significance.[61]

Alternative Cardiovascular Autonomic Function Tests

As there are difficulties in testing cardiovascular autonomic function using bedside tests, various other methods have been used in addition to HRV. One study[68] reported significantly lower cardioacceleration in response to body movements during sleep in patients with AD, in comparison with healthy controls, suggesting sympathetic underactivity. They were not able to demonstrate a difference in parasympathetic activity as reflected by the ratio of absolute R-R intervals between wakefulness, and various stages of sleep. However, the numbers were small, and absolute R-R interval is not as a reliable an indicator of parasympathetic activity as is beat-to-beat variability.

Szili-Torok et al.[89] measured baroreflex sensitivity by the spontaneous sequences method during rest and found reduced baroreflex sensitivity in AD patients. Baseline heart rate was also increased, which may indicate reduced parasympathetic tone. A disturbance of central autonomic mechanisms was postulated by the authors.

Non-cardiovascular Autonomic Function Tests

The most extensively investigated non-cardiovascular autonomic test is the pupillary response to topical tropicamide, a cholinergic antagonist. The purpose of most these studies was to develop a potential non-invasive neurobiological test for AD, following an initial report of its potential usefulness.[90] These studies have been extensively reviewed.[91, 92] In summary, at least five studies have shown increased mydriasis in response to tropicamide in AD patients in comparison with controls.[90, 93–96] This could be due to upregulation of cholinergic receptors in response to a cholinergic deficit. However, 13 studies have found no statistically significant differences between groups,[97–108] and one found a reduction in mydriasis in the AD patients.[109] Other studies have examined light and darkness reflexes rather than response to tropicamide, and have shown reduced pupil diameter and impairment of some pupillary reflexes in AD.[92, 109–111] In summary, although tropicamide has not proved a useful test for Alzheimer's disease, there is some evidence that parasympathetic cholinergic pupillary deficits occur. No studies of pupillary responses in VaD or DLB and no comparative studies of AD, DLB, and VaD were identified for the purpose of this review.

Studies of non-cardiovascular autonomic functions in dementia, other than in the pupil, have included small numbers of AD patients.[112–115] Two studies showed a reduction in skin blood-vessel reactivity to iontophoresis of pharmacological agents,[113, 114] which could indicate the presence of either a preganglionic or postganglionic autonomic deficit. A study[112] of sweat gland responses to choline and carbachol found evidence of deficits in sympathetic cholinergic activity, but a study of muscarinic receptor binding in sweat glands did not find any reduction in AD.[115] Three studies examined the sympathetic skin response in AD. Two of these found no differences between AD and healthy age-matched controls,[32, 73] and one found abnormalities in most AD patients.[78]

Neurally Mediated Syncope

Only two studies have examined vasovagal responses to prolonged head-up tilt in dementia patients. The first of these was a small study of eight AD patients and six healthy controls.[76] Participants underwent tilt testing after placebo, acute oral xanomeline (a muscarinic agonist), and three days' administration of xanomeline. There were no differences between AD and controls in hemodynamic changes or catecholamine responses to injection of placebo or xanomeline. Two healthy, and none of the AD, subjects developed vasovagal response to placebo tilt, with a greater decline in blood pressure in controls. Xanomeline reversed the apparently greater orthostatic tolerance in the AD patients, four of whom had a vasovagal response to xanomeline tilt in comparison with three healthy controls. Peripheral blockade of xanomeline with methoscopolamine did not prevent syncope. The second study[65] demonstrated a positive response to a prolonged passive head-up tilt in 7% of 30 patients with DLB and none of the 35 AD patients. As noted previously, this was an uncontrolled study, and so the prevalence of vasovagal syncope may not be greater than that found in healthy controls.[116]

In two prospective studies, the prevalence of cardio-inhibitory carotid sinus hypersensitivity (CSH) in DLB was 41% and 31%, respectively.[65, 117] This was significantly higher than in AD (28% and 11%, respectively), and a healthy control group (3.2%). In the second of these studies, vasodepressor CSH occurred in 38% DLB, 26% AD, and 37% controls, and was not significantly more common in any group compared with the others. The magnitude of blood pressure fall was significantly greater in DLB patients than AD patients.[117] However, the mean age of the control group was significantly lower than that of both patient groups, and the AD group was older than the DLB group in this study. Another study has described carotid sinus hypersensitivity in only two of 30 AD patients, but this study also lacked controls.[118]

Cardiac ^{123}I-Meta-iodobenzylguanidine scintigraphy

Two studies have examined cardiac uptake of ^{123}I MIBG in DLB in comparison with AD. In the first study,[45] a healthy control group was included. The heart/mediastinum (H/M) ratio of MIBG uptake in all patients with DLB was significantly lower than that in the patients with AD and control subjects. The H/M ratio in the patients with AD was indistinguishable from that in the control subjects. The second showed a pathological reduction in cardiac uptake of ^{123}I MIBG in DLB but not AD.[67] Both groups concluded that the findings indicated the loss of local myocardial sympathetic innervation, and postulated that cardiac uptake of MIBG is a more reliable marker of DLB than an orthostatic test. This test has now been included as a supportive feature in the most recent diagnostic criteria for DLB.[55] Oka et al. also showed that cardiac uptake of ^{123}I MIBG in DLB was reduced in comparison with controls with confirmed autonomic dysfunction.[63]

Summary of the Current Evidence Regarding Autonomic Dysfunction in Dementia

The above discussions highlight the conflicting nature of the studies of autonomic function in dementia, many of which have been plagued by small numbers, lack of appropriate control groups, and other methodological difficulties. However, a consensus appears to be emerging that significant autonomic dysfunction is least often found in AD, despite some evidence that autonomic areas can be affected by typical AD neuropathology at post mortem. However, this does not rule out the possibility that autonomic dysfunction may occur in a small number of AD cases, particularly as the disease progresses. Whether this is due to the simultaneous occurrence of non-AD pathology is less clear. Where autonomic dysfunction does occur in AD, it has been proposed that this is more likely to be associated with neurofibrillary tangle pathology within the insular cortex than with brainstem autonomic nuclei, in contrast to the Lewy body disorders.[119] The insular cortex is affected early in the course of AD, from Braak stage II;[120] it exerts higher-level control of autonomic responses, and therefore pathology in these areas may account for the findings that responses to cognitive and emotional stimuli are impaired in AD.[69, 81]

In VaD, there is less evidence and much more conflict in the evidence, but it seems likely that, although autonomic dysfunction is not a typical feature, it probably does occur more commonly than in AD. This is not incompatible with evidence of post-stroke autonomic dysfunction.[121] What does seem clear is that autonomic dysfunction is extremely common and a typical feature of DLB. This is not unduly surprising, as DLB is one the Lewy body disorders, which are well known to be associated with autonomic dysfunction (see below). There are several reported cases of DLB presenting with pure autonomic failure as a first symptom.[44, 45] In view of this expanding body of evidence, autonomic dysfunction is now given much more weight in the third set of consensus criteria for the diagnosis of DLB.[55]

Autonomic Dysfunction in Other Neurological Conditions

Parkinson's Disease

Parkinson's disease (PD) is a well known cause of primary autonomic failure.[1] Autonomic dysfunction was initially thought to be a less common feature of PD, but an increasing amount of evidence supports the view that it is actually extremely common. Indeed the finding of reduced cardiac uptake of ^{123}I MIBG has been shown to be highly specific for differentiating PD from other extrapyramidal disorders, although there may be fewer autonomic symptoms in the early stages of the disease.[25, 122] As in dementia, estimates of the prevalence of OH in Parkinson's disease vary according to patient selection and methodology. In a study of patients with *de novo* PD, the prevalence has been found to be as low as 14%,[123] whereas studies including patients with a range of durations of illness have found prevalence of 45% to 58%.[124–126] It has been suggested that OH is more commonly found in PD patients with the phenotype of gait and balance disturbance than in those with tremor dominance.[127] In detailed studies of cardiovascular autonomic function using bedside tests and HRV techniques, it has been shown that impairments are more pronounced in those with hypokinesia and rigidity as an initial symptom, in comparison with those with the initial symptom of tremor.[128, 129] These findings are significant because this phenotype is thought to be associated with a poorer prognosis.[130] The early occurrence of autonomic symptoms in PD may, therefore, be an adverse prognostic feature, and there are several studies that suggest that autonomic dysfunction is more severe in the later stages of PD, particularly when dementia is present.[131, 132]

Lewy bodies and alpha synuclein staining have been reported in locus coeruleus, substantia nigra, preganglionic parasympathetic cells and sympathetic ganglia at autopsy in cases of pure autonomic failure, and in both the peripheral and central autonomic nervous systems in Parkinson's disease.[38, 133–136] Lewy bodies are not confined to the cardiovascular autonomic nervous system, also having been found in the enteric nervous system.[137, 138] Braak has proposed a staging procedure for the classification of neuropathological findings in sporadic PD, noting that the pathological process appears to target specific induction sites: "Lesions initially occur in the dorsal motor nucleus of the glossopharyngeal and vagal nerves and anterior olfactory nucleus. Thereafter, less vulnerable nuclear grays and cortical areas gradually become affected. The disease process in the brain stem pursues an ascending course with little interindividual variation." This ascending course is thought to proceed towards the neocortex.[40] In one study, a series of cases with confirmed neocortical Lewy body disease at autopsy all showed Parkinsonism, dementia, and autonomic failure in life, as did many with limbic-type disease.[38] Those with brainstem-type disease alone had autonomic failure (diagnosed from case notes) but without dementia. The finding that alpha synuclein aggregates may be present in gastric autonomic plexuses[139] or in the abdominopelvic plexuses resected from surgical patients without any known neurodegenerative disease, and that this is associated with cardiac sympathetic denervation and impaired responses to the Valsalva maneuver,[140] has led some investigators have suggested that Lewy body disease may actually begin peripherally, potentially being due to an environmental pathogen affecting the peripheral autonomic nerves, with retrograde transmission towards the central nervous system. If this is the case, early identification of autonomic involvement might be a means of finding individuals who would benefit from new neuroprotective treatments.

Multiple System Atrophy

Multiple system atrophy (MSA) is also a well-known cause of primary autonomic failure,[1] and the disease frequently begins with autonomic symptoms, particularly urinary symptoms and erectile dysfunction in males. A neuropathological diagnosis of definite MSA requires the presence of widespread and abundant alpha synuclein positive glial cytoplasmic inclusions in the central nervous system associated with neurodegenerative changes in striatonigral or olivopontocerebellar structures.[141] Marked neuronal cell loss and gliosis occur in the basal ganglia, pontine nuclei, inferior olives, cerebellar Purkinje cells, and intermediolateral gray columns of the spinal cord.

The second consensus statement on the diagnosis of MSA requires definite autonomic failure for a probable diagnosis and at least one feature suggesting autonomic dysfunction for a possible diagnosis.[141] This is associated with poorly levodopa-responsive Parkinsonism (MSA-P) or a cerebellar syndrome (MSA-C). MSA-P is the more common form, and the motor features progress more rapidly than in PD, with early postural instability.[142] The autonomic failure of MSA is thought to be central in origin, and there is usually no evidence of cardiac sympathetic denervation on myocardial scintigraphy.[26] Postganglionic sympathetic neurons are usually neuropathologically spared, as is the cerebral cortex.

Progressive Supranuclear Palsy

Progressive supranuclear palsy (PSP) is an extrapyramidal syndrome similar to PD, but with atypical features, including increased axial tone, pseudobulbar palsy, neck hyperextension, and supranuclear gaze palsy. The neuropathological features of PSP include widespread neurofibrillary degeneration with neuronal loss and gliosis in subcortical areas, particularly the subthalamic nucleus, substantia nigra, brainstem tegmentum, and dentate nuclei. The cerebral cortex is not usually substantially involved. Autonomic dysfunction is not usually considered to be a feature of PSP, but as in AD, this is somewhat controversial. Some small studies have failed to find any evidence, or only minor evidence, of dysautonomia, using bedside clinical autonomic function tests[143–146] and HRV techniques.[147, 148] However, there are also some positive studies using clinical methods[149] and measurement of baroreflex sensitivity using HRV techniques.[150] As these studies have all been small, it seems that the prevalence of autonomic dysfunction in PSP is not yet established.

Stroke

Acute stroke commonly causes changes in autonomic function, most easily seen in disturbance of blood pressure regulation and ECG abnormalities such as arrhythmias, prolonged QT intervals, and ST segment and T wave changes. ECG changes usually revert to normal within two weeks,[151] but subtler autonomic abnormalities can be detected using HRV techniques six months after a hemispheric infarction.[121, 152] This can be associated with a worse functional prognosis.[152, 153] In addition to cardiovascular autonomic sequelae, there may be more widespread autonomic disturbance, including urogenital, gastrointestinal, and thermoregulatory dysfunction. There may also be a reciprocal relationship between autonomic dysfunction and stroke.[154] Hypertension causes impairment of baroreflex sensitivity and increased blood pressure variability, including nocturnal non-dipping of blood pressure, both themselves risk factors for stroke. An extensive review of the interrelationships between stroke and the autonomic nervous system is beyond the scope of this review, but this should not minimize their importance. While control of hypertension for the prevention of stroke is well established, the long-term effects of hypotension and OH secondary to autonomic dysfunction and antihypertensive treatments remain unclear.

Implications of Autonomic Nervous System Dysfunction in Neurological Disorders

Syncope and Falls

Syncope and falls are particularly important symptoms of autonomic dysfunction because of their adverse consequences. Orthostatic hypotension, autonomic dysfunction, and neurally mediated syncope have been shown to account for a significant proportion of cases referred to secondary care for the investigation of syncope, accounting for 47% of adult referrals in one unit.[155] Older people have been shown to have inaccurate recall of falls and may therefore be unable to give an accurate history of events.[156] In addition, up to 30% are unable to recall loss of consciousness, even immediately after it has been witnessed.[157] In older people, therefore, the history of syncope and falls may overlap.[158] Falls (defined as an event whereby a person comes to lie on the ground or another lower level with or without loss of consciousness) are a significant cause of injuries, loss of confidence, increased morbidity, institutionalization, and mortality in older people.[159, 160] Autonomic dysfunction has not been extensively studied as a risk factor for falls in any older population, but there is some indirect evidence from studies that have examined orthostatic hypotension. Orthostatic hypotension has been shown to be a risk factor for falls in intermediate or long term care settings,[161, 162] and as a risk factor for recurrent falls in the community,[163] in residences for the elderly,[164] and in nursing homes,[165] although other studies based in the community[166–171] and residential care[172] have not shown an association with OH. Some of the successful multifactorial intervention trials for the prevention of falls have addressed orthostatic hypotension as one of the interventions,[173–175] suggesting that appropriate management of orthostatic hypotension may contribute to successful prevention of falls in older people, and this may include older people with neurological conditions such as dementia and Parkinson's disease.

In people with dementia, falls are a significant cause of increased morbidity, institutionalization, and mortality.[176, 177] Patients with dementia recover less well after a fall than those without dementia.[178] However, the role that autonomic dysfunction might play in causing falls and syncope in dementia is likely to be a complex one, depending on its interactions with other risk factors for falls in dementia.[50–53] It is likely that falls in dementia are multifactorial in origin, with risk factors similar to those in the older population as a whole, but there have been few previous studies of the risk factors for falling within the population with dementia. Of the twelve studies identified in this review,[51, 53, 179–188] most studies of specific dementia subtypes included only patients with AD. Two studies found increased risk of falls in DLB in comparison with AD.[51, 53] Although only one of these studies included assessment of orthostatic hypotension,[51] it is possible that OH may be a significant contributor to falls in DLB, in combination with gait and balance disturbance. Only one previous multifactorial intervention study has exclusively recruited participants with dementia. Interventions were based upon those used in successful trials in people without dementia and included treatment of OH. This study did not show a significant reduction in falls or number of fallers.[189] However, 70% of the participants in this trial lived in institutional settings, most had moderate to severe cognitive impairment, and all had already presented to hospital with a fall. It is possible that multifactorial interventions, including management of OH and autonomic dysfunction, would be successful in patients with less severe dementia. There are several non-pharmacological interventions for orthostatic hypotension, which include avoidance of precipitating factors for low blood pressure, physical counter maneuvers,[190] elevation of the head of the bed at night,[191]and application of graduated pressure with support garments.[192] Recommended pharmacological interventions include fludrocortisone,[193] midodrine,[194, 195] desmopressin (DDAVP), and octreotide.[196] All drug treatment for orthostatic hypotension requires frequent monitoring for supine hypertension, electrolyte imbalance, and congestive heart failure.

Cognitive Function

In addition to the potential risk of falls, autonomic dysfunction may have implications for the progression of cognitive decline in people with neurological disorders. In older people without neurological disorders, there is accumulating evidence that hypotension and OH are associated with cognitive decline, and that systemic blood pressure falls prior to the onset of dementia.[197] There is some evidence that a fall in systolic blood pressure of greater than 30 mmHg on standing in patients with neurodegenerative disorders is associated with a greater risk of significant white matter hyperintensities in basal ganglia and deep white matter on magnetic resonance imaging.[198] In DLB the magnitude of blood pressure fall on carotid sinus massage has been shown to be correlated with the severity of deep white matter hyperintensities on MRI.[117] In both these studies, it was suggested that greater severity of white matter disease would have negative implications for cognitive function.

There is emerging evidence that OH is associated with impairment of cognitive function in Parkinson's disease both without and without dementia. In cross-sectional studies, significant impairment of attentional function assessed by computerized methods was found in PD patients with OH compared with those without OH[199] and in Parkinson's disease dementia (PD), scores achieved on an attentional task declined on head-up tilt, to a degree correlated with fall in BP, although this finding was not present in PD without dementia.[132] Interestingly, cognitive impairment in MSA is mild, suggesting that autonomic dysfunction may have a more complex relationship with cognitive impairment in PD, perhaps related to age of onset and degree of concomitant cortical pathology.[200]

Perceptual, attentional, and executive functioning deficits can be found following a stroke even in those without post-stroke cognitive impairment or dementia, and it has been hypothesized that these may be due to small vessel disease.[201] It is possible that the deficits seen in individuals with postural hypotension or hypertension, similar to those seen following a stroke, may be due to lacunar infarcts occurring in watershed areas of the cerebral circulation. The pattern of neuropsychological deficits in non-memory domains has been noted to occur within the spectrum of vascular cognitive impairment (vascular CIND [cognitive impairment, no dementia], VaD and mixed AD/VaD).[202] However, the etiology of cognitive impairment cannot always be imputed from the domains affected. There are no studies specifically examining autonomic failure and cognitive impairment after stroke.

Unfortunately, the significance of autonomic dysfunction and OH in relation to dementia has not been extensively examined in longitudinal studies. One recent study has shown that low diastolic blood pressure increased the risk of conversion of MCI to dementia,[203] but the role of orthostatic hypotension in the development of MCI or progression of MCI to dementia has not been established. The significance of the severity or duration of orthostatic hypotension is also unclear. It is possible that autonomic dysfunction may influence cognition differently in the various neurological conditions, and this may be substantially related to age of onset and comorbidities. Clearly, well-designed longitudinal studies are required to further elucidate these relationships.

Mortality

Orthostatic hypotension has also been reported to be associated with excess mortality in a prospective study of older adults,[204] and there is evidence to suggest that dysautonomia is associated with excess mortality, particularly sudden death.[205] Autonomic neuropathy is known to be a risk factor for increased mortality in diabetes,[206] and reduced HRV has been shown to be a risk factor for increased mortality after myocardial infarction,[7, 207] for increased all-cause mortality in an elderly population,[208] and also cardiac death or sudden cardiac death.[209] This may be due to an excess of sudden deaths due to arrhythmias, and it has been postulated that this is a potential therapeutic target in cardiovascular disease.[205] Impaired baroreflex sensitivity is predictive of long-term mortality after stroke.[151] It has also been suggested that neurodegenerative disease in the insular cortex may account for excess mortality due to arrhythmias.[119] In neurological disorders, there is some evidence that autonomic dysfunction may also be associated with excess mortality in PD and AD.[210]

Conclusions

In this review, substantial evidence has been reported that emphasizes the importance of autonomic dysfunction in neurological conditions, but particularly the Lewy body disorders and other alphasynucleinopathies. However, although there have been many cross-sectional studies, there are many fewer longitudinal studies, and the long-term sequelae of autonomic dysfunction are not yet understood. There are virtually no interventional studies to assess whether adverse events such as falls and syncope or cognitive decline can be prevented, and therefore current management of autonomic dysfunction in neurological disorders should primarily be guided by symptoms. There is much work still to be done.

Notes

1. Bannister R, Mathias C. Introduction and classification of autonomic disorders. In Mathias CJ, Bannister R (Eds.), *Autonomic failure. A textbook of clinical disorders of the autonomic nervous system* (pp. xviii–xxii). Oxford, UK: Oxford University Press, 1999.
2. Shepherd RFJ, Shepherd JT. *Control of blood pressure and the circulation in man.* Oxford, UK: Oxford University Press, 1999.
3. Eckberg D, Sleight P. *Human baroreflexes in health and disease.* Oxford, UK: Clarendon Press, 1992.

4. Walter PF, Crawley S, Dorney WR. Carotid sinus hypersensitivity and syncope. *Am J Cardiol*. 1978;42:396–403.
5. McLeod JG, Tuck RR. Disorders of the autonomic nervous system: Part 1. Pathophysiology and clinical features. *Ann Neurol*. 1987;21(5):419–430.
6. Pang CC. Autonomic control of the venous system in health and disease: Effects of drugs. *Pharmacol Ther*. 2001;90(2–3):179–230.
7. Kleiger RE, Miller JP, Bigger JT, Jr., Moss AJ. Decreased heart rate variability and its association with increased mortality after acute myocardial infarction. *Am J Cardiol*. 1987;59(4):256–262.
8. Gribbin B, Pickering TG, Sleight P. Decrease in baroreflex sensitivity with increasing arterial pressure and with increasing age. *Br Heart J*. 1969;31(6):791–798.
9. Gribbin B, Pickering TG, Sleight P, Peto R. Effect of age and high blood pressure on baroreflex sensitivity in man. *Circ Res*. 1971;29(4):424–431.
10. Janig W. In Schmidt RF, Thews G (Eds.), *Physiologie des menschen*. 26th ed. (pp. 340–369). Heidelberg/Berlin: Springer Verlag, 1995.
11. Low PA, Opfer-Gehrking TL, McPhee BR, et al. Prospective evaluation of clinical characteristics of orthostatic hypotension. *Mayo Clin Proc*. 1995;70(7):617–622.
12. Mathias CJ, Bannister R. Investigation of autonomic disorders. In Mathias CJ, Bannister R (Eds.), *Autonomic Failure: A textbook of clinical disorders of the autonomic nervous system*, 4th ed. (pp. 169–195). Oxford, UK: Oxford University Press, 1999.
13. McKeith IG, Dickson DW, Lowe J, et al. Diagnosis and management of dementia with Lewy bodies: Third report of the DLB Consortium. *Neurology*. 2005;65(12):1863–1872.
14. Anonymous. Assessment: Clinical autonomic testing report of the Therapeutics and Technology Assessment Subcommittee of the American Academy of Neurology. *Neurology*. 1996;46(3):873–880.
15. Anonymous. Consensus statement on the definition of orthostatic hypotension, pure autonomic failure, and multiple system atrophy. *J Neurol Sci*. 1996;144(1–2):218–219.
16. Hale WA, Chambliss ML. Should primary care patients be screened for orthostatic hypotension? *J Fam Pract*. 1999;48(7):547–552.
17. Ewing DJ, Martyn CN, Young RJ, Clarke BF. The value of cardiovascular autonomic function tests: 10 years' experience in diabetes. *Diabetes Care*. 1985;8(5):491–498.
18. Low PA. Composite autonomic scoring scale for laboratory quantification of generalized autonomic failure. *Mayo Clin Proc*. 1993;68(8):748–752.
19. Smirne S, Ferini SL, Zucconi M, Pinto P, Franceschi M. Cardiac autonomic dysfunction during sleep in some neurological diseases. *Neurophysiol Clin*. 1990;20(2):131–136.
20. Kenny RA. Neurally mediated syncope. *Clin Geriatr Med*. 2002;18(2):191–210, vi.
21. Akselrod S, Gordon D, Ubel FA, Shannon DC, Berger AC, Cohen RJ. Power spectrum analysis of heart rate fluctuation: A quantitative probe of beat-to-beat cardiovascular control. *Science*. 1981;213(4504):220–222.
22. Anonymous. Heart rate variability: Standards of measurement, physiological interpretation and clinical use. Task Force of the European Society of Cardiology and the North American Society of Pacing and Electrophysiology. *Circulation*. 1996;93(5):1043–1065.
23. Malliani A, Pagani M, Lombardi F, Cerutti S. Cardiovascular neural regulation explored in the frequency domain. *Circulation*. 1991;84(2):482–492.
24. Bellavere F, Balzani I, De Masi G, et al. Power spectral analysis of heart-rate variations improves assessment of diabetic cardiac autonomic neuropathy. *Diabetes*. 1992;41(5): 633–640.

25. Orimo S, Ozawa E, Nakade S, Sugimoto T, Mizusawa H. (123)I-metaiodobenzylguanidine myocardial scintigraphy in Parkinson's disease. *J Neurol Neurosurg Psychiatry.* 1999;67(2):189–194.
26. Orimo S, Oka T, Miura H, et al. Sympathetic cardiac denervation in Parkinson's disease and pure autonomic failure but not in multiple system atrophy. *J Neurol Neurosurg Psychiatry.* 2002;73(6):776–777.
27. Yoshita M. Loss of 123I-metaiodobenzylguanidine uptake by the heart in Parkinson's disease. *J Nucl Med.* 2000;41(8):1442.
28. Perry EK, Tomlinson BE, Blessed G, Bergmann K, Gibson PH, Perry RH. Correlation of cholinergic abnormalities with senile plaques and mental test scores in senile dementia. *BMJ.* 1978;2(6150):1457–1459.
29. Perry EK, Marshall E, Perry RH, et al. Cholinergic and dopaminergic activities in senile dementia of Lewy body type. *Alzheimer Dis Assoc Disord.* 1990;4(2):87–95.
30. Aharon-Peretz J, Harel T, Revach M, Ben-Haim SA. Increased sympathetic and decreased parasympathetic cardiac innervation in patients with Alzheimer's disease. *Arch Neurol.* 9/1992 1992;49(9):919–922.
31. Elmstahl S, Petersson M, Lilja B, Samuelsson SM, Rosen I, Bjuno L. Autonomic cardiovascular responses to tilting in patients with Alzheimer's disease and in healthy elderly women. *Age Aging.* 7/1992 1992;21(4):301–307.
32. Algotsson A, Viitanen M, Winblad B, Solders G. Autonomic dysfunction in Alzheimer's disease. *Acta Neurol Scand.* 1/1995 1995;91(1):14–18.
33. Rub U, Del Tredici K, Schultz C, Thal DR, Braak E, Braak H. The autonomic higher-order processing nuclei of the lower brain stem are among the early targets of the Alzheimer's disease-related cytoskeletal pathology. *Acta Neuropathol.* 2001;101(6):555–564.
34. Wakabayashi K, Hayashi S, Morita T, Shibasaki Y, Watanabe Y, Takahashi. Neurofibrillary tangles in the peripheral sympathetic ganglia of non-Alzheimer elderly individuals. *Clin Neuropathol.* 7/1999 1999;18(4):171–175.
35. Martignoni E, Pacchetti C, Godi L, Micieli G, Nappi G. Autonomic disorders in Parkinson's disease. *J Neural Trans Suppl.* 1995;45:11–19.
36. Koike Y, Takahashi A. Autonomic dysfunction in Parkinson's disease. *Eur Neurol.* 1997;38(Suppl 2):8–12.
37. Chaudhuri KR. Autonomic dysfunction in movement disorders. *Curr Opin Neurol.* 2001;14(4):505–511.
38. Hishikawa N, Hashizume Y, Yoshida M, Sobue G. Clinical and neuropathological correlates of Lewy body disease.[*see comment*]. *Acta Neuropath.* 2003;105(4):341–350.
39. Braak H, Ghebremedhin E, Rub U, Bratzke H, Del Tredici K. Stages in the development of Parkinson's disease-related pathology. *Cell Tissue Res.* 2004;318(1):121–134.
40. Braak H, Del Tredici K, Rub U, de Vos RA, Jansen Steur EN, Braak E. Staging of brain pathology related to sporadic Parkinson's disease. *Neurobiol Aging.* 2003;24(2):197–211.
41. Tsuboi Y, Dickson DW. Dementia with Lewy bodies and Parkinson's disease with dementia: Are they different? *Parkinsonism Relat Disord.* 2005;11 Suppl 1:S47–51.
42. Yamamoto R, Iseki E, Marui W, et al. Non-uniformity in the regional pattern of Lewy pathology in brains of dementia with Lewy bodies. *Neuropathology.* 2005;25(3):188–194.
43. Jellinger KA. Lewy body-related alpha-synucleinopathy in the aged human brain. *J Neural Trans.* 2004;111(10–11):1219–1235.
44. Kuzuhara S, Yoshimura M. Clinical and neuropathological aspects of diffuse Lewy body disease in the elderly. *Adv Neurol.* 1993;60:464–469.

45. Watanabe H, Ieda T, Katayama T, et al. Cardiac (123)I-meta-iodobenzylguanidine (MIBG) uptake in dementia with Lewy bodies: Comparison with Alzheimer's disease. *J Neurol Neurosurg Psychiatry*. 2001;70(6):781–783.
46. Horimoto Y, Matsumoto M, Akatsu H, et al. Autonomic dysfunctions in dementia with Lewy bodies. *J Neurol*. 2003;250(5):530–533.
47. Jellinger KA, Horimoto Y, Matsumoto M, et al. Neuropathological spectrum of synucleinopathies: Autonomic dysfunctions in dementia with Lewy bodies. *Move Disord*. 2003;18(6):530–533.
48. Del Ser T, Hachinski V, Merskey H, Munoz DG. Clinical and pathologic features of two groups of patients with dementia with Lewy bodies: Effect of coexisting Alzheimer-type lesion load. *Alzheimer Dis Assoc Disord*. 2001;15(1):31–44.
49. Del-Ser T, Munoz DG, Hachinski V. Temporal pattern of cognitive decline and incontinence is different in Alzheimer's disease and diffuse Lewy body disease. *Neurology*. 1996;46(3):682–686.
50. Ballard CG, O'Brien J, Lowery K, et al. A prospective study of dementia with Lewy bodies. *Age Aging*. 1998;27(5):631–636.
51. Ballard CG, Shaw F, Lowery K, McKeith I, Kenny R. The prevalence, assessment and associations of falls in dementia with Lewy bodies and Alzheimer's disease. *Dement Geriatr Cogn Disord*. 1999;10(2):97–103.
52. Del Ser T, McKeith I, Anand R, Cicin-Sain A, Ferrara R, Spiegel R. Dementia with Lewy bodies: Findings from an international multicentre study. *Int J Geriatr Psychiatry*. 2000;15(11):1034–1045.
53. Imamura T, Hirono N, Hashimoto M, et al. Fall-related injuries in dementia with Lewy bodies (DLB) and Alzheimer's disease. *Eur J Neurol*. 2000;7(1):77–79.
54. McKeith IG, Perry EK, Perry RH. Report of the second dementia with Lewy body international workshop: Diagnosis and treatment. Consortium on Dementia with Lewy Bodies. *Neurology*. 1999;53(5):902–905.
55. McKeith IG, Dickson DW, Lowe J, et al. Diagnosis and management of dementia with Lewy bodies: Third report of the DLB Consortium. *Neurology*. 2005;65(12):1863–1872.
56. Landin K, Blennow K, Wallin A, Gottfries CG. Low blood pressure and blood glucose levels in Alzheimer's disease. Evidence for a hypometabolic disorder? *J Int Med*. 1993;233(4): 357–363.
57. Guo Z, Viitanen M, Fratiglioni L, Winblad B. Low blood pressure and dementia in elderly people: The Kungsholmen project. *BMJ*. 1996;312(7034):805–808.
58. Londos E, Passant U, Gustafson L. Blood pressure and drug treatment in clinically diagnosed Lewy body dementia and Alzheimer's disease. *Arch Gerontol Geriatr*. 2000;30(1):35–46.
59. Idiaquez J, Rios L, Sandoval E. Postprandial hypotension in Alzheimer's disease. *Clin Auton Res*. 1997;7(3):119–120.
60. Siennicki-Lantz A, Lilja B, Elmstahl S. Orthostatic hypotension in Alzheimer's disease: Result or cause of brain dysfunction? *Aging (Milano)*. 1999;11(3):155–160.
61. Allan L, Ballard C, Allen J, et al. Autonomic dysfunction in dementia. *J Neurol Neurosurg Psychiatry*. 2007;78(7):671–677.
62. Andersson M, Hansson O, Minthon L, Ballard CG, Londos E. The period of hypotension following orthostatic challenge is prolonged in dementia with Lewy bodies. *Int J Geriatr Psychiatry*. 2008;23(2):192–198.
63. Oka H, Morita M, Onouchi K, Yoshioka M, Mochio S, Inoue K. Cardiovascular autonomic dysfunction in dementia with Lewy bodies and Parkinson's disease. *J Neurol Sci*. 2007;254(1–2):72–77.

64. Passant U, Warkentin S, Gustafson L. Orthostatic hypotension and low blood pressure in organic dementia: A study of prevalence and related clinical characteristics. *Int J Geriatr Psychiatry*. 1997;12(3):395–403.
65. Ballard C, Shaw F, McKeith I, Kenny R. High prevalence of neurovascular instability in neurodegenerative dementias. *Neurology*. 1998;51(6):1760–1762.
66. Lebert F, Mouly C, Pasquier F. Tolerance to tacrine, arterial hypotension and leuko-araiosis in Alzheimer's disease. *Age Aging*. 1998;27(5):654.
67. Yoshita M, Taki J, Yamada M. A clinical role for [(123)I]MIBG myocardial scintigraphy in the distinction between dementia of the Alzheimer's-type and dementia with Lewy bodies. *J Neurol Neurosurg Psychiatry*. 2001;71(5):583–588.
68. Franceschi M, Ferini-Strambi L, Minicucci F, Sferrazza-Papa A, Smirne S. Signs of cardiac autonomic dysfunction during sleep in patients with Alzheimer's disease. *Gerontology*. 1986;32(6):327–334.
69. Borson S, Barnes RF, Veith RC, Halter JB, Raskind MA. Impaired sympathetic nervous system response to cognitive effort in early Alzheimer's disease. *J Gerontol*. 1989;44(1):M8–12.
70. Yamamoto T, Shimazu K, Tamura N, Watanabe S, Hamaguchi K. Autonomic nervous functions in Alzheimer type and multi-infarct dementia—a hemodynamic study. *Rinsho Shinkeigaku Clin Neurol*. 1990;30(9):1020–1022.
71. Pomara N, Deptula D, Singh R. Pretreatment postural blood pressure drop as a possible predictor of response to the cholinesterase inhibitor velnacrine (HP 029) in Alzheimer's disease. *Psychopharmacol Bull*. 1991;27(3):301–307.
72. Vitiello B, Veith RC, Molchan SE, et al. Autonomic dysfunction in patients with dementia of the Alzheimer type. *Biol Psychiatry*. 1993;34(7):428–433.
73. Wang SJ, Liao KK, Fuh JL, Yamada M. Cardiovascular autonomic functions in Alzheimer's disease. *Age Aging*. 1994;23(5):400–404.
74. Jhee SS, Sramek JJ, Wardle TS, Cutler NR. Orthostasis in Alzheimer disease: A retrospective analysis. *Alzheimer Dis Assoc Disord*. 1995;9(4):243–246.
75. Watanabe M, Nishimura R, Ito H, Mano K, Watanabe H. Clinical significance of orthostatic blood pressure decline in patients with Binswanger-type infarction. *Rinsho Shinkeigaku Clin Neurol*. 1997;37(10):868–872.
76. Medina A, Bodick N, Goldberger AL, Mac MM, Lipsitz, LA. Effects of central muscarinic-1 receptor stimulation on blood pressure regulation. *Hypertension*. 1997;29(3):828–834.
77. Giubilei F, Strano S, Imbimbo BP, et al. Cardiac autonomic dysfunction in patients with Alzheimer disease: possible pathogenetic mechanisms. *Alzheimer Dis Assoc Disord*. 1998;12(4):356–361.
78. Paradowski B, Bilinska M, Koszewicz M, Pokryszko A. Evaluation of cardiovascular and sudomotor functions in Alzheimer's disease. *Polski Merkuriusz Lekarski*. 1999;7(40): 180–184.
79. Niimi Y, Watanabe M, Nishimura R, Mano K, Watanabe H. Baroreflex function in patients with Binswanger's encephalopathy. *Rinsho Shinkeigaku Clin Neurol*. 1999;39(7):700–704.
80. Idiaquez J, Sandoval E. High prevalence of neurovascular instability in neurodegenerative dementias. *Neurology*. 1999;53(7):1610.
81. Rainero I, Vighetti S, Bergamasco B, Pinessi L, Benedetti F. Autonomic responses and pain perception in Alzheimer's disease. *Eur J Pain*. 2000;4(3):267–274.
82. Pascualy M, Petrie EC, Brodkin K, Peskind ER, Wilkinson CW, Raskind MA. Hypothalamic pituitary adrenocortical and sympathetic nervous system responses to the cold pressor test in Alzheimer's disease. *Biol Psychiatry*. 2000;48(3):247–254.

83. Watanabe M, Niimi Y, Koike Y, Sugiyama Y. Power spectrum analysis of heart rate variability to orthostatic challenge in cases of Binswanger's encephalopathy. *Rinsho Shinkeigaku Clin Neurol*. 2000;40(6):551–555.
84. Idiaquez J, Sandoval E, Seguel A. Association between neuropsychiatric and autonomic dysfunction in Alzheimer's disease. *Clin Auton Res*. 2002;12(1):43–46.
85. Kalman J, Szakacs R, Torok T, et al. Decreased cutaneous vasodilatation to isometric handgrip exercise in Alzheimer's disease. *Int J Geriatr Psychiatry*. 2002;17(4):371–374.
86. Allan L. Orthostatic Hypotension and Autonomic Dysfunction. In Ballard C (Ed.), *Parkinson's Dementia* (pp. 99–110). Delray Beach, FL: Carma Publishing, 2007.
87. Allan LM, Kerr SR, Ballard CG, et al. Autonomic function assessed by heart rate variability is normal in Alzheimer's disease and vascular dementia. *Dement Geriatr Cogn Dis*. 2005;19(2–3):140–144.
88. de Vilhena Toledo MA, Junqueira LF Jr. Cardiac sympathovagal modulation evaluated by short-term heart interval variability is subtly impaired in Alzheimer's disease. *Geriatr Gerontol Int*. 2008;8(2):109–118.
89. Szili-Torok T, Kalman J, Paprika D, Dibo G, Rozsa Z, Rudas L. Depressed baroreflex sensitivity in patients with Alzheimer's and Parkinson's disease. *Neurobiol Aging*. 2001;22(3):435–438.
90. Scinto LF, Daffner KR, Dressler D, et al. A potential noninvasive neurobiological test for Alzheimer's disease. *Science*. 1994;266(5187):1051–1054.
91. Kardon RH. Drop the Alzheimer's drop test. *Neurology*. 1998;50(3):588–591.
92. Granholm E, Morris S, Galasko D, Shults C, Rogers E, Vukov B. Tropicamide effects on pupil size and pupillary light reflexes in Alzheimer's and Parkinson's disease. *Int J Psychophysiol*. 2003;47(2):95–115.
93. Gomez-Tortosa E, del Barrio A, Jimenez-Alfaro I. Pupil response to tropicamide in Alzheimer's disease and other neurodegenerative disorders. *Acta Neurol Scand*. 1996;94(2):104–109.
94. Kono K, Miyao M, Ishihara S, et al. Hypersensitivity in the pupil dilation response to a cholinergic antagonist in patients with Alzheimer's disease and Down's syndrome. *Nippon Ronen Igakkai Zasshi*. 1996;33(11):829–834.
95. Arai H, Terajima M, Nakagawa T, Higuchi S, Mochizuki H, Sasaki H. Pupil dilatation assay by tropicamide is modulated by apolipoprotein E epsilon 4 allele dosage in Alzheimer's disease. *Neuroreport*. 1996;7(4):918–920.
96. Higuchi S, Matsushita S, Hasegawa Y, Muramatsu T, Arai H. Pupillary response to tropicamide in Japanese patients with alcoholic dementia, Alzheimer's disease, and vascular dementia. *Exp Neurol*. 1997;144(1):199–201.
97. Fridh M, Havelius U, Elofsson G, Hindfelt B. The pupillary response to tropicamide in Alzheimer's disease. *Acta Ophthalmol Scand*. 1996;74(3):276–279.
98. Litvan I, FitzGibbon EJ. Can tropicamide eye drop response differentiate patients with progressive supranuclear palsy and Alzheimer's disease from healthy control subjects? *Neurology*. 1996;47(5):1324–1326.
99. Loupe DN, Newman NJ, Green RC, et al. Pupillary response to tropicamide in patients with Alzheimer disease. *Ophthalmology*. 1996;103(3):495–503.
100. Robles A, Tourino R, Sesar A, Suarez P, Noya M. Experience with pupil tropicamide test in Alzheimer's disease. *Revista de Neurologia*. 1996;24(125):65–68.
101. Treloar AJ, Assin M, Macdonald AJ. Pupillary response to topical tropicamide as a marker for Alzheimer's disease. *Br J Clin Pharmacol*. 1996;41(3):256–257.

102. FitzSimon JS, Waring SC, Kokmen E, McLaren JW, Brubaker RF. Response of the pupil to tropicamide is not a reliable test for Alzheimer disease. *Arch Neurol*. 1997;54(2):155–159.
103. Graff-Radford NR, Lin SC, Brazis PW, et al. Tropicamide eyedrops cannot be used for reliable diagnosis of Alzheimer's disease. *Mayo Clin Proc*. 1997;72(6):495–504.
104. Growdon JH, Graefe K, Tennis M, Hayden D, Schoenfeld D, Wray SH. Pupil dilation to tropicamide is not specific for Alzheimer disease. *Arch Neurol*. 1997;54(7):841–844.
105. Kalman J, Kanka A, Magloczky E, Szoke A, Jardanhazy T, Janka Z. Increased mydriatic response to tropicamide is a sign of cholinergic hypersensitivity but not specific to late-onset sporadic type of Alzheimer's dementia. *Biol Psychiatry*. 1997;41(8):909–911.
106. Kurz A, Marquard R, Fremke S, Leipert KP. Pupil dilation response to tropicamide: A biological test for Alzheimer's disease? *Pharmacopsychiatry*. 1997;30(1):12–15.
107. Reitner A, Baumgartner I, Thuile C, et al. The mydriatic effect of tropicamide and its diagnostic use in Alzheimer's disease. *Vision Res*. 1997;37(1):165–168.
108. Kaneyuki H, Mitsuno S, Nishida T, Yamada M. Enhanced miotic response to topical dilute pilocarpine in patients with Alzheimer's disease. *Neurology*. 1998;50(3):802–804.
109. Ferrario E, Molaschi M, Villa L, Varetto O, Bogetto C, Nuzzi R. Is videopupillography useful in the diagnosis of Alzheimer's disease? *Neurology*. 1998;50(3):642–644.
110. Prettyman R, Bitsios P, Szabadi E. Altered pupillary size and darkness and light reflexes in Alzheimer's disease. *J Neurol Neurosurg Psychiatry*. 1997;62(6):665–668.
111. Fotiou F, Fountoulakis KN, Tsolaki M, Goulas A, Palikaras A. Changes in pupil reaction to light in Alzheimer's disease patients: A preliminary report. *Int J Psychophysiol*. 2000;37(1):111–120.
112. Lamb K, Bradshaw CM, Szabadi E. The responsiveness of human eccrine sweat glands to choline and carbachol. Application to the study of peripheral cholinergic functioning in Alzheimer-type dementia. *Eur J Clin Pharmacol*. 1983;24(1):55–62.
113. Hornqvist R, Henriksson R, Back O, Bucht G, Winblad B. Iontophoretic study of adrenergic and cholinergic skin vessel reactivity in normal aging and Alzheimer's disease. *Gerontology*. 1987;33(6):374–379.
114. Algotsson A, Nordberg A, Almkvist O, Winblad B. Skin vessel reactivity is impaired in Alzheimer's disease. *Neurobiol Aging*. 1995;16(4):577–582.
115. Ryer HI, Katz SE, Serby M. Muscarinic receptors on human eccrine sweat gland in aging and Alzheimer's disease. *Biol Psychiatry*. 1995;37(4):259–264.
116. Kumar NP, Youde JH, Ruse C, et al. Responses to the prolonged head-up tilt followed by sublingual nitrate provocation in asymptomatic older adults. *Age Aging*. 2000;29(5): 419–424.
117. Kenny RA, Shaw FE, O'Brien JT, Scheltens PH, Kalaria R, Ballard C. Carotid sinus syndrome is common in dementia with Lewy bodies and correlates with deep white matter lesions. *J Neurol Neurosurg Psychiatry*. 2004;75(7):966–971.
118. Bordier P, Colsy M, Robert F, et al. Prevalence of positive carotid sinus massage and related risk of syncope in patients with Alzheimer's disease. *Europace*. 2007;9(9):829–834.
119. Royall DR, Gao JH, Kellogg DL, Jr. Insular Alzheimer's disease pathology as a cause of "age-related" autonomic dysfunction and mortality in the non-demented elderly. *Med Hypotheses*. 2006;67(4):747–758.
120. Braak H, Braak E. Evolution of neuronal changes in the course of Alzheimer's disease. *J Neural Trans Suppl*. 1998;53:127–140.
121. McLaren A, Kerr S, Allan L, et al. Autonomic function is impaired in elderly stroke survivors. *Stroke*. 2005;36(5):1026–1030.
122. Taki J, Yoshita M, Yamada M, Tonami N. Significance of ^{123}I-MIBG scintigraphy as a pathophysiological indicator in the assessment of Parkinson's disease and related

disorders: It can be a specific marker for Lewy body disease. *Ann Nucl Med*. 2004;18(6): 453–461.

123. Bonuccelli U, Lucetti C, Del Dotto P, et al. Orthostatic hypotension in de novo Parkinson disease. *Arch Neurol*. 2003;60(10):1400–1404.
124. Senard JM, Rai S, Lapeyre-Mestre M, et al. Prevalence of orthostatic hypotension in Parkinson's disease. *J Neurol Neurosurg Psychiatry*. 1997;63(5):584–589.
125. Wood BH, Bilclough JA, Bowron A, Walker RW. Incidence and prediction of falls in Parkinson's disease: A prospective multidisciplinary study. *J Neurol Neurosurg Psychiatry*. 2002;72(6):721–725.
126. Allcock LM, Ullyart K, Kenny RA, Burn DJ. Frequency of orthostatic hypotension in a community based cohort of patients with Parkinson's disease. *J Neurol Neurosurg Psychiatry*. 2004;75(10):1470–1471.
127. Allcock LM, Kenny RA, Burn DJ. Clinical phenotype of subjects with Parkinson's disease and orthostatic hypotension: Autonomic symptom and demographic comparison. *Mov Disord*. 2006;21(11):1851–1855.
128. Kallio M, Haapaniemi T, Turkka J, et al. Heart rate variability in patients with untreated Parkinson's disease. *Eur J Neurol*. 2000;7(6):667–672.
129. Haapaniemi TH, Pursiainen V, Korpelainen JT, Huikuri HV, Sotaniemi KA, Myllyla VV. Ambulatory ECG and analysis of heart rate variability in Parkinson's disease. *J Neurol Neurosurg Psychiatry*. 2001;70(3):305–310.
130. Jankovic J, McDermott M, Carter J, et al. Variable expression of Parkinson's disease: A base-line analysis of the DATATOP cohort. The Parkinson Study Group. *Neurology*. 1990;40(10):1529–1534.
131. van Dijk JG, Haan J, Zwinderman K, Kremer B, van Hilten BJ, Roos RA. Autonomic nervous system dysfunction in Parkinson's disease: Relationships with age, medication, duration, and severity. *J Neurol Neurosurg Psychiatry*. 1993;56(10):1090–1095.
132. Peralta C, Stampfer-Kountchev M, Karner E, et al. Orthostatic hypotension and attention in Parkinson's disease with and without dementia. *J Neural Trans*. 2007;114(5):585–588.
133. Arai K, Kato N, Kashiwado K, Hattori T. Pure autonomic failure in association with human alpha-synucleinopathy. *Neurosci Lett*. 2000;296(2–3):171–173.
134. Iwanaga K, Wakabayashi K, Yoshimoto M, et al. Lewy body-type degeneration in cardiac plexus in Parkinson's and incidental Lewy body diseases. *Neurology*. 4/12/1999 1999;52(6):1269–1271.
135. Hague K, Lento P, Morgello S, Caro S, Kaufmann H. The distribution of Lewy bodies in pure autonomic failure: Autopsy findings and review of the literature. *Acta Neuropath*. 1997;94(2):192–196.
136. Wakabayashi K, Takahashi H. Neuropathology of autonomic nervous system in Parkinson's disease. *Eur Neurol*. 1997;38(Suppl 2):2–7.
137. Wakabayashi K, Takahashi H, Ohama E, Takeda S, Ikuta F. Lewy bodies in the visceral autonomic nervous system in Parkinson's disease. *Adv Neurol*. 1993;60:609–612.
138. Wakabayashi K, Takahashi H, Ohama E, Ikuta F. Parkinson's disease: An immunohistochemical study of Lewy body-containing neurons in the enteric nervous system. *Acta Neuropath*. 1990;79(6):581–583.
139. Braak H, de Vos RA, Bohl J, et al. Gastric alpha-synuclein immunoreactive inclusions in Meissner's and Auerbach's plexuses in cases staged for Parkinson's disease-related brain pathology. *Neurosci Lett*. 2006;396(1):67–72.
140. Minguez-Castellanos A, Chamorro CE, Escamilla-Sevilla F, et al. Do alpha-synuclein aggregates in autonomic plexuses predate Lewy body disorders? A cohort study. *Neurology*. 2007;68(23):2012–2018.

141. Gilman S, Wenning GK, Low PA, et al. Second consensus statement on the diagnosis of multiple system atrophy. *Neurology*. 2008;71(9):670–676.
142. Seppi K, Yekhlef F, Diem A, et al. Progression of Parkinsonism in multiple system atrophy. *J Neurol*. 2005;252(1):91–96.
143. Sandroni P, Ahlskog JE, Fealey RD, Low PA. Autonomic involvement in extrapyramidal and cerebellar disorders. *Clin Auton Res*. 1991;1(2):147–155.
144. Gutrecht JA. Autonomic cardiovascular reflexes in progressive supranuclear palsy. *J Auton Nerv Sys*. 1992;39(1):29–35.
145. Deguchi K, Sasaki I, Tsukaguchi M, et al. Abnormalities of rate-corrected QT intervals in Parkinson's disease—a comparison with multiple system atrophy and progressive supranuclear palsy. *J Neurol Sci*. 2002;199(1–2):31–37.
146. Kimber J, Mathias CJ, Lees AJ, et al. Physiological, pharmacological and neurohormonal assessment of autonomic function in progressive supranuclear palsy. *Brain*. 2000;123 (Pt 7):1422–1430.
147. Brefel-Courbon C, Thalamas C, Rascol O, Montastruc JL, Senard JM. Lack of autonomic nervous dysfunction in progressive supranuclear palsy, a study of blood pressure variability. *Clin Auton Res*. 2000;10(5):309–312.
148. Holmberg B, Kallio M, Johnels B, Elam M. Cardiovascular reflex testing contributes to clinical evaluation and differential diagnosis of Parkinsonian syndromes. *Mov Disord*. 2001;16(2):217–225.
149. van Dijk JG, Haan J, Koenderink M, Roos RA. Autonomic nervous function in progressive supranuclear palsy. *Arch Neurol*. 1991;48(10):1083–1084.
150. Friedrich C, Rudiger H, Schmidt C, et al. Baroreflex sensitivity and power spectral analysis in different extrapyramidal syndromes. *J Neural Trans*. 2008;115(11):1527–1536.
151. Korpelainen JT, Sotaniemi KA, Myllyla VV. Autonomic nervous system disorders in stroke. *Clin Auton Res*. 1999;9(6):325–333.
152. Korpelainen JT, Sotaniemi KA, Huikuri HV, Myllya VV. Abnormal heart rate variability as a manifestation of autonomic dysfunction in hemispheric brain infarction. *Stroke*. 1996;27(11):2059–2063.
153. Bassi A, Colivicchi F, Santini M, Caltagirone C. Cardiac autonomic dysfunction and functional outcome after ischaemic stroke. *Eur J Neurol*. 2007;14(8):917–922.
154. Micieli G, Cavallini A. The autonomic nervous system and ischemic stroke: A reciprocal interdependence. *Clin Auton Res*. 2008;18(6):308–317.
155. Mathias CJ, Deguchi K, Schatz I. Observations on recurrent syncope and presyncope in 641 patients. *Lancet*. 2001;357(9253):348–353.
156. Cummings SR, Nevitt MC, Kidd S. Forgetting falls. The limited accuracy of recall of falls in the elderly. *J Am Geriatr Soc*. 1988;36(7):613–616.
157. McIntosh SJ, Lawson J, Kenny RA. Clinical characteristics of vasodepressor, cardioinhibitory, and mixed carotid sinus syndrome in the elderly. *Am J Med*. 1993;95(2):203–208.
158. Shaw FE, Kenny RA. The overlap between syncope and falls in the elderly. *Postgrad Med J*. 1997;73(864):635–639.
159. Tinetti ME, Inouye SK, Gill TM, Doucette JT. Shared risk factors for falls, incontinence, and functional dependence. Unifying the approach to geriatric syndromes. *J Am Med Assoc*. 1995;273(17):1348–1353.
160. Tinetti ME, Williams CS. Falls, injuries due to falls, and the risk of admission to a nursing home. *N Engl J Med*. 1997;337(18):1279–1284.
161. Tinetti ME, Williams TF, Mayewski R. Fall risk index for elderly patients based on number of chronic disabilities. *Am J Med*. 1986;80(3):429–434.

162. Lipsitz LA, Jonsson PV, Kelley MM, et al. Causes and correlates of recurrent falls in ambulatory frail elderly. *J Gerontol*. 1991;46(4):M114–122.
163. Rutan GH, Hermanson B, Bild DE, Kittner SJ, LaBaw F, Tell GS. Orthostatic hypotension in older adults. The Cardiovascular Health Study. CHS Collaborative Research Group. *Hypertension*. 1992;19(6 Pt 1):508–519.
164. Graafmans WC, Ooms ME, Hofstee HM, et al. Falls in the elderly: A prospective study of risk factors and risk profiles. *Am J Epidemiol*. 1996;143(11):1129–1136.
165. Ooi WL, Hossain M, Lipsitz LA. The association between orthostatic hypotension and recurrent falls in nursing home residents. *Am J Med*. 2000;108(2):106–111.
166. Tinetti ME, Speechley M, Ginter SF. Risk factors for falls among elderly persons living in the community. *N Engl J Med*. 1988;319(26):1701–1707.
167. Campbell AJ, Borrie MJ, Spears GF. Risk factors for falls in a community-based prospective study of people 70 years and older. *J Gerontol*. 1989;44(4):M112–117.
168. Robbins AS, Rubenstein LZ, Josephson KR, et al. Predictors of falls among elderly people. Results of two population-based studies. *Arch Intern Med*. 1989;149(7):1628–1633.
169. Liu BA, Topper AK, Reeves RA, et al. Falls among older people: Relationship to medication use and orthostatic hypotension. *J Am Geriatr Soc*. 1995;43(10):1141–1145.
170. Lord SR, Anstey KJ, Williams P, et al. Psychoactive medication use, sensori-motor function and falls in older women. *Br J Clin Pharmacol*. 1995;39(3):227–234.
171. Maurer MS, Cohen S, Cheng H. The degree and timing of orthostatic blood pressure changes in relation to falls in nursing home residents. *J Am Med Dir Assoc*. 2004;5(4):233–238.
172. Clark RD, Lord SR, Webster IW. Clinical parameters associated with falls in an elderly population. *Gerontology*. 1993;39(2):117–123.
173. Tinetti ME, Baker DI, McAvay G, et al. A multifactorial intervention to reduce the risk of falling among elderly people living in the community. *N Engl J Med*. 1994;331(13): 821–827.
174. Close J, Ellis M, Hooper R, et al. Prevention of falls in the elderly trial (PROFET): A randomised controlled trial. *Lancet*. 1999;353(9147):93–97.
175. Davison J, Bond J, Dawson P, Steen IN, Kenny RA. Patients with recurrent falls attending Accident and Emergency benefit from multifactorial intervention—a randomised controlled trial. *Age Aging*. 2005;34(2):162–168.
176. Morris JC, Rubin EH, Morris EJ, Mandel SA. Senile dementia of the Alzheimer's type: An important risk factor for serious falls. *J Gerontol*. 1987;42(4):412–417.
177. van Doorn C, Gruber-Baldini AL, Zimmerman S, et al. Dementia as a risk factor for falls and fall injuries among nursing home residents. *J Am Geriatr Soc*. 2003;51(9): 1213–1218.
178. Shaw FE. Falls in cognitive impairment and dementia. *Clin Geriatr Med*. 2002;18(2): 159–173.
179. Buchner DM, Larson EB. Falls and fractures in patients with Alzheimer-type dementia. *J Am Med Assoc*. 1987;257(11):1492–1495.
180. van Dijk PT, Meulenberg OG, van de Sande HJ, Habbema JD. Falls in dementia patients. *Gerontologist*. 1993;33(2):200–204.
181. Nakamura T, Meguro K, Sasaki H. Relationship between falls and stride length variability in senile dementia of the Alzheimer type. *Gerontology*. 1996;42(2):108–113.
182. Asada T, Kariya T, Kinoshita T, et al. Predictors of fall-related injuries among community-dwelling elderly people with dementia. *Age Aging*. 1996;25(1):22–28.
183. Lowery K, Buri H, Ballard C. What is the prevalence of environmental hazards in the homes of dementia sufferers and are they associated with falls. *Int J Geriatr Psychiatry*. 2000;15(10):883–886.

184. Camicioli R, Licis L. Motor impairment predicts falls in specialized Alzheimer care units. *Alzheimer Dis Assoc Disord*. 2004;18(4):214–218.
185. Katz IR, Rupnow M, Kozma C, Schneider L. Risperidone and falls in ambulatory nursing home residents with dementia and psychosis or agitation: Secondary analysis of a double-blind, placebo-controlled trial. *Am J Geriatr Psychiatry*. 2004;12(5):499–508.
186. Sato Y, Kanoko T, Satoh K, Iwamoto J. Risk factors for hip fracture among elderly patients with Alzheimer's disease. *J Neurol Sci*. 2004;223(2):107–112.
187. Olsson RH, Jr., Wambold S, Brock B, Waugh D, Sprague H. Visual spatial abilities and fall risk: An assessment tool for individuals with dementia. *J Gerontol Nurs*. 2005;31(9):45–51; quiz, 52–43.
188. Horikawa E, Matsui T, Arai H, Seki T, Iwasaki K, Sasaki H. Risk of falls in Alzheimer's disease: A prospective study. *Int Med*. 2005;44(7):717–721.
189. Shaw FE, Bond J, Richardson DA, et al. Multifactorial intervention after a fall in older people with cognitive impairment and dementia presenting to the accident and emergency department: Randomised controlled trial. *BMJ*. 2003;326(7380):73.
190. Bouvette CM, McPhee BR, Opfer-Gehrking TL, Low PA. Role of physical countermaneuvers in the management of orthostatic hypotension: Efficacy and biofeedback augmentation. *Mayo Clin Proc*. 1996;71(9):847–853.
191. Ten Harkel AD, Van Lieshout JJ, Wieling W. Treatment of orthostatic hypotension with sleeping in the head-up tilt position, alone and in combination with fludrocortisone. *J Int Med*. 1992;232(2):139–145.
192. Denq JC, Opfer-Gehrking TL, Giuliani M, et al. Efficacy of compression of different capacitance beds in the amelioration of orthostatic hypotension. *Clin Auton Res*. 1997;7(6):321–326.
193. Hussain RM, McIntosh SJ, Lawson J, Kenny RA. Fludrocortisone in the treatment of hypotensive disorders in the elderly. *Heart*. 1996;76(6):507–509.
194. Low PA, Gilden JL, Freeman R, Sheng KN, McElligott MA. Efficacy of midodrine vs placebo in neurogenic orthostatic hypotension. A randomized, double-blind multicenter study. Midodrine Study Group. *J Am Med Assoc*. 1997;277(13):1046–1051.
195. Wright RA, Kaufmann HC, Perera R, et al. A double-blind, dose-response study of midodrine in neurogenic orthostatic hypotension. *Neurology*. 1998;51(1):120–124.
196. Bordet R, Benhadjali J, Libersa C, Destee A. Octreotide in the management of orthostatic hypotension in multiple system atrophy: Pilot trial of chronic administration. *Clin Neuropharmacol*. 1994;17(4):380–383.
197. Moretti R, Torre P, Antonello RM, et al. Risk factors for vascular dementia: Hypotension as a key point. *Vasc Health Risk Manag*. 2008;4(2):395–402.
198. Ballard C, O'Brien J, Barber B, et al. Neurocardiovascular instability, hypotensive episodes, and MRI lesions in neurodegenerative dementia. *Ann N Y Acad Sci*. 2000;903:442–445.
199. Allcock LM, Kenny RA, Mosimann UP, et al. Orthostatic hypotension in Parkinson's disease: Association with cognitive decline? *Int J Geriatr Psychiatry*. 2006;21(8):778–783.
200. Bak TH, Crawford LM, Hearn VC, Mathuranath PS, Hodges JR. Subcortical dementia revisited: Similarities and differences in cognitive function between progressive supranuclear palsy (PSP), corticobasal degeneration (CBD) and multiple system atrophy (MSA). *Neurocase*. 2005;11(4):268–273.
201. Stephens S, Kenny RA, Rowan E, et al. Neuropsychological characteristics of mild vascular cognitive impairment and dementia after stroke. *Int J Geriatr Psychiatry*. 2004;19(11):1053–1057.
202. Rockwood K, Howard K, MacKnight C, Darvesh S. Spectrum of disease in vascular cognitive impairment. *Neuroepidemiology*. 1999;18(5):248–254.

203. Ravaglia G, Forti P, Maioli F, et al. Conversion of mild cognitive impairment to dementia: Predictive role of mild cognitive impairment subtypes and vascular risk factors. *Dement Geriatr Cogn Dis Disorders*. 2006;21(1):51–58.
204. Masaki KH, Schatz IJ, Burchfiel CM, et al. Orthostatic hypotension predicts mortality in elderly men: The Honolulu Heart Program. *Circulation*. 1998;98(21):2290–2295.
205. Routledge HC, Chowdhary S, Townend JN. Heart rate variability—a therapeutic target? *J Clin Pharm Ther*. 2002;27(2):85–92.
206. Ewing DJ, Campbell IW, Clarke BF. Mortality in diabetic autonomic neuropathy. *Lancet*. 1976;1(7960):601–603.
207. Zuanetti G, Neilson JM, Latini R, Santoro E, Maggioni AP, Ewing DJ. Prognostic significance of heart rate variability in post-myocardial infarction patients in the fibrinolytic era. The GISSI-2 results. Gruppo Italiano per lo Studio della Sopravvivenza nell' Infarto Miocardico. *Circulation*. 1996;94(3):432–436.
208. Tsuji H, Venditti FJ Jr., Manders ES, et al. Reduced heart rate variability and mortality risk in an elderly cohort. The Framingham Heart Study. *Circulation*. 1994;90(2):878–883.
209. Makikallio TH, Huikuri HV, Makikallio A, et al. Prediction of sudden cardiac death by fractal analysis of heart rate variability in elderly subjects. *J Am Coll Cardiol*. 2001;37(5):1395–1402.
210. Ishizaki F, Harada T, Yoshinaga H, Nakayama T, Yamamura Y, Nakamura S. Prolonged QTc intervals in Parkinson's disease—relation to sudden death and autonomic dysfunction. *Brain Nerve*. 1996;48(5):443–448.
211. Brignole M, Menozzi C, Del Rosso A, et al. New classification of haemodynamics of vasovagal syncope: Beyond the VASIS classification. Analysis of the pre-syncopal phase of the tilt test without and with nitroglycerin challenge. Vasovagal Syncope International Study. *Europace*. 2000;2(1):66–76.
212. Kenny RA, O'Shea D, Parry SW. The Newcastle protocols for head-up tilt table testing in the diagnosis of vasovagal syncope, carotid sinus hypersensitivity, and related disorders. *Heart*. 2000;83(5):564–569.

18

STRUCTURAL AND METABOLIC MAGNETIC RESONANCE IMAGING AND VASCULAR RISK FACTORS

Istvan Csapo, Troy Russell, Jared Price, Daniel McCaffrey, Jeffrey Dewey, Ekta Sem, and David F. Tate

Magnetic resonance imaging (MRI) technologies have seen dramatic improvement over the past decade, resulting in widespread use in clinical and research settings. MRI has been used successfully to examine a range of neurological disorders, developmental abnormalities, as well as typical aging patterns *in vivo*. These studies greatly inform our understanding of the relationships between a wide variety of clinical factors affecting the central nervous system (CNS) and have unique potential for examining vascular-related changes in patients with accumulating vascular risk factors (see Table 18-1 for a summary of reasons to examine CVD patients). For example, neuroimaging markers of pathological vascular changes in the cerebral white matter (WM) are frequently detected by structural MRI (see below). These findings are observed in both asymptomatic and cognitively impaired patients and, if present in sufficient numbers, can lead to vascular dementia (VaD). In fact, cerebrovascular disease (CVD) is the second leading cause of dementia after Alzheimer's disease (AD)[1] and is associated with the accumulation of signal abnormalities found in the cerebral white matter.

The objective of this chapter is to give an overview of *in vivo* structural and metabolic imaging findings associated with vascular risk factors and underlying CVD in the CNS. We begin the chapter by briefly discussing the pathological consequences of vascular dysfunction and basic MRI physics for structural and metabolic imaging. We then discuss the common clinical and quantitative MRI findings associated with established vascular disease risk factors. We end the chapter by suggesting future directions for research.

Pathological Consequences

Identifying the mechanisms responsible for injury to the brain parenchyma is important for understanding the MRI manifestations and the evolution of such injury. CVD-related

Table 18-1 Summary of the current clinical and research objectives of MRI examination in CVD patients experiencing cognitive changes

Make a diagnosis of vascular-related changes
1. Screen or rule out the possibility of other neurologic complications.
2. Understand disease etiology/pathogenesis.
3. Assess disease severity (a single MRI exam allows examination of the amount of CNS involvement).
4. Monitor progression (serial MRI provides markers of progression—translation of vascular activity into neurodegeneration).
5. Potentially inform treatment by assessing effect (both CNS-specific treatment as well as generic treatment to the extent that neurodegeneration is a covariate of general progression).

brain injury covers a plethora of conditions; however, the most common underlying cause for patients "at risk" for developing vascular dementia is ischemic brain injury. In ischemia, the cerebral blood flow (CBF) is reduced enough to cause functional or metabolic deficits that can lead to overt brain damage. The reduction in CBF is usually secondary to diminished arterial flow or vascular obstruction, but it may also be caused by increased intracranial or tissue pressure that in turn results in decreased perfusion.[2] This reduction not only affects the delivery of essential substrates, such as oxygen and glucose, to the parenchyma, but may also lead to the accumulation of neurotoxic metabolic by-products,[2] a change in the permeability of the blood–brain barrier (BBB),[3,4] and the failure of autoregulatory mechanisms necessary for maintaining consistent blood flow to the brain.[5,6] The ensuing cascade of events produces detectable changes on several MRI sequences that follow a unique time course (see below).

In moderate ischemia, oxygen delivery is reduced enough to perturb metabolic operations necessary to sustain normal synaptic activity, but not sufficient to jeopardize cell survival.[2] The resulting symptoms resemble those observed in severe hypoxia; however, the affected tissue may recover. A similar situation is thought to exist in the tissues outside of the central core of a focal ischemic lesion.[7,8] More severe degrees of ischemia (with CBF reduced to about 20% of control) can trigger bioenergetic failure and start a sequence of events that results in cell death. Neurons are especially vulnerable to such an event, even if the duration is limited to four to six minutes.[2] In addition to bioenergetic failure, reduced CBF might not be sufficient to remove toxic metabolic waste products and can also trigger a potentially harmful interaction between endothelial cells and blood-borne elements. This interaction not only physically hinders perfusion but also elicits an inflammatory response. The resulting immune response adversely affects BBB function and microvascular tone (autoregulation), further compromising cerebral perfusion.

In spite of fluctuations in blood flow and systemic pressure changes, the brain has a set of compensatory mechanisms to sustain consistent arterial pressure. This mechanism—often termed *autoregulation*—can maintain CBF within a certain range of arterial pressure, given its ability to rapidly counter pressure fluctuations.[9] However, it is believed that this autoregulatory mechanism can be compromised for patients who have chronic untreated or undetected hypertension.[10] In the context of hypertension, autoregulation is thought to be disturbed, especially in small microvessels, via injury to the endothelial cells of the blood vessel walls. Consequently, it becomes increasingly difficult for endothelial cells to respond to sudden shifts in blood pressure. This type of injury to the endothelial cells is particularly relevant in patients with small-vessel disease, which makes them more vulnerable to sudden fluctuations in blood pressure. In particular, damage to the autoregulatory function due to hypertension renders patients more susceptible to the effects of hypotension or ischemic events.

Alteration of endothelial permeability is another possible mechanism for brain injury. With decreased permeability, found in certain small-vessel diseases, the ensuing effects are similar to that of ischemia: Even though CBF remains normal, nutrients cannot efficiently reach the parenchyma, and metabolic by-products are not removed. Severe damage to the endothelium can lead to the disintegration of the microvessel walls and result in increased permeability that enables blood-borne neurotoxic agents to cross the blood–brain barrier.[11] There is little evidence, however, that the change in the permeability of the vessel walls is the primary component of CVD-related histopathological brain injury.

It is important to note that the extent of tissue damage, the clinical manifestations, and MRI findings associated with ischemic injury depend on the severity, duration, and location of the injury. However, due to the relative morphological homogeneity of white matter, there is a limited range of structural responses to a number of pathological conditions.[12] CVD indirectly affects white matter through reduced blood flow, ischemia, accumulation of neurotoxic by-products, and alteration of vessel-wall permeability. This leads to the accumulation of several basic pathological components of CVD-related white matter injury, including loss of parenchymal elements (myelin, axons, and glial cells), increase in glial cells (gliosis), edema, vascular changes, gross and regional atrophy, and necrosis with scarring or cavitation.[12] Though the etiological specificity of MRI is limited, it is possible to examine these pathological changes *in vivo*. For example, demyelination, gliosis, and vasogenic edema all appear as hyperintense (bright) regions on T2-weighted (T2w) MRI images. If combined with information from other MRI sequences, poor specificity can be improved, and subtle differences in pathology (e.g., difference between cytotoxic and vasogenic edema) can be examined.

Common Quantitative Structural Neuroimaging Findings

Several different types of MRI sequences exist that provide unique types of tissue contrast that improve sensitivity of the imaging to various pathological processes. MRI contrast is based on the relative density of protons in tissue and the different physical and chemical environments they experience. Though MRI physics is too complicated to be discussed in depth here, Table 18-2 contains a brief description of common structural and metabolic sequences used to examine vascular disease in the CNS, as well as common MRI findings associated with each sequence.

In the following section, we examine several of the most common findings associated with vascular disease. Additionally, we examine these MRI abnormalities and their association with various cerebrovascular risk factors.

White Matter Signal Abnormalities or White Matter Hyperintensities

By far, the most common imaging finding among patients with vascular risk factors or patients with vascular-related dementia is white matter signal abnormalities (WMSA). WMSA are most apparent in the T2-weighted or fluid attenuated inversion recovery (FLAIR) images (see Fig. 18-1), where they appear as bright (hyperintense) regions that can appear as well-defined concentric or confluent regions (see Fig. 18-12). In contrast, WMSA are not readily seen in T1-weighted images. However, especially hyperintense abnormalities on the T2/FLAIR images can be seen as hypointense regions in the T1 image. WMSA

Table 18-2 Common MRI pulse sequences and their sensitivity to pathology.

Sequence	Brief Description	Common Finding
T1 (MPRAGE, SPGR, etc)	Anatomical sequence with excellent contrast between gray and white matter.	Lacunes, microbleeds, and small lesions. Typically used to measure global and regional atrophy.
T2, T2*	Excellent visualization of CSF/fluid filed spaces though quite poor contrast between gray and white matter.	Excellent for detecting and quantifying ventricles, surface CSF, and WMSAs.
Proton Density	Often used to identify different water components. Can be used to measure total and myelin water content.	Signal is unaffected in early stroke, though as vasogenic edema increases, signal is attenuated. There is a high correlation between signal change in PD and T2.
FLAIR (fluid attenuated inversion recovery)	T2-weighted sequence, with the signal from the CSF suppressed.	Excellent for detecting WMSAs.
Diffusion-Weighted Imaging and Diffusion Tensor Imaging (DWI, DTI)	Is capable of characterizing and quantifying the movement of water molecules in living tissue. Is a measure of structural integrity and tissue connectivity.	Diffusion imaging is particularly sensitive to early ischemic changes.
Magnetic Resonance Spectroscopy (MRS)	Examines metabolic changes associated with injury and common cellular processes.	Inflammatory metabolites, cell membrane turnover, and increased energy metabolism are common findings though more research is clearly needed.

are commonly found in older patient populations, with nearly 100% of patients over the age of 85 having observable WMSA.[13, 14] These findings are more common or exacerbated among patients with vascular risk factors and are required for a diagnosis of vascular dementia.

Typically, the incidental age-related WMSA findings produce either no symptoms or only mild, nonspecific symptoms. However, with the accumulation of WMSA over time, there can be a significant increase in neurologic, psychiatric, or medical dysfunction.[15, 16] There are studies that have documented increased volume and incidence of WMSA in dementia patients[15, 16] as well as patients with increased gait impairments and falls.[17, 18]

Microbleeds and Lacunes

In addition to WMSA, vascular disease patients often have a significant number of microbleeds and/or lacunes. Microbleeds can be characterized as "small, homogenous, round foci of low signal intensity on magnetic resonance imaging gradient echo T2 sequences."[19] Lacunes are the result of occlusion in small arteries and can essentially be described as miniature strokes. These discrete findings are best observed in T2-weighted images and can be found throughout the brain (see Fig. 18-3). However, there appears to be a predilection for the subcortical nuclei (basal ganglia and thalamus) that is generally thought to be due to the unique structural aspects of the blood vessels in these

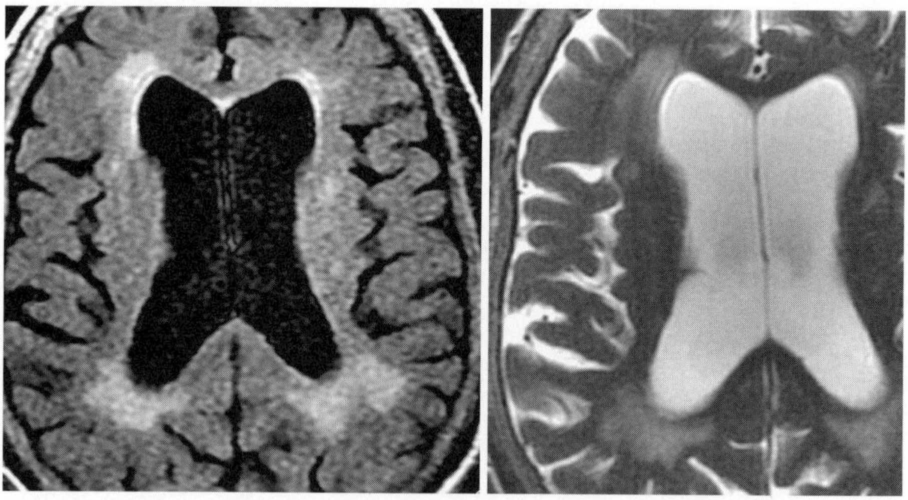

Figure 18-1 A FLAIR (left) and T2-weighted image (right) seen from a chronic uncontrolled hypertension patient show lateral ventricle expansion, a prominent feature of global white matter atrophy, and white matter signal abnormalities.

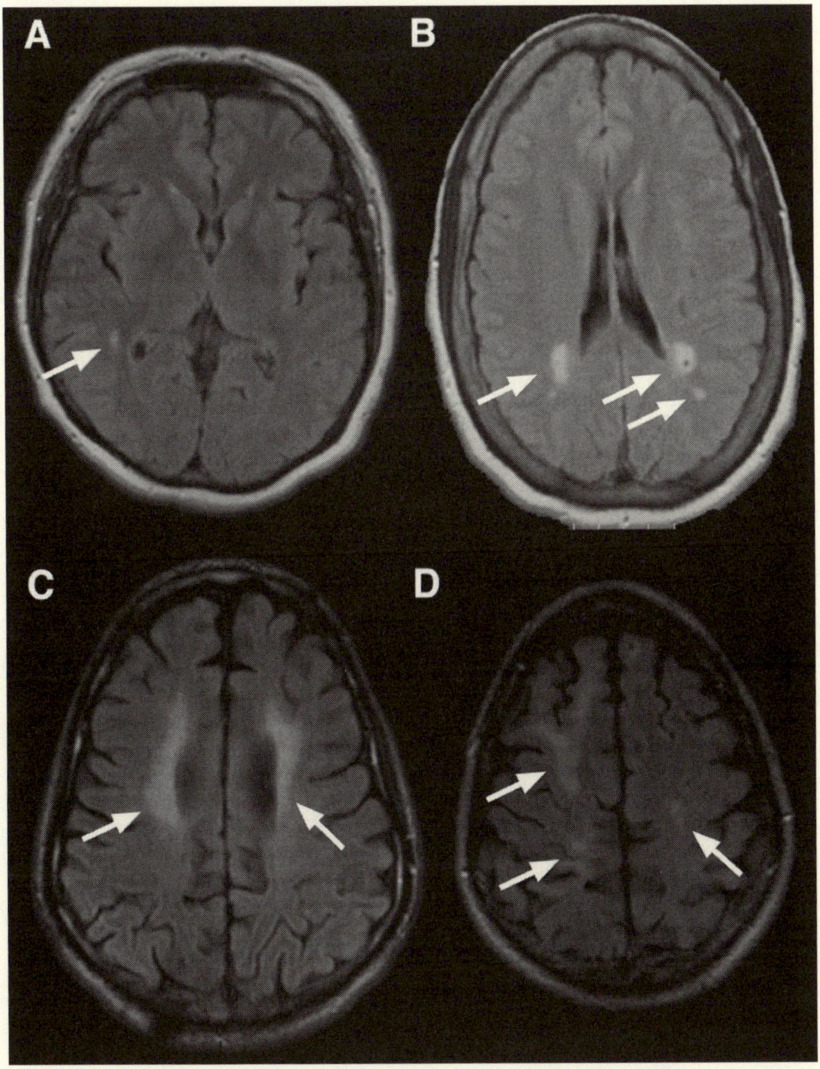

Figure 18-2 Axial slices showing small focal (A-B) and confluent diffuse (C-D) white matter signal abnormalities.

areas. These middle cerebral-artery vessels (lenticulostriate and thalamocortical) do not anastomose and as a result bear the burden of blood pressure changes over a lifetime. The vulnerability of the arteries in these areas and the accumulating injuries associated with vascular disease may well underlie the cognitive dysfunction observed in vascular dementia patients. Though cognitive symptoms in vascular dementia vary, most researchers and clinicians characterize the cognitive symptoms as "subcortical" in nature.

Diffusion Abnormalities

Although diffusion-weighted imaging (DWI) has not been widely used in clinical settings, there is an increasing number of studies successfully using this sensitive imaging method. In particular, it appears that DWI is quite sensitive in detecting strokes early in the acute phase, due to its ability to quantify the gross movement of water on a microscopic level over short periods of time. For example, using animal models, several labs have described a consistent temporal evolution and progression of diffusion.[20–22] In the initial stages of an occlusion, there is a sharp decline in apparent diffusion metrics, even within minutes of the occlusion. Following reperfusion, the diffusion metrics return to normal, and then over the next several weeks, sharp increases in the apparent diffusion metric are observed. In contrast, structural imaging sequences do not show any significant changes during the initial stages of occlusion. DWI allows for better delineation

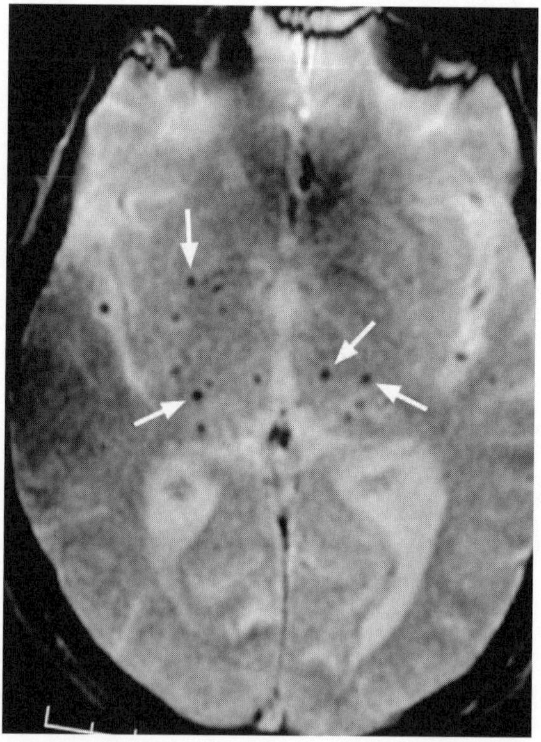

Figure 18-3 Signal-intensity loss in a T2-weighted image, displayed as black dots indicated by white arrows, represents microbleeds, a common occurrence resulting from intracerebral hemorrhage in cardiovascular disease.

of affected areas in stroke and is capable of predicting areas of potential permanent damage.

Global and Regional Atrophy

Other well-known MRI findings associated with vascular disease and risk factors are global atrophy, enlarging ventricles, and/or widening sulci. These are found especially in patients with vascular dementia, though the presence of one or more cardiac risk factors has also been shown to be associated with global atrophy. Regional atrophy typically occurs in patients with overt strokes and is most commonly found in subcortical structures, such as the basal ganglia and the thalamus. This can lead to changes in local anatomy surrounding the area of the stroke and, as such, influence the symptom manifestation.

Summary

Although there are other MRI abnormalities present in CVD patients, WMSA, lacunes/microbleeds, alterations in diffusion, and atrophy are the primary manifestations. We now discuss these findings with respect to various vascular risk factors.

Vascular Risk Factors and MRI Findings

Many vascular risk factors have been identified in the literature. In particular, epidemiological studies have been useful in identifying several risk factors, including hypertension, atherosclerosis, smoking, diabetes, endothelial function, systemic perfusion, and even a few genetic risk factors. Though this is not an exhaustive list, we will review a few of the more prominent risk factors and the associated MRI findings.

Hypertension

Next to age, hypertension (HTN) has been identified as one of the most common risk factors for the accumulation of WMSA. This association has been demonstrated in both cross-sectional and longitudinal imaging studies.[23, 24] Even when using a conservative criterion for defining HTN (systolic >160 mmHg, diastolic >90 mmHg), studies have demonstrated associations between the accumulation of WMSA and HTN.[25, 26] Additionally, it appears that patients who are on successful treatment for HTN present with significantly fewer WMSA.[27]

Accumulating evidence suggests that chronic elevations in blood pressure exacerbate the effects of aging on the brain,[28–31] possibly by inducing small-vessel disease. Chronic distention of the endothelium of the blood vessels may result in injury that renders the endothelial cells unable to respond quickly to changes in blood pressure. In particular, elevated midlife blood pressure appears to be predictive of an increase in the WMSA volume of patients later in life, independent of age.[24, 32]

Atherosclerosis

Atherosclerosis constitutes another vascular risk factor that has been examined in relation to abnormal MRI findings. As a risk factor, it is one of the leading contributors to cerebral abnormalities and risk of morbidity (70% of CVD deaths are attributed to atherosclerosis).[33] Studies demonstrate that the detectability of white matter lesions (WML) and microbleeds in atherosclerotic ischemic attacks may vary by such factors as age, severity, and symptom trends.[34]

Two independent studies following homozygous familial hypercholesterolemia (FH), a direct accelerator of atherosclerosis, examined the predictability of WMSA detection later in life in two different patient age populations. Neither the young (median age of 23 years, ranging from 12–36 years old) nor middle-aged (ages 48–64 years old) FH participants manifested detectable subcortical WMSA. Young FH subjects did not show WMSA even in high resolution 3 Tesla T2-weighted or FLAIR images.[35] Middle-aged FH patients did not exhibit WMSA differences from similar-aged control patients despite the FH subjects' years of atherosclerotic carotid artery disease. When subsequent scans were compared to sequences performed approximately two decades earlier, older participants displayed significant associations between the severity of aortic atherosclerosis and periventricular WMSA.[35, 36] Further investigation of the middle-aged patient population over a longer duration will identify more accurate trends in WMSA detectability and their associated cognitive impairments caused by atherosclerosis.[37]

While high resolution MRI has been established to be more sensitive in identifying more discrete and/or earlier asymptomatic atherosclerotic plaques not detectable by X-ray angiography,[38] the MRI modalities differ greatly in their usefulness in detecting the ischemic attacks based on atherosclerosis. DWI has been shown to be almost twice as sensitive in detecting acute ischemic stroke lesions and more than three times as sensitive in hyperacute cases (0–6 hours) compared to T2-weighted FLAIR under all conditions.[39] When used without the DWI, follow-up T2-weighted sequences were deemed insufficient to rule out small infarctions.[40] The ability of DWI to detect atherosclerotic ischemic tissue injury within minutes of symptom manifestation allows researchers to recognize 76.3% of the original transient ischemic attack-related DWI abnormalities that will persist as permanent WMSA as seen in follow-up DWI scans two weeks later.[39, 40]

Alongside WMSA, microbleeds have also been shown to be important in recognizing atherosclerotic microangiopathy. The presence of cerebral microbleeds suggests an increase in the likelihood of intracranial bleeding, and consequently an increased risk of thrombolytic or antiplatelet treatment complications.[41] Different sensitivities of imaging sequences used to identify microbleeds has caused some disparity between their expected incidence in the general population and those suffering from atherosclerotic microangiopathy and other CVD. Though T1-weighted sequences allow easy detection of microbleeds as linear structures (never dots) and symmetrical shapes in the subcortical structures, 3D T2*GRE (T2 star Gradient Echo) sequences are significantly more sensitive to cerebral microbleeds in CVD and general populations.[41, 42]

C-Reactive Protein, Homocysteine, and Other Inflammatory Markers

More than 20 studies demonstrate C-reactive protein (CRP) to be an independent predictor of future cardiovascular events; however, it remains unclear whether CRP acts simply as an inflammatory biomarker or as an integral part of the inflammatory mechanism.[43] The Rotterdam Scan Study findings have shown CRP levels to be tightly regulated, to have little short-term fluctuation, and to demonstrate positive relationships with the presence and progression of WMSA.[44, 45] When adjusted for age, sex, and carotid atherosclerosis and other cardiovascular risk factors, higher CRP levels were shown to correlate with severe periventricular and subcortical WMSA and lacunar infarcts at baseline in T2-weighted and proton density (PD)-weighted images.[44] Axial T2 and PD imaging comparison studies provide evidence that CRP is involved in the onset stages in larger-vessel atherosclerosis. However, conflicting results in cerebral small-vessel disease suggest additional studies are required to confirm the current perspective of little to no CRP association.[46]

MRI imaging of the proinflammatory and prothrombotic effects of homocysteine (Hcy) implicate its role in brain aging, small-vessel disease, and other vascular diseases.[47–50] Many researchers admit there is no clear consensus on whether Hcy levels have predictive clinical value for WMSA, due to the cross-sectional nature of many studies.[49, 51–53] Several earlier studies provide evidence that, when accounting for socio-demographic variation and vascular risk factors, plasma Hcy level is a risk factor for T2-weighted WMSA.[50, 54, 55] In addition, Hcy levels seemed to have an ethnic component, shown by the higher prevalence of detectable WMSA in blacks (40%) compared to whites (20%) and Hispanics (24%), suggesting a possible genetic susceptibility to WM damage.[53] However, while confirming previous reports of higher Hcy levels in healthy adults' being associated with smaller brain volumes (total intracranial volume) and silent brain infarcts, investigators were unable to confirm any significant plasma Hcy and WMSA associations.[51, 52] Results from a large study of 622 elderly participants confirm these findings by suggesting that increased WMSA and high plasma Hcy levels may be a result of previous and prevalent transient ischemic attacks or stroke and not a consequence of a direct relationship.[52]

Researchers are hesitant to directly attribute WMSA findings to high levels of CRP, Hcy, or any other inflammatory agent.[43, 56] Though not consistently found among studies, interleukin-6, CD40 ligand, soluble intracellular adhesion molecule-1, monocyte chemoattractant protein-1, myeloperoxidase, osteoprotegerin, P-selectin, tumor necrosis factor-α, and tumor necrosis factor receptor II, as well as many others have been implicated as biomarkers in complex pathways and mechanisms associated with WMSA.[57–59] Studies utilizing younger, healthier subjects did not find WMSA associations, while older populations manifested the more widely accepted association of inflammation and atherosclerosis.[44, 58, 60, 61]

Diabetes

A moderate, but expanding, body of literature has convincingly demonstrated a link between diabetes and pathological MRI findings. Because of heterogeneous diabetic pathology and the known connection between diabetes and other conditions such as HTN and CVD, it is difficult to know for certain how much of this pathology is due directly to aberrant glucose metabolism and how much is due to comorbid vascular disease.

Diabetes has been linked at statistically significant levels to deep WML,[62] microbleeds,[19] reduced regional CBF,[63] lacunar infarcts,[64] and generalized and localized gray matter atrophy.[65] However, there is considerable variability in the robustness and reproducibility of these associations across studies. A 2006 systematic review of brain imaging findings in diabetes concluded that strong evidence exists linking diabetes to cerebral atrophy and lacunar infarcts, but that evidence linking diabetes to WMSA is inconsistent.[64] This analysis included 46 MRI and/or CT studies and employed meta-analyses where possible.

A study published in 2007 reported decreased global white matter ($p = 0.006$), decreased global gray matter ($p = 0.001$), and increased CSF volume ($P < 0.0001$) in patients with type 2 diabetes compared to controls.[63] They also reported regional loss of white matter in the frontal region of the brain and regional loss of gray matter in the parieto-occipital region.[63] Global gray matter atrophy is a finding that is fairly consistent across studies.[64] However, there can be wide variation in the location of gray matter atrophy across different patient populations. For example, a study published in 2008 also reported global gray matter atrophy in patients with type 2 diabetes but reported regional losses in the anterior cingulate and orbitofrontal regions after global gray matter loss was controlled.[65] Interpretation of these results may be confounded somewhat by a recent study that reported that obesity, as measured by BMI, can be linked to both global and regional losses in gray matter independently of diabetes, although this result was only significant in males.[66, 67]

Markers of CVD, particularly WMSA and microbleeds, have been found in diabetic patients. A systematic review of spontaneous brain microbleeds reports a significant association between these MRI findings and diabetes (OR 2.2, 95% CI 1.2–4.2) in otherwise healthy adults.[19]

DWI has been used to study subclinical cerebral edema in children with diabetic ketoacidosis.[68] In this analysis, elevated apparent diffusion coefficient metrics provided evidence of vasogenic edema.[68] DWI has also been used to analyze susceptibility of tissue to ischemic stress.[69] MRS studies have revealed an elevated myo-inositol–creatine ratio and a reduced N-acetylaspartate–creatine ratio in diabetic patients[64] and are being used to deduce the mechanism of insulin resistance in humans.[70] Increased BBB permeability has been detected in diabetic patients through the use of MR imaging using intravenous gadolinium diethylenetriamine pentaacetic acid (Gd-DTPA) contrast.[71]

MRI has also been useful when diagnosing central diabetes insipidus. Researchers and clinicians have noted that in a normal T1-weighted image, the posterior lobe of the pituitary gland has a characteristic hyperintense signal. This signal is due to the normal accumulation of neurosecretory granules in patients without diabetes and is consistently absent in patients with central diabetes insipidus.[72]

Smoking

Despite strong evidence that chronic cigarette smoking results in nervous system pathology, neuroimaging studies among this group are relatively rare and often confounded by simultaneous abuse of other substances. Despite these limitations, evidence exists that certain abnormal MRI findings are associated with chronic smoking.

One study concluded that smokers exhibit reduced gray matter volume and density in certain regions of the frontal, occipital, and temporal lobes.[73] Additionally, children whose mothers smoked during gestation exhibited reduced global cortical volume and parenchymal volume as well as a reduced head circumference in comparison to controls when these measures were taken 10 to 14 years after birth,[74] even when correcting for the effect of additional substances of abuse. In fact, smoking was the only factor that remained significant after this correction,[74] suggesting an independent effect of smoking on the developing brain. An association between smoking and silent cerebral infarcts has also been reported.[75]

Imaging has not only been used to study the direct pathological effects of smoking, but also to study the effect of smoking on the progression of other diseases. For example, smoking appears to significantly increase the progression of multiple sclerosis.[76] In this study, smokers who presented with a clinically isolated syndrome were found to be more likely to progress to a diagnosis of multiple sclerosis than those who did not smoke.[76] Smoking was also associated with cerebral atrophy in areas that are associated with early Alzheimer's disease.[77] Structural imaging has further been used to demonstrate an additional reduction in gray matter among alcoholics with a significant smoking history.[78]

Diffusion tensor imaging was recently used to examine the microstructural integrity of white matter in smokers and nonsmokers. Chronic smokers showed reduced microstructural integrity in the corpus callosum as measured by fractional anisotropy, compared to nonsmokers.[79]

Using MRS, Gazdzinski et al. demonstrated that smoking is associated with slower recovery to metabolic normalcy in recovering alcoholics as measured by using MRS to track N-acetylaspartate and choline-containing compounds.[80] MRS has also been used to show that chronic cigarette smoking has both independent and additive effects on the cell death and reduction in membrane integrity exhibited in alcoholic cohorts.[81]

Systemic Cardiac Function and Cerebral Blood Flow

A growing, but still limited, amount of research is available linking systemic measures of cardiac function to neuroimaging findings. In a study of elderly patients (mean age 71.5) with a history of cardiac disease, low cardiac output was found to be regionally associated with increased WMSA volume in and around subcortical gray matter structures (basal ganglia, thalamus), as detected on FLAIR images. In contrast, WMSA occurring elsewhere in the white matter parenchyma exhibited no significant associations with cardiac output.[82]

In another investigation using MRS, parietal white matter creatine levels were found to be severely diminished in patients with decreased ejection fraction due to advanced congestive heart failure. Choline, N-acetylaspartate, and myo-inositol were also diminished in the occipital gray matter of these patients. These metabolic abnormalities were visible on MRS images despite normal appearance on T1-weighted MRI, suggesting that MRS may be a more sensitive tool for detecting the effects of diminished cardiac function in the brain.[83]

In both of the above studies, decreased cardiac function is thought to result in reductions in CBF. There may be some evidence for a hypoperfusion model from a recent post-mortem histological study, which demonstrated that tissue molecular markers of hypoxia were localized to regions of hyperintense WMSA identified by pre-dissection MRI.[84] This relationship has also been demonstrated *in vivo*. Using perfusion-weighted MRI, Marstrand et al. compared the local CBF in hyperintense regions of WM with that of normal-appearing white matter in a group of elderly patients.[85] The authors found that CBF, along with mean transit time and vascular reactivity, were locally diminished in hyperintense white matter relative to adjacent areas of normal-appearing white matter.[85]

In addition to WMSA, cortical atrophy has also been correlated with decreased CBF. In a of cohort elderly patients exhibiting mild cognitive impairment (mean age 69.3), levels of cortical atrophy in the medial temporal lobe were shown to be inversely correlated to global CBF.[86] Similarly, Appelman et al. found that subcortical brain atrophy was associated with decreased CBF.[87] However, the correlation was only significant in patients exhibiting WMSA, suggesting a common underlying cause for these pathologies.[87]

Despite the apparent connection between hypoperfusion and brain abnormalities, causal relationships are difficult to establish, due to the multitude of factors that determine systemic and cerebral perfusion. However, further support has been given to the role of systemic hypoperfusion by investigation of neuroimaging correlates of various cardiac disease states. In a group of randomly selected elderly subjects (ages 60–90), cross-sectional analysis revealed a direct relationship between the presence of atrial fibrillation at the time of testing and observed periventricular WMSA. A five-year follow-up showed a significant increase in WMSA volume in patients with persistent atrial fibrillation. Both of these effects remained when corrected for other risk factors, including hypertension and atherosclerosis. Notably, no relationship was found between atrial fibrillation and the presence of subcortical WMSA.[88] In a study of patients diagnosed with mitochondrial cardiomyopathies, four out of seven examined by MRI or CT scans exhibited abnormalities, most commonly lesions of the basal ganglia and cortical degeneration.[89] Similar findings were obtained from a group of older patients (mean age

51 years) diagnosed with heart failure, with the atrophy extended to the thalamus and right cingulate gyrus, among other structures.[90]

Even though MRS can identify abnormal regions of decreased metabolism in the brain, it is unclear yet whether decreased perfusion is the primary cause of tissue damage or a secondary result of decreased demand in these cases, limiting the conclusions that can be drawn from MRS findings.[83, 91] Diffusion-weighted MRI has been shown to be more sensitive than traditional structural MRI sequences for detecting ischemic lesions during chronic and acute stroke.[39, 92] Additionally, in a study of multiple sclerosis patients, DWI revealed regions of hypoperfusion-induced WM degeneration in areas of the corpus callosum that appeared normal in perfusion-weighted MR images.[93] Together, these findings suggest that DWI may prove to be the most useful tool for identifying areas of decreased CBF in patients at risk for CVD.

Endothelial Function

In addition to standard cardiovascular risk factors, dysfunction of the vascular endothelium has been implicated, both directly and indirectly, in the progression of CVD and its associated pathologies. Conditions that may lead to endothelial dysfunction in the cerebral vasculature include the previously mentioned diabetes, atherosclerosis, and hypertension, all of which are well-recognized risk factors for CVD as well.[94]

As mentioned above, cerebrovascular endothelial dysfunction can be directly visualized through T1-weighted MRI in conjunction with intravenous gadolinium-DTPA (Gd-DTPA) injection. Studies using this technique have performed scans at set intervals, beginning at the time of the injection, to assess the degree of gadolinium diffusion through the BBB. By subtracting the initial image from each subsequent image, any changes in signal intensity can be quantified. A greater mean signal intensity and/or a more rapid change in signal intensity indicate that the integrity of the BBB has been compromised.[71, 95, 96]

The frequent presence of WML in patients with endothelial dysfunction, identified as leukoariosis, has been significantly correlated to decreased vasomotor reactivity to hypercapnia and the level of WMLs in elderly patients.[5] A similar study confirmed these results, demonstrating that diminished endothelium-dependent vasodilation was significantly associated with increased WMSA volume, after controlling for the effects of age and cardiovascular risk factors. Defects in endothelium-independent vasodilation were not associated with WMSA volume in this study.[97] A longitudinal study of randomly selected patients, aged 50 to 75, showed that an increase in circulating levels of intercellular adhesion molecule 1 (ICAM) and thrombomodulin were correlated with an increase in WMSA volume at three- and six-year follow-ups. ICAM and TM expression are upregulated on activated endothelial cells, and increased circulating plasma levels of these molecules indicate endothelial activation or damage.[98] Together, these findings imply an active role for the vascular endothelium in the progression of WMSA.

Endothelial dysfunction has also been implicated as a contributor to various stroke conditions, most notably lacunar infarctions. In a study examining elderly patients presenting with symptomatic lacunar infarct and asymptomatic patients at high risk for ischemic stroke (based on cardiovascular risk factors), plasma levels of von Willebrand factor (vWF) were found to be significantly elevated in patients exhibiting five or more subclinical infarcts, as compared with those exhibiting one or two. Both vWF and thrombomodulin levels were elevated in symptomatic patients compared with non-lacunar patients.[95] Additionally, the endothelial integrity of lacunar stroke patients has been shown to be significantly decreased when compared with that of cortical stroke patients, suggesting a specific role for endothelial dysfunction in this stroke subtype.[96]

In the studies cited above, and indeed in most of the existing literature, both WMSA and lacunar infarcts are identified as hyperintensities on T2-weighted MR images. However, diffusion-weighted MR imaging has been shown to be superior to T2-weighted images in some respects. Leukoariosis and lacunar stroke both manifest as WM axonal degeneration, making them ideal candidates for DWI. Both of these pathologies appear as areas of diminished or abolished anisotropy, reflecting loss of directionality due to demyelination and increased water levels in the affected tissues.[99] The sensitivity of DWI allows for areas of acute and chronic lacunar infarction, as well as leukoariosis, to be differentiated—and the severity of the latter determined—by examining variations in the average diffusion coefficient values. Moreover, the researchers in this study were able to identify leukoariosis in white matter that appeared normal in T2-weighted images.[100] DW identification of WMLs has also been shown to be a more sensitive and accurate predictor of cognitive decline in patients with lacunar stroke and leukoariosis than T2, T1, or FLAIR sequences.[101] These findings demonstrate that DWI is a useful tool for the analysis of symptom progression in patients with endothelial dysfunction and at risk for associated pathologies.

Genetic Risk Factors

Biomedical research has had limited success in identifying CVD risk-factor genes. This is primarily due to the small effect sizes of common CVD risk alleles, probably complicated by one of several gene-by-gene and gene-by-environment interactions.[102] In spite of these limitations, there are have been a few genes identified that appear to confer additional risk in developing stroke (PDE4D, ALOx5AP)[103, 104] or other related neurodegenerative diseases such as Alzheimer's disease (APOE4).[105] Genetic research combined with brain MRI has been able to identify heritable endophenotypes associated with CVD, such as stroke and dementia.[106–110]

The Boston University Medical Center and the Framingham Heart study conducted a genome-wide associate and linkage analysis study to explore specific endophenotypes. In the community-based sample of 705 dementia-stroke-free participants, the single nucleotide polymorphisms (SNPs) PDE4D, LTA4H, and VLDLR were linked with MRI and cognitive endophenotypes that displayed increase risk for both stroke and dementia.[111] Two of these SNPs, PDE4D and LTA4H, have previously been associated with stroke,[103, 112] and VLDLR has been associated with an increased risk of dementia in the presence of vascular risk factors.[113] An additional interesting finding from the

Framingham Heart study was support for a linkage of white matter hyperintensities on chromosome 4.[111] These results suggest that genes associated with clinical neurological disease also have detectable effects on subclinical phenotypes.

Summary of Findings and Future Directions Toward Pathological Specificity

Though there have been advancements in the study of neurocognitive factors in cardiovascular patients, there are still many unanswered questions about behavioral and cognitive consequences of the disease. There are several ways that the clinical assessment and treatment of cardiovascular patients might be improved by neuroimaging. One significant improvement that will advance the CVD literature will be larger, prospective studies. To date, the vast majority of imaging studies are cross-sectional in design or use samples taken from epidemiological studies. There are a few notable exceptions, though these studies are often limited to smaller cohorts and/or limited time points (not more than two time points). One major advantage of prospective studies is the improved statistical power when using participants as their own controls. There has been much work recently reported in the literature regarding time-series analyses of prospective imaging data among several different patient populations.[114, 115] The interest in this type of imaging data has resulted in a growing set of methods for dealing with longitudinal data, including subtraction imaging, time-series analyses, etc. For example, in a study

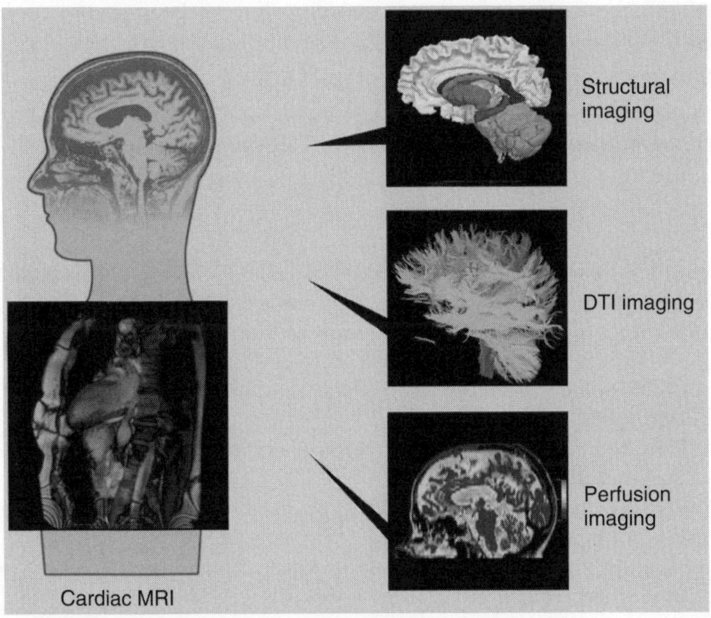

Figure 18-4 The combination of different imaging modalities should greatly enhance pathological specificity.

of multiple sclerosis patients, the level of disease activity varies greatly among individuals, as does the severity and rate of progression. Morphological change is reflected in focal lesions (a common finding in CVD patients) as well as global and regional atrophy, with both brain and spinal cord affected. Occurrence, duration, and residual of individual MS lesions are often stochastic, potentially confounding associations with clinical outcomes. Additionally, emerging longitudinal studies of Alzheimer's disease have revealed significant variability in the rate and progression of neuroimaging abnormalities. Morphological alteration in AD is reflected in global and regional atrophy as well as specific anatomical abnormalities such as hippocampal atrophy. Despite this complexity, there has been encouraging success in modeling lesion variability in MS patients[115] and global/regional atrophy rates in AD patients,[116, 117] which might also be applied to CVD patients. Monitoring the literature for advances in longitudinal methods among other patient populations will most certainly reveal additional ways of examining HIV-associated CNS injury and/or treatment efficacy.

What should be clear from the current neuroimaging research literature is the fact that MRI variables in isolation provide limited pathological specificity. Future studies of CVD-associated CNS injury would benefit from the use of multi-modal imaging methods that exploit the complementary and unique sensitivities of different imaging modalities (see Fig. 18-4). Studies designed to maximize the dissociative qualities of different imaging modalities have the best potential of establishing pathological specificity not afforded by clinical and/or cognitive variables. Additionally, studies directly assessing cardiac and CNS function/integrity simultaneously should be undertaken. These types of studies would be able to increase our understanding of the impact of cardiovascular function on CNS abnormalities in perfusion, function, and/or structure. Though there is still much to be learned about CVD-associated CNS injury, it is obvious that MRI and other associated imaging modalities hold significant promise for evaluating the evolution, progression, and treatment effects among CVD patients.

Notes

1. Prencipe M, Ferretti C, Casini AR, Santini M, Giubilei F, Culasso F. Stroke, disability, and dementia: Results of a population survey. *Stroke*. 1997;28(3):531–536.
2. Siesjö BK, Kristián T, Katsura K-I. Overview of bioenergetic failure and metabolic cascades in brain ischemia. In Ginsberg MD, Bogousslavsky J (Eds.), *Cerebrovascular disease: Pathophysiology, diagnosis, and management*, vol.1 (pp. 3–13). Blackwell Science, Malden, MA 1998.
3. Kalaria RN. The blood–brain barrier and cerebrovascular pathology in Alzheimer's disease. *Ann N Y Acad Sci*. 1999;893:113–125.
4. Wardlaw JM, Sandercock PAG, Dennis MS, Starr J. Is breakdown of the blood–brain barrier responsible for lacunar stroke, leukoaraiosis, and dementia? *Stroke*. 2003;34(3):806–812.
5. Bakker SL, de Leeuw FE, de Groot JC, Hofman A, Koudstaal PJ, Breteler MM. Cerebral vasomotor reactivity and cerebral white matter lesions in the elderly. *Neurology*. 1999;52(3):578–583.
6. Terborg C, Gora F, Weiller C, Rother J. Reduced vasomotor reactivity in cerebral microangiopathy: A study with near-infrared spectroscopy and transcranial Doppler sonography. *Stroke*. 2000;31(4):924–929.

7. Davis SM, Donnan GA. Advances in penumbra imaging with MR. *Cerebrovasc Dis.* 2004;17(Suppl 3):23–27.
8. Ginsberg MD, Pulsinelli WA. The ischemic penumbra, injury thresholds, and the therapeutic window for acute stroke. *Ann Neurol.* 1994;36(4):553–554.
9. Paulson OB, Strandgaard S, Edvinsson L. Cerebral autoregulation. *Cerebrovasc Brain Metab Rev.* Summer 1990;2(2):161–192.
10. Strandgaard S, Paulson OB. Cerebrovascular damage in hypertension. *J Cardiovasc Risk.* 1995;2(1):34–39.
11. Pantoni L, Garcia JH. Pathogenesis of leukoaraiosis: A review. *Stroke.* 1997;28(3):652–659.
12. Bronge L, Wahlund LO. White matter changes in dementia: Does radiology matter? *Br J Radiol.* 2007;80(Spec. No. 2):S115–S120.
13. Awad IA, Johnson PC, Spetzler RF, Hodak JA. Incidental subcortical lesions identified on magnetic resonance imaging in the elderly. II: Postmortem pathological correlations. *Stroke.* 1986;17(6):1090–1097.
14. Kertesz A, Black SE, Tokar G, Benke T, Carr T, Nicholson L. Periventricular and subcortical hyperintensities on magnetic resonance imaging. "Rims, caps, and unidentified bright objects." *Arch Neurol.* 1988;45(4):404–408.
15. Kidwell CS, Saver JL. Progress in understanding white matter hyperintensities. *Stroke.* 1996;27(12):2338.
16. de Groot JC, de Leeuw FE, Oudkerk M, et al. Cerebral white matter lesions and cognitive function: The Rotterdam Scan Study. *Ann Neurol.* 2000;47(2):145–151.
17. Baloh RW, Yue Q, Socotch TM, Jacobson KM. White matter lesions and disequilibrium in older people. I: Case-control comparison. *Arch Neurol.* 1995;52(10):970–974.
18. Price TR, Manolio TA, Kronmal RA, et al. Silent brain infarction on magnetic resonance imaging and neurological abnormalities in community-dwelling older adults. The Cardiovascular Health Study. CHS Collaborative Research Group. *Stroke.* 1997;28(6): 1158–1164.
19. Cordonnier C, Al-Shahi Salman R, Wardlaw J. Spontaneous brain microbleeds: Systematic review, subgroup analyses and standards for study design and reporting. *Brain.* 2007;130 (Pt 8):1988–2003.
20. Mintorovitch J, Moseley ME, Chileuitt L, Shimizu H, Cohen Y, Weinstein PR. Comparison of diffusion- and T2-weighted MRI for the early detection of cerebral ischemia and reperfusion in rats. *Magn Reson Med.* 1991;18(1):39–50.
21. Moseley ME, Cohen Y, Mintorovitch J, et al. Early detection of regional cerebral ischemia in cats: Comparison of diffusion- and T2-weighted MRI and spectroscopy. *Magn Reson Med.* 1990;14(2):330–346.
22. Moonen CT, Pekar J, de Vleeschouwer MH, van Gelderen P, van Zijl PC, DesPres D. Restricted and anisotropic displacement of water in healthy cat brain and in stroke studied by NMR diffusion imaging. *Magn Reson Med.* 1991;19(2):327–332.
23. Pantoni L, Garcia JH. The significance of cerebral white matter abnormalities 100 years after Binswanger's report. A review. *Stroke.* 1995;26(7):1293–1301.
24. Dufouil C, de Kersaint-Gilly A, Besancon V, et al. Longitudinal study of blood pressure and white matter hyperintensities: The EVA MRI Cohort. *Neurology.* 2001;56(7):921–926.
25. Longstreth WT, Jr., Manolio TA, Arnold A, et al. Clinical correlates of white matter findings on cranial magnetic resonance imaging of 3301 elderly people. The Cardiovascular Health Study. *Stroke.* 1996;27(8):1274–1282.
26. Breteler MM, van Swieten JC, Bots ML, et al. Cerebral white matter lesions, vascular risk factors, and cognitive function in a population-based study: The Rotterdam Study. *Neurology.* 1994;44(7):1246–1252.

27. van Dijk EJ, Breteler MMB, Schmidt R, et al. The association between blood pressure, hypertension, and cerebral white matter lesions: Cardiovascular determinants of dementia study. *Hypertension*. 2004;44(5):625–630.
28. de Leeuw FE, de Groot JC, van Gijn J. [Cerebral white matter lesions in the elderly: Vascular risk factors and cognitive consequences]. *Ned Tijdschr Geneeskd*. 2001;145(43): 2067–2071.
29. Raz N, Rodrigue KM, Acker JD. Hypertension and the brain: Vulnerability of the prefrontal regions and executive functions. *Behav Neurosci*. 2003;117(6):1169–1180.
30. Goldstein IB, Bartzokis G, Guthrie D, Shapiro D. Ambulatory blood pressure and brain atrophy in the healthy elderly. *Neurology*. 2002;59(5):713–719.
31. Goldstein IB, Bartzokis G, Guthrie D, Shapiro D. Ambulatory blood pressure and the brain: A 5-year follow-up. *Neurology*. 2005;64(11):1846–1852.
32. Swan GE, DeCarli C, Miller BL, et al. Association of midlife blood pressure to late-life cognitive decline and brain morphology. *Neurology*. 1998;51(4):986–993.
33. Yuan C, Kerwin WS. MRI of atherosclerosis. *J Magn Reson Imaging*. 2004;19(6):710–719.
34. Maillard P, Delcroix N, Crivello F, et al. An automated procedure for the assessment of white matter hyperintensities by multispectral (T1, T2, PD) MRI and an evaluation of its between-centre reproducibility based on two large community databases. *Neuroradiology*. 2008;50(1):31–42.
35. Schmitz SA, O'Regan DP, Fitzpatrick J, et al. MRI at 3 Tesla detects no evidence for ischemic brain damage in intensively treated patients with homozygous familial hypercholesterolemia. *Neuroradiology*. 2007;49(11):927–931.
36. de Leeuw FE, De Groot JC, Oudkerk M, et al. Aortic atherosclerosis at middle age predicts cerebral white matter lesions in the elderly. *Stroke*. 2000;31(2):425–429.
37. Bombois S, Debette S, Bruandet A, et al. Vascular subcortical hyperintensities predict conversion to vascular and mixed dementia in MCI patients. *Stroke*. 2008;39(7):2046–2051.
38. Corti R, Fuster V, Fayad ZA, et al. Lipid lowering by simvastatin induces regression of human atherosclerotic lesions: Two years' follow-up by high-resolution noninvasive magnetic resonance imaging. *Circulation*. 2002;106(23):2884–2887.
39. Perkins CJ, Kahya E, Roque CT, Roche PE, Newman GC. Fluid-attenuated inversion recovery and diffusion- and perfusion-weighted MRI abnormalities in 117 consecutive patients with stroke symptoms. *Stroke*. 2001;32(12):2774–2781.
40. Oppenheim C, Lamy C, Touze E, et al. Do transient ischemic attacks with diffusion-weighted imaging abnormalities correspond to brain infarctions? *Am J Neuroradiol*. 2006;27(8):1782–1787.
41. Vernooij MW, Ikram MA, Wielopolski PA, Krestin GP, Breteler MM, van der Lugt A. Cerebral microbleeds: accelerated 3D T2*-weighted GRE MR imaging versus conventional 2D T2*-weighted GRE MR imaging for detection. *Radiology*. 2008;248(1):272–277.
42. Vernooij MW, van der Lugt A, Ikram MA, et al. Prevalence and risk factors of cerebral microbleeds: The Rotterdam Scan Study. *Neurology*. 2008;70(14):1208–1214.
43. Ridker PM. C-reactive protein and the prediction of cardiovascular events among those at intermediate risk: Moving an inflammatory hypothesis toward consensus. *J Am Coll Cardiol*. 2007;49(21):2129–2138.
44. van Dijk EJ, Prins ND, Vermeer SE, et al. C-reactive protein and cerebral small-vessel disease: The Rotterdam Scan Study. *Circulation*. 2005;112(6):900–905.
45. Macy EM, Hayes TE, Tracy RP. Variability in the measurement of C-reactive protein in healthy subjects: Implications for reference intervals and epidemiological applications. *Clin Chem*. 1997;43(1):52–58.

46. Schmidt R, Schmidt H, Pichler M, et al. C-reactive protein, carotid atherosclerosis, and cerebral small-vessel disease: Results of the Austrian Stroke Prevention Study. *Stroke*. 2006; 37(12):2910–2916.
47. Harker LA, Ross R, Slichter SJ, Scott CR. Homocystine-induced arteriosclerosis. The role of endothelial cell injury and platelet response in its genesis. *J Clin Invest*. 1976;58(3): 731–741.
48. Hajjar KA. Homocysteine-induced modulation of tissue plasminogen activator binding to its endothelial cell membrane receptor. *J Clin Invest*. 1993;91(6):2873–2879.
49. Hankey GJ. Is homocysteine a causal and treatable risk factor for vascular diseases of the brain (cognitive impairment and stroke)? *Ann Neurol*. 2002;51(3):279–281.
50. Vermeer SE, van Dijk EJ, Koudstaal PJ, et al. Homocysteine, silent brain infarcts, and white matter lesions: The Rotterdam Scan Study. *Ann Neurol*. 2002;51(3):285–289.
51. Seshadri S, Wolf PA, Beiser AS, et al. Association of plasma total homocysteine levels with subclinical brain injury: Cerebral volumes, white matter hyperintensity, and silent brain infarcts at volumetric magnetic resonance imaging in the Framingham Offspring Study. *Arch Neurol*. 2008;65(5):642–649.
52. Longstreth WT, Jr., Katz R, Olson J, et al. Plasma total homocysteine levels and cranial magnetic resonance imaging findings in elderly persons: The Cardiovascular Health Study. *Arch Neurol*. 2004;61(1):67–72.
53. Wright CB, Paik MC, Brown TR, et al. Total homocysteine is associated with white matter hyperintensity volume: The Northern Manhattan Study. *Stroke*. 2005;36(6):1207–1211.
54. Sachdev P. Homocysteine, cerebrovascular disease and brain atrophy. *J Neurol Sci*. 2004; 226(1–2):25–29.
55. Dufouil C, Alperovitch A, Ducros V, Tzourio C. Homocysteine, white matter hyperintensities, and cognition in healthy elderly people. *Ann Neurol*. 2003;53(2):214–221.
56. Willerson JT, Ridker PM. Inflammation as a cardiovascular risk factor. *Circulation*. 2004; 109(21)(Suppl 1):II2–10.
57. Engelhart MJ, Geerlings MI, Meijer J, et al. Inflammatory proteins in plasma and the risk of dementia: The Rotterdam study. *Arch Neurol*. 2004;61(5):668–672.
58. Jefferson AL, Poppas A, Paul RH, Cohen RA. Systemic hypoperfusion is associated with executive dysfunction in geriatric cardiac patients. *Neurobiol Aging*. 2007;28(3):477–483.
59. Pepys MB, Hirschfield GM, Tennent GA, et al. Targeting C-reactive protein for the treatment of cardiovascular disease. *Nature*. 2006;440(7088):1217–1221.
60. Libby P, Ridker PM, Maseri A. Inflammation and atherosclerosis. *Circulation*. 2002; 105(9):1135–1143.
61. Packard RR, Libby P. Inflammation in atherosclerosis: From vascular biology to biomarker discovery and risk prediction. *Clin Chem*. 2008;54(1):24–38.
62. Manschot SM, Brands AM, van der Grond J, et al. Brain magnetic resonance imaging correlates of impaired cognition in patients with type 2 diabetes. *Diabetes*. 2006;55(4): 1106–1113.
63. Last D, Alsop DC, Abduljalil AM, et al. Global and regional effects of type 2 diabetes on brain tissue volumes and cerebral vasoreactivity. *Diabetes Care*. 2007;30(5):1193–1199.
64. van Harten B, de Leeuw FE, Weinstein HC, Scheltens P, Biessels GJ. Brain imaging in patients with diabetes: A systematic review. *Diabetes Care*. 2006;29(11):2539–2548.
65. Kumar A, Haroon E, Darwin C, et al. Gray matter prefrontal changes in type 2 diabetes detected using MRI. *J Magn Reson Imaging*. 2008;27(1):14–19.
66. Taki Y, Kinomura S, Sato K, et al. Relationship between body mass index and gray matter volume in 1,428 healthy individuals. *Obesity (Silver Spring)*. 2008;16(1):119–124.

67. Gunstad J, Paul RH, Cohen RA, et al. Relationship between body mass index and brain volume in healthy adults. *Int J Neurosci*. 2008;118(11):1582–1593.
68. Figueroa RE, Hoffman WH, Momin Z, Pancholy A, Passmore GG, Allison J. Study of subclinical cerebral edema in diabetic ketoacidosis by magnetic resonance imaging T2 relaxometry to apparent diffusion coefficient maps. *Endocr Res*. 2005;31(4):345–355.
69. Ay H, Koroshetz WJ, Vangel M, et al. Conversion of ischemic brain tissue into infarction increases with age. *Stroke*. 2005;36(12):2632–2636.
70. Shulman GI. Unraveling the cellular mechanism of insulin resistance in humans: New insights from magnetic resonance spectroscopy. *Physiology (Bethesda)*. 2004;19:183–190.
71. Starr JM, Wardlaw J, Ferguson K, MacLullich A, Deary IJ, Marshall I. Increased blood–brain barrier permeability in type II diabetes demonstrated by gadolinium magnetic resonance imaging. *J Neurol Neurosurg Psychiatry*. 2003;74(1):70–76.
72. Fujisawa I, Uokawa K, Horii N, et al. Bright pituitary stalk on MR T1-weighted image: Damming up phenomenon of the neurosecretory granules. *Endocr J*. 2002;49(2):165–173.
73. Gallinat J, Meisenzahl E, Jacobsen LK, et al. Smoking and structural brain deficits: A volumetric MR investigation. *Eur J Neurosci*. 2006;24(6):1744–1750.
74. Rivkin MJ, Davis PE, Lemaster JL, et al. Volumetric MRI study of brain in children with intrauterine exposure to cocaine, alcohol, tobacco, and marijuana. *Pediatrics*. 2008;121(4):741–750.
75. Howard G, Wagenknecht LE, Cai J, Cooper L, Kraut MA, Toole JF. Cigarette smoking and other risk factors for silent cerebral infarction in the general population. *Stroke*. 1998;29(5):913–917.
76. Di Pauli F, Reindl M, Ehling R, et al. Smoking is a risk factor for early conversion to clinically definite multiple sclerosis. *Mult Scler*. 2008;14(8):1026–1030.
77. Almeida OP, Garrido GJ, Lautenschlager NT, Hulse GK, Jamrozik K, Flicker L. Smoking is associated with reduced cortical regional gray matter density in brain regions associated with incipient Alzheimer disease. *Am J Geriatr Psychiatry*. 2008;16(1):92–98.
78. Gazdzinski S, Durazzo TC, Studholme C, Song E, Banys P, Meyerhoff DJ. Quantitative brain MRI in alcohol dependence: Preliminary evidence for effects of concurrent chronic cigarette smoking on regional brain volumes. *Alcohol Clin Exp Res*. 2005;29(8):1484–1495.
79. Paul RH, Grieve SM, Niaura R, et al. Chronic cigarette smoking and the microstructural integrity of white matter in healthy adults: A diffusion tensor imaging study. *Nicotine Tob Res*. 2008;10(1):137–147.
80. Gazdzinski S, Durazzo TC, Yeh PH, Hardin D, Banys P, Meyerhoff DJ. Chronic cigarette smoking modulates injury and short-term recovery of the medial temporal lobe in alcoholics. *Psychiatry Res*. 2008;162(2):133–145.
81. Durazzo TC, Gazdzinski S, Banys P, Meyerhoff DJ. Cigarette smoking exacerbates chronic alcohol-induced brain damage: A preliminary metabolite imaging study. *Alcohol Clin Exp Res*. 2004;28(12):1849–1860.
82. Jefferson AL, Tate DF, Poppas A, et al. Lower cardiac output is associated with greater white matter hyperintensities in older adults with cardiovascular disease. *J Am Geriatr Soc*. 2007;55(7):1044–1048.
83. Lee CW, Lee JH, Kim JJ, et al. Cerebral metabolic abnormalities in congestive heart failure detected by proton magnetic resonance spectroscopy. *J Am Coll Cardiol*. 1999;33(5):1196–1202.
84. Fernando MS, Simpson JE, Matthews F, et al. White matter lesions in an unselected cohort of the elderly: Molecular pathology suggests origin from chronic hypoperfusion injury. *Stroke*. 2006;37(6):1391–1398.

85. Marstrand JR, Garde E, Rostrup E, et al. Cerebral perfusion and cerebrovascular reactivity are reduced in white matter hyperintensities. *Stroke*. 2002;33(4):972–976.
86. Caroli A, Testa C, Geroldi C, et al. Brain perfusion correlates of medial temporal lobe atrophy and white matter hyperintensities in mild cognitive impairment. *J Neurol*. 2007;254(8):1000–1008.
87. Appelman AP, van der Graaf Y, Vincken KL, et al. Total cerebral blood flow, white matter lesions and brain atrophy: The SMART-MR study. *J Cereb Blood Flow Metab*. 2008;28(3):633–639.
88. de Leeuw FE, de Groot JC, Oudkerk M, et al. Atrial fibrillation and the risk of cerebral white matter lesions. *Neurology*. 2000;54(9):1795–1801.
89. Lev D, Nissenkorn A, Leshinsky-Silver E, et al. Clinical presentations of mitochondrial cardiomyopathies. *Pediatr Cardiol*. 2004;25(5):443–450.
90. Woo MA, Macey PM, Fonarow GC, Hamilton MA, Harper RM. Regional brain gray matter loss in heart failure. *J Appl Physiol*. 2003;95(2):677–684.
91. Malloy CR. Correlation of cerebral metabolites with clinical outcome among patients with severe congestive heart failure. *Circulation*. 2001;103(23):2771–2772.
92. Gass A, Ay H, Szabo K, Koroshetz WJ. Diffusion-weighted MRI for the "small stuff": The details of acute cerebral ischaemia. *Lancet Neurol*. 2004;3(1):39–45.
93. Saindane AM, Law M, Ge Y, Johnson G, Babb JS, Grossman RI. Correlation of diffusion tensor and dynamic perfusion MR imaging metrics in normal-appearing corpus callosum: Support for primary hypoperfusion in multiple sclerosis. *Am J Neuroradiol*. 2007;28(4): 767–772.
94. Munzel T, Sinning C, Post F, Warnholtz A, Schulz E. Pathophysiology, diagnosis and prognostic implications of endothelial dysfunction. *Ann Med*. 2008;40(3):180–196.
95. Kario K, Matsuo T, Kobayashi H, Asada R, Matsuo M. "Silent" cerebral infarction is associated with hypercoagulability, endothelial cell damage, and high Lp(a) levels in elderly Japanese. *Arterioscler Thromb Vasc Biol*. 1996;16(6):734–741.
96. Wardlaw JM, Farrall A, Armitage PA, et al. Changes in background blood–brain barrier integrity between lacunar and cortical ischemic stroke subtypes. *Stroke*. 2008;39(4): 1327–1332.
97. Hoth KF, Tate DF, Poppas A, et al. Endothelial function and white matter hyperintensities in older adults with cardiovascular disease. *Stroke*. 2007;38(2):308–312.
98. Markus HS, Hunt B, Palmer K, Enzinger C, Schmidt H, Schmidt R. Markers of endothelial and hemostatic activation and progression of cerebral white matter hyperintensities: Longitudinal results of the Austrian Stroke Prevention Study. *Stroke*. 2005;36(7):1410–1414.
99. Jones DK, Lythgoe D, Horsfield MA, Simmons A, Williams SC, Markus HS. Characterization of white matter damage in ischemic leukoaraiosis with diffusion tensor MRI. *Stroke*. 1999;30(2):393–397.
100. Helenius J, Soinne L, Salonen O, Kaste M, Tatlisumak T. Leukoaraiosis, ischemic stroke, and normal white matter on diffusion-weighted MRI. *Stroke*. 2002;33(1):45–50.
101. Nitkunan A, Barrick TR, Charlton RA, Clark CA, Markus HS. Multimodal MRI in cerebral small vessel disease: Its relationship with cognition and sensitivity to change over time. *Stroke*. 2008;39(7):1999–2005.
102. Mitchell BD, McArdle PF, Shen H, et al. The genetic response to short-term interventions affecting cardiovascular function: Rationale and design of the Heredity and Phenotype Intervention (HAPI) Heart Study. *Am Heart J*. 2008;155(5):823–828.
103. Gretarsdottir S, Thorleifsson G, Reynisdottir ST, et al. The gene encoding phosphodiesterase 4D confers risk of ischemic stroke. *Nat Genet*. 2003;35(2):131–138.
104. Dichgans M. Genetics of ischaemic stroke. *Lancet Neurol*. 2007;6(2):149–161.

105. Corder EH, Saunders AM, Strittmatter WJ, et al. Gene dose of apolipoprotein E type 4 allele and the risk of Alzheimer's disease in late onset families. *Science*. 1993;261(5123): 921–923.
106. DeCarli C, Massaro J, Harvey D, et al. Measures of brain morphology and infarction in the Framingham Heart Study: Establishing what is normal. *Neurobiol Aging*. 2005;26(4): 491–510.
107. Seshadri S, Wolf PA, Beiser A, et al. Stroke risk profile, brain volume, and cognitive function: The Framingham Offspring Study. *Neurology*. 2004;63(9):1591–1599.
108. Vermeer SE, Hollander M, van Dijk EJ, Hofman A, Koudstaal PJ, Breteler MM. Silent brain infarcts and white matter lesions increase stroke risk in the general population: The Rotterdam Scan Study. *Stroke*. 2003;34(5):1126–1129.
109. Jack CR, Jr., Shiung MM, Weigand SD, et al. Brain atrophy rates predict subsequent clinical conversion in normal elderly and amnestic MCI. *Neurology*. 25 2005;65(8):1227–1231.
110. Jack CR, Jr., Petersen RC, Xu YC, et al. Hippocampal atrophy and apolipoprotein E genotype are independently associated with Alzheimer's disease. *Ann Neurol*. 1998; 43(3):303–310.
111. Seshadri S, DeStefano AL, Au R, et al. Genetic correlates of brain aging on MRI and cognitive test measures: A genome-wide association and linkage analysis in the Framingham Study. *BMC Med Genet*. 2007;8(Suppl 1):S15.
112. Helgadottir A, Manolescu A, Thorleifsson G, et al. The gene encoding 5-lipoxygenase activating protein confers risk of myocardial infarction and stroke. *Nat Genet*. 2004; 36(3):233–239.
113. Helbecque N, Berr C, Cottel D, et al. VLDL receptor polymorphism, cognitive impairment, and dementia. *Neurology*. 2001;56(9):1183–1188.
114. Leow A, Klunder A, Jr CJ, et al. Longitudinal stability of MRI for mapping brain change using tensor-based morphometry. *Neuroimage*. 2006;31(2):627–640.
115. Meier DS, Guttmann CR. MRI time series modeling of MS lesion development. *Neuroimage*. 2006;32(2):531–537.
116. Barnes J, Lewis E, Scahill R, et al. Automated measurement of hippocampal atrophy using fluid-registered serial MRI in AD and controls. *J Comput Assist Tomogr*. 2007; 31(4):581–587.
117. Bradley K, Bydder G, Budge M, et al. Serial brain MRI at 3–6 month intervals as a surrogate marker for Alzheimer's disease. *Br J Radiol*. 2002;(75):894.

19

FUNCTIONAL NEUROIMAGING IN CARDIOVASCULAR DISEASE

Lawrence H. Sweet, Andreana P. Haley, and Ronald A. Cohen

Structural brain imaging methods such as magnetic resonance imaging (MRI) and computerized tomography (CT) are neurodiagnostic procedures that have been well established as the standard of care in the assessment of many neurological disorders, including cardioembolic stroke. These routine examinations are excellent for detecting and evaluating brain abnormalities secondary to infarction of large cerebral vessels. However, they are less useful for distinguishing healthy from abnormal brain function in the absence of a major stroke, or for informing us about the impact of structural abnormalities on mood, cognition, and behavior. These factors are particularly relevant to neurobehavioral and cognitive difficulties secondary to microvascular disease and chronic cerebral hypoperfusion often experienced by patients with severe cardiovascular disease.

While large-vessel stroke and microvascular disturbances are both associated with cardiovascular disease, the occurrence of a single large infarction is usually obvious to the patient, their family, and their doctors. In contrast, smaller infarctions, white matter disease, and associated subtle cognitive dysfunction often go undetected. Patients with chronic cardiovascular disease are particularly susceptible to microvascular disturbances that affect the brain's white matter and subcortical systems. In most cases, the detection of a single event such as an evolving infarction is impossible. Small lacunar infarctions are frequently detected; however, the effects are often subtle and fall below the threshold for clinical concern. Similarly, insidious cerebral abnormalities secondary to chronic cerebral hypoperfusion without obvious infarction are difficult to discern based on a single structural imaging assessment.

Dramatic advances in functional neuroimaging methods have occurred over the last two decades. Although these methods have considerable potential value for diagnosis, prognosis, and treatment of neurological disorders, they are rarely used in clinical practice. In this chapter, we will describe the information that can be derived through functional neuroimaging and review research using these methods to study cerebrovascular dysfunction.

Functional neuroimaging refers to techniques such as functional MRI (FMRI) and positron emission tomography (PET) that enable the visualization and quantification of brain function over time. The targets are usually neural networks associated with discrete cognitive challenges, broadly defined to include emotional, motivational, sensory, and motor processes. It is important to note that many functional neuroimaging methods, including FMRI and $H_2{}^{15}O$PET, actually measure cerebrovascular response to neural activity in systems elicited by these cognitive challenges. Thus, these methods typically rely on hemodynamic measurements that are spatially and temporally coupled with the underlying neural activity under normal circumstances. This basic assumption, however, requires further investigation in conditions associated with vascular dysfunction, such as cardiovascular disease.

Prior to the development of FMRI, PET and single photon emission computed tomography (SPECT) were the primary functional imaging methods available. These methods rely on the detection of radioactive contrast agents administered through intravenous infusion. Blood-oxygen-level-dependent (BOLD) FMRI, on the other hand, relies on endogenous contrast created by rapid changes in the ratio of oxygenated to deoxygenated hemoglobin induced by the increased oxygen demands of firing neurons. Thus, while FMRI, PET, and SPECT overlap somewhat in the information they provide, they also offer unique profiles of advantages and disadvantages, and each allows quantification of unique information about brain function and cerebral hemodynamics. Table 19-1 summarizes the types of information that can be most directly derived from functional brain imaging methods, along with key advantages and limitations.

In the remainder of this chapter, we will provide an overview of functional imaging techniques using MRI, summarizing underlying assumptions and basic methods, describing limitations that affect their clinical application, reviewing efforts to apply these methods to the study of cerebrovascular dysfunction, and discussing how these methods could be applied in the future for the study and clinical assessment of cardiovascular disease. We will present existing data from studies of cardiovascular disease and chronic cerebrovascular diseases. Since relatively few studies have applied these methods directly to cardiovascular disease, we will first discuss the application of these methods to studying function in healthy older samples, and also in neurological disorders, such as stroke.

BOLD FMRI

FMRI is an exciting tool for noninvasive examination of brain function. FMRI research has grown rapidly, and clinical applications have been developed.[1] The rapid growth of FMRI is reflected in the number of publications indexed on the NIH PubMed search engine with "FMRI" in the title or abstract. This number has increased from just two in 1993, the first year they appeared, to 1941 in the year 2008 (see Fig. 19-1). Although this is an underestimate of the total number of publications on FMRI, it demonstrates the increase over time. With such rapid growth in research and clinical settings, it has become critical to identify potential applications and limitations of this technology.

Table 19-1 Techniques used to measure brain response to experimental challenges over time

Type	Resolution		Cost	Advantages	Disadvantages
SPECT	cm	min	High	Absolute blood flow, specific molecules, clinical uses, out of scanner paradigms possible	Radioactive tracers, invasive, design limits—availability of PET/cyclotron
PET	mm	min	Higher		
EEG	Poor	ms	Low	Non invasive, clinical uses flexible experimental design	Spatial resolution, especially subcortical structures
MEG	mm	ms	Higher	Non invasive, flexible experimental design	Availability, subcortical resolution, strong magnetic field
BOLD FMRI	mm	sec	High	Non invasive, availability, other MRI scans available, flexible experimental design	Movement and susceptibility artifact, noise, space, strong magnetic field and RF waves, response lag—partial brain only in ASL
ASL FMRI	mm	sec	High		
NIRS	Poor	sec	Low	Non invasive, portable, flexible experimental design	limited to relatively small areas of brain surface

Abbreviations: SPECT = single photon emission computed tomography, PET = positron emission tomography, EEG = electroencephalography, MEG = magnetoencephalography, BOLD = blood oxygen dependent, FMRI = functional magnetic resonance imaging, ASL = arterial spin labeling, NIRS = near infrared spectroscopy, min = minutes, sec = seconds, ms = milliseconds, RF = radio frequency.

For instance, highly relevant to cardiovascular disease, there is substantial evidence that the sensitivity of BOLD FMRI may vary as a function of cerebrovascular health.

BOLD is the most common FMRI method. It uses the magnetic properties of hemoglobin for use as an endogenous contrast agent. This method takes advantage of the fact that deoxyhemoglobin is paramagnetic, while oxyhemoglobin is not, and the observation that neural activity reliably leads to the delivery of an excess of oxyhemoglobin. A smaller deoxyhemoglobin–oxyhemoglobin ratio in the capillary beds surrounding active neurons yields a more homogenous magnetic field and a greater MR signal. While it is known that increased neural activity results in vasodilation and greater delivery of an excess of oxygen-rich blood, the intervening mechanisms have been not well established.

BOLD FMRI enables cognitive neuroscientists to measure brain response to various cognitive, behavioral, and emotional challenges. While the goal of traditional MRI is to acquire high-resolution images of brain anatomy and structural abnormalities, the goal of FMRI is to detect variations in MRI signal that occur over time and map them with relatively high spatial resolution. When rapid MRI acquisitions using echoplanar T2* sequences sensitive to paramagnetic distortions of deoxyhemoglobin are repeated,

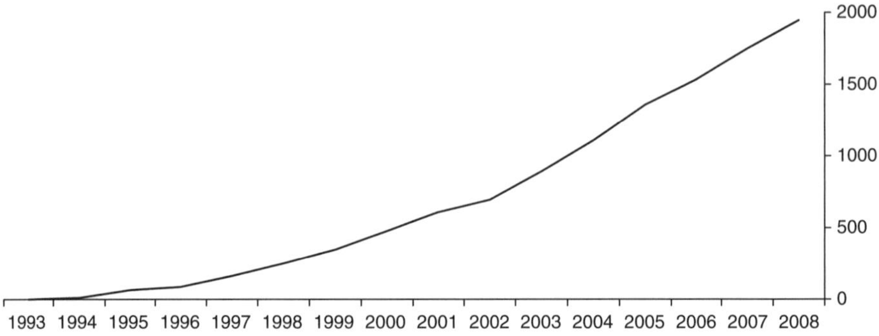

Figure 19-1 Annual totals of Medline indexed publications with "FMRI" in title or abstract.

a time series including both spatial and temporal information is obtained. When this is coupled with precise experimental challenges that enable this variation to be fractionated by different cognitive conditions, it is possible to obtain data that reflect changes in brain function associated with specific processes.

FMRI data acquisition sessions involve stimulus presentation and usually some type of behavioral response. BOLD signal is sampled in repeated acquisitions of a brain volume during a carefully designed stimulus presentation protocol. Brain volumes may include the whole brain or selected slices in any plane. For example, one whole-brain volume of 48 contiguous 3 mm-thick axial slices might be acquired every three seconds. These resulting raw data undergo several preprocessing steps to yield a time-dependent signal course for each voxel (i.e., the smallest unit of three-dimensional spatial resolution within each imaging slice).

The raw BOLD signal obtained from each voxel of an individual is typically converted to a standardized metric to allow comparison across subjects or time. For example, a simple method is subtracting an individual's mean baseline signal from mean signal during the experimental condition. These mean difference scores may be compared to a hypothetical mean of zero (i.e., the null hypothesis) using a one-sample student's t-test for each voxel. Other methods such as cross-correlation and multiple regression can be used to determine how closely each voxel's time course is related to the time course of the stimulation. Thus, individual datasets are assigned a value per voxel that corresponds to the voxel's intensity change between conditions or relatedness to the stimulus presentation over time.

The term *activation* is usually used to denote voxels in which intensity of the BOLD signal, or the relatedness of the BOLD signal to the task presentation, exceeds a significance threshold that is usually corrected for multiple comparisons. Deactivation usually denotes significant decreases in activity relative to baseline. Volumes of activation may also be quantified by counting the number of voxels exceeding the threshold. Grouped statistical comparisons are performed once the dependent variable is calculated for each individual, and the region of interest is specified. Voxel-wise and regional analyses are typically conducted following stereotaxic standardization and spatial blurring to compensate for individual differences in functional anatomy. Associated behavioral data, if recorded, are used to validate that participants adequately performed the task and to test performance-related experimental hypotheses.

The early BOLD FMRI experiments used subtraction and cross-correlation analyses of block designs to demonstrate task-associated BOLD response in primary motor or visual processing areas. For example Bandetini and colleagues[2] identified brain voxels most related to the time course of a self-paced finger-tapping task. FMRI studies of higher-order cognitive processes, such as language[3] and executive functions,[4] began to appear soon after using similar cross-correlation methods. Early studies typically did not examine the whole brain and tended to include small sample sizes. However, these methods were soon applied to experiments employing whole-brain imaging and larger sample sizes. For example, Rao and colleagues[5] reported a whole-brain network of cortical and subcortical brain structures that exhibited activity associated with a conceptual reasoning paradigm among eleven healthy adults. Another major advance in FMRI was the development of linear multiple regression methods to identify activity associated with rapid presentation of stimulus trials.[6–9] This advance grew out of the findings that BOLD responses could be detected following very brief stimuli (<1 second),[2, 10] and that responses to such stimuli were additive and approximately linear.[8, 11] These were significant advances, because event-related designs could be developed that did not require long inter-stimulus intervals to allow the hemodynamic BOLD response to return to baseline.[8] Event-related designs also provided more flexibility than the blocked design, which had been the neuroimaging paradigm used in PET and FMRI research. Other advantages of event-related design include observation of the evolution of activity over short periods of time (e.g., 10 seconds)[12] and the ability to retrospectively bin stimulus events into different conditions based upon performance.[13]

While these BOLD FMRI studies have contributed immensely to the understanding of healthy brain function, they have also laid a methodological and theoretical foundation with which we may contrast patient populations. The methods and findings of FMRI studies of stroke, Alzheimer's disease, and healthy geriatric populations are of particular relevance in guiding future studies of patients with chronic cerebrovascular disease.

BOLD FMRI Research Findings Related to Cardiovascular Disease

Since the first report of non-contrast echoplanar BOLD[14] and the application to human experiments[15–17] in the early 1990s, BOLD FMRI has rapidly diversified in terms of cognitive domains and populations studied. The earliest studies examined primary visual and motor cortices among healthy participants; however, the technique was soon applied to investigations of higher-order cognitive functions of every cognitive domain (e.g., memory, language, attention, and emotional functioning). Within a decade, FMRI investigators had directed their attention to participants of all ages and a variety of psychiatric and neurological populations. Healthy cognitive functioning,[18–27] as well as developmental disorders, such as epilepsy,[28–32] dyslexia,[33–40] and ADHD,[41–43] have been studied among children. Psychiatric disorders studied include substance abuse (cocaine,[44–48] nicotine,[49–52] alcohol[53–58]), anxiety disorders (phobias,[59–61] obsessive-compulsive disorder[62–63]), schizophrenia,[64–71] and personality disorders (antisocial[72]). Neurological populations studied included multiple sclerosis,[73–76] Parkinson's disease,[77–84] and Alzheimer's disease patients.[85–89]

Studies of cardiovascular disease have only just begun to appear in the FMRI literature;[90] however, other chronic cerebrovascular disorders have been studied more extensively. These include acute stroke and stroke recovery,[91–96] arteriovenous malformation,[97–98] migraine headaches,[99–100] and Cerebral Autosomal Dominant Arteriopathy with Sub-cortical Infarcts and Leukoencephalopathy (CADASIL).[101] Interesting recent FMRI research has also been conducted on healthy groups at risk for hypertension[102] and Alzheimer's disease.[103–104]

Cardiovascular disease FMRI studies in patients with chronic cardiovascular disease without stroke have only recently begun to emerge. In a study of peripheral vascular health and BOLD, Haley et al.[90] demonstrated that, FMRI may be sensitive to early vascular disease processes that lead to cognitive impairment. The study reported that, among non-demented patients with cardiovascular disease, higher burden of atherosclerosis, as measured by carotid artery intima-media thickness, was associated with lower signal intensity in the right-middle frontal gyrus in response to a verbal working-memory task (Fig. 19-2). Selective attention, executive ability, and psychomotor speed are all crucial to our ability to maintain and process verbal information in working memory.[105] These skills are also compromised in elderly patients with cardiovascular disease even if their global cognitive functioning is intact,[106] presumably due to small-vessel disease. Interestingly, the relationship between BOLD response to cognition and level of atherosclerosis in the Haley et al. study was independent of age and small-vessel disease, indicating that hypoperfusion due to small-vessel disease does not account for all the observed variance in the BOLD response to cognition. Task-related activation intensity in the same region was positively correlated with task performance (accuracy). Since the posterior-middle frontal gyri are involved in subvocal rehearsal, with the right side recruited in conditions of increased working-memory demand,[107] atherosclerosis appears to be associated with dysfunction specifically in brain areas responsible for articulatory rehearsal and executive processes crucial for successful verbal working-memory functioning. This possibility was supported by the strong positive relationship between performance accuracy and task-related brain activity the right premotor area. Therefore, large-vessel atherosclerosis may be another mechanism contributing to brain dysfunction in patients with cardiovascular disease. The BOLD contrast also appeared to be highly sensitive to peripheral vascular health as measured by carotid artery intima-media thickness. Considering that the correlation between intima-media thickness and activation intensity remained significant after controlling for task performance (response accuracy), it appears that FMRI may detect vascular-related changes in brain function early in the disease process, before cognitive performance is substantially impaired.

This idea is further supported by reported differences in the hemodynamic response to working memory in healthy young adults at risk for hypertension recently observed by Haley and colleagues.[102] This study examined the relationship between a family history of hypertension and brain response to a working-memory challenge in healthy young adults with intact working-memory performance. The results showed that family history of hypertension, a marker of increased genetic risk for developing the disease, was associated with lower task-related activation in the right-inferior parietal lobule and right-inferior temporal gyrus as well as with substantially greater deactivation of the posterior cingulate. These results fit well with a growing body of clinical research literature indicating that FMRI is able to detect altered brain function among individuals at risk, before clinical symptoms or behavioral deficits are present.[73–74, 103, 108] Unlike those prior studies, however, the alterations reported in the hypertension study[102] consisted of lower, rather than higher, BOLD response to a cognitive challenge in the population at risk. The authors hypothesized that these differences are significant and indicative of a different underlying mechanism. For example, in individuals at risk for vascular cognitive impairment, changes in BOLD response to cognitive function may be related to cerebral hypoperfusion. In individuals at risk for cognitive impairment related to multiple sclerosis,[73–74] HIV,[108] or genetic risk for Alzheimer's disease[103–104], the other hand, changes in BOLD response to cognitive challenges may be related to inflammatory or other non-vascular processes. The task-related deactivations in the posterior cingulate observed in the participants with a positive family history of hypertension are also very interesting, and consistent with the opinion that lower BOLD response to a cognitive challenge in a population at risk for vascular disease provides evidence of subclinical

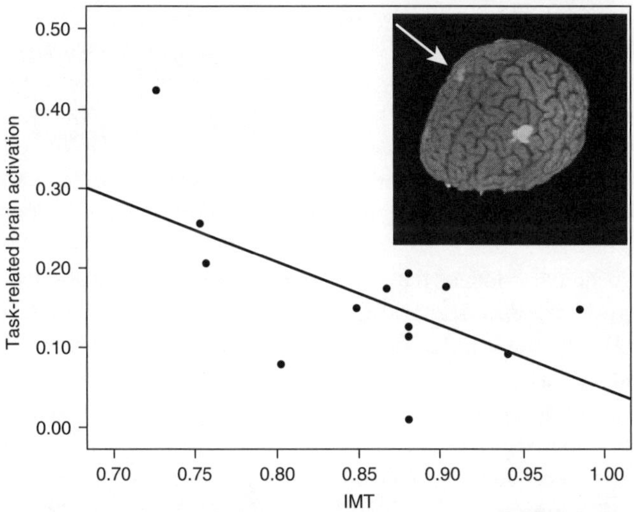

Figure 19-2 BOLD response to a verbal working-memory challenge among cardiovascular disease patients as a function of atherosclerosis (inta-media thickness).

cognitive impairment. Task-related deactivations in several brain regions including the posterior cingulate have been increasingly reported in imaging studies.[109–111] These deactivations, indicating higher neural activity during the baseline/low-demand conditions as opposed to the experimental/high-demand conditions, appear to be associated with internally generated thoughts involving episodic memory, planning, problem solving, processing emotions, and self-monitoring.[112–113] Task-related deactivations have been shown to increase in magnitude (i.e., deactivate further) with increasing task difficulty, giving rise to the hypothesis that selective withdrawal of attention from self-referential, stimulus-independent thought in favor of more challenging cognitive tasks may be a compensatory mechanism employed by participants who are struggling to complete the task at hand.[113–114] Withdrawal of resources from this so-called default-mode brain network responsible for stream-of-consciousness type mental images and thoughts[112] has also been associated with nicotine-induced enhancement of visual spatial attention.[115] Therefore, while in some contexts, withdrawal of resources from self-referential thought may indicate more efficient concentration and better performance, in other cases, where participants are maintaining normal cognitive performance in suboptimal conditions (e.g., reduced cerebral perfusion), this increased withdrawal of resources from irrelevant brain areas seems to indicate a passive compensatory mechanism that allows patients at risk to maintain normal cognitive functioning.

In sum, although very few FMRI studies of chronic cardiovascular disease have been published, the results are intriguing and beg for further investigation. They also suggest the utility of FMRI as a potentially clinically useful tool for identifying and treating individuals at risk for future cognitive impairment before clinical symptoms compromise their everyday functioning.

Older adults Several FMRI studies of older adults have appeared since the mid 1990s[116–137] that may be useful to help us differentiate expected from unexpected hemodynamic changes among older adults. This is crucial because controlled studies of cerebrovascular disease may identify FMRI changes among older participants that are related to aging rather than cardiovascular disease *per se*. On the other hand, the vascular cognitive impairment associated with cardiovascular disease may simply represent an extreme example of normal aging that is qualitatively similar, but quantitatively extreme.

There is substantial evidence that the age-related vascular changes that occur among older adults are likely to influence BOLD response independently of cognition. For instance, BOLD response is influenced by several hemodynamic factors, such as vascular tone, vascular dilation, blood pressure, blood flow, blood volume, and blood perfusion rates that are known to vary with age.[135] It has been demonstrated that, even among younger adults, blood volume and flow influence BOLD signal.[140] The finding that older adults experience slower peripheral capillary refill rates[141] is particularly relevant because a significant portion of the BOLD response is due to changes at the capillary level.[142] These age-related vascular factors directly affect the likelihood that changes in BOLD signal are detected, identified as significantly active within an individual, or considered significantly different when compared to those in younger groups. Moreover, there is substantial direct evidence that BOLD signal itself changes with age. Some studies have directly assessed BOLD response among older participants. These have revealed slower, less intense, and more variable hemodynamic responses among older adults.[126, 128, 134–135] Specifically, FMRI studies of visual and motor functions among older adults have revealed longer hemodynamic lags, later peak intensity, more inter-subject variability, and lower signal-to-noise ratios.[116, 126, 128] Lower BOLD signal has also been confirmed with near-infrared spectroscopy,[136–137] suggesting that it is not a FMRI methodological artifact. Attenuated hypercapnic BOLD signal response among older participants compared younger participants has also been observed during a finger-tapping task, suggesting that the older cerebral vessels may not respond normally to FMRI challenges.[123] Together, these findings suggest that BOLD response may be affected by the integrity of cerebral hemodynamics, independently of cognitive function.

There is growing evidence that older adults exhibit different patterns of BOLD response compared to younger adults during sensory stimulation, simple motor movement, and higher-order cognitive tasks.[116, 126, 128, 133–134, 141] Studies of basic perception, such as vision and olfaction, have reported less associated activity compared to younger control participants.[126–128] Perception of more complex facial emotion has also been associated with less activity in regions activated among younger controls.[129–130] However, one of these studies also reported relatively greater left frontal activity.[130]

A robust finding among studies of motor function is that older adults demonstrate decreased BOLD activation within primary motor and somatosensory areas during self-paced motor tasks, such as finger-tapping.[123–124] This finding has been replicated during paced (i.e., matched) finger and wrist flexion/extension paradigms, but also resulted in greater supplementary motor area (SMA) activation compared to younger controls.[125]

Other FMRI studies of older adults have focused on cognitive domains in which elderly patients typically demonstrate declining function. These include memory, executive function, and psychomotor speed.[131–133]

FMRI studies of memory encoding have reported less prefrontal activity compared to younger control participants regardless of matching for performance.[116–117] However, more bilateral activity has been reported in these studies, particularly if older participants performed equally to younger participants.[117–120] In contrast, greater prefrontal activity has been reported among older adults who performed well during verbal working-memory tasks.[121–122]

Dual task performance has yielded similar patterns of activity in younger and older groups; however, each task alone continued to elicit dorsolateral prefrontal cortex activation among the older group, but not the younger group.[131] Attentional interference tasks have shown a pattern of increased and more bilateral prefrontal and parietal activation pattern among equal performers[132] and produced less frontal and parietal activity among older participants with lower scores.[133]

Taken together, the major findings of FMRI studies of older adults suggest BOLD signal declines with age-related declines in cognitive performance and perception.

Furthermore, a compensatory bilateral frontal activation pattern emerges, particularly when participants are matched to younger controls for performance. These trends in FMRI studies of older adults point to the importance of understanding normal changes in aging brain function that may be mistaken for the result of pathological processes. The cognitive domains studied among older adults (executive, memory, and motor functioning) provide an excellent foundation of what to expect in studies of cardiovascular disease since they happen to be areas of deficit in this population.[195–200] Alternatively, cardiovascular disease manifestations in the brain may represent a pathological process very different from accelerated aging and may require an entirely different approach to prevention and treatment. Considering the progressive aging of the population and the impending health care crisis with exponentially increasing numbers of cognitively impaired elderly, research on these issues is of utmost importance.

Stroke Most FMRI studies of stroke populations focus on recovery of language and motor functions subsequent to large-vessel infarcts. The few studies of stroke patients who have aphasia have demonstrated that their language dysfunction is associated with greater contralateral and perilesional activation than expected from healthy control groups. Furthermore, greater bilateral activity and greater perilesional activity was associated with better language recovery.[91–92]

The most consistent finding from investigations of recovery of motor functions (typically hemiparestic patients) is increased ipsilateral primary somatosensory area activity compared to healthy control participants.[93–96] An interesting finding is that this ipsilateral recruitment effect has been enhanced by a single dose of fluoxetine.[95] These findings also suggest that greater bilateral activity may be transient if the infarct has not cause significant damage to the primary motor areas (i.e., becomes lateralized again once patients recover function).[96]

One group studied motor function among CADASIL patients without hemiparesis or other focal motor symptoms.[101] They found decreased laterality in the primary motor area compared to control participants and an inverse relationship between white matter injury and laterality. Therefore, ipsilateral recruitment of motor areas may not be limited patients exhibiting hemiparesis.

Summary In sum, the major findings of FMRI studies of older adults suggest BOLD signal declines with normal aging, possibly due to normal cerebrovascular changes, and this decline may be independent of performance. Compensatory activation patterns may also appear, particularly when participants are matched to younger controls on performance measures. This compensatory activity may occur in prefrontal regions and contralateral homologues of expected regions of interest (ROIs). FMRI studies of stroke patients have demonstrated that stroke-related language dysfunction is often associated with greater contralateral and perilesional activation relative to healthy controls, with greater bilateral and perilesional activity indicative of better language recovery. Stroke-related motor dysfunction has been associated with greater activity in ipsilateral primary somatosensory cortex relative to healthy controls. Studies of chronic cardiovascular disease and risk for cardiovascular disease, on the other hand, have indicated lower BOLD response to working memory in the dorsolateral prefrontal cortex, inferior parietal lobule, and inferior temporal gyrus. Greater deactivation in the posterior cingulate gyrus was also reported, possibly indicating a passive withdrawal of resources from self-referential processes to maintain normal cognitive performance.

Strengths and Limitations of BOLD FMRI

FMRI has several advantages over other functional neuroimaging techniques, which include greater feasibility, better resolution, more design flexibility, and greater availability. FMRI, as typically performed, already has the inherent advantages of investigating concurrent relationships between BOLD response, behavioral response, and structural morphometry as observed on high-resolution T1-weighted images. Moreover, additional MR scans may be acquired during the FMRI session (e.g., T2, perfusion, and diffusion-weighted scans, fluid attenuated inversion recovery [FLAIR], and magnetic resonance spectroscopy [MRS]) with little additional inconvenience to the patient (i.e., more time). BOLD FMRI is also noninvasive, repeatable, and less expensive than PET, allowing more design flexibility, including repeated measures and studies of children. While typical FMRI spatial resolution is 3 mm^3 to 5 mm^3 for whole brain studies with temporal resolution of two to four seconds, spatial resolution less than 1mm^3, and temporal resolution below one second can be achieved with specialized sequences. A good balance of spatial and temporal resolution is chosen based on the study questions, with an inherent trade-off between these two parameters and the extent of brain coverage. Thus, smaller regions and more transient cognitive processes can be observed using FMRI compared to other functional neuroimaging techniques. FMRI designs have been evolving, providing greater flexibility, especially after the introduction of event-related designs in the late 1990s. Finally, FMRI has the advantage of the proliferation of MRI systems in most large medical settings. Standard clinical MRI scanners are technically capable of running FMRI sequences; however, a contract with the scanner manufacturer to use this capability is usually necessary, which adds to costs.

At the same time, there are several special considerations in FMRI experiments including cardiovascular disease patients. Subject screening and selection must be more carefully considered than with younger and healthier adults. For example, cardiovascular disease patients tend to have more health issues and experience more medical interventions leading to MR contraindications, including implanted cardiac stents and magnetically activated devices such as pacemakers. Safety is also a special consideration with cognitively impaired patients who many be unable to follow instructions or may forget to disclose important information. Additionally, eyesight, movement, comfort level, and body morphometry (size and shape) in general tend to be greater issues in older adults and patients.

When studying any clinical population, investigators must be particularly sensitive to the effects of loud scanner noise, the potential danger of a magnetic environment, motion artifacts, claustrophobia, and susceptibility artifacts. Scanner noise in conjunction with hearing difficulties may make verbal responding impossible and may require more sophisticated responding and stimulus presentation paradigms. These paradigms may be more confusing to patients with cognitive problems than standard neuropsychological testing. Other stimulus presentation issues include the need for MR-compatible equipment (safe and functional) and the ability to present stimuli to participants who are lying in a narrow MRI bore. Averaging and temporal smoothing of BOLD signal is necessary to gain reliable data, because observed signal changes are typically less than 10%, even during the more robust response to motor and visual stimulation paradigms. Generalizability of findings may be a problem because acquisition, preprocessing, statistical analysis, thresholding of significant effects, and technology differ from site to site. Finally, FMRI research with patient populations is expensive. It depends on specialized equipment and highly trained personnel from several different disciplines, such as clinicians, radiologists, biomedical engineers, physicists, statisticians, neuroscientists, programmers, computer information technologists, and scanner technologists.

FMRI of chronic cardiovascular disease patients remains a topic of little research, yet there is great potential. It is very likely that similar deviations in brain function will be discovered in patients with cardiovascular disease as have been reported among other patient populations. However, verification of the validity of BOLD studies among this population is particularly important given the compromise of cerebrovasculature and our incomplete understanding of the mechanisms underlying the BOLD response. This may involve replication of studies of healthy controls, research aimed at a better understanding the effects of healthy aging on BOLD signal, and clarification of the meaning of relatively greater or less signal among patients in general (e.g., successful compensation or inefficient activity). FMRI of patients also provides an excellent method to evaluate models of brain dysfunction and the efficacy of medications.

Technical advances such as application of non-echoplanar sequences to reduce susceptibility artifacts, higher-field-strength magnets, and more powerful (and more uniform) preprocessing and statistical analysis techniques may produce significant advances in our understanding of chronic cerebrovascular disease. With the emerging finding of BOLD signal decline among older healthy adults due to hemodynamic factors, it is crucial to understand how much of the BOLD signal decline is related to these factors in patients with disorders directly affecting hemodynamics. Understanding of these intervening hemodynamic mechanisms will be crucial to interpreting BOLD data from patients with compromised cerebrovascular systems.

Perfusion Imaging

Perfusion-weighted imaging uses fast gradient-echo or spin-echo pulse sequences to observe the movement of a paramagnetic contrast agent through capillaries over time. The most common perfusion MRI technique is dynamic susceptibility contrast (DSC) imaging, which involves intravenous administration of a bolus of an exogenous non-ionizing contrast agent such as gadolinium. This leads to magnetic field inhomogenieties, and therefore greater T2* signal attenuation in brain regions with greater blood perfusion. DSC provides a means of measuring cerebral blood perfusion in specific regions of interest.

Noninvasive methods have also been developed that magnetically label blood to be used as an endogenous contrast agent.[142–147] This is done by manipulating proton spins before the blood reaches the region of interest. These methods are typically named "arterial spin labeling" (ASL). ASL provides quantitative perfusion data of cerebral blood flow (CBF) with relatively high spatial resolution. Image contrast in ASL is obtained by magnetically labeling blood-water spins flowing into the slice of interest. Two images are acquired; one with the flow-labeling present and one with labeling absent. The labeled image is then subtracted from the non-labeled image, and the resulting image is converted to CBF in units of (ml blood)/(ml tissue)/minute from measured blood spin-lattice relaxation time (T1B) and the relaxed magnetization of arterial blood (M0B).

Perfusion MRI provides excellent measures of resting cerebrovascular perfusion. Several perfusion characteristics can be derived from DSC and ASL MRI. These include cerebral blood volume (CBV; the ratio of blood volume to tissue volume), CBF (the volume of blood delivered to the tissue volume per minute), and mean transit time (MTT; the average time it takes the contrast to pass through the tissue).

While typical perfusion MRI methods provide a reliable snapshot of cerebrovascular dynamics using repeated sampling in a resting state, sampling may also be performed over time during cognitive, behavioral, emotional, or pharmacological challenges. Thus, ASL may be used as a noninvasive perfusion FMRI technique. Because ASL uses endogenous contrasts, it can be practically used to measure the brain response over periods of time that are useful for the investigation of discrete, repeated neural stimulation. This development in perfusion MRI allows clinical researchers, and eventually clinicians, to evaluate the brain response of specific functional systems to targeted challenges.

Perfusion MRI applied to neurological disorders is a growing field of research with a growing list of clinical applications. For example, it is useful in predicting neurological outcome in head injury,[148] cardiac surgery,[149–150] and epilepsy.[151] However, studies of stroke have been the most common experimental and clinical application, and several studies of patients with brain tumors and internal carotid artery occlusion have also been reported.

These studies have shown that perfusion MRI is useful in the diagnosis of stroke, identification of ischemic tissue, prediction of infarct volume, and evaluation of treatment outcome.[152–160] Specifically, increased CBF, increased CBV, and decreased MTT suggest that tissue is involved in acute ischemia,[156, 161] while CBF and CBV have been shown to predict final infarct volume.[154–156, 161] In individual unilateral stroke patients, perfusion values from the affected hemisphere are often compared to these measures from the unaffected hemisphere to identify and determine the volume of ischemic tissue. When the DSC-identified abnormal tissue volume exceeds the volume identified by diffusion-weighted imaging, the excess tissue has been shown to be in danger of permanent infarct.[160–167] Thus DSC can be used in addition to diffusion imaging to identify ischemic tissue in danger of infarct, and when combined, both methods are more sensitive and specific than either alone. However, DSC has been shown to have unique value in identifying transient ischemic attacks and subarachnoid hemorrhage.[168]

Abnormal perfusion findings have been associated with chronic occlusive carotid artery disease in a series of studies.[169–172] In these studies, perfusion response rate (time to peak response) was found to be a more reliable marker of carotid disease severity than cerebral blood volume. Therefore, perfusion MRI can be used as a reliable indicator of chronic occlusive carotid artery disease. Another study, of giant aneurisms of the intracranial internal carotid artery, found that less cerebral blood flow and more variable blood volume were strong predictors of recovery on functional measures after bypass surgery.[173] Studies of this type show how perfusion MRI can be applied beyond acute stroke to the study of chronic cerebrovascular disease.

Of special relevance to hypoperfusion mechanisms in cardiovascular disease is a perfusion study of eight patients with ischemic leukoaraiosis. Patients exhibited less resting CBF in white matter regions of interest and greater resting CBV in gray matter ROIs compared to healthy control participants. MTTs were longer among the patients in superior white matter. The authors concluded that white matter hypoperfusion may underlie leukoaraiosis.[174]

Previous studies have demonstrated the diagnostic utility of DSC and ASL among Alzheimer's patients. One group compared 19 Alzheimer's disease patients to 18 age-matched healthy control participants. They demonstrated less bilateral temporopatietal DSC-CBV among the patients and diagnosed with a sensitivity of 88% to 95% and specificity of 96%.[175–177] Alsop and colleagues[178] demonstrated less ASL-measured CBF in temporal, parietal, and frontal cortices among 18 Alzheimer's disease patients compared to 11 age-matched control subjects. These investigations concluded that perfusion MRI is a good alternative to SPECT and PET in this population. It is noteworthy that these Alzheimer's disease patients exhibited cortical hypoperfusion, while leukoaraiosis patients[174] exhibited white matter hypoperfusion.

Although functional imaging studies of brain perfusion in cardiovascular disease have not yet been published, recent studies have been reported on the use of functional ASL in aging, mild cognitive impairment, and Alzheimer's dementia that suggest future utility among older adults with cardiovascular disease. For instance, results from two recent studies contrasting older (70s) and younger (20s) groups suggest a decoupling of BOLD signal and neural function in the medial temporal lobe during memory encoding.[179–180] Specifically, resting CBF was lower among the older groups, but increases were significantly greater in response to the paradigm compared to the younger groups. In one of the studies,[179] task performance was significantly related to ASL measured CBF, but not BOLD. This suggests that ASL perfusion may be a more sensitive indicator of brain response among older adults than the BOLD response. The authors also reported that stroke risk on the Framingham Stroke Risk Profile[181] was not related to performance, but was positively related to both BOLD and ASL response. Although this group was not at high risk for stroke according to this profile, functional ASL and BOLD may be more sensitive to this risk than measures of cognitive performance. In a similar study of individuals at genetic risk for AD,[182] a greater resting perfusion and a decreased CBF and BOLD response to a memory encoding paradigm was observed, which resulted in no significant differences relative to the control group in absolute CBF response to the paradigm. Another functional ASL study of 12 mild cognitive impairment patients also revealed significant CBF hypoperfusion in the cuneus and precuneus that decreased further and expanded to include the posterior cingulate.[183] In contrast, patients did not exhibit a CBF increase in the right parahippocampus that was observed among the age-matched control participants. These recent findings suggest that hemodynamic changes associated with normal aging may be dissociated from pathological processes using multi-modal MRI.

In sum, the utility of DSC perfusion MRI in identifying ischemic tissue is evident in its growing use in clinical settings. It appears to have the potential to better identify ischemic events not identified by other imaging methods such as diffusion-weighted imaging and may therefore be of special value in the study and clinical treatment of cardiovascular disease. ASL provides a promising alternative to DSC, and holds additional promise as a method to observe response to specific FMRI challenges.

Compared to PET, SPECT, and structural MRI, perfusion MRI has been demonstrated to be as sensitive and specific to several neurological disorders (e.g., Alzheimer's disease, stroke). In some instances, perfusion MRI better detects and differentiates pathology (e.g., tumor, transient ischemia). Advantages of ASL over traditional methods include availability, lower cost, lack of ionizing radiation, noninvasiveness, and the ability to measure brain response to specific functional challenges over time.

Relatively few clinical studies using arterial spin labeling have been published[151, 182–184] compared to DSC perfusion and BOLD FMRI; however, they represent a promising and growing future direction. Although ASL techniques are noninvasive and may technically be implemented on typical MR scanners, they are less frequently used due to the lack of availability of pulse sequences, lower signal-to-noise ratios, more complicated data analysis pipelines, and partial brain coverage.

Future Directions

Functional neuroimaging has proven useful in localization of neural functions among healthy and clinical populations, and in the further investigation of neural and cerebrovascular dysfunction in these identified regions. This has been useful in understanding behavioral manifestations of neural abnormalities and neural manifestations of physiological abnormalities. Functional neuroimaging has great potential in the assessment of the severity of cognitive effects, prognosis of cognitive function and disease course, the search for effective treatments, and a better understanding of neural mechanisms in general as they begin to fail. The great utility of functional neuroimaging in clinical research is only beginning to extend into clinical practice. An excellent example of this is the use of BOLD FMRI in presurgical mapping for epilepsy.[1] Language and motor systems are mapped with selective behavioral challenges and avoided during surgery. As functional ASL and MRS, that is, in 3D+time, become more practical, there are many potential clinical applications.

In addition to the factors described above (e.g., temporal and spatial resolution, availability), MRI has a major advantage over electroencephalograpic, radiological, and optical functional neuroimaging techniques in that many MRI sequences are available for use in the same imaging session. Each of these other MRI sequences can be used in combination to gather structural (e.g., T1, T2, FLAIR), functional (BOLD, ASL), and even chemical (MRS) information during the same exam. As some of these exciting complementary techniques are combined with functional neuroimaging in clinical research, substantial leaps in our understanding of brain disorders are certain to follow. The revolutionary impact of T1, T2, and FLAIR MRI on diagnostics in disorders such as multiple sclerosis and stroke is clear. However, we are now able to further capitalize on these advances by precisely mapping function and dysfunction to structural lesion locations and volumes. Complimentary MRI techniques are described in the following sections, along with how they may be used in functional neuroimaging as applied to cardiovascular disease research.

Multi-Modal MRI

One of the most intriguing lines of research has evolved from efforts to characterize the relationships between systemic vascular disease, cerebrovascular perfusion, and associated brain function. With rapidly growing experimental and clinical applications, it is important to demonstrate the validity and reliability of the BOLD FMRI technique among groups where cerebral hemodynamics may be altered. This is crucial among populations with known alterations of vascular integrity and subsequent hemodynamic responsivity (e.g., older adults and patients with stroke and carotid artery stenosis). Cardiovascular disease without large-vessel stroke is a model system for studying such hemodynamic functions.

The link between cardiovascular disease and cognitive dysfunction has been demonstrated,[195–199] and the link between cognitive performance and BOLD FMRI among cardiovascular disease patients, including the negative impact of poor systemic vascular health on cognition and BOLD FMRI, has also been reported.[90, 200–201] Although links have been confirmed between cardiovascular disease, cerebrovascular perfusion, cognitive performance, and BOLD response to cognitive function, they have not yet been examined together. Therefore, future work is needed that is aimed at examining the interrelationship between the neural (cognitive) and hemodynamic consequences of severe cardiovascular disease, their underlying mechanisms, and their impact on our ability to assess cardiovascular disease patients.

We have proposed a model in which systemic hypoperfusion secondary to severe cardiovascular disease leads to cerebrovascular hypoperfusion (Fig. 19-3, bottom). We predict that cerebrovascular hypoperfusion then leads to an altered BOLD response to cognitive challenges via two mechanisms. The *first* is a neural mechanism by which hypoperfusion leads to neuronal damage and dysfunction. This, in turn, results in cognitive impairment as observed by lower cognitive performance and lower BOLD response to cognitive challenges. This is the typical model of coupled neural and hemodynamic response assumed when results of FMRI studies of patients are reported (Fig. 19-3, top). The *second*, alternative mechanism can be tested by measuring how acute hemodynamic response is altered (BOLD reactivity and cerebrovascular hypoperfusion) independently of cognitive performance, or even cognitive demands. Central to the assumed versus alternative distinction is the differentiation between chronic and acute effects of hypoperfosion, followed by the determination if normally excessive acute hemodynamic responses are sufficient to support neural demands. Thus, we expect significant decoupling of the normal task-related BOLD response among subsamples of cardiovascular disease patients that extends beyond the chronic effects of hypoperfusion on neuronal integrity. In this group, increases in oxygen consumption ratios are likely due to decreased, but sufficient volume of BOLD response for normal cognitive function.

Investigation of this model requires multi-modal MRI, including functional ASL, BOLD FMRI, and consideration of structural impact of the disease via high-resolution FLAIR and T1 imaging. These sequences, when combined with targeted cognitive and physiological challenges (e.g., hypercapnia) can yield the necessary information to calculate baseline perfusion rates, BOLD and perfusion response to the challenges, oxygen consumption rates, white and gray matter structural integrity, and concurrent cognitive performance. While experimental design, data analysis and integration of results pose substantial challenges, this invaluable set of information may be acquired in a single scanning session.

Diffusion Tensor Imaging

Diffusion tensor imaging (DTI) is based on the fact that water diffusion in the brain has the property of being directionally dependent or organized in directional pathways (directional anisotropy). Since white matter fibers are highly organized, the direction and magnitude of restricted diffusion along white matter tissue can be imaged to

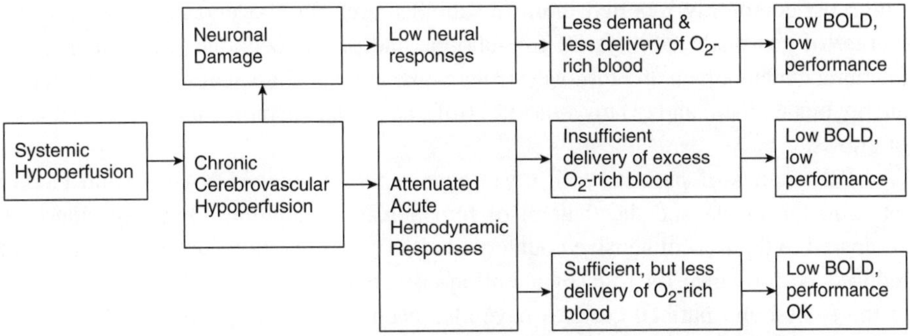

Figure 19-3 Effects of cardiovascular disease on relationships between hemodynamic and cognitive functions.

provide additional information regarding the integrity and connectivity of white matter pathways within the brain. DTI provides an index of the directional coherence of the particular pathways being imaged, called *fractional anisotropy* (FA). This measure of directional coherence provides information about how highly organized the pathway is, and also its integrity. DTI data can also be analyzed to determine the correlation of spatial orientation between different regions of brain tissue. This value, called the lattice anisotropy (LA) coefficient, provides another way of examining the integrity of the white matter pathways and interconnected brain systems.

Clinical researchers have directed considerable attention to DTI to gain insights into the characteristics of diseased and injured brain tissue. These efforts are likely to contribute important complementary information to functional and structural imaging research, and vice versa. This is because, relative to traditional MRI methods, DTI offers a means of better characterizing subtle changes associated with cognitive decline and exploring the integrity of white matter tracts connecting cortical regions that exhibit abnormal hemodynamic responses.

The sensitivity of diffusion imaging to the fundamental pathophysiological changes that occur in a variety of disease states related to cardiovascular disease suggests its utility in multi-modal research aimed at the examination of relationships between structure and function. Over the next several years, it is expected that more studies in cardiovascular disease will be conducted using diffusion imaging because measuring diffusivity and anisotropy has the potential to distinguish between subtle types of microstructural damage in types of dementia previously conceptualized as being etiologically different. Additionally, regional analyses of white matter involvement in cardiovascular disease are likely to demonstrate differences between dementia types, which could lead to more specific classification of dementia as well as affect its treatment.

Magnetic Resonance Spectroscopy

Proton magnetic resonance spectroscopy (^{1}H MRS) is another MR modality that allows researchers and clinicians to observe changes in brain chemistry to metabolism *in vivo*. The most commonly reported brain metabolites are: (1) N-acetylaspartate (NAA), a marker of neuronal viability; (2) free choline and phosphocholine (Cho), markers of membrane metabolism and turnover; (3) creatine and phosphocreatine (Cr), markers of energy metabolism; and (4) myo-inositol (mI), an organic osmolite and possible marker of gliosis.

MRS studies of patients with CVD have reported reduced NAA/Cr and Cho/Cr ratios in the insula and the thalami of hypertensive community-dwelling elderly as compared to their normotensive counterparts.[185] These reductions were correlated with reduced performance on tests of attention-executive function. Reduced NAA levels in the frontal and parietal cortices have also been reported in patients with subcortical ischemic vascular dementia relative to healthy controls,[186] patients with subjective memory complaints,[187] and patients with Alzheimer's disease.[188] Reported decreases in the gray and white matter NAA of vascular dementia patients have been associated with white matter lesions as well as the number of lacunes.[188–189] Extensive and large white matter lesions in patients with ischemic vascular dementia have also been associated with increased Cho and lower Cr levels relative to contralateral, normal-appearing white matter.[190] Acute cerebral infarctions, on the other hand, have been associated with significantly increased lactate concentrations in addition to reduced NAA.[191–192] One study reported that spectroscopic changes, namely increased lactate, could be detected in areas of the brain where infarction subsequently occurred, suggesting that MRS may have greater sensitivity than conventional MR imaging to detect stroke risk.[193] Stroke recovery has also been studied with indications that MRS may be sensitive to stroke-related diaschisis in the cerebral hemisphere ipsilateral to the infarction.[194]

Summary and Integration

Mounting evidence suggest that the cumulative effects of chronic cardiovascular disease on brain structure and function are significant, particularly as people reach advanced age. Elderly patients with severe chronic cardiovascular disease, who have heart failure and endothelial dysfunction, develop functional impairments. Cardiovascular disease-associated brain changes appear to increase over time, and there is compelling evidence that systemic vascular factors contribute to these changes.

Relatively few of these methods have been adopted for routine clinical use, although it is likely that they will play a greater role in the future. At this time, only SPECT is widely used in clinical studies of dementia. DSC is used in clinical stroke studies, and will probably be used to an even greater extent as new drugs are tested and efforts are made to study the evolution of infarction. ASL is becoming a feasible noninvasive alternative to standard DSC. Advanced imaging methods such as DTI, MRS, and FMRI using ASL and BOLD hold promise for future efforts to evaluate patients with cardiovascular disease, particularly when combined with each other, and recent advances in analyses of more traditional structural imaging sequences (T1, T2, FLAIR) that quantify white and gray matter volumes and lesions and cortical thickness. However, much more research is needed to develop standardized methods for clinical use, to gain a full understanding of how cardiovascular disease patients respond on these tasks, and to establish normative data upon which clinical decision making can be based.

Many important questions remain. First, what is the clinical and functional significance of the neuroimaging findings that have emerged from initial studies of cardiovascular disease? Although we have observed relationships between brain response to FMRI challenges, systemic measures of vascular disease, and cognitive function, the extent to which these relationships are clinically important requires further exploration.

Second, preliminary pilot data regarding DTI and ASL findings in cardiovascular disease indicate the need for additional studies to examine the relationship between systemic vascular function and cerebral measures of perfusion and ischemia. The relationship between systemic vascular disturbance as measured by brachial artery response, intima-media thickness, cardiac output, blood pressure variability, and cerebrovascular abnormalities such as cerebral hypoperfusion is largely unknown at this point. While intuitively it would seem that cerebrovascular disease should evolve from the same pathophysiological mechanisms that cause cardiac and systemic vascular disease, there is not necessarily a one-to-one relationship between these disorders, as is apparent from the fact that not all patients with cardiovascular disease experience brain impairments. The occurrence of cerebrovascular disease and subsequent brain dysfunction seems to depend on a complex interaction between cardiac-systemic factors and cerebral hemodynamics. This interaction is only now beginning to be studied through neuroimaging methods.

Third, age-associated changes in neurocognitive function occur independently of the presence of comorbidity. Cardiovascular disease may affect the rate of decline that would be expected over time, though to date there are relatively few longitudinal data from which to model these expected change effects. Therefore, it is now difficult to factor information regarding neuroimaging abnormalities into existing knowledge regarding functional brain abnormalities associated with normal aging for clinical decision-making. Finally, despite evidence that cognitive impairments associated with cardiovascular disease correspond with structural brain abnormalities (e.g., subcortical white matter hyperintensities, reduced structural brain volumes), these relationships have not been directly linked to the cerebrovascular abnormalities evident through neuroimaging methods.

Functional brain imaging methods have great clinical potential, but they also have certain limitations. With few exceptions, these methods are not now available as routine clinical tests, nor are they reimbursed by insurance companies. Functional brain imaging requires sophisticated infrastructure and considerable expertise, including specialists to translate these methods for clinical use. Furthermore, the cost today of routinely obtaining functional brain imaging for patients with heart disease is prohibitive. Decision rules will need to be developed to achieve greater efficiency and reduce costs.

Another consideration is reliability. The fact that variability exists across scanners of the same magnetic field strength, and even across imaging sessions when the same scanner is used, complicates interpretation of data across sites. This variability is not a major problem for routine structural MRI in which signal-to-noise ratios are relatively large. In contrast, FMRI capitalizes on minor variation in BOLD signal over time (i.e., less than 10%). Variability across scanners can result in differences in signal intensity and localization.

Another standardization issue relates to the fact that adequate normative data are not available for most brain neuroimaging methods. For example, FMRI studies have employed paradigms derived from a wide range of different cognitive tasks, but for the most part have employed relatively small sample sizes. Most of these studies were not conducted with goal of developing normative data for how the brain responds during particular paradigms. With only limited efforts to date to establish normative databases, with reliability and validity data for people across different age groups, it is very difficult to interpret findings from a single patient. Statistically significant group differences in brain activity may reflect relatively subtle effects that are not readily apparent in the results from a single patient. Accordingly, before most techniques can become clinically useful, there is much standardization that needs to be accomplished for each of the functional brain imaging methods.

Additional safety measures must be implemented, and MRI is contraindicated for many patients. MRI-based methods are much safer than invasive methods that require the use of radiation, but pose problems for patients with metal implants or metal-related injuries. Also, patients who require oxygen tanks, wheelchairs, and other assistive devices require special provisions for assessment in the scanner. The issue of implants is a particularly difficult one, as increasingly pacemakers are being used to enhance ventricular function in patients with severe heart disease. Historically, it has been difficult to perform MRI imaging after pacemaker implantation because of the metal contained in the pacemakers, and also concern about the magnet's interfering with the electrical signals from the pacemakers. Some breakthroughs have occurred in the development of MRI-safe pacemaker devices.

Finally, there are limitations related to patient comfort and other practical considerations. FMRI is particularly sensitive to movement artifact. Therefore patients who cannot lie still during the exam may not yield reliable data. Patients with claustrophobia cannot be administered anxiolytic medication to help ease their response to the confined scanner space, due to confounding effects on the cognitive and emotional processes under investigation. Large patients may not fit into the scanner. For brain scans the patient's head must be located at the center of a tube typically about 55 cm in diameter.

In conclusion, several functional and structural brain imaging methods have been discussed in this chapter that have potential value for the study and clinical management of cardiovascular disease. Clinical research has been presented that demonstrates the utility of these neuroimaging methods in providing information about early brain dysfunction among patients with cardiovascular disease in the absence of stroke and dementia. These findings are very encouraging and raise the possibility that in the future these methods may provide early biomarkers of brain dysfunction secondary to heart disease. Yet this research is only in its infancy. There is a need for neuroimaging studies that combine methods such as FMRI, DTI, and MRS to characterize the interactions between the structural, functional, and metabolic disturbances over time to better understand the evolution of cognitive impairment in patients with cardiovascular disease.

Notes

1. Matthews PM, Honey GD, Bullmore ET. Applications of fMRI in translational medicine and clinical practice. *Nat Rev Neurosci.* 2006;7(9):732–744.
2. Bandettini PA, Jesmanowicz A, Wong EC, Hyde JS. Processing strategies for time-course data sets in functional MRI of the human brain. *Magn Reson Med.* 1993;30(2):161–173.
3. Binder JR, Rao SM, Hammeke TA, Yetkin FZ, Jesmanowicz A, Bandettini PA, Wong EC, Estkowski LD, Goldstein MD, Haughton VM, et al. Functional magnetic resonance imaging of human auditory cortex. *Ann Neurol.* 1994;35(6):662–672.
4. D'Esposito M, Detre JA, Alsop DC, et al. The neural basis of the central executive system of working memory. *Nature*, 1995;378:279–281.

5. Rao SM, Bobholz JA, Hammeke TA, Rosen AC, Woodley SJ, Cunningham JM, Cox RW, Stein EA, and Binder JR. Functional evidence for subcortical participation in conceptual reasoning skills. *Neuroreport*, 1997;8:1987–1993.
6. Buckner RL, Bandettini PA, O'Craven KM, Savoy RL, Petersen SE, Raichle ME, Rosen BR. Detection of cortical activation during averaged single trials of a cognitive task using functional magnetic resonance imaging. *Proc Natl Acad Sci USA*. 1996;93(25):14878–14883.
7. Zahran E, Aguire G, D'Esposito M. A trial-based experimental design for fMRI. *Neuroimage*. 1997;6:122–138.
8. Dale AM, and Buckner RL. Selective averaging of rapidly presented individual trials using fMRI. *Hum Brain Mapp*. 1997;5:329–340.
9. Josephs O, Turner R, and Friston K. Event-related fMRI. *Hum Brain Mapp*. 1997; 5:243–248.
10. Savoy RL, Bandettini PA, O'Craven KM, Kwong KK, Davis TL, Baker JR, Weisskoff RM, Rosen BR. "Pushing the temporal resolution of fMRI: Studies of very brief visual stimuli, onset variability and asynchrony, and stimulus-correlated changes in noise." Presented at the Annual Meeting of the Society of Magnetic Resonance in Nice, France, August 1995.
11. Boynton GM, Engel SA, Glover GH, Heeger DJ. Linear systems analysis of functional magnetic resonance imaging in human V1. *J Neurosci*. 1996;16(13):4207–4221.
12. Cohen JD, Perlstein WM, Braver TS, et al. Temporal dynamics of brain activation during a working memory task. *Nature*. 1997;386:604–607.
13. Wagner AD, Schacter DL, Rotte M, Koutstaal W, Maril A, Dale AM, Rosen BR, Buckner RL. Building memories: Remembering and forgetting of verbal experiences as predicted by brain activity. *Science*. 1998;281(5380):1188–1191.
14. Ogawa S, Lee TM, Nayak AS, et al. Oxygenation-sensitive contrast in magnetic resonance image of rodent brain at high magnetic fields. *Magn Reson Med*. 1990;14: 68–78.
15. Ogawa S, Tank DW, Menon R, Ellermann JM, Kim SG, Merkle H, Ugurbil K. Intrinsic signal changes accompanying sensory stimulation: Functional brain mapping with magnetic resonance imaging. *Proc Natl Acad Sci USA*. 1992;89(13):5951–5955.
16. Bandettini PA, Wong EC, Hinks RS, Tikofsky RS, Hyde JS. Time course EPI of human brain function during task activation. *Magn Reson Med*. 1992;25(2):390–397.
17. Kwong KK, Belliveau JW, Chesler DA, Goldberg I.E., Weisskoff RM, Poncelet BP, Kennedy DN, Hoppel BE, Cohen MS, Turner R, Cheng H, Brady TJ, Rosen BR. Dynamic magnetic resonance imaging of human brain activity during primary sensory stimulation. *Proc Natl Acad Sci USA*. 1992;89(12):5675–5679.
18. Ahmad Z, Balsamo LM, Sachs BC, Xu B, Gaillard WD. Auditory comprehension of language in young children: Neural networks identified with fMRI. *Neurology*. 2003;60(10):1598–1605.
19. Gaillard WD, Sachs BC, Whitnah JR, Ahmad Z, Balsamo LM, Petrella JR, Braniecki SH, McKinney CM, Hunter K, Xu B, Grandin CB. Developmental aspects of language processing: FMRI of verbal fluency in children and adults. *Hum Brain Mapp*. 2003;18(3): 176–185.
20. Gaillard WD, Balsamo LM, Ibrahim Z, Sachs BC, Xu B. fMRI identifies regional specialization of neural networks for reading in young children. *Neurology*. 2003;60(1):94–100.
21. Peterson BS, Vohr B, Kane MJ, Whalen DH, Schneider KC, Katz KH, Zhang H, Duncan CC, Makuch R, Gore JC, Ment LR.A functional magnetic resonance imaging study of language processing and its cognitive correlates in prematurely born children. *Pediatrics*. 2002;110(6):1153–1162.
22. Adleman NE, Menon V, Blasey CM, White CD, Warsofsky IS, Glover GH, Reiss AL. A developmental fMRI study of the Stroop color-word task. *Neuroimage*. 2002;16(1):61–75.

23. Bunge SA, Dudukovic NM, Thomason ME, Vaidya CJ, Gabrieli JD. Immature frontal lobe contributions to cognitive control in children: Evidence from fMRI. *Neuron*. 2002;33(2): 301–311.
24. Klingberg T, Forssberg H, Westerberg H. Increased brain activity in frontal and parietal cortex underlies the development of visuospatial working memory capacity during childhood. *J Cogn Neurosci*. 2002;14(1):1–10.
25. Holland SK, Plante E, Weber Byars A, Strawsburg RH, Schmithorst VJ, Ball WS Jr. Normal fMRI brain activation patterns in children performing a verb generation task. *Neuroimage*. 2001;14(4):837–843.
26. Gaillard WD, Pugliese M, Grandin CB, Braniecki SH, Kondapaneni P, Hunter K, Xu B, Petrella JR, Balsamo L, Basso G. Cortical localization of reading in normal children: An fMRI language study. *Neurology*. 2001;57(1):47–54.
27. Serafini S, Steury K, Richards T, Corina D, Abbott R, Dager SR, Berninger V. Comparison of fMRI and PEPSI during language processing in children. *Magn Reson Med*. 2001;45(2): 217–225.
28. Boor S, Vucurevic G, Pfleiderer C, Stoeter P, Kutschke G, Boor R. EEG-related functional MRI in benign childhood epilepsy with centrotemporal spikes. *Epilepsia*. 2003;44(5): 688–692.
29. Liegeois F, Connelly A, Salmond CH, Gadian DG, Vargha-Khadem F, Baldeweg T. A direct test for lateralization of language activation using fMRI: Comparison with invasive assessments in children with epilepsy. *Neuroimage*. 2002;17(4):1861–1867.
30. Holloway V, Gadian DG, Vargha-Khadem F, Porter DA, Boyd SG, Connelly A. The reorganization of sensorimotor function in children after hemispherectomy. A functional MRI and somatosensory evoked potential study. *Brain*. 2000;123(Pt 12):2432–2444.
31. Graveline CJ, Mikulis DJ, Crawley AP, Hwang PA. Regionalized sensorimotor plasticity after hemispherectomy fMRI evaluation. *Pediatr Neurol*. 1998;19(5):337–342.
32. Stapleton SR, Kiriakopoulos E, Mikulis D, Drake JM, Hoffman HJ, Humphreys R, Hwang P, Otsubo H, Holowka S, Logan W, Rutka JT. Combined utility of functional MRI, cortical mapping, and frameless stereotaxy in the resection of lesions in eloquent areas of brain in children. *Pediatr Neurosurg*. 1997;26(2):68–82.
33. Aylward EH, Richards TL, Berninger VW, Nagy WE, Field KM, Grimme AC, Richards AL, Thomson JB, Cramer SC. Instructional treatment associated with changes in brain activation in children with dyslexia. *Neurology*. 2003;61(2):212–219.
34. Shaywitz BA, Shaywitz SE, Pugh KR, Mencl WE, Fulbright RK, Skudlarski P, Constable RT, Marchione KE, Fletcher JM, Lyon GR, Gore JC. Disruption of posterior brain systems for reading in children with developmental dyslexia. *Biol Psychiatry*. 2002;52(2): 101–110.
35. Georgiewa P, Rzanny R, Gaser C, Gerhard UJ, Vieweg U, Freesmeyer D, Mentzel HJ, Kaiser WA, Blanz B. Phonological processing in dyslexic children: A study combining functional imaging and event-related potentials. *Neurosci Lett*. 2002;318(1):5–8.
36. Seki A, Koeda T, Sugihara S, Kamba M, Hirata Y, Ogawa T, Takeshita K. A functional magnetic resonance imaging study during sentence reading in Japanese dyslexic children. *Brain Dev*. 2001;23(5):312–316.
37. Corina DP, Richards TL, Serafini S, Richards AL, Steury K, Abbott RD, Echelard DR, Maravilla KR, Berninger VW. fMRI auditory language differences between dyslexic and able reading children. *Neuroreport*. 2001;12(6):1195–1201.
38. Temple E, Poldrack RA, Salidis J, Deutsch GK, Tallal P, Merzenich MM, Gabrieli JD. Disrupted neural responses to phonological and orthographic processing in dyslexic children: An fMRI study. *Neuroreport*. 2001;12(2):299–307.

39. Georgiewa P, Rzanny R, Hopf JM, Knab R, Glauche V, Kaiser WA, Blanz B. fMRI during word processing in dyslexic and normal reading children. *Neuroreport*. 1999;10(16):3459–3465.
40. Levin HS, Scheller J, Rickard T, Grafman J, Martinkowski K, Winslow M, Mirvis S. Dyscalculia and dyslexia after right hemisphere injury in infancy. *Arch Neurol*. 1996;53(1):88–96.
41. Durston S, Tottenham NT, Thomas KM, Davidson MC, Eigsti IM, Yang Y, Ulug AM, Casey BJ. Differential patterns of striatal activation in young children with and without ADHD. *Biol Psychiatry*. 2003;53(10):871–878.
42. Anderson CM, Polcari A, Lowen SB, Renshaw PF, Teicher MH. Effects of methylphenidate on functional magnetic resonance relaxometry of the cerebellar vermis in boys with ADHD. *Am J Psychiatry*. 2002;159(8):1322–1328.
43. Bush G, Frazier JA, Rauch SL, Seidman LJ, Whalen PJ, Jenike MA, Rosen BR, Biederman J. Anterior cingulate cortex dysfunction in attention-deficit/hyperactivity disorder revealed by fMRI and the Counting Stroop. *Biol Psychiatry*. 1999;45(12):1542–1552.
44. Lee JH, Telang FW, Springer CS Jr, Volkow ND. Abnormal brain activation to visual stimulation in cocaine abusers. *Life Sci*. 2003;73(15):1953–1961.
45. Wexler BE, Gottschalk CH, Fulbright RK, Prohovnik I, Lacadie CM, Rounsaville BJ, Gore JC. Functional magnetic resonance imaging of cocaine craving. *Am J Psychiatry*. 2001;158(1):86–95.
46. Li SJ, Biswal B, Li Z, Risinger R, Rainey C, Cho JK, Salmeron BJ, Stein EA. Cocaine administration decreases functional connectivity in human primary visual and motor cortex as detected by functional MRI. *Magn Reson Med*. 2000;43(1):45–51.
47. Gollub RL, Breiter HC, Kantor H, Kennedy D, Gastfriend D, Mathew RT, Makris N, Guimaraes A, Riorden J, Campbell T, Foley M, Hyman SE, Rosen B, Weisskoff R. Cocaine decreases cortical cerebral blood flow but does not obscure regional activation in functional magnetic resonance imaging in human subjects. *J Cereb Blood Flow Metab*. 1998;18(7):724–734.
48. Breiter HC, Gollub RL, Weisskoff RM, Kennedy DN, Makris N, Berke JD, Goodman JM, Kantor HL, Gastfriend DR, Riorden JP, Mathew RT, Rosen BR, Hyman SE. Acute effects of cocaine on human brain activity and emotion. *Neuron*. 1997;19(3):591–611.
49. Kumari V, Gray JA, Ffytche DH, Mitterschiffthaler MT, Das M, Zachariah E, Vythelingum GN, Williams SC, Simmons A, Sharma T. Cognitive effects of nicotine in humans: An fMRI study. *Neuroimage*. 2003;19(3):1002–1013.
50. Due DL, Huettel SA, Hall WG, Rubin DC. Activation in mesolimbic and visuospatial neural circuits elicited by smoking cues: Evidence from functional magnetic resonance imaging. *Am J Psychiatry*. 2002;159(6):954–960.
51. Jacobsen LK, Gore JC, Skudlarski P, Lacadie CM, Jatlow P, Krystal JH. Impact of intravenous nicotine on BOLD signal response to photic stimulation. *Magn Reson Imaging*. 2002;20(2):141–145.
52. Bloom AS, Hoffmann RG, Fuller SA, Pankiewicz J, Harsch HH, Stein EA. Determination of drug-induced changes in functional MRI signal using a pharmacokinetic model. *Hum Brain Mapp*. 1999;8(4):235–244.
53. Parks MH, Morgan VL, Pickens DR, Price RR, Dietrich MS, Nickel MK, Martin PR. Brain FMRI activation associated with self-paced finger tapping in chronic alcohol-dependent patients. *Alcohol Clin Exp Res*. 2003;27(4):704–711.
54. Wrase J, Grusser SM, Klein S, Diener C, Hermann D, Flor H, Mann K, Braus DF, Heinz A. Development of alcohol-associated cues and cue-induced brain activation in alcoholics. *Eur Psychiatry*. 2002;17(5):287–291.

55. Schneider F, Habel U, Wagner M, Franke P, Salloum JB, Shah NJ, Toni I, Sulzbach C, Honig K, Maier W, Gaebel W, Zilles K. Subcortical correlates of craving in recently abstinent alcoholic patients. *Am J Psychiatry*. 2001;158(7):1075–1083.
56. George MS, Anton RF, Bloomer C, Teneback C, Drobes DJ, Lorberbaum JP, Nahas Z, Vincent DJ. Activation of prefrontal cortex and anterior thalamus in alcoholic subjects on exposure to alcohol-specific cues. *Arch Gen Psychiatry*. 2001;58(4):345–352.
57. Tapert SF, Brown GG, Kindermann SS, Cheung EH, Frank LR, Brown SA. fMRI measurement of brain dysfunction in alcohol-dependent young women. *Alcohol Clin Exp Res*. 2001;25(2):236–245.
58. Levin JM, Ross MH, Mendelson JH, Kaufman MJ, Lange N, Maas LC, Mello NK, Cohen BM, Renshaw PF. Reduction in BOLD fMRI response to primary visual stimulation following alcohol ingestion. *Psychiatry Res*. 1998;82(3):135–146.
59. Paquette V, Levesque J, Mensour B, Leroux JM, Beaudoin G, Bourgouin P, Beauregard M. "Change the mind and you change the brain": Effects of cognitive-behavioral therapy on the neural correlates of spider phobia. *Neuroimage*. 2003;18(2):401–409.
60. Schneider F, Weiss U, Kessler C, Muller-Gartner HW, Posse S, Salloum JB, Grodd W, Himmelmann F, Gaebel W, Birbaumer N. Subcortical correlates of differential classical conditioning of aversive emotional reactions in social phobia. *Biol Psychiatry*. 1999;45(7): 863–871.
61. Birbaumer N, Grodd W, Diedrich O, Klose U, Erb M, Lotze M, Schneider F, Weiss U, Flor H. fMRI reveals amygdala activation to human faces in social phobics. *Neuroreport*. 1998;9(6):1223–1226.
62. Adler CM, McDonough-Ryan P, Sax KW, Holland SK, Arndt S, Strakowski SM. fMRI of neuronal activation with symptom provocation in unmedicated patients with obsessive compulsive disorder. *J Psychiatr Res*. 2000;34(4–5):317–324.
63. Levine JB, Gruber SA, Baird AA, Yurgelun-Todd D. Obsessive-compulsive disorder among schizophrenic patients: An exploratory study using functional magnetic resonance imaging data. *Compr Psychiatry*. 1998;39(5):308–311.
64. Schlosser R, Gesierich T, Kaufmann B, Vucurevic G, Hunsche S, Gawehn J, Stoeter P. Altered effective connectivity during working memory performance in schizophrenia: A study with fMRI and structural equation modeling. *Neuroimage*. 2003;19(3):751–763.
65. Jessen F, Scheef L, Germeshausen L, Tawo Y, Kockler M, Kuhn KU, Maier W, Schild HH, Heun R. Reduced hippocampal activation during encoding and recognition of words in schizophrenia patients. *Am J Psychiatry*. 2003;160(7):1305–1312.
66. Walter H, Wunderlich AP, Blankenhorn M, Schafer S, Tomczak R, Spitzer M, Gron G. No hypofrontality, but absence of prefrontal lateralization comparing verbal and spatial working memory in schizophrenia. *Schizophr Res*. 2003;61(2–3):175–184.
67. Hofer A, Weiss EM, Golaszewski SM, Siedentopf CM, Brinkhoff C, Kremser C, Felber S, Fleischhacker WW. An FMRI study of episodic encoding and recognition of words in patients with schizophrenia in remission. *Am J Psychiatry*. 2003;160(5):911–918.
68. Lawrie SM, Whalley HC, Job DE, Johnstone EC. Structural and functional abnormalities of the amygdala in schizophrenia. *Ann N Y Acad Sci*. 2003;985:445–460.
69. Schroder J, Wenz F, Schad LR, Baudendistel K, Knopp MV. Sensorimotor cortex and supplementary motor area changes in schizophrenia. A study with functional magnetic resonance imaging. *Br J Psychiatry*. 1995;167(2):197–201.
70. Volz HP, Gaser C, Hager F, Rzanny R, Mentzel HJ, Kreitschmann-Andermahr I, Kaiser WA, Sauer H. Brain activation during cognitive stimulation with the Wisconsin Card Sorting Test—A functional MRI study on healthy volunteers and schizophrenics. *Psychiatry Res*. 1997;75(3):145–157.

71. Callicott JH, Ramsey NF, Tallent K, Bertolino A, Knable MB, Coppola R, Goldberg T, van Gelderen P, Mattay VS, Frank JA, Moonen CT, Weinberger DR. Functional magnetic resonance imaging brain mapping in psychiatry: Methodological issues illustrated in a study of working memory in schizophrenia. *Neuropsychopharmacology*. 1998;18(3):186–196.
72. Schneider F, Habel U, Kessler C, Posse S, Grodd W, Muller-Gartner HW. Functional imaging of conditioned aversive emotional responses in antisocial personality disorder. *Neuropsychobiology*. 2000;42(4):192–201.
73. Sweet L, Rao S, Primeau P, Mayer A, and Cohen R. Functional magnetic resonance imaging of working memory among multiple sclerosis patients. *J Neuroimaging*. 2004;14(2): 150–157.
74. Sweet L, Rao S, Primeau P, Durgerian S, and Cohen R. FMRI response to increased verbal working memory demands among patients with multiple sclerosis. *Hum Brain Mapp*. 2006;27(1):28–36.
75. Penner IK, Rausch M, Kappos L, Opwis K, Radu EW. Analysis of impairment-related functional architecture in MS patients during performance of different attention tasks. *J Neurol*. 2003;250(4):461–472.
76. Staffen W, Mair A, Zauner H, Unterrainer J, Niederhofer H, Kutzelnigg A, Ritter S, Golaszewski S, Iglseder B, Ladurner G. Cognitive function and fMRI in patients with multiple sclerosis: Evidence for compensatory cortical activation during an attention task. *Brain*. 2002;125(Pt 6):1275–1282.
77. Lewis SJ, Dove A, Robbins TW, Barker RA, Owen AM. Cognitive impairments in early Parkinson's disease are accompanied by reductions in activity in frontostriatal neural circuitry. *J Neurosci*. 2003;23(15):6351–6356.
78. Peters S, Suchan B, Rusin J, Daum I, Koster O, Przuntek H, Muller T, Schmid G. Apomorphine reduces BOLD signal in fMRI during voluntary movement in Parkinsonian patients. *Neuroreport*. 2003;14(6):809–812.
79. Werheid K, Zysset S, Muller A, Reuter M, von Cramon DY. Rule learning in a serial reaction time task: An fMRI study on patients with early Parkinson's disease. *Brain Res Cogn Brain Res*. 2003;16(2):273–284.
80. Grossman M, Cooke A, DeVita C, Lee C, Alsop D, Detre J, Gee J, Chen W, Stern MB, Hurtig HI. Grammatical and resource components of sentence processing in Parkinson's disease: An fMRI study. *Neurology*. 2003;60(5):775–781.
81. Rowe J, Stephan KE, Friston K, Frackowiak R, Lees A, Passingham R. Attention to action in Parkinson's disease: Impaired effective connectivity among frontal cortical regions. *Brain*. 2002;125(Pt 2):276–289.
82. Jech R, Urgosik D, Tintera J, Nebuzelsky A, Krasensky J, Liscak R, Roth J, Ruzicka E. Functional magnetic resonance imaging during deep brain stimulation: A pilot study in four patients with Parkinson's disease. *Mov Disord*. 2001;16(6):1126–1132.
83. Haslinger B, Erhard P, Kampfe N, Boecker H, Rummeny E, Schwaiger M, Conrad B, Ceballos-Baumann AO. Event-related functional magnetic resonance imaging in Parkinson's disease before and after levodopa. *Brain*. 2001;124(Pt 3):558–570.
84. Sabatini U, Boulanouar K, Fabre N, Martin F, Carel C, Colonnese C, Bozzao L, Berry I, Montastruc JL, Chollet F, Rascol O. Cortical motor reorganization in akinetic patients with Parkinson's disease: A functional MRI study. *Brain*. 2000;123(Pt 2):394–403.
85. Kato T, Knopman D, Liu H. Dissociation of regional activation in mild AD during visual encoding: A functional MRI study. *Neurology*. 2001;57(5):812–816.
86. Small SA, Nava AS, Perera GM, Delapaz R, Stern Y. Evaluating the function of hippocampal subregions with high-resolution MRI in Alzheimer's disease and aging. *Microsc Res Tech*. 2000;51(1):101–108.

87. Sperling RA, Bates JF, Chua EF, Cocchiarella AJ, Rentz DM, Rosen BR, Schacter DL, Albert MS. fMRI studies of associative encoding in young and elderly controls and mild Alzheimer's disease. *J Neurol Neurosurg Psychiatry*. 2003;74(1):44–50.
88. Prvulovic D, Hubl D, Sack AT, Melillo L, Maurer K, Frolich L, Lanfermann H, Zanella FE, Goebel R, Linden DE, Dierks T. Functional imaging of visuospatial processing in Alzheimer's disease. *Neuroimage*. 2002;17(3):1403–1414.
89. Johnson SC, Saykin AJ, Baxter LC, Flashman LA, Santulli RB, McAllister TW, Mamourian AC. The relationship between fMRI activation and cerebral atrophy: Comparison of normal aging and Alzheimer disease. *Neuroimage*. 2000;11(3):179–187.
90. Haley AP, Sweet LH, Gunstad J, Forman DE, Poppas A, Paul RH, Tate DF, Cohen RA. Verbal working memory and atherosclerosis in patients with cardiovascular disease: An fMRI study. *J Neuroimaging* 2007;17:227–233.
91. Cao Y, Vikingstad EM, George KP, Johnson AF, Welch KM. Cortical language activation in stroke patients recovering from aphasia with functional MRI. *Stroke*. 1999;30(11): 2331–2340.
92. Zahn R, Huber W, Drews E, Specht K, Kemeny S, Reith W, Willmes K, Schwarz M. Recovery of semantic word processing in transcortical sensory aphasia: A functional magnetic resonance imaging study. *Neurocase*. 2002;8(5):376–386.
93. Johansen-Berg H, Rushworth MF, Bogdanovic MD, Kischka U, Wimalaratna S, Matthews PM. The role of ipsilateral premotor cortex in hand movement after stroke. *Proc Natl Acad Sci USA*. 2002;99(22):14518–23.
94. Marshall RS, Perera GM, Lazar RM, Krakauer JW, Constantine RC, De La Paz RL. Evolution of cortical activation during recovery from corticospinal tract infarction. *Stroke*. 2000;31(3):656–661.
95. Pariente J, Loubinoux I, Carel C, Albucher JF, Leger A, Manelfe C, Rascol O, Chollet F. Fluoxetine modulates motor performance and cerebral activation of patients recovering from stroke. *Ann Neurol*. 2001;50(6):718–729.
96. Feydy A, Carlier R, Roby-Brami A, Bussel B, Cazalis F, Pierot L, Burnod Y, Maier MA. Longitudinal study of motor recovery after stroke: Recruitment and focusing of brain activation. *Stroke*. 2002;33(6):1610–1617.
97. Ozdoba C, Nirkko AC, Remonda L, Lovblad KO, Schroth G. Whole-brain functional magnetic resonance imaging of cerebral arteriovenous malformations involving the motor pathways. *Neuroradiology*. 2002;44(1):1–10.
98. Lazar RM, Marshall RS, Pile-Spellman J, Duong HC, Mohr JP, Young WL, Solomon RL, Perera GM, De La Paz RL. Interhemispheric transfer of language in patients with left frontal cerebral arteriovenous malformation. *Neuropsychologia*. 2000;38(10):1325–1332.
99. Cao Y, Aurora SK, Nagesh V, Patel SC, Welch KM. Functional MRI-BOLD of brainstem structures during visually triggered migraine. *Neurology*. 2002;59(1):72–78.
100. Smith M, Cros D, Sheen V. Hyperperfusion with vasogenic leakage by fMRI in migraine with prolonged aura. *Neurology*. 2002;58(8):1308–1310.
101. Reddy H, De Stefano N, Mortilla M, Federico A, Matthews PM. Functional reorganization of motor cortex increases with greater axonal injury from CADASIL. *Stroke*. 2002;33(2): 502–508.
102. Haley AP, Gunstad J, Cohen RA, Jerskey BA, Mulligan R, Sweet LH. Neural correlates of visuospatial working memory in healthy young adults at risk for hypertension. *Brain Imag Behav* 2008;2:192–199.
103. Bookheimer SY, Strojwas MH, Cohen MS, Saunders AM, Pericak-Vance MA, Mazziotta JC, Small GW. Patterns of brain activation in people at risk for Alzheimer's disease. *N Engl J Med*. 2000;343:450–456.

104. Fleisher AS, Podraza KM, Bangen KJ, Taylor C, Sherzai A, Sidhar K, Liu TT, Dale AM, Buxton RB. Cerebral perfusion and oxygenation differences in Alzheimer's disease risk. *Neurobiology of Aging*, in press.
105. Baddeley A. *Human memory*. Neddham Heights, MA: Allyn & Bacon, 1998.
106. Haley AP, Forman DE, Poppas A, Hoth KF, Gunstad J, Jefferson AL, Paul RH, Ler AS, Sweet LH, Cohen RA. Carotid artery intima-media thickness and cognition in cardiovascular disease. *Int J Cardiol*. 2007;121:148–154.
107. Smith EE, Jonides J. Working memory: A view from neuroimaging. *Cognit. Psychol.* 1997;33:5–42.
108. Chang L, Speck O, Miller EN, Braun J, Jovicich J, Koch C, Itti L, Ernst T. Neural correlates of attention and working memory deficits in HIV patients. *Neurology*. 2001;57:1001–1007.
109. Binder JR, Frost JA, Hammeke TA, Bellgowan PS, Rao SM, Cox RW. Conceptual processing during the conscious resting state. A functional MRI study. *J. Cogn Neurosci.* 1999;11:80–95.
110. Mazoyer B, Zago L, Mellet E, Bricogne S, Etard O, Houde O, Crivello F, Joliot M, Petit L, Tzourio-Mazoyer N. Cortical networks for working memory and executive functions sustain the conscious resting state in man. *Brain Res. Bull.* 2001;54:287–298.
111. Shulman GL, Fiez JA, Corbetta M, Buckner RL, Miezin FM, Raichle ME, Petersen SE. Common blood flow changes across visual tasks. 2. Decreases in cerebral cortex. *J Cogn Neurosci* 1997;9:648–663.
112. Greicius MD, Menon V. Default-mode activity during a passive sensory task: Uncoupled from deactivation but impacting activation. *J Cogn Neurosci*. 2004;16:1484–1492.
113. McKiernan KA, Kaufman JN, Kucera-Thompson J, Binder JR. A parametric manipulation of factors affecting task-induced deactivation in functional neuroimaging. *J Cogn Neurosci*. 2003;15:394–408.
114. Sweet LH, Paskavitz JF, Haley AP, Gunstad JJ, Mulligan RC, Nyalakanti PK, Cohen RA. Imaging phonological similarity effects on verbal working memory. *Neuropsychologia*. 2008;46(4):1114–1123. Epub, 2007 Nov. 9.
115. Hahn B, Ross TJ, Yang YH, Kim I, Huestis MA, Stein EA. Nicotine enhances visuospatial attention by deactivating areas of the resting brain default network. *J Neurosci*. 2007;27:3477–3489.
116. Stebbins GT, Carrillo MC, Dorfman J, Dirksen C, Desmond JE, Turner DA, Bennett DA, Wilson RS, Glover G, Gabrieli JD. Aging effects on memory encoding in the frontal lobes. *Psychol Aging*. 2002;17(1):44–55.
117. Rosen AC, Prull MW, O'Hara R, Race EA, Desmond JE, Glover GH, Yesavage JA, Gabrieli JD. Variable effects of aging on frontal lobe contributions to memory. *Neuroreport*. 2002;13(18):2425–2428.
118. Morcom AM, Good CD, Frackowiak RS, Rugg MD. Age effects on the neural correlates of successful memory encoding. *Brain*. 2003;126(Pt 1):213–229.
119. Cabeza R, Anderson ND, Locantore JK, McIntosh AR. Aging gracefully: Compensatory brain activity in high-performing older adults. *Neuroimage*. 2002;17(3):1394–1402.
120. Cabeza R. Cognitive neuroscience of aging: Contributions of functional neuroimaging. *Scand J Psychol*. 2001;42(3):277–286.
121. Mencl WE, Pugh KR, Shaywitz SE, Shaywitz BA, Fulbright RK, Constable RT, Skudlarski P, Katz L, Marchione KE, Lacadie C, Gore JC. Network analysis of brain activations in working memory: Behavior and age relationships. *Microsc Res Tech*. 2000;51(1):64–74.

122. Grossman M, Cooke A, DeVita C, Alsop D, Detre J, Chen W, Gee J. Age-related changes in working memory during sentence comprehension: An fMRI study. *Neuroimage.* 2002;15(2):302–317.
123. Riecker A, Grodd W, Klose U, Schulz JB, Groschel K, Erb M, Ackermann H, Kastrup A. Relation between regional functional MRI activation and vascular reactivity to carbon dioxide during normal aging. *J Cereb Blood Flow Metab.* 2003;23(5):565-D73.
124. Hesselmann V, Zaro Weber O, Wedekind C, Krings T, Schulte O, Kugel H, Krug B, Klug N, Lackner KJ. Age-related signal decrease in functional magnetic resonance imaging during motor stimulation in humans. *Neurosci Lett.* 2001;308(3):141–144.
125. Hutchinson S, Kobayashi M, Horkan CM, Pascual-Leone A, Alexander MP, Schlaug G. Age-related differences in movement representation. *Neuroimage.* 2002;17(4):1720–1728.
126. Huettel SA, Singerman JD, McCarthy G. The effects of aging upon the hemodynamic response measured by functional MRI. *Neuroimage.* 2001;13(1):161–175.
127. Suzuki Y, Critchley HD, Suckling J, Fukuda R, Williams SC, Andrew C, Howard R, Ouldred E, Bryant C, Swift CG, Jackson SH. Functional magnetic resonance imaging of odor identification: The effect of aging. *J Gerontol A Biol Sci Med Sci.* 2001;56(12):M756–M760.
128. Ross MH, Yurgelun-Todd DA, Renshaw PF, Maas LC, Mendelson JH, Mello NK, Cohen BM, Levin JM. Age-related reduction in functional MRI response to photic stimulation. *Neurology.* 1997;48(1):173–176.
129. Gunning-Dixon FM, Gur RC, Perkins AC, Schroeder L, Turner T, Turetsky BI, Chan RM, Loughead JW, Alsop DC, Maldjian J, Gur RE. Age-related differences in brain activation during emotional face processing. *Neurobiol Aging.* 2003;24(2):285–295.
130. Lidaka T, Sadato N, Yamada H, Murata T, Omori M, Yonekura Y. An fMRI study of the functional neuroanatomy of picture encoding in younger and older adults. *Brain Res Cogn Brain Res.* 2001;11(1):1–11.
131. DiGirolamo GJ, Kramer AF, Barad V, Cepeda NJ, Weissman DH, Milham MP, Wszalek TM, Cohen NJ, Banich MT, Webb A, Belopolsky AV, McAuley E. General and task-specific frontal lobe recruitment in older adults during executive processes: A fMRI investigation of task-switching. *Neuroreport.* 2001;12(9):2065–2071.
132. Nielson KA, Langenecker SA, Garavan H. Differences in the functional neuroanatomy of inhibitory control across the adult life span. *Psychol Aging.* 2002;17(1):56–71.
133. Milham MP, Erickson KI, Banich MT, Kramer AF, Webb A, Wszalek T, Cohen NJ. Attentional control in the aging brain: Insights from an fMRI study of the Stroop task. *Brain Cogn.* 2002;49(3):277–296.
134. Taoka T, Iwasaki S, Uchida H, Fukusumi A, Nakagawa H, Kichikawa K, Takayama K, Yoshioka T, Takewa M, Ohishi H. Age correlation of the time lag in signal change on EPI-fMRI. *J Comput Assist Tomogr.* 1998;22(4):514–517.
135. D'Esposito M, Zarahn E, Aguirre GK, Rypma B. The effect of normal aging on the coupling of neural activity to the bold hemodynamic response. *Neuroimage.* 1999;10(1):6–14.
136. Mehagnoul-Schipper DJ, van der Kallen BF, Colier WN, van der Sluijs MC, van Erning LJ, Thijssen HO, Oeseburg B, Hoefnagels WH, Jansen RW. Simultaneous measurements of cerebral oxygenation changes during brain activation by near-infrared spectroscopy and functional magnetic resonance imaging in healthy young and elderly subjects. *Hum Brain Mapp.* 2002;16(1):14–23.
137. Hock C, Müller-Spahn F, Schuh-Hofer S, et al. Age dependency of changes in cerebral hemoglobin oxygenation during brain activation: A near-infrared spectroscopy study. *J Cereb Blood Flow Metab.* 1995;15(6):1103–1108.
138. Buxton RB, Frank LR. A model for the coupling between cerebral blood flow and oxygen metabolism during neural stimulation. *J Cereb Blood Flow Metab.* 1997;17(1):64–72.

139. Schriger DL, Barav LJ. Defining normal capillary refill: Variation with age, sex and temperature. *Ann Emerg Med* 1988;17:932–935.
140. Menon RS, Ogowa S, Hu X, Strupp JP, Anderson P, and Ugurbil K. BOLD based functional MRI at 4 Tesla includes a capillary bed contribution. *Magn Reson Med*, 1995;33(3): 453–445.
141. Garavan H, Fassbender C, Murphy K, Sweet L, Rao S, and Stein E, Quantitative age-related differences in functional recruitment in a working memory task. *Neuroimage.* 2001;13(6):S404.
142. Detre J, Zhang W, Roberts D, Silva A, Williams DS, Grandis DJ, et al. Tissue specific perfusion imaging using arterial spin labeling. *NMR Biomed.* 1994;7:75–82.
143. Wong EC, Luh WM, Liu TT. Turbo ASL: Arterial spin labeling with higher SNR and temporal resolution. *Magn Reson Med.* 2000;44(4):511–515.
144. Wong EC, Buxton RB, Frank LR. Quantitative perfusion imaging using arterial spin labeling. *Neuroimaging Clin N Am.* May 1999;9(2):333–342.
145. Wong E, Buxton RB, Frank LR. Quantitative imaging of perfusion using a single subtraction (QUIPSS and QUIPSSII). *Magn Reson Med.* 1998;39:702–708.
146. Luh WM, Wong EC, Bandettini PA, Hyde JS. QUIPSS II with thin-slice TI1 periodic saturation: A method for improving accuracy of quantitative perfusion imaging using pulsed arterial spin labeling. *Magn Reson Med.* 1999;41(6):1246–1254.
147. Wong EC, Buxton RB, Frank LR. Implementation of quantitative perfusion imaging techniques for functional brain mapping using pulsed arterial spin labeling. *NMR Biomed.* 1997;10(4–5):237–249.
148. Garnett MR, Blamire AM, Corkill RG, Rajagopalan B, Young JD, Cadoux-Hudson TA, Styles P. Abnormal cerebral blood volume in regions of contused and normal-appearing brain following traumatic brain injury using perfusion magnetic resonance imaging. *J Neurotrauma.* 2001;18(6):585–593.
149. Wityk RJ, Goldsborough MA, Hillis A, Beauchamp N, Barker PB, Borowicz LM Jr, McKhann GM. Diffusion- and perfusion-weighted brain magnetic resonance imaging in patients with neurological complications after cardiac surgery. *Arch Neurol.* 2001;58(4):571–576.
150. Restrepo L, Wityk RJ, Grega MA, Borowicz L Jr, Barker PB, Jacobs MA, Beauchamp NJ, Hillis AE, McKhann GM. Diffusion- and perfusion-weighted magnetic resonance imaging of the brain before and after coronary artery bypass grafting surgery. *Stroke.* 2002;33(12):2909–2915.
151. Wolf RL, Alsop DC, Levy-Reis I, Meyer PT, Maldjian JA, Gonzalez-Atavales J, French JA, Alavi A, Detre JA. Detection of mesial temporal lobe hypoperfusion in patients with temporal lobe epilepsy by use of arterial spin labeled perfusion MR imaging. *Am J Neuroradiol.* 2001;22(7):1334–1341.
152. Kidwell CS, Saver JL, Mattiello J, Starkman S, Vinuela F, Duckwiler G, Gobin YP, Jahan R, Vespa P, Kalafut M, Alger JR. Thrombolytic reversal of acute human cerebral ischemic injury shown by diffusion/perfusion magnetic resonance imaging. *Ann Neurol.* 2000;47(4):462–469.
153. Singer OC, de Rochemont Rdu M, Foerch C, Stengel A, Lanfermann H, Sitzer M, Neumann-Haefelin T. Relation between relative cerebral blood flow, relative cerebral blood volume, and mean transit time in patients with acute ischemic stroke determined by perfusion-weighted MRI. *J Cereb Blood Flow Metab.* 2003;23(5):605–611.
154. Zhu M, Dai J, Li S. Cerebral angiography and MR perfusion images in patients with ischemic cerebral vascular disease. *Chin Med J (Engl).* 2002;115(11):1687–1691.

155. Schaefer PW, Romero JM, Grant PE, Wu O, Sorensen AG, Koroshetz W, Gonzalez RG. Perfusion magnetic resonance imaging of acute ischemic stroke. *Semin Roentgenol.* 2002;37(3):230–236.
156. Flacke S, Urbach H, Folkers PJ, Keller E, van den Brink JS, Traber F, Block W, Gieseke J, Schild HH. Ultra-fast three-dimensional MR perfusion imaging of the entire brain in acute stroke assessment. *J Magn Reson Imag.* 2000;11(3):250–259.
157. Rordorf G, Koroshetz WJ, Copen WA, Cramer SC, Schaefer PW, Budzik RF Jr, Schwamm LH, Buonanno F, Sorensen AG, Gonzalez G. Regional ischemia and ischemic injury in patients with acute middle cerebral artery stroke as defined by early diffusion-weighted and perfusion-weighted MRI. *Stroke.* 1998;29(5):939–943.
158. Arenillas JF, Rovira A, Molina CA, Grive E, Montaner J, Alvarez-Sabin J. Prediction of early neurological deterioration using diffusion- and perfusion-weighted imaging in hyperacute middle cerebral artery ischemic stroke. *Stroke.* 2002;33(9):2197–2203.
159. Sorensen AG, Copen WA, Ostergaard L, et al. Hyperacute stroke: Simultaneous measurement of relative cerebral blood volume, relative cerebral blood flow, and mean tissue transit time. *Radiology.* 1999;210:519–527.
160. Beaulieu C, de Crespigny A, Tong DC, et al. Longitudinal magnetic resonance imaging study of perfusion and diffusion in stroke: Evolution of lesion volume and correlation with clinical outcome. *Ann Neurol.* 1999;46:568–578.
161. Parsons MW, Yang Q, Barber PA, Darby DG, Desmond PM, Gerraty RP, Tress BM, Davis SM. Perfusion magnetic resonance imaging maps in hyperacute stroke: Relative cerebral blood flow most accurately identifies tissue destined to infarct. *Stroke.* 2001;32(7):1581–1587.
162. Wu O, Koroshetz WJ, Ostergaard L, Buonanno FS, Copen WA, Gonzalez RG, Rordorf G, Rosen BR, Schwamm LH, Weisskoff RM, Sorensen AG. Predicting tissue outcome in acute human cerebral ischemia using combined diffusion- and perfusion-weighted MR imaging. *Stroke.* 2001;32(4):933–942.
163. Uno M, Harada M, Yoneda K, Matsubara S, Satoh K, Nagahiro S. Can diffusion- and perfusion-weighted magnetic resonance imaging evaluate the efficacy of acute thrombolysis in patients with internal carotid artery or middle cerebral artery occlusion? *Neurosurgery.* 2002;50(1):28–34;discussion, 34–5.
164. Baird AE, Benfield A, Schlaug G, et al. Enlargement of human cerebral ischemic lesion volumes measured by diffusion-weighted magnetic resonance imaging. *Ann Neurol.* 1997;41:581–589.
165. Barber PA, Darby DG, Desmond PM, et al. Prediction of stroke outcome with echoplanar perfusion- and diffusion-weighted MRI. *Neurology.* 1998;51:418–426.
166. Neumann-Haefelin T, Wittsack HJ, Wenserski F, et al. Diffusion- and perfusion-weighted MRI: The DWI/PWI mismatch region in acute stroke. *Stroke.* 1999;30:1591–1597.
167. Karonen JO, Vanninen RL, Liu Y, et al. Combined diffusion and perfusion MRI with correlation to single-photon emission CT in acute ischemic stroke: Ischemic penumbra predicts infarct growth. *Stroke.* 1999;30:1583–1590.
168. Rordorf G, Koroshetz WJ, Copen WA, et al. Diffusion- and perfusion-weighted imaging in vasospasm after subarachnoid hemorrhage. *Stroke.* 1999;30:599–605.
169. Kajimoto K, Moriwaki H, Yamada N, Hayashida K, Kobayashi J, Miyashita K, Naritomi H. Cerebral hemodynamic evaluation using perfusion-weighted magnetic resonance imaging: Comparison with positron emission tomography values in chronic occlusive carotid disease. *Stroke.* 2003;34(7):1662–1666. Epub, 2003 Jun. 05.
170. van Osch MJ, Rutgers DR, Vonken EP, van Huffelen AC, Klijn CJ, Bakker CJ, van der Grond J. Quantitative cerebral perfusion MRI and CO_2 reactivity measurements in patients with symptomatic internal carotid artery occlusion. *Neuroimage.* 2002;17(1):469–478.

171. Kim JH, Lee EJ, Lee SJ, Choi NC, Lim BH, Shin T. Reliability of perfusion MR imaging in symptomatic carotid occlusive disease. Cerebral blood volume, mean transit time and time-to-peak. *Acta Radiol.* 2002;43(4):360–364.
172. Kikuchi K, Murase K, Miki H, Kikuchi T, Sugawara Y, Mochizuki T, Ikezoe J, Ohue S. Measurement of cerebral hemodynamics with perfusion-weighted MR imaging: Comparison with pre- and post-acetazolamide 133Xe-SPECT in occlusive carotid disease. *Am J Neuroradiol.* 2001;22(2):248–254.
173. Caramia F, Santoro A, Pantano P, Passacantilli E, Guidetti G, Pierallini A, Fantozzi LM, Cantore GP, Bozzao L. Cerebral hemodynamics on MR perfusion images before and after bypass surgery in patients with giant intracranial aneurysms. *Am J Neuroradiol.* 2001;22(9):1704–1710.
174. Markus HS, Lythgoe DJ, Ostegaard L, O'Sullivan M, Williams SC. Reduced cerebral blood flow in white matter in ischaemic leukoaraiosis demonstrated using quantitative exogenous contrast based perfusion MRI. *J Neurol Neurosurg Psychiatry.* 2000;69(1):48–53.
175. Maas LC, Harris GJ, Satlin A, English CD, Lewis RF, Renshaw PF. Regional cerebral blood volume measured by dynamic susceptibility contrast MR imaging in Alzheimer's disease: A principal components analysis. *J Magn Reson Imaging.* 1997;7(1):215–219.
176. Harris GJ, Lewis RF, Satlin A, English CD, Scott TM, Yurgelun-Todd DA, Renshaw PF. Dynamic susceptibility contrast MRI of regional cerebral blood volume in Alzheimer's disease. *Am J Psychiatry.* 1996;153(5):721–724.
177. Harris GJ, Lewis RF, Satlin A, English CD, Scott TM, Yurgelun-Todd DA, Renshaw PF. Dynamic susceptibility contrast MR imaging of regional cerebral blood volume in Alzheimer disease: A promising alternative to nuclear medicine. *Am J Neuroradiol.* 1998;19(9): 1727–1732.
178. Alsop DC, Detre JA, Grossman M. Assessment of cerebral blood flow in Alzheimer's disease by spin-labeled magnetic resonance imaging. *Ann Neurol.* 2000;47(1):93–100.
179. Bangen KJ, Restom K, Liu TT, Jak AJ, Wierenga CE, Salmon DP, Bondi MW. Differential age effects on cerebral blood flow and BOLD response to encoding: Associations with cognition and stroke risk. *Neurobiol Aging.* 2007 Dec. 19 Epub ahead of print.
180. Restom K, Bangen KJ, Bondi MW, Perthen JE, Liu TT. Cerebral blood flow and BOLD responses to a memory encoding task: A comparison between healthy young and elderly adults. *Neuroimage.* 2007;37(2):430–439. Epub, 2007 May 25.
181. D'Agostino RB, Wolf PA, Belanger AJ, Kannel WB. Stroke risk profile: Adjustment for antihypertensive medication. The Framingham Study. *Stroke.* 1994;25(1):40–43.
182. Fleisher AS, Podraza KM, Bangen KJ, Taylor C, Sherzai A, Sidhar K, Liu TT, Dale AM, Buxton RB. Cerebral perfusion and oxygenation differences in Alzheimer's disease risk. *Neurobiol Aging.* In press.
183. Xu G, Antuono PG, Jones J, Xu Y, Wu G, Ward D, Li SJ. Perfusion fMRI detects deficits in regional CBF during memory-encoding tasks in MCI subjects. *Neurology.* 2007;69(17):1650–1656.
184. Detre JA, Alsop DC, Vives LR, et al. Noninvasive MRI evaluation of cerebral blood flow in cerebrovascular disease. *Neurology.* 1998;50:633–641.
185. Ben Salem D, Walker PM, Bejot Y, Aho SL, Tavernier B, Rouaud O, Ricolfi F, Brunotte F. N-acetylaspartate/creatine and choline/creatine ratios in the thalami, insular cortex and white matter as markers of hypertension and cognitive impairment in the elderly. *Hypertens Res.* 2008;31(10):1851–1857.
186. MacKay S, Meyerhoff DJ, Constans JM, Norman D, Fein G, Weiner MW. Regional gray and white matter metabolite differences in subjects with AD, with subcortical ischemic

vascular dementia, and elderly controls with 1H magnetic resonance spectroscopic imaging. *Arch Neurol*. 1996;53(2):167–174.

187. Weiss U, Bacher R, Vonbank H, Kemmler G, Lingg A, Marksteiner J. Cognitive impairment: Assessment with brain magnetic resonance imaging and proton magnetic resonance spectroscopy. *J Clin Psychiatry*. 2003;64(3):235–242.
188. Schuff N, Capizzano AA, Du AT, Amend DL, O'Neill J, Norman D, Jagust WJ, Chui HC, Kramer JH, Reed BR, Miller BL, Yaffe K, Weiner MW. Different patterns of N-acetylaspartate loss in subcortical ischemic vascular dementia and AD. *Neurology*. 2003;61(3):358–364.
189. Capizzano AA, Schuff N, Amend DL, Tanabe JL, Norman D, Maudsley AA, Jagust W, Chui HC, Fein G, Segal MR, Weiner MW. Subcortical ischemic vascular dementia: Assessment with quantitative MR imaging and 1H MR spectroscopy. *Am J Neuroradiol*. 2000;21(4):621–630.
190. Constans JM, Meyerhoff DJ, Gerson J, MacKay S, Norman D, Fein G, Weiner MW. H-1 MR spectroscopic imaging of white matter signal hyperintensities: Alzheimer disease and ischemic vascular dementia. *Radiology*. 1995;197(2):517–523.
191. Sappey-Marinier D, Calabrese G, Hetherington HP, Fisher SN, Deicken R, Van Dyke C, Fein G, Weiner MW. Proton magnetic resonance spectroscopy of human brain: Applications to normal white matter, chronic infarction, and MRI white matter signal hyperintensities. *Magn Reson Med*. 1992;26(2):313–327.
192. Gillard JH, Barker PB, van Zijl PC, Bryan RN, Oppenheimer SM. Proton MR spectroscopy in acute middle cerebral artery stroke. *Am J Neuroradiol*. 1996;17(5):873–886.
193. Barker PB, Gillard JH, van Zijl PC, Soher BJ, Hanley DF, Agildere AM, Oppenheimer SM, Bryan RN. Acute stroke: Evaluation with serial proton MR spectroscopic imaging. *Radiology*. 1994;192(3):723–732.
194. Chu WJ, Mason GF, Pan JW, Hetherington HP, Liu HG, San Pedro EC, Mountz JM. Regional cerebral blood flow and magnetic resonance spectroscopic imaging findings in diaschisis from stroke. *Stroke*. 2002;33(5):1243–1248.
195. Cohen R, Moser D, Clark M, Aloia M, Cargill B, Stefanik S, Albrecht A, Tilkemeier P, Forman D. (1999). Neurocognitive functioning and improvement in quality of life following participation in cardiac rehabilitation. *Am J Cardiol*, 83, 1374–1378.
196. Paul R, Gunstad J, Poppas A, Tate D, Forman D, Brickman A, Jefferson A, Hoth K, Cohen R. (in press). Neuroimaging and cardiac correlates of cognitive function among patients with cardiac disease. *Cerebrovasc Dis*.
197. Gunstad J, MacGregor K, Paul R, Poppas A, Jefferson A, Todaro J, Cohen R. (in press). Cardiac rehabilitation improves cognitive performance in older adults with cardiovascular disease. *J Cardiopulm Rehabil*.
198. Moser D, Cohen R, Clark M, Aloia M, Tate B, Stefanik S, Forman D, Tilkemeier P. Neuropsychological functioning among cardiac rehabilitation patients. *J Cardiopulm Rehabil*. 1999;19:91–97.
199. Cohen RA, Poppas A, Forman DE, Hoth KF, Haley AP, Gunstad J, Jefferson AL, Tate DF, Paul RH, Sweet LH, Ono M, Jerskey BA, Gerhard-Herman M. Vascular and cognitive functions associated with cardiovascular disease in the elderly. *J Clin Exp Neuropsychol*. 2009;31(1):96–110. Epub, 2008 Jun. 16.
200. Sweet LH, Gunstad J, MacGregor K, Paul R, and Cohen R. Age-related FMRI activation differences among older adults during a difficult verbal working memory task: abstract. *J Int Neuropsych Soc*., Feb. 2005.
201. Gunstad J, Sweet LH, Paul R, Poppas A, Tate D, MacGregor K, and Cohen R. Reduced fMRI activation and task performance in cardiovascular disease. *NeuroImage*. 2005;26:S1, S56.

20

THE DYSEXECUTIVE SYNDROME ASSOCIATED WITH SUBCORTICAL WHITE MATTER DISEASE AND RELATED WHITE MATTER PATHOLOGY

Melissa Lamar, Cate C. Price, Tania Giovannetti, Rod Swenson, and David J. Libon

Interest in the neuropsychological and behavioral alterations associated with cerebrovascular pathology is usually traced to the work of Otto Binswanger[1] who introduced the idea that white matter atrophy, caused by vascular insufficiency, can result in cognitive impairment. In support of this proposal, Binswanger described a small series of patients who experienced a slowly progressive course of mental deterioration in combination with focal neurological signs; enlarged ventricles, particularly around the temporal and occipital horns; and substantial loss of corresponding white matter with a general sparing of the cortex.[1] Although he never provided detailed microscopic information, the disorder is thought to have included small focal lesions in the internal capsule, lenticular nuclei, and pyramidal areas around the pons.[1, 2] In subsequent research, Alois Alzheimer substantiated Binswanger's original observations,[3] re-labeling the disorder *Binswanger's disease*. By the turn of the twentieth century, cerebrovascular dementia was a well-established clinical syndrome. Indeed, Alzheimer himself wrote many more papers on vascular dementia (VaD) than the illness that now bears his name and anticipated many of the controversies that continue to be associated with vascular dementia.[4]

The modern history of cerebrovascular pathology, more specifically VaD, dates from the seminal work of Hachinski[5] who introduced the concept of multi-infarct dementia (MID) to explain the interrelationship between cerebral atherosclerosis and cognitive decline often seen in older adults.[5, 6] The concept of MID quickly became synonymous with most vascular dementia syndromes. The introduction of diagnostic criteria for vascular dementia from the Alzheimer's Disease Diagnostic and Treatment Centers[7] (ADDTC) and the National Institute of Neurological and Communicative Disorders and Stroke—Association Internationale pour la Recherché et l'Enseignement en Neurosciences (NINDS-AIREN criteria,[3] have helped redefine the impact of cerebrovascular disease in pathological aging. Furthermore, the acknowledgement of the role of cerebrovascular disease as related to mild or subtle vascular cognitive impairment[8, 9] belies its importance in normal aging and risk for dementia.

Despite these advances, state-of-the-art neuroimaging techniques and large-scale autopsy studies suggest that not all structural brain alterations associated with cerebrovascular disease fit under a common diagnostic rubric. In fact, among some patients, there may be overlap with respect to the neuropathology underlying the clinical presentation of their specific neurodegenerative, e.g., dementia, syndrome.[10–12] For example, over 30% of patients diagnosed with VaD have concomitant AD,[13] while upwards of 40% of pathologically confirmed AD cases also present with significant white matter alterations.[14, 15] In addition to the vascular-mediated damage that may be associated with dementia, other age-related neurodegenerative processes complicated by cognitive decline like dementia associated with Parkinson's disease point to importance of considering various forms of subcortical white matter involvement when considering a profile of impairment. Taken together, this suggests that the presence of subcortical white matter neuropathology influences the symptoms, signs, and course of a dementia, irrespective of dementia subtype.[11, 16–19]

Over the past twenty years, we have documented the neuropsychological presentation of subcortical white matter pathology. This has led to an empirical understanding of three core concepts that promote the larger dysexecutive syndrome in white matter disease: pathological inertia, mental bradyphrenia and disengagement, and temporal reordering. Taken together, this work suggests that white matter alterations impair executive functioning. Thus, a detailed analysis of the dysexecutive phenotype associated with subcortical vascular disease and other age-related neurodegenerative processes involving subcortical structures regardless of dementia subtype is key to our understanding of cerebrovascular pathology and its associated behaviors. The remainder of this chapter will demonstrate that the dysexecutive phenotype associated with subcortical white matter pathology is related to fundamental impairments of gating subserved by basal ganglia-thalamic pathways within and across various dementia syndromes.

The Dysexecutive Phenotype of Subcortical Vascular Disease

Pathological Inertia and Maintaining Mental Set

Similar to ideas put forth by other researchers,[20, 21] we define the ability to establish and maintain a mental set as the ability to appreciate and understand the nature of a task and to respond within the context of that task until the task is completed. When the ability to maintain a proper mental set is impaired, errors in performance may manifest as perseverations such as being "stuck in set,"[22] or a complete inability to engage at the level of task demands. When examined in detail, the presence of subcortical vascular disease can significantly impact the degree to which these errors reflect a specific dementia diagnosis and its putative underlying neuropathology.

We have shown that patients diagnosed with VaD associated with MRI evidence of subcortical vascular disease produce significantly more perseverative errors than patients diagnosed with AD. Equally, if not more, important, the perseverations produced by patients with VaD are distinctly different from the perseverations produced by their AD counterparts.[23] This was illustrated by examining the perseverations produced by dementia patients on the Graphical Sequence Test—Dementia Version (GST-D),[23, 24] a task based on the observations of A.R. Luria,[25] designed to induce various types of motor perseverative behavior (Fig. 20-1).

Patients diagnosed with VaD disproportionately generate *hyperkinetic/interminable* perseverative errors indicative of persistent motor responses, while patients with AD

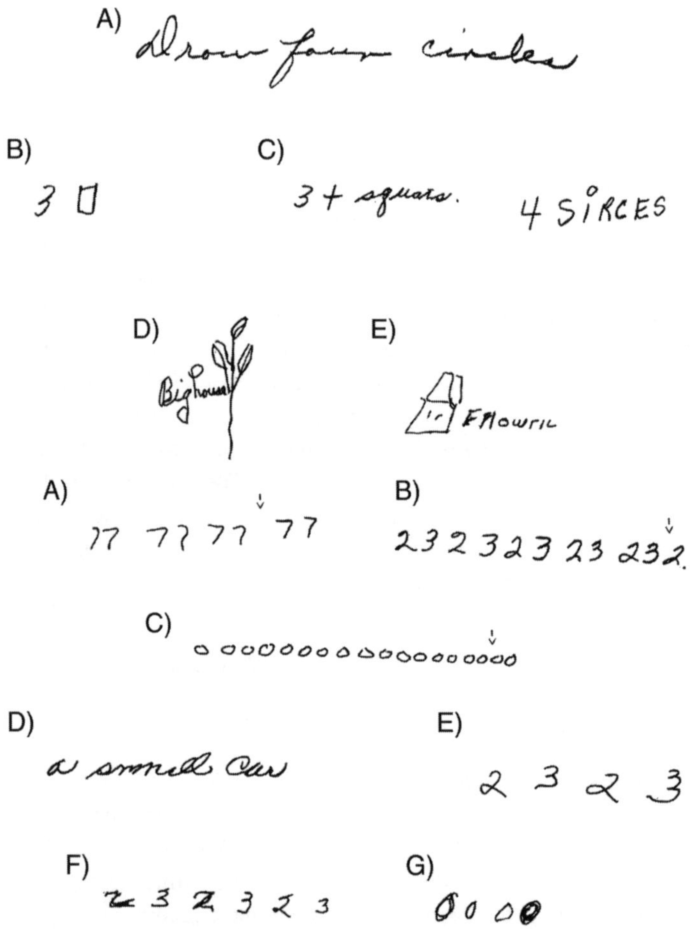

Figure 20-1 Left panel displays various hyperkinetic perseverations (A–G) made by individuals with vascular dementia associated with white matter alterations. Right panel displays various semantic perseverations (A–E) made by individuals with Alzheimer's disease and little to no white matter alterations.

display conceptual confusion over distinct forms of motor output resulting in *semantically* based perseverations. Thus, after the command series, "Draw a circle, draw a circle, draw a circle," individuals with VaD continue to produce circles beyond the number required even though the examiner has ceased to ask that more be drawn (Fig. 20-1: left panel). This pattern of VaD performance, pervasive across the entire GST-D, correlated with poorer performance on tests of executive and motor functioning. In contrast, when asked to *write* the sentence "three squares and two circles," AD patients might *draw* three squares and two circles; or when asked to *draw* a house to the right of a flower, AD patients often *write* the word "house" next to the picture of a flower, or vice versa (Fig. 20-1: right panel). This AD pattern of performance correlated with tests of naming and semantic knowledge. It appears that the subcortical vascular disease associated with VaD promotes a more severe impairment of the conscious termination of a simple motor behavior when compared to the more conceptual mistakes produced in the presence of little MRI white matter hyperintensities but significant AD neuropathology.

Higher-level conceptual versus lower-level pervasive difficulties in establishing and maintaining mental set are also noted on verbal tests. This was seen when zero-point responses produced on the WAIS-R Similarities subtest,[26] a test of verbal concept formation, were recoded to reflect patients' ability to attain mental set even at a superordinate level. Individuals with VaD who presented with at least a moderate degree of MRI white matter alterations produced *out of* set errors that were blatantly incorrect (e.g., *dog–lion—one barks and the other growls*) and associated with other executive deficits. By contrast, patients with AD who presented with little MRI white matter alterations produced zero-point errors that were vague, but nonetheless superficially related to the given word pair (e.g., *dog–lion—they're alive*). The errors produced by patients with AD were associated with poor performance on measures of language and semantic knowledge.[27] Taken together, both studies suggest that greater underlying subcortical vascular disease like that associated with VaD promotes a *dysexecutive* profile characterized by a pervasive impairment in the engagement and/or termination of behavior in compliance with task demands.

Not only does subcortical vascular disease promote a more severe form of dysexecutive deficits in patients' ability to establish and maintain a proper mental set, but vascular ities like hypertension and diabetes that promote various forms of subcortical vascular disease including "silent" strokes, white matter hyperintensities,[28] and cerebral small vessel disease[29] also result in more severe dysexecutive behavior. African Americans with AD and hypertension show significantly poorer performance on executive indices from the Mattis Dementia Rating Scale reflecting initiation and perseveration as well as abstract concept formation when compared to normotensive African Americans with AD.[30] Regardless of race, increasing numbers of vascular comorbidities combined with mild to moderate AD are associated with decreasing verbal reasoning and set shifting skills.[31] Furthermore, increasing numbers of vascular comorbidities in patients with AD were associated with increasing numbers of *out of* set zero-point error responses on the WAIS-III Similarities subtest;[32, 33] a pattern of impairment previously attributed to the subcortical vascular disease underlying VaD.[27] Taken together, this work suggests that vascular comorbidities associated with MRI evidence of subcortical vascular disease may subtly alter the cognitive phenotype of AD toward a more dysexecutive profile.

The unique pattern of perseverations seen in our research is consistent with the pathological inertia seen following prefrontal lesions that extend into associated structures of the basal ganglia.[25] Regardless of whether the patient is asked to respond physically or verbally, the inability to establish or maintain the proper mental set under the simplest of conditions (e.g., "draw a circle," or "how are a fork and a spoon alike?") suggests continual repetition of an ineffective response style; repetition seen following prefrontal lesions that involve the structural or functional integrity of the basal ganglia.[25] In whatever form, pathological inertia as seen in conjunction with a moderate degree of subcortical vascular disease (as well as other pathological disorders impacting subcortical regions of the basal ganglia), prohibits behavior once initiated from being appropriately terminated and prevents the inhibition of irrelevant responses. Thus, vascular disease and associated vascularities that promote white matter alterations in dementia result in mechanistic or lower-level processing that contributes to a core dysexecutive phenotype involving pathological inertia. It is as if there were a decoupling between the production of a response and the monitoring or gating of that response during and after task completion.

Cognitive Control and Mental Bradyphrenia

Cognitive control requires aspects of interference inhibition and flexibility of response selection, as well as sustained attention. When impaired, patients may be unable to inhibit irrelevant responses, and commit errors of commission, overlook appropriate responses in the form of omission errors, or become unable to sustain performance across a specific period. When examined in detail, the presence of subcortical vascular disease appears to selectively affect the production of these errors as well as the natural progression of behavioral performance over a specified period.

Errors of commission and omission appear to be differentially affected by MRI evidence of subcortical vascular disease. This was observed in a study examining performance on simple and more complex mental-control tasks derived, in part, from the Wechsler Memory Scale (WMS) Mental Control subtest.[34] Patients with VaD associated with MRI evidence of subcortical white matter disease not only made more total errors than their AD counterparts regardless of the complexity of the task, the greatest proportion of errors produced in VaD were errors of commission. In contrast, patients with AD tended to make more omission errors but only on the most complex mental control tests.[35] The pattern of impairment in VaD was most evident at the beginning and end of each mental control task, whereas errors in AD were equally distributed across time points of the task.[35] This suggests that subcortical vascular disease underlying VaD impedes the ability to select appropriate targets and, more important, to inhibit erroneous ones, suggesting a more severe dysexecutive deficit.

Testing of disease-specific patterns of cognitive control across a specified time period was also analyzed by investigating response production across the four 15-second quadrants from tests of letter fluency (letters "FAS"). When controlled for total output, patients with VaD associated with MRI evidence of subcortical vascular disease, as well as dementia patients with Parkinson's disease (dPD), which also impacts subcortical white matter regions including the basal ganglia, generated a larger percentage of words during the first 15 seconds when compared to individuals with little to no MRI evidence of subcortical vascular disease or basal ganglia involvement, including patients with AD and healthy controls[35] (Fig. 20-2). However, after the first 15-second epoch, dPD and VaD output dropped precipitously below that seen in AD. In contrast, patients with AD were no different from healthy controls in terms of the percentage of output for the remainder of the task. Much like the performance of individuals with subcortical vascular disease and dementia, patients with subcortical white matter pathology (i.e., dPD) were unable to maintain a consistent level of performance throughout the length of the letter fluency task.

Both the production and temporal nature of the cognitive control deficits associated with MRI evidence of subcortical vascular disease and/or basal ganglia involvement suggests an inability to actively engage inhibitory mechanisms, as well as a more overarching difficulty initiating and maintaining cognitive control for the duration of performance. The fact that most errors on these tasks were errors of commission suggests that individuals with VaD associated with at least a moderate degree of MRI white

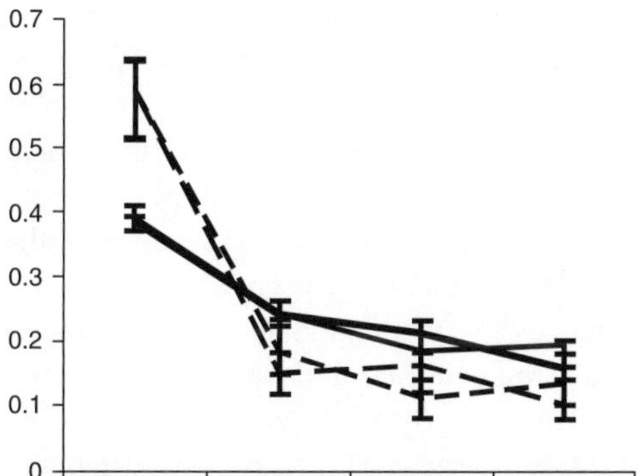

	1st Qtr	2nd Qtr	3rd Qtr	4th Qtr
NC	0.38	0.24	0.19	0.19
AD	0.39	0.24	0.21	0.16
IVD	0.58	0.15	0.16	0.11
PD	0.57	0.19	0.11	0.13

Figure 20-2 Displays the proportion of letter S output per 15-second epoch.

matter alterations were unable to accurately monitor and inhibit irrelevant responses. That these errors occurred at the beginning and end of the task, coupled with the fact that, under a time-limited procedure such as letter ("FAS") fluency, these same patients produced most their responses at the beginning of the task, suggests that differential impairment in cognitive control in VaD is not due to response latency but to differences in response styles. Not only were individuals with VaD associated with MRI evidence of subcortical white matter disease unable to maintain adequate performance for more than a short period, their response style was also seen in patients with dPD, a neurodegenerative disease with concomitant subcortical vascular disease and basal ganglia involvement.

Thus, individuals with at least a moderate degree of MRI white matter pathology appear to be unable to sustain the necessary engagement over an extended period. The phenomenon of knowing *what to do* was impeded by an inability of knowing *how to do*; somewhat akin to the deficits in motor initiation and execution or the bradyphrenia seen in Parkinson's disease. It is possible that a *mental* bradyphrenia—not a cognitive slowing or lengthened response latency per se—but a state of fleeting cognitive and temporal control of behavior is at work in VaD and dPD. In conjunction with increased commission errors secondary to an inability to adequately engage inhibitory mechanisms, this mental bradyphrenia contributes to the dysexecutive syndrome of cognitive control seen in subcortical vascular disease.

Disengagement and Temporal Re-Ordering

Working memory is a key component of executive functioning, much like encoding is a key component of memory. Baddeley's model of working memory[36] proposes that the brain has lower-level, modality-specific buffer systems that store and rehearse information and a higher-level central executive responsible both for overseeing these buffer systems and for executing processes like the manipulation of information.[37] No investigation into the dsyexecutive phenotype associated with subcortical white matter pathology is complete without an assessment of these components of working memory. We have found that the aspects of Baddeley's model that are particularly impaired in the presence of subcortical vascular disease include the search and manipulation of retrieved information; i.e., the core concept of disengagement and temporal reordering.[38]

In a recent study, we designed a new Backward Digit Task (BDT) similar to the WAIS-III Digit Span Backward subtest to tease apart specific components of Baddeley's model of working memory. The BDT[39] requires participants to repeat three-, four-, and five-span trials in reverse order; however, the variables of interest distinguish lower-level short-term storage and rehearsal deficits from higher-level disengagement and temporal reordering deficits. Interestingly, lower-level skills involving short-term storage and rehearsal were equivalent across dementia participants regardless of the presence or absence of MRI subcortical vascular disease. In contrast, patients with dementia associated with at least a moderate degree of MRI white matter alterations displayed significant deficits in higher-level disengagement and temporal reordering.[39] A closer inspection of these errors revealed that dementia patients with MRI evidence of subcortical vascular disease showed impaired working memory, due in part to an inability to disengage from or inhibit over-learned and automatic memories.[23, 40]

We have recently devised a visual analogue to the verbally mediated BDT called the Object Span Test (OST), where patients are shown a series of two, three, and four simple two-dimensional shapes and asked to draw the objects in the order they were presented. Performance in patients with dementia and concomitant white matter alterations on the OST was consistent with the disengagement and temporal reordering deficits seen with the BDT.[41] Furthermore, the OST elicited motor perseverations in patients with MRI white matter alterations, regardless of dementia subtype, similar to those seen on the GST-D in VaD.[23] Taken together, the patterns of performance seen on both the BDT and OST suggest a pervasive level of impairment across verbal as well as visual working-memory abilities in the presence of subcortical vascular disease, regardless of dementia subtype. These working-memory deficits may be due, in part, to the inability to inhibit automatic or irrelevant responses.[40]

By limiting our working-memory tasks to two to five items, we capitalized on the ability of our participants to perform lower-level storage and rehearsal while taxing them on higher-level disengagement and temporal reordering skills. It is primarily these latter processes that are thought to be heavily dependent, not only on the normal functioning of the higher-level central executive,[42] but also on the normal functioning of white matter connections associated with the dorsolateral prefrontal cortex.[42, 43, 45] In addition to the prefrontal cortex and associated white matter tracts, structures of the basal ganglia, including the caudate and the dorsomedial nucleus of the thalamus, participate in the networks of cortical-striato-thalamo-cortical loops that interact with the dorsolateral frontal lobe. When the core concepts of pathological inertia, mental bradyphrenia and disengagement, and temporal reordering that make up the dysexecutive phenotype associated with subcortical vascular disease, and neurodegenerative disorders that are associated with the basal ganglia-thalamic pathways are considered together, we begin to see that white matter neuropathology may alter or derail how subcortical gray matter structures gate information back to the frontal lobes.

Theoretical and Neuroanatomical Considerations

When viewed as a whole, the clinical presentations outlined above suggest that the dysexecutive syndrome associated with subcortical vascular disease as seen in VaD, and neurodegenerative disorders involving subcortical regions as seen in dPD, is rather pandemic: involving such core concepts as pathological inertia, mental bradyphrenia and disengagement, and temporal reordering deficits. In contrast, the executive control deficits associated with a more cortical, gray matter disease state, such as AD or minimal subcortical vascular disease, are restricted and context-specific related to lexical and semantic operations. The core constructs impacted by subcortical white matter pathology appear to have two things in common: (1) they result in a pervasive executive impairment, and (2) they involve an inability to "gate" or filter information back to the frontal lobes. In determining possible neuroanatomical underpinnings of this dysexecutive phenotype, an assumption about the impact of white matter connectivity must be considered.

First put forth by Luria[25] and later advanced by others,[24, 46] is the notion that certain aspects of executive functioning are related to specific, higher-level disorders of cognition, while other aspects of behaviors are more rudimentary and pervasive. It follows that the severity, as well as the specificity, of executive dysfunction is determined by whether a lesion actually resides in the frontal lobes and/or disrupts important connections between the frontal lobes and other areas of the brain. These conclusions support the idea that subcortical vascular disease, as well as neurodegenerative disorders involving subcortical regions (while not directly involving the frontal lobes), negatively impact executive functioning at a rather significant and pervasive level by means of their direct impact on important connections between the frontal lobes and associated white matter structures.

From a diagnostic point of view, the neuropathology of VaD often involves alterations in the basal ganglia, thalamus, and white matter tracts leading to and from the frontal lobes. This suggests that disruption of these prefrontal-basal ganglia-thalamic pathways[47] may explain the rather pervasive dysexecutive syndrome seen in dementia patients with MRI evidence of subcortical white matter disease. It is important to note, however, that vascular diseases present in individuals with AD, as well as other disorders involving subcortical white matter pathology of the basal ganglia (i.e., dPD), also produced a dysexecutive syndrome similar to that seen in the presence of at least a moderate degree of MRI white matter alterations, suggesting the need for a more encompassing, less diagnostically driven approach to this dysexecutive syndrome.

When considered regardless of dementia diagnosis, but as its own neurodegenerative process associated with dementia, white matter neuropathology appears to negatively impact a specific group of cognitive concepts associated with operations ultimately governed by the frontal lobes. These concepts, while seemingly separate (e.g., pathological inertia, mental bradyphrenia, disengagement and temporal reordering) show interrelated deficits in the face of subcortical involvement. That is, white matter neuropathology appears to prohibit adequate engagement in task demands, and when engaged, not only prohibits the behavior initiated from being preserved but also appears to prohibit the inhibition of irrelevant responses; in essence, decoupling the production of responses from the monitoring of responses during and after task completion.

Subcortical vascular disease and related white matter pathology in neurodegeneration and dementia regardless of diagnosis involves the white matter tracts projecting from subcortical structures like the basal ganglia and thalamus into the prefrontal cortex. In fact, even the earliest neuroanatomical conceptualizations of subcortical vascular disease were thought to have included small focal lesions in the internal capsule, lenticular nuclei, and pyramidal areas around the pons.[1, 2] The role of the afferent and efferent connections between these subcortical structures and the prefrontal cortex, as well as the role of the basal ganglia and thalamus as major structures involved in cognition, should be explored as they relate to the dysexecutive syndrome outlined above.

Across animal and human investigations, the notion of a gating mechanism responsible for the selection and subsequent production of appropriate responses has relied heavily on subcortical structures and their intimate connections with the prefrontal cortex. Within the animal literature, derailment in the production of responses based on internal representation and inhibitory control are related to the prefrontal cortex,[48] with resulting behaviors mediated through different regions of the caudate nucleus.[49] Across animal and human studies, the thalamus is thought to have a major regulatory role in the cortical synchronization of behavior via the basal ganglia.[50] Several researchers have speculated that the inhibitory actions of the basal ganglia serve as a selective gating mechanism that updates and directs operations that are then fed back to the frontal lobes through the thalamus.[51, 52] When these structures are damaged, directly or indirectly through white matter pathology (e.g., disconnectivity), the frontal lobes cannot effectively function to meet the needs that may be required when task demands change or become complex.

Thalamic disruption has been used to explain impaired executive behavior in a number of human studies.[53, 54] Furthermore, neuroimaging studies suggest that automatic and over-learned behavioral sequences are housed within the basal ganglia and thalamus.[55] It is possible that white matter damage in dementia releases these automatic behaviors, making them more capable of interfering in cognition and resulting in the core conceptual deficits described as the dysexecutive phenotype within this chapter. Clearly, more directed neuroanatomical investigations need to be done to elucidate the notion that an impaired gating mechanism of the basal ganglia-thalamic pathway may be responsible for the dysexecutive syndrome associated with subcortical vascular disease and related white matter neuropathology in dementia. However, we argue that such white matter damage, regardless of dementia subtype, may prove a surrogate for the role played by the basal ganglia and thalamus in monitoring the release of appropriate responses, thus weakening a subcortical gating mechanism.

Conclusions

The research reviewed in this chapter suggests that the dysexecutive syndrome associated with subcortical vascular disease and related white matter pathology in dementia is caused by a derailment in three distinct but interrelated cognitive concepts (i.e., pathological inertia, mental bradyphrenia, disengagement and temporal reordering). As described above, this dysexecutive syndrome tends to be pervasive regardless of the task at hand or the modality used. More specifically, subcortical vascular disease and related white matter neuropathology in dementia regardless of subtype appears to prohibit adequate engagement in task demands, and when engaged, prohibits the preservation of relevant behavior and the inhibition of irrelevant responses. This decoupling of response production from response monitoring is seen, not only on executive tests, but also when patients with subcortical vascular disease and related white matter neuropathology are asked to copy the Rey Osterietth Complex Figure,[56] to draw a clock to command and copy,[57] and to retrieve information as assessed with a verbal serial list-learning tasks.[58] In this sense, the pervasiveness of the dysexecutive syndrome associated with subcortical vascular disease and related white matter neuropathology in dementia appears to intrude into other aspects of cognition.

In describing the dysexecutive phenotype associated with subcortical vascular disease and related white matter neuropathology in dementia, we have put forth a hypothesis that elements of this syndrome may be caused by a derailed basal ganglia/thalamic gating mechanism regardless of dementia subtype. The disruption of frontal lobe-basal ganglia-thalamic pathways secondary to increasing white matter damage probably weakens gating mechanisms and ultimately may be the etiology of both of the pervasiveness and the poor regulation of executive control deficits.[47, 59] New technologies such as advances in white matter tractography afforded by diffusion tensor imaging, as well as recently applied methods of magnetization transfer imaging and deep brain stimulation, may be able to give us additional information regarding how white matter connectivity (and disconnectivity) produced dysexecutive behavior in dementia.

Notes

1. Blass JP, Hoyer S, Nitsch R. A translation of Otto Binswanger's 1894 article, "The delineation of the generalized progressive paralyses." *Arch Neurol.* 1991;48(9):961–972.
2. Filley CM. *The behavioral neurology of white matter* (pp. 146–150;154–157). New York: Oxford University Press, 2001.
3. Roman GC, Tatemichi TK, Erkinjuntti T, Cummings JL, Masdeu JC, Garcia JH, et al. Vascular dementia: Diagnostic criteria for research studies. Report of the NINDS-AIREN International Workshop. *Neurology.* 1993;43(2):250–260.
4. Libon DJ, Price CC, Heilman KM, Grossman M. Alzheimer's "other dementia." *Cogn Behav Neurol.* 2006;19(2):112–116.
5. Hachinski VC, Lassen NA, Marshall J. Multi-infarct dementia. A cause of mental deterioration in the elderly. *Lancet.* 1974;2(7874):207–210.
6. Hachinski VC, Iliff LD, Zilhka E, Du Boulay GH, McAllister VL, Marshall J, et al. Cerebral blood flow in dementia. *Arch Neurol.* 1975;32(9):632–637.
7. Chui HC, Victoroff JI, Margolin D, Jagust W, Shankle R, Katzman R. Criteria for the diagnosis of ischemic vascular dementia proposed by the State of California Alzheimer's Disease Diagnostic and Treatment Centers. *Neurology.* 1992;42(3 Pt 1):473–480.
8. Bowler JV, Hachinski V. Vascular cognitive impairment: A new approach to vascular dementia. *Baillieres Clinical Neurology.* 1995;4(2):357–376.
9. Bowler JV, Steenhuis R, Hachinski V. Conceptual background to vascular cognitive impairment. *Alzheimer Disease and Associated Disorders.* 1999;13(Suppl 3):S30–37.
10. Cosentino SA, Jefferson AL, Carey M, Price CC, Davis-Garrett K, Swenson R, et al. The clinical diagnosis of vascular dementia: A comparison among four classification systems and a proposal for a new paradigm. *Clin Neuropsychol.* 2004;18(1):6–21.
11. Jellinger KA. Alzheimer disease and cerebrovascular pathology: An update. *J Neural Transmission.* 2002a;109(5–6):813–836.
12. Pantoni L, Garcia JH. Pathogenesis of leukoaraiosis: A review. *Stroke.* 1997;*28*(3):652–659.
13. Kalaria RN, Ballard C. Overlap between pathology of Alzheimer disease and vascular dementia. *Alzheimer Disease Association and Related Disorders.* 1999;13 Suppl 3:S115–123.
14. Merino JG, Hachinski V. Leukoaraiosis: Reifying rarefaction. *Arch Neurol.* 2000;*57*(7): 925–926.

15. Yip AG, McKee AC, Green RC, Wells J, Young H, Cupples LA, et al. APOE, vascular pathology, and the AD brain. *Neurology*. 2005;65(2):259–265.
16. Jellinger KA. The pathology of ischemic-vascular dementia: An update. *J Neurol Sci. 2002*b; 203–204:153–157.
17. Libon DJ, Price CC, Giovannetti T, Swenson R, Bettcher BM, Heilman KM, et al. Linking MRI hyperintensities with patterns of neuropsychological impairment: Evidence for a threshold effect. *Stroke*. 2008;39(3):806–813.
18. Luchsinger JA, Reitz C, Honig AS, Tang MX, Shea S, Mayeux R. Aggregation of vascular risk factors and risk of incident Alzheimer's disease. *Neurology*. 2005;65:545–551.
19. Price CC, Jefferson AL, Merino JG, Heilman KM, Libon DJ. Subcortical vascular dementia: Integrating neuropsychological and neuroradiologic data. *Neurology*. 2005;*65*(3):376–382.
20. Dias R, Robbins TW., Roberts AC. Dissociable forms of inhibitory control, within prefrontal cortex with an analog of the Wisconsin Card Sorting Test: Restrictions to novel situations and independence from "on-line" processing. *J Neurosci* 1997;17 (23):9285–9297.
21. Rogers RD., Andrews TC., Grasby PM., Brooks DJ., and Robbins TW. Contrasting cortical and subcortical activations produced by attentional-set shifting and reversal learning in humans. *J Cogn Neurosci*. 2000;12 (1):142–162.
22. Sandson J, Albert ML. Varieties of perseveration. *Neuropsychologia*. 1984;22(6):715–732.
23. Lamar M, Podell K, Carew TG, Cloud BS, Resh R, Kennedy C, et al. Perseverative behavior in Alzheimer's disease and subcortical ischemic vascular dementia. *Neuropsychology*. 1997;11(4):523–534.
24. Goldberg E. Varieties of perseveration: A comparison of two taxonomies. *J Clin Exp Neuropsychol*. 1986;8(6):710–726.
25. Luria AR. *Higher cortical functions* (pp. 246–360). New York: Basic Books, 1980.
26. Wechsler DA. *The Wechsler Adult Intelligence Scale–III*. San Antonio TX: Psychology Corporation, 1997.
27. Giovannetti T, Lamar M, Cloud BS, Swenson R, Fein D, Kaplan E, et al. Different underlying mechanisms for deficits in concept formation in dementia. *Arch Clin Neuropsychol*. 2001;16(6):547–560.
28. Schmidt R, Schmidt H, Fazekas F. Vascular risk factors in dementia. *J Neurol*. 2000; 247(2):81–87.
29. Frisoni GB, Galluzzi S, Pantoni L, Filippi M. The effect of white matter lesions on cognition in the elderly—small but detectable. *Nat Clin Pract Neurol*. 2007;3(11):620–627.
30. Goldstein FC, Ashley AV, Freedman LJ, Penix L, Lah JJ, Hanfelt J, et al. Hypertension and cognitive performance in African Americans with Alzheimer disease. *Neurology*. 2005; 64(5):899–901.
31. Goldstein FC, Ashley AV, Endeshaw YW, Hanfelt J, Lah JJ, Levey AI. (in press). Effects of hypertension and hypercholesterolemia on cognitive functioning in patients with Alzheimer's disease. *Alzheimer Dis Assoc Disord*.
32. Lamar M, Goldstein FC, Libon DJ, Ashley AV, Lah JJ, Levey AI. The impact of vascular risk on concept formation in Alzheimer's disease. Paper presented at the 10th annual International Research Conference on Alzheimer's Disease and Related Disorders, Madrid, Spain, 2006.
33. Lamar M, Libon D, Ashley AV, Lah JJ, Levey AI, Goldstein FC (under review). The impact of vascular comorbidity on abstract reasoning and concept formation in Alzheimer's disease.
34. Wechsler DA. A standardized memory scale for clinical use. *J Psychol*. 1945;19:87–95.
35. Lamar M, Price CC, Davis KL, Kaplan E, Libon DJ. Capacity to maintain mental set in dementia. *Neuropsychologia*. 2002;40(4):435–445.
36. Baddeley A, Logie R, Bressi S, Della Sala S, Spinnler H. Dementia and working memory. *Q J Exp Psychol*: *A*. 1986;38(4):603–618.

37. Baddeley A, Hitch G. Developments in the concept of working memory. *Neuropsychology*. 1994;8:485–493.
38. Lamar M, Swenson R, Kaplan E, Libon DJ. Characterizing alterations in executive functioning across distinct subtypes of cortical and subcortical dementia. *Clin Neuropsychol*. 2004;18(1):22–31.
39. Lamar M, Price CC, Libon DJ, Penney DL, Kaplan E, Grossman M, et al. Alterations in working memory as a function of leukoaraiosis in dementia. *Neuropsychologia*. 2007;45(2): 245–254.
40. Stuss DT, Shallice T, Alexander MP, Picton TW. A multidisciplinary approach to anterior attentional functions. *Ann N Y Acad Sci*. 1995;769:191–211.
41. Lamar M, Price CC, Heilman KM, Penney DL, Libon DJ. Assessing executive control deficits in patients with subcortical vascular disease: The impact of region specific leukoaraiosis on working memory deficits. The 3rd Congress of the International Society for Vascular Behavioral and Cognitive Disorders. San Antonio, Texas, 2007.
42. Hester RL, Kinsella GJ, Ong B. Effect of age on forward and backward span tasks. *J Int Neuropsychol Soc*. 2004;10(4):475–481.
43. Charlton RA, Morris RG, Nitkunan A, Markus HS. The cognitive profiles of CADASIL and sporadic small vessel disease. *Neurology*. 2006;66(10):1523–1526.
44. Collette F, Van der Linden M, Bechet S, Salmon E. Phonological loop and central executive functioning in Alzheimer's disease. *Neuropsychologia*. 1999;37(8):905–918.
45. D'Esposito M, Aguirre GK, Zarahn E, Ballard D, Shin RK, Lease J. Functional MRI studies of spatial and nonspatial working memory. *Cogn Brain Res*. 1998;7(1):1–13.
46. Goldberg E, Bilder R. The frontal lobes and hierarchical organization of cognitive control. In E. Perecman (Ed.), *The frontal lobes revised*. New York: IRBN Press, 1987.
47. Alexander GE, DeLong MR, Strick PL. Parallel organization of functionally segregated circuits linking basal ganglia and cortex. *Ann Rev Neurosci*. 1986;9:357–381.
48. Fuster JM. *The prefrontal cortex-anatomy, physiology and neuropsychology of the frontal lobe*, 3rd ed. Philadelphia, PA: Lippincott-Raven, 1997.
49. Calabresi P, De Murtas M, Bernardi G. The neostriatum beyond the motor function: Experimental and clinical evidence. *Neuroscience*. 1997;78(1):39–60.
50. Benarroch EE. The midline and intralaminar thalamic nuclei: Anatomic and functional specificity and implications in neurologic disease. *Neurology*. 2008;71(12):944–949.
51. Beiser DG, Houk JC. Model of cortical-basal ganglionic processing: Encoding the serial order of sensory events. *J Neurophysiol*. 1998;79(6):3168–3188.
52. Frank MJ, Loughry B, O'Reilly RC. Interactions between frontal cortex and basal ganglia in working memory: A computational model. *Cogn Affect Behav Neurosci*. 2001;1(2): 137–160.
53. Hudson AJ. Perseveration. *Brain*. 1968;91(3):571–582.
54. Ojemann GA. Language and the thalamus: Object naming and recall during and after thalamic stimulation. *Brain Lang*. 1975;2(1):101–120.
55. Grafton ST, Mazziotta JC, Presty S, Friston KJ, Frackowiak RS, Phelps ME. Functional anatomy of human procedural learning determined with regional cerebral blood flow and PET. *J Neurosci*. 1992;12(7):2542–2548.
56. Freeman RQ, Giovannetti T, Lamar M, Cloud BS, Stern RA, Kaplan E, et al. Visuoconstructional problems in dementia: Contribution of executive systems functions. *Neuropsychology*. 2000;14(3):415–426.
57. Cosentino SA., Jefferson A, Chute DL, Kaplan E, Libon DJ. Clock drawing errors in dementia: Neuropsychological and neuroanatomical considerations. *Cogn Behav Neurol*. 2004;17(2):74–84.

58. Davis KL, Price CC, Kaplan E, Libon DJ. Error analysis of the nine-word California Verbal Learning Test (CVLT-9) among older adults with and without dementia. *Clin Neuropsychol.* 2002;16(1):81–89.
59. Sultzer DL, Mahler ME, Cummings JL, Van Gorp WG, Hinkin CH, Brown C. Cortical abnormalities associated with subcortical lesions in vascular dementia. Clinical and position emission tomographic findings. *Arch Neurol.* 1995;52(8):773–780.

INDEX